D1609019

Perioperative Nursing

Perioperative Nursing
Principles and Practice
Second Edition

Susan S. Fairchild, R.N.C., Ed.D(c)., M.S.N., C.N.O.R.
Assistant Professor, Barry University School of Nursing,
Miami Shores, Florida

Little, Brown and Company
Boston   New York   Toronto   London

Copyright © 1996 by Little, Brown and Company (Inc.)

Second Edition

Previous edition copyright © 1993 by Jones and
Bartlett Publishers, Inc.

All rights reserved. No part of this book may be
reproduced in any form or by any electronic or
mechanical means, including information storage
and retrieval systems, without permission in writing
from the publisher, except by a reviewer who may
quote brief passages in a review.

Library of Congress Cataloging-in-Publication Data

Perioperative nursing : principles and practice / Susan S.
　Fairchild.—2nd ed.
　　　p.—cm.
　　Rev. ed. of: Perioperative nursing / Susan S. Fairchild. c1993.
　　Includes bibliographical references and index.
　　ISBN 0-316-25969-1
　　1. Operating room nursing.　I. Fairchild, Susan S.
　　[DNLM:　1. Operating Room Nursing.　WY 162 P4447 1996]
　RD32.3.F35　1996
　610.73'677—dc20
　DNLM/DLC
　for Library of Congress　　　　　　　　95-50442
　　　　　　　　　　　　　　　　　　　　　CIP

Printed in the United States of America

KP

Editorial: Evan R. Schnittman, Richard L. Wilcox
Indexer: Nanette Cardon
Production Supervisor/Designer: Louis C. Bruno, Jr.
Cover Designer: Linda Dana Willis

The material contained in this book is endorsed by
　　RN as a useful component in the ongoing
　　　　　ocess of perioperative nurses.

Contents

Contributing Authors

Kathleen Blais, Ed.D., R.N.
Associate Professor, Florida International University, School of Nursing, Miami

Mary Ann Brooks, R.N., M.S.H.S.A.
Director of Central Services, Cedars Medical Center, Miami

Susan S. Fairchild, R.N.C., Ed.D.(c)., M.S.N., C.N.O.R.
Assistant Professor, Barry University School of Nursing, Miami Shores, Florida

Alfredo Ferrari, M.D., P.A.
Anesthesiologist, Surgical Services and Anesthesia, Imperial Point Medical Center, Fort Lauderdale, Florida

Daniel James Little, R.N., M.S.N., M.B.A.
Former Associate Professor of Nursing, Miami Dade Community College, Miami

James Mulchay, R.N., C.R.N.A., A.R.N.P.
Anesthesia Practitioner, Anesthesia Associates, Fort Lauderdale, Florida

Linda Cruz Agustin Simunek, R.N., Ph.D., J.D.
Dean, Florida International University, School of Nursing, Miami

Sandra L. Hunter Sword, R.N., M.S., C.N.O.R.
Assistant Administrator of Surgical Services, Olympia Fields Hospital and Medical Center, Olympia Fields, Illinois

Consultant/Review Board

Mary Boyle, R.N., C.N.O.R.
Director, Department of Surgical Services, Mount Sinai Medical Center, New York

Robin Chard, R.N., C.N.O.R., R.N.F.A
Staff Nurse, Department of Surgery, Broward General Medical Center, Fort Lauderdale, Florida

Maria Lourdes Viado Lizardo, R.N., M.S.N.
Assistant Professor, Department of Nursing, Florida International University, North Miami, Florida

Nan D. Register, R.N., C.N.O.R., R.N.F.A.
Independent Practitioner, Registered Nurse First Assistant, Palm Beach Gardens, Florida

Brenda C. Ulmer, R.N., C.N.O.R.
Clinical Educator, Department of Surgical Services, Eastside Medical Center, Stone Mountain, Georgia

Norman Wolford, Ed.D., R.N., C.R.N.A.
Director, Master of Science Anesthesia Practitioner Program, Barry University, Miami Shores, Florida

Preface

The purpose of *Perioperative Nursing: Principles and Practice*, Second Edition, is to provide a succinct, yet comprehensive, exploration of the core material (*critical elements*) for entry-level practitioners and nurses seeking to update current perioperative nursing practices. Through the integration of biophysical and behavioral sciences, the *nursing process*, and a systems approach to surgical procedures, this text is applicable to any facet of perioperative nursing practice, regardless of the level of experience or practice setting.

The second edition, as the first, emphasizes both the technical skills and behavioral aspects of perioperative nursing practice. In today's age of high technology, computerized nurses' notes, and expanded areas of practice, it is important to consider the fundamental responsibilities of the perioperative nurse during the three phases of surgical intervention: Preoperative, Intraoperative, and Postoperative.

The Standards for Clinical Practice and Professional Performance, along with the Recommended Practices for the perioperative nurse, were developed by the members of the **Association of Operating Room Nurses (AORN)**, who represent perioperative nurses throughout the United States and abroad. Adherence to these standards and recommended practices can help to create and maintain a safe, therapeutic environment for the patient undergoing surgical intervention and the staff rendering the care within this rapidly changing and technologically advancing specialty area.

The text is divided into **five Modules** (specific content areas of related information and tasks). Each module provides the reader with a variety of learning experiences. Self-assessment Exercises are included throughout each chapter as well as Questions for Review at the conclusion of each module.

Module I explores the historical development of operating room nursing to the present practice of perioperative nursing. The module provides an orientation to the surgical setting and a look at the organizational structure and management of the Department of Surgical Services and examines the Standards for Perioperative Nursing Practice according to the AORN.

Module II reviews the biophysical sciences and the impact they have on the surgical client. In addition, this module describes how the sciences interrelate with the practice of nursing in the operating room including microbiology, epidemiology, wound healing, surgical pharmacology, anesthesia, and hemodynamics.

Module III focuses on the creation and maintenance of an aseptic environment. Perioperative nursing implications related to aseptic technique, preparation of supplies and equipment, and monitoring activities required to maintain a safe, therapeutic environment during surgery are stressed in this module.

Module IV explores the nursing process as it applies to perioperative nursing and its impact on the care and management of a client during the perioperative period. Additionally, the module discusses the ethical and legal implications related to this specialized area of nursing practice.

Module V presents a surgical anthology and related perioperative nursing considerations for a variety of surgical procedures by using a systems approach. The module also examines nursing theories and advanced areas of clinical practice of the perioperative nurse in today's complex and expanding practice settings.

Although the format for this edition remains the same, some key areas have been revised to provide the latest theories and concepts related to the practice of perioperative nursing. These areas include

- legal and ethical dimensions of perioperative nursing practice
- preparation of surgical supplies and equipment
- anesthesia and hemodynamic monitoring
- nursing theories and concepts applied to perioperative nursing practice
- expanded roles and education of the perioperative nurse

Perioperative Nursing, Second Edition, intends to dispel the idea that the practice of nursing in the operating room is merely a mechanical, task-oriented process. Effective perioperative nursing care requires that the client be seen as an *individual*, and stresses the importance of the client as a holistic being who requires scientifically based, skilled professional nursing care during all three phases of surgical intervention.

To this end, *Perioperative Nursing: Principles and Practice*, Second Edition, was created as both a directed or self-directed learning tool to assist the practitioner in understanding and implementing safe, efficient nursing care during the perioperative period.

To those persons and institutions who have provided invaluable help and support while creating this text; to my **Students**, past, present, and future; and to my colleagues who practice **Perioperative Nursing**, this book is dedicated.

S.S.F.

MODULE I

Perioperative Nursing
Specialists in Caring

Chapter Outline

1. Introduction to Perioperative Nursing
2. The Surgical Setting
   Unit 1: Environmental Orientation
   Unit 2: Organizational Structure: The Team Concept
3. Standards for Perioperative Nursing Practice
Questions for Review for Module I
Glossary
Bibliography for Module I
Answers for Module I

Content Overview

This module reviews the historical development and eventual specialization from the original practice of operating room nursing to the perioperative nursing role of today's practitioner.

Additionally, the module describes the physical environment and organizational structure of the Department of Surgery, and examines the Standards of Perioperative Nursing Practice.

Module Objectives

Upon completion of this module, you will be able to:

1. Compare and contrast the initial role of the operating room nurse to the practice of today's perioperative nurse.
2. Discuss the philosophy and organizational structure of the Department of Surgery, including the management of the daily workings of the department.
3. Describe the physical layout and components that make up the surgical suite.
4. Relate the role of the perioperative nurse with the Association of Operating Room Nurses Standards of Practice during all three phases of surgical intervention.

Notice

The indications and dosages of all drugs in this book have been recommended in the medical literature and conform to the practices of the general medical community. The medications described do not necessarily have specific approval by the Food and Drug Administration for use in the diseases and dosages for which they are recommended. The package insert for each drug should be consulted for use and dosage as approved by the FDA. Because standards for usage change, it is advisable to keep abreast of revised recommendations, particularly those concerning new drugs.

1 Introduction to Perioperative Nursing

When I want to understand what is happening today, or try to decide what will happen tomorrow, I look back.

—Oliver Wendell Holmes, Jr.

Surgery is a unique human experience. Unique, because it is unlike any other form of therapy, and human, because it requires holistic nursing care to be effective.

Surgery has been described as a planned alteration of the human body designed to (1) arrest, (2) alleviate, or (3) eradicate some pathologic process, but this does not adequately define the surgical experience since it does not address the biosocial or psychologic aspects of patient care.

Nursing intervention, however, has made this definition complete, since as a specialty perioperative nursing has become an important, vital factor in the success of the planned surgical intervention.

Perioperative nursing is a natural outgrowth of operating room (OR) nursing as it was practiced in its early years. But unlike its predecessor, perioperative nursing practice involves caring for the surgical patient during all three phases of surgical intervention.

Perioperative nursing is *patient-centered* rather than task-oriented, combining both the physiologic and psychosocial aspects of nursing, which ultimately benefits both the patient and the nurse.

OR nursing is the oldest nursing specialty on record. It dates back to 1875 with the first lecture to nurses, entitled "Surgical Instrument Preparation for Surgery." The lecture was given at Johns Hopkins University in Baltimore, the first institution to open its doors to student nurses for a tour of duty in surgery.[1]

Much of the early history of operating room nursing is limited; however, it is known that by the late 1800s the following description concerning the qualities of an operating room nurse stated that the individual must

> possess a level head, keen eyes; ever watchful for all that may be required, a mind not easily irritated or confused, combined with the faculty of keeping out of the way, yet, still being of the greatest help.[2]

As the practice of surgery increased, nursing students were rotated to the operating theater for lessons in anatomy, aseptic technique, and general housekeeping duties relating to the surgical suite. However, patient care and the preparation of surgical supplies were not yet part of the nurses' role.

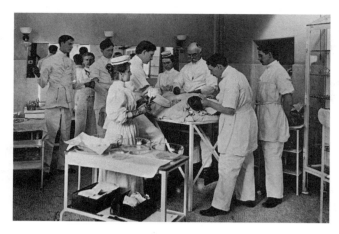

Operating room, 1901 (The Bettman Archive)

Following a request of the Chief Operating Room nurse at Boston Training School (Massachusetts General Hospital), student nurses were sent to assist with Saturday operations (since this would not interfere with their weekday assignments or classes), and, following a class in scrubbing, they were allowed to participate in the operation in a limited fashion.

In this way, new nurses were being trained to perform in surgery while they were still learning the art and science of nursing. The scrub role, however, was usually performed by the junior or senior level nurses, since the belief at that time was that the more experienced student should be assisting the surgeon, while the fundamental students could perform the general duty tasks, such as cleaning, restocking, and "fetching" items that were needed during the procedure. Neither a position description nor a delineation of the scrub/circulator roles had as yet been developed or defined, since no great distinction was made between the activities performed.

As the number of cases increased, surgeons began to recognize the importance of having nurses in the operating room. Along with this recognition came a more active and consistent role in the daily schedule, but still no definite role description had been created.

In answer to this, Martha Luce, acting Chief Nurse of Surgery at Boston Training School, wrote a brief description of what the nurse was to do when assigned to surgery:

> Nurses are not there to see the operation . . . but to make their presence realized by the quiet way in which all wants are foreseen or supplied during surgery.[3]

Since the number of nurses trained for surgery was limited, nurses came with their patients from the ward to assist in performing the general tasks needed during the operation, leaving the more seasoned nurse for the actual assisting role and the teaching of student nurses rotating in surgery. Upon completion of the procedure, the same nurse who brought the patient to surgery accompanied the patient back to the ward and cared for the patient until he or she was discharged from the hospital. The student would then prepare the operating room for the next procedure, and the cycle repeated itself throughout the day.

As years went by, a Scottish surgeon, Dr. Joseph Bell, began to recognize the importance of specialized training for the nurses assisting in the OR, and thus began the specialty of operating room nursing. However, it was not until the early 1900s that hospital-based nursing programs added a surgery component to their generic curricula, providing students an opportunity to spend 3 to 4 months in the OR as part of their initial clinical experience.

THE TEAM CONCEPT IS ESTABLISHED

In 1894, at the request of Dr. Hunter Robb, a surgeon at Johns Hopkins, the "Team Concept" for surgical procedures was first introduced as a means for providing quality patient care in the surgical suite.

The team consisted of a senior nurse in the scrub role, a junior nurse or student to assist with dispensing sterile supplies to the surgical field, and a physician's assistant, usually an intern, trained to assist the attending surgeon, depending on the type of procedure being performed. The senior nurse, who was more experienced in procedures and tasks, became the scrub or instrument nurse, while the junior nurse/student performed all other duties required within the procedure room (circulating nurse). This team concept remained in effect until 1910, when the American Nurses Association (ANA) wrote a paper describing the need for the senior nurse to function in the circulating role, since the duties required a "more experienced nurse in patient care and aseptic technique."

In this paper, the ANA also said the role of the scrub nurse required less experience, since the duties were technically oriented and somewhat mechanical, and did not require any vast nursing experience in surgery. To this day, the role of the circulating nurse is delegated to the professional registered nurse (RN), while the role of the scrub nurse is performed by either an RN or a surgical technician.

In 1919, the National League for Nursing-Education Committee, who wrote and approved nursing school curricula, established the OR rotation as a "worthwhile clinical area" and included in their standard curricula a section on OR technique, consisting of 10 hours of theory, 20 hours of bacteriology and surgical diseases, and a 2- to 3-month rotation in surgery, depending on the student/hospital needs.

Formal training of the student nurse for surgery did not exist, however, since most of the clinical training was performed by the OR supervisor, with most of the concepts passed on to the student based on previous practices. By 1933, the National League for Nursing (NLN) had outlined a master curriculum plan for advanced courses in OR theory and technique, which served as a model for training OR nurses during the next decade.

1940 to 1945: The War Years

World War II was a turning point for OR nursing and for hospitals in general. With nurses leaving the hospitals and joining the Armed Forces, an acute shortage of nurses was felt, especially in critical areas such as surgery.

Hospitals were finding it necessary to train ancillary personnel to take the place of the nurses, bringing about the emergence of nursing aides and orderlies. In the OR, changes were also occurring at a rapid rate. Since the war had recruited most of the experienced nurses, leaving ORs with inadequate personnel for both the scrub and circulating roles, a new member of the OR team was created: the surgical technician, who was instructed to assist in surgical procedures through an on-the-job training program. Today, although their education has increased to a 12- to 14-month program that includes basic science courses in addition to OR technique, these technicians continue to function in their original role, with slight expansion depending on the needs of the institution.

In the field hospitals and on board hospital ships, medical corpsmen were being trained to assist the physicians as well as the surgeons. Nurses were fulfilling roles that in civilian life they would not have been expected to perform, such as administering anesthesia during surgery and acting as first assistant during a procedure.

At the end of the war, the majority of corpsmen who had performed as assistants in surgery returned to civilian life and assumed the role of the surgical technician, while others went on to become physician's assistants (PAs).

It was during this time, and with this new definition of roles, that RNs began to look more closely at the role of the nurse in surgery.

Since many nursing positions had been filled with nonnursing personnel during the war years, and since the shortage of patient-care nurses still existed, the shift from general practitioners to specialists began to emerge in an attempt to capture lost professional

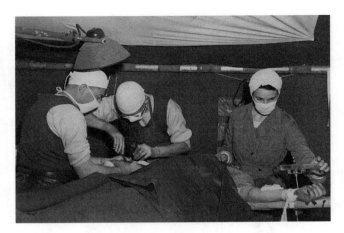

World War II nurse (right) (UPI/Bettman)

positions within the hospital and ORs. Nurses in surgery began to see their roles as leaders, supervisors, and teachers, and as professional nurses who accepted the responsibility for all nursing activities performed in the procedure room. By the late 1940s, OR nurses managed not only the care of the patient during surgical intervention, but also became managers and administrators of surgical departments, while the role of scrub nurse transferred to the surgical technician.

1946 to 1960: Post-War Changes

The changes that had started during the immediate post-war years were beginning to affect the future of OR nursing, in both the professional and educational arenas. Since surgical technicians could perform the routine duties of the scrub nurse, under the supervision of an RN, the need to train nurses for the OR became the lowest priority of the NLN. Consequently, the OR rotation was phased out, until, by 1949, the OR rotation was eliminated from the nursing curriculum and was maintained only by those schools that were hospital-based and/or by instructors who believed it would be beneficial. Even then, it was only for observational purposes; OR nursing was no longer a mandatory subject or area of clinical practice.

THE EMERGENCE OF OPERATING ROOM NURSING AS A SPECIALTY

In January 1949, while the number of nurses specifically trained for surgery was being reduced and as their new role in surgery was emerging, many OR nurses believed that it was time to create an organization for their specialty designed to exchange knowledge and ideas.

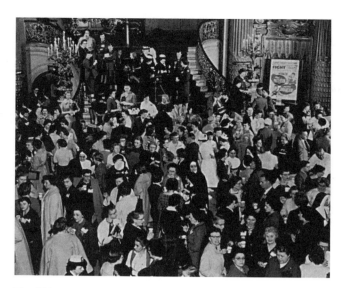

Twelfth AORN Congress, New York, 1965 (Reprinted with permission from Driscoll, J. *Preserving the Legacy: AORN 1949–1989.* Denver, CO: AORN, Inc., 1990. P. 11.)

To this end, 17 OR supervisors from New York City met to establish such an organization, to be called the Association of Operating Room Nurses (AORN), which would eventually stimulate OR nurses around the country to form similar groups; to share knowledge; motivate experienced OR nurses to teach the neophyte; and promote and benefit professional OR nursing to a level of specialization.

Because the parent organization, American Nurses Association (ANA), was unwilling to support or offer suggestions for this group, it became apparent that to create an organization that would benefit the OR nurse, some independent alternatives had to be found. Edith Dee Hall, one of the original 17 nurses and founder of the association, was elected as the first President of the New York Chapter, and by 1950, through the work of this group, 26 chapters had been formed around the country.

In 1956, just 5 short years later, the AORN was ready to become a separate professional organization, dedicated to improving professional nursing care in the operating room.

In that same year, Hall met with ANA again to ask for an affiliation with that group so that the AORN could hold its own annual meeting, and again the request was denied. But that didn't stop this young group of dedicated nurses, for in 1954, despite all efforts of ANA to prevent it from happening, the first national conference of the Association of Operating Room Nurses was held in New York City.

In 1957, following another unsuccessful meeting with the ANA Board of Directors, it was decided that the AORN should draft a separate charter, making it an independent professional nursing organization with its own national officers and Board of Directors. This decision eventually led to the incorporation of AORN the following year, with a national membership of 3200 OR nurses.

Concerned for the future of OR nurses, and realizing they were about to face their greatest challenge, the AORN began to attempt to change the overall perspective of OR nursing, from the task-oriented profession it had been to a patient-centered profession, and, with input from the ANA, the association created the original Standards of Practice: OR as a basis for safe and effective clinical practice.

As the professional OR nurses' activities expanded, further clarification of the role was needed, and in 1976, a proposal to define further the role of nurses in the OR was approved by the AORN Board of Directors. Two years later (1978), via the efforts of a task force selected by the members, the term "perioperative" was first used to describe the role of the professional nurse during the three phases of surgical intervention: preoperative, intraoperative, and postoperative.

PERIOPERATIVE NURSING PRACTICE

In 1978 the first description of perioperative nursing practice was presented to the AORN members at the 25th National AORN Congress, stating:

> The RN specializing in Perioperative Nursing practice performs nursing activities in the preoperative, intraoperative, and postoperative phases of the patients' surgical experience.[4]

In addition to the newly defined role, the Nursing Practice Committee of the AORN was charged with the responsibility of reviewing and revising the original standards to reflect the new dimension of the perioperative nurses' role. It is these standards that govern and guide the nurse when rendering patient care during the perioperative period.

In 1982, the standards were revised as requested, and the definition of perioperative nursing practice was expanded to its current content, stating that perioperative nursing practice begins at an entry level based on clinical expertise and continues on to an expanded level of practice, recognized today as Certification in Perioperative Nursing Practice (CNOR).

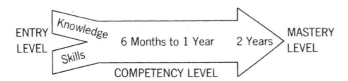

Fig. 1-1. Perioperative nursing continuum (phase I)

The Perioperative Nurses' Role

In 1984 and 1985, the Nursing Practice Committee of the AORN redefined perioperative nursing practice to reflect more accurately the scope of nursing practice in the OR (Fig. 1-1):[5]

> The registered nurse specializing in perioperative nursing practice performs nursing activities in the preoperative, intraoperative and postoperative phases of the patient's surgical experience. Registered nurses enter perioperative nursing practice at a beginning level depending on their expertise and competency to practice. As they gain knowledge and skills, they progress on a continuum to an advanced level of practice.

Based on the Standards and Recommended Practices for Perioperative Nursing—AORN, the OR nurse provides a continuity of care throughout the perioperative period, using scientific and behavioral practices with the eventual goal of meeting the individual needs of the patient undergoing surgical intervention. This process is dynamic and continuous, and requires constant reevaluation of individual nursing practice in the OR.

Perioperative nursing represents a multifaceted challenge to today's OR nurse. In this role, the nurse has an opportunity to (1) prepare the patient and family for surgery, (2) provide comfort and support to patient and family, and (3) use sound nursing judgment and problem-solving techniques to assure a safe and effective surgical experience.

Whether scrubbing, circulating, or supervising other team members, the perioperative nurse is always aware of the total environment, as well as the patient's reaction to the environment and the care given during all three phases of surgical intervention. The perioperative nurse is knowledgeable about aseptic technique, patient safety, legal aspects of nursing, and the management of nursing activities associated with the specific surgical procedure being performed.

Perioperative nursing is unique: it provides a specialty service during the perioperative period that stresses the need for continuity of care and respect for the individuality of the patient's needs.

The Perioperative Nurses' Duties and Responsibilities

The perioperative nurse is responsible and accountable for the major nursing activities occurring in the surgical suite. These include but are not limited to,

1. Assessing of the patient's physiologic and psychological status before, during, and after surgery.
2. Identifying priorities and implementing care based on sound nursing judgment and individual patient needs.
3. Functioning as a role model of a professional perioperative nurse for students and colleagues.
4. Functioning as a patient advocate by protecting the patient from incompetent, unethical, or illegal practices during the perioperative period.
5. Coordinating all activities associated with the implementation of nursing care by other members of the health-care team.
6. Demonstrating a thorough knowledge of aseptic principles and techniques to maintain a safe and therapeutic surgical environment.
7. Directing or assisting with the care and handling of all supplies, equipment, and instruments, to ensure their economic and efficient function for the patient and personnel under both normal and hazardous conditions.
8. Performing as the scrub, circulating nurse, or RNFA as needed, based on knowledge and expertise for a specific procedure.
9. Participating in continuing education programs directed toward personal and professional growth and development.
10. Participating in professional organizational and research activities that support and enhance perioperative nursing practice.

PROFESSIONALISM AND PERIOPERATIVE NURSING

> Nursing is an independent, autonomous, self-regulating profession with the primary function that of helping each person attain the highest possible level of general health . . .
>
> —*M. Schlotfeldt, 1973*

In 1978, perioperative nursing practice took on a different look because of a reevaluation of professional nursing practice in the OR and the practice of nursing in general. Society continued to depict nurses as dependent individuals, even though great strides had been accomplished to change that image.

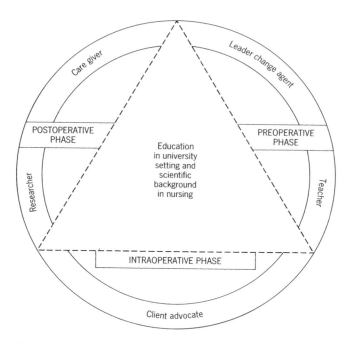

Fig. 1-2. Perioperative nursing practice—multiple roles

Toward this effort, nursing as a profession moved from an *occupation* to a profession, which is distinguished by cognitive, normative, and evaluative dimensions.

As part of this change, nursing has defined the characteristics and behaviors that are necessary for a profession, including the entry level requirements for nursing education in a university setting.

Increased higher education has become a prerequisite for many nurses, including those wishing to practice perioperative nursing.

A model for professional perioperative nursing practice has been created to depict the characteristics and attributes inherent in the practice of professional nursing during the perioperative period. The model is designed as a wheel. The center or hub represents the educational preparation for professional nursing practice. The spokes of the wheel depict the characteristics, interchanging roles, and attributes inherent in the practice of professional perioperative nursing (Fig. 1-2).

THE PRESENT: SURGERY AND ANESTHESIA SERVICES

In 1985, the Joint Commission for Accreditation of Healthcare Organizations (JCAHO), in their accreditation manual, required hospitals to establish a mechanism to assure that quality patient care was being performed in accordance with the standards of practice currently in force for all nursing areas.

In response to this, the AORN developed a credentialing model which was used by the JCAHO as a basis for nursing practice in the surgical unit, and in 1987 a new chapter was added to the manual, entitled "Sur-

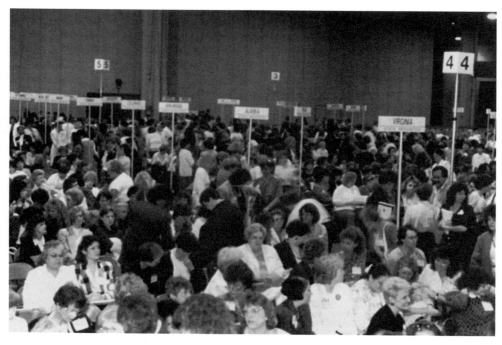

AORN Congress, Dallas, TX, 1991—House of Delegate meeting (Photograph by David Zeiger)

gery and Anesthesia Services," addressing most of the key issues presented by the AORN. This chapter was intended to serve as a guideline for acceptable, minimal levels of practice, but each OR and each perioperative nurse is ultimately responsible for assuring quality patient care, the central core of all nursing practice.

These basic competency statements were not confined to the hospitalized patient, but to any patient, in any setting, who was about to undergo surgical intervention and/or invasive procedures, including freestanding ambulatory surgical facilities.

Additionally, the JCAHO issued a separate manual for ambulatory care facilities in 1984, and it too reflects current recommendations for safe, therapeutic nursing intervention for the surgical patient.

THE ASSOCIATION OF OPERATING ROOM NURSES (AORN) AND PERIOPERATIVE NURSING TODAY

Today AORN is an international body of concerned professional nurses. As of October 1995, AORN represents over 48,000 nurses serving in a variety of roles and clinical settings. As of January, 1995, AORN is composed of over 380 chapters in all 50 states and around the world. These chapters and its members make up the heart and soul of the organization. AORN is dedicated to providing education, representation, and standards of quality patient care through a unified, voluntary professional organization.

Specialty Certification: Perioperative Nursing

In 1979, AORN created a voluntary certification program to demonstrate professional achievement in perioperative nursing practice. Nurses who successfully complete the certification examination are recognized by the letters "CNOR" following their titles. CNOR certification is the first step on the perioperative clinical ladder, and is recognized by most hospitals and institutions around the country as a mark of excellence in practice.

In 1992, at the request of the membership, and the changing roles of the perioperative nurse, the National Certification Board: Perioperative Nursing, Inc., (NCB: PNI) provided the first voluntary certification examination for those nurses who successfully completed the *RN First Assistant* (CRNFA) program; an expanded role of perioperative nursing. (See Chap. 15 for further discussion of the RNFA.) As of 1995, there are over 26,000 certified (CNOR) nurses and over 400 CRNFAs.[6]

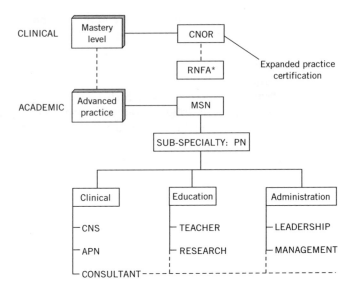

Certification eligibility will require BSN in 1998

Fig. 1-3. Perioperative nursing continuum (phase II)

ADVANCED PRACTICE: PERIOPERATIVE NURSING

In 1994, the AORN Board of Directors issued a statement regarding advanced practice in perioperative nursing. The statement developed as a result of an in-depth research study conducted by the National Research Committee-AORN. The study sampled 62 AORN members currently practicing in advanced roles (i.e., CNS, nurse practitioner, RNFA). (See Fig. 1-3.) The following is the approved definition of Advanced Practice Nursing (APN) in perioperative nursing.

The perioperative advanced practice nurse (APN) is a registered professional nurse who uses specialized knowledge and skills in the care of patients and families undergoing operative and other invasive procedures. The APN possesses a graduate degree in nursing that forms the foundation for an advanced role. The perioperative APN conducts comprehensive health assessments and demonstrates autonomy and skill in diagnosing and treating complex responses of clients (i.e., patient, family, community) to actual and potential health problems that are related to the prospect or performance of operative or other invasive procedures. The perioperative APN formulates clinical decisions to manage acute and chronic illness by assessing, diagnosing, and prescribing treatment modalities, including pharmacological agents. The perioperative APN promotes wellness. The perioperative APN integrates clinical practice, education, research, management, leadership, and consultation into a single role. The perioperative APN functions in a collegial relationship with nurses, physicians, and others who influence the health environment.[7]

In addition to the APN statement, the AORN Nursing Practice Committee established nursing competencies for this advanced practice role, which includes areas related to management, interpersonal relations, teaching and counseling, collaborative practice, leadership, and research.[8]

As the impact of this specialized nursing practice increases due to new and advanced technology, the perioperative nurse must continue to perform as the guardian of quality patient care. By achieving specialized certification and advanced practice in perioperative nursing, a statement has been made: Perioperative nursing promotes excellence in practice, while providing specialized services to those entrusted to their care during surgical and invasive procedures.

Self-assessment Exercise 1

Directions: Complete the following exercises. The answers are given at the end of this module.

1. Explain why the term *perioperative nurse* is a more comprehensive description than *operating room nurse.*

2. The scope of perioperative nursing practice consists of nursing activities during the three phases of surgical intervention.

    True   False

3. Perioperative nurses provide a wide range of services in locations other than acute care facilities.

    True   False

4. Perioperative nursing is a natural extension of the operating room nurses' role as originally practiced.

    True   False

5. Perioperative nursing practice is _____ centered rather than _____ oriented.

References

1. Steward I. Education of nurses. New York: Macmillan, 1944. P. 84.
2. Francis ME. Asepsis for the nurse. July, 1889.
3. Lukes E. Lectures on general nursing. London, 1887.
4. AORN. Standards and recommended practices. Denver: The Association, 1995. P. 70.
5. Ibid., p. I:1–2.
6. National Certification Board: Perioperative Nursing Inc. Denver, 1995 (conversation with the National Certification Board: Perioperative Nursing [NCB:PNI]): Certification specialist (1995 Congress).
7. House of Delegates 42nd Annual AORN Congress, 1995. *AORN J.* Editorial (June 1995) 6:6, 958.
8. AORN. Standards and recommended practices. Denver: The Association, 1995. Pp. 87–92.

2 The Surgical Setting

Sandra L. Hunter Sword

Demographics of the Surgical Suite
Surgical Suite Design Concepts
Environmental Safety
Infection Control: Principles and Practices
Environmental Sanitation
The Department of Surgery
Functions of the Surgical Team
Nursing Management
Role Assessment: An Administrator's Perception

UNIT 1

Environmental Orientation

The beginning practitioner usually conceives the operating room (OR) as a mysterious or forbidden area of the hospital, with signs on its doors stating "Restricted Area. Authorized Personnel Only."

This unit will attempt to unlock the mystery of the surgical suite and provide an orientation to the physical environment in which surgery is performed.

The modern surgical suite serves four fundamental purposes, and the activities that occur in this area have one common goal: to provide a safe therapeutic environment for the patient undergoing surgical intervention. These purposes are described as:

1. To obtain geographic isolation within the hospital, protected from unauthorized persons.
2. To obtain bacteriologic isolation through specific practices, attire, delivery, and disposal systems, in order to prevent cross-contamination from other areas of the hospital.

3. To centralize equipment and supplies, providing immediate access to specific items needed for surgery without leaving the protected area.
4. To centralize specialty personnel, since modern surgery requires the combined efforts of many groups to perform a variety of specialized tasks.

These four fundamental functions permit surgery to be performed in an isolated, restricted, yet flexible environment, dedicated to the safety of the surgical patient and the personnel working within the suite.

DEMOGRAPHICS OF THE SURGICAL SUITE

The surgical suite consists of specific areas in which selected tasks are performed. These are the *procedure rooms* (ORs), *storage areas* (sterile and non-sterile), and *ancillary support areas*, such as the preoperative holding/admission area, the postanesthesia care unit (recovery room), satellite pathology labs, and pharmacy dispensaries within the suite.

The overall floor plan of a surgical suite is divided into three areas, or zones, which are directly or indirectly involved with the operative procedure, equipment, supplies, or personnel. For descriptive purposes, the zones represent the type of activities, dress code, or restrictions for that zone, and each person working within the suite must abide by the policies and procedures related to the zone.

The Three-Zone Concept

The Unrestricted (Non-restricted) Area

The unrestricted area provides an entrance and exit from the surgical suite for personnel, equipment, and patients. Depending on the physical design of the surgical suite, the holding/admission area, and the postanesthesia care unit may be found in this zone, along with dressing rooms, lounges, offices, and receiving/storage areas for supplies to be used within the surgical suite.

Street clothes are permitted in this area, and the area provides access to communication with personnel within the suite and with personnel and patient's families outside the suite.

The Semirestricted Area

The semirestricted area provides access to the procedure rooms and peripheral support areas within the surgical suite. Personnel entering this area must be in proper OR attire, and traffic control must be designed to prevent violation of this area by unauthorized personnel or persons improperly attired for this zone. Peripheral support areas consist of storage areas for clean and sterile supplies; a sterilization, processing, and distribution area for instruments and nondisposable equipment; and corridors leading to procedure rooms and substerile utility areas.

The Restricted Area

The restricted area includes the procedure room where surgery is performed and adjacent substerile areas where the scrub sinks and autoclaves are located. Additional storage for immediate use by the adjacent procedure rooms is also found in the substerile areas, such as blanket/solution warmers, solutions, and so on. Personnel working in this area must be in proper OR attire, including a mask, since this area requires maximum protection from possible contamination.

In addition to the three zones just described, a central administration area, located in any of the three areas, acts as the coordinator for all activities performed within the suite. This area, commonly referred to as the nursing core desk or surgery desk, provides continuity, coordination, and communication within the surgical suite.

SURGICAL SUITE DESIGN CONCEPTS

The design and size of the surgical suite is usually determined by the functions and needs of the institution and the community it serves. For example, a small rural hospital may not need a large surgical suite and may need only five or six rooms, which do not require complicated equipment for cardiovascular and neurosurgery, while a large metropolitan hospital, serving a larger population, may require 14 to 18 procedure rooms within its suite.

A rule of thumb used when planning a surgical suite is based on a formula that recommends that the number of procedure rooms should equal 5 percent of the total number of surgical beds. Additional considerations could include:

1. Types of surgery being performed
2. Type of hospital (teaching, county, private)
3. Emergency department services provided
4. Number of surgeries being performed and the hours in which the service is provided

Physical Layout and Design

The surgical suite layout must conform to the three-zone concept discussed earlier, yet must be able to support the services' needs through established traffic patterns.

There are four basic designs for a modern surgical suite:

1. Central corridor (single corridor)
2. Double corridor (U or T shape)
3. Peripheral corridor (inner core/outer core)
4. Cluster, pod, or modular design

Central Corridor (Single Corridor)

The central corridor design is usually used when two to four procedure rooms are required; both the procedure rooms and the ancillary area function off of one central corridor (Fig. 2-1).

Double Corridor (U or T Shape)

Usually designed in an open or closed U or T shape, this design can accommodate 5 to 15 procedure rooms

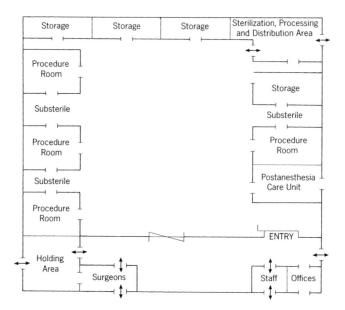

Fig. 2-1. Central (single) corridor design (usually reserved for small ORs)

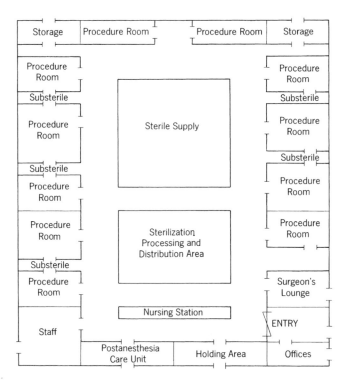

Fig. 2-2. Double corridor design (working area confined to central area in this design)

along the periphery of the area, with a central core usually designated as the "work area" of the surgical suite, housing the sterilization distribution and supply (SPD) area, storage rooms for supplies and equipment, and ancillary areas (Fig. 2-2).

Peripheral Corridor (Inner Core/Outer Core)

The peripheral corridor design calls for a corridor or hallway around the outside of the surgical suite (outer core), and a hallway inside the suite (inner core). The sterile/clean area is located in the inner core with the procedure rooms, while the outer core provides entry and exit to ancillary areas not requiring strict isolation, such as the holding area, postanesthesia recovery room, and so on. This design usually demands a large area and an elaborate traffic pattern design (Fig. 2-3).

Cluster, Pod, or Modular Design

The newest of surgical suite designs, the cluster consists of four procedure rooms attached to a central core area with pass-through windows or doors to allow for distribution of supplies. A technician is stationed in each core to service the attached rooms, and a peripheral corridor surrounds the entire suite to allow for entrance and exit of staff and patients. This design is advantageous when future expansion is contemplated, since the cluster or pod area will not disrupt the existing facilities. Each suite could conceivably contain three to five pods, or clusters, depending on the total area of the suite (Fig. 2-4).

Traffic Patterns: Controlling the Environment

Regardless of the design or age of the hospital, specific traffic patterns for personnel, patients, and supplies and equipment must be established to maintain an

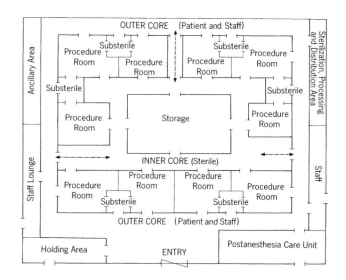

Fig. 2-3. Peripheral corridor design (created around inner core/outer core concept)

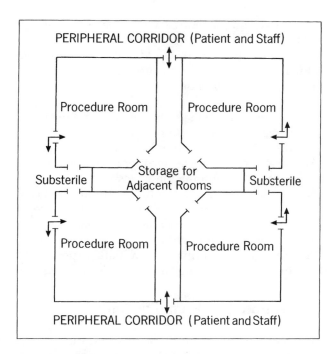

Fig. 2-4. Cluster, pod, or modular design (ideal for additions to existing structures)

aseptic environment and provide the services needed to perform safe and effective surgery.

According to the AORN recommended practices for traffic patterns within the surgical suite:[1]

1. The practice setting should be designed to facilitate movement of patients and personnel through, into, and out of defined areas within the suite.
2. Movement of personnel should be kept to a minimum while surgery is in progress.
3. The movement of clean and sterile supplies and equipment should be separated as much as possible from contaminated supplies, equipment, and waste by space, time, or traffic patterns.[2]

Traffic flow within the surgical suite is based on the principles of asepsis and infection control. The flow of traffic both in and out of the surgical suite will depend on the surgical suite design, but within a specific area the flow must be established according to principles that maintain an aseptic environment. Signs should clearly mark the area and the environmental controls and/or restrictions required.

Ideally, each pattern is unidirectional; that is, the flow of traffic is from entry to exit and from clean to dirty. However, this concept is ideal, and flexibility, based on acceptable principles, is required to achieve the ultimate goal: *the prevention of cross-contamination from one area to another.*

Before entering the surgical suite, visible signs should be posted restricting the area to authorized personnel only, thus reducing the number of persons within the actual suite to those who are directly involved with the activities occurring within the suite.

Once inside the suite, traffic patterns should prevent the mixing of clean, sterile, and dirty supplies by maintaining the institution's policies involving patients, equipment, and personnel.

Patients usually enter the suite through the unrestricted area, that is, the holding area, and will wait in that area while preoperative activities are performed, such as the preoperative assessment, the shave prep if ordered, starting preoperative intravenous infusions, and so on.

Before entering the semirestricted area, the patient's hair should be covered by a cap, then transported through this area to the restricted area of the suite. Since the patient does not wear a mask in the procedure room, the sterile set-up should be well away from both the head of the table and the entrance to the room, since respiratory droplets, which could lead to contamination of the sterile set-up, travel less than 10 feet, even with forced exhalation.

After surgery, the patient will again travel through the semirestricted area to the postanesthesia care unit (PACU), which in some institutions is considered both semirestricted and unrestricted, depending on its proximity to outside hallways within the institution.

If the suite is designed with an inner core/outer core layout, the patient should never be moved through the inner core.

Supplies and Equipment

Supplies and equipment entering or moving within the surgical suite should also follow a designated traffic pattern. Separation of clean and dirty items is essential to maintain the aseptic environment, just as clean and sterile items must be separated.

Items should be removed from corrugated paper boxes and outside shipping cartons before they enter the surgical suite, since they can be a source for dust and possible vermin, and because the containers have been handled and transported by common carriers working outside the protected area.

Equipment coming from outside the area should be damp-dusted with the recommended germicidal solution before entering into the semirestricted area of the suite. If clean or sterile supplies are coming from another area (central service), they should be transported to the suite on covered carts; the cover is removed prior to entry into the semirestricted areas.

Soiled instruments and items used during a surgical

procedure that require reprocessing must leave the procedure room covered or contained in some manner to prevent cross-contamination during transport to the designated area. Soiled items and instruments should never be left next to clean or sterile items for any length of time, and should be decontaminated immediately upon arrival into the decontamination area.

Items such as linen and trash should be double-bagged for proper containment, sealed and tied, and taken to a designated area for pick-up and disposal by appropriate personnel.

Most important in the prevention and control of infection is the practice of good handwashing technique by all members of the surgical staff, both between cases and before reentry into the suite from an outside area. This practice serves to protect both the person and the people working outside the surgical suite.

ENVIRONMENTAL SAFETY

Environmental safety is the responsibility of all personnel, and with on-going safety programs and diligent observation and detection methods, the surgical suite can remain a safe environment for both patients and staff. Five important considerations concerning the internal environment of the surgical suite directly relate to patient safety and infection control:

1. The size of the procedure room
2. Temperature and humidity control
3. Ventilation and air exchange systems
4. Electrical safety
5. Communication systems

Size of the Procedure Room

The standard procedure room is usually rectangular or square in shape, and should be 20 × 20 × 10 (or similar dimensions) to provide a minimum floor space of 360 square feet, exclusive of fixed cabinets and built-in shelves. The design of the suite should allow for two to four procedure rooms to share a substerile area and scrub facilities, depending on the actual floor plan.

Procedure rooms designed for services requiring additional equipment, such as open heart surgery, neurosurgery, or orthopedic surgery, will require a 20 × 30 × 10 area or a floor space of 600 square feet. For services requiring less equipment, such as endoscopy, a minimum of 250 square feet of floor space is recommended. Ceiling heights should be approximately 10 feet to accommodate ceiling-mounted lighting fixtures, and room lighting should be flush-mounted,

as close to ceiling without leaving space for dust accumulation.[3]

Each procedure room should have at minimum the following equipment to ensure maximum efficiency and safety for both patient and staff:[4]

1. Communication system, internal and external
2. Oxygen and vacuum outlets
3. Mechanical ventilation assistance equipment
4. Respiratory and cardiac monitoring equipment
5. X-ray film illumination boxes
6. Cardiac defibrillator with synchronization capability (adequate number to service the suite)
7. High-efficiency particulate air filters
8. Adequate room lighting
9. Emergency lighting system (battery-powered)
10. Entry and exit from substerile area for personnel

Temperature and Humidity Control

Since most pathogenic bacteria grow best in temperatures close to 98.6°F (37°C), the temperature in a procedure room should be maintained between 70°F and 75°F, with humidity levels kept between 50 and 60 percent at all times. Controlling the internal temperature and humidity at this constant level greatly reduces the chance of growth of microorganisms or the production of static electricity, thus providing a safe environment for both patient and staff. One exception to this temperature guideline involves preparation for pediatric surgery, which requires that the room be as warm as possible, at least 10 to 15 minutes before the arrival of the patient, since children rapidly lose body heat.

Ventilation and Air Exchange Systems

Airborne contamination can occur in a procedure room; therefore, an effective ventilation and filtration system is one that minimizes this threat to patients and staff.

Current recommendations for designing a new procedure room state that the air exchange in each procedure room should be at least 25 air exchanges every hour, and that 5 of these exchanges should be fresh air. A high-filtration particulate filter, working at 95 percent efficiency, is recommended. Inlet vents should be located as close to the ceiling as possible, while outlet vents should be located close to the floor.

Each procedure room should be maintained with positive pressure, which forces the old air out of the room and prevents the air from surrounding areas from entering into the procedure room. To maintain this positive pressure and reduce the risk of airborne contamination, the doors to the procedure rooms should *always* remain closed.

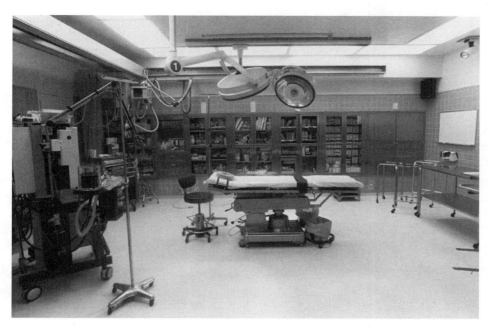

Procedure room with essential furniture and equipment

The anesthesia machine should contain an effective scavenging system to rid the air of escaped gases, thus eliminating the exposure of personnel and patient to a low concentration of vapors trapped in the room.

If hazardous solutions or materials are required during surgery, a separate evacuation system must be used to eliminate possible exposure to that material or waste product.

Electrical Safety

Although the use of combustible anesthetic gases has been eliminated from most surgical suites, the possibility of a spark from a piece of electrical equipment is still a major safety concern. The three most common hazards associated with electricity are fire, burns, and electric shock. The risk of each of these potentially dangerous situations can be greatly reduced by following recommended practices during the preparation, performance, and termination of a surgical procedure.

Faulty wiring, excessive use of extension cords, poorly maintained equipment, and a lack of current safety measures are just some of the hazardous factors that must be constantly checked for by all members of the staff whether they are directly or indirectly involved with patient care activities.

Through the institution of an effective safety program and monitoring of equipment by the biomedical engineering department, the suite can be monitored and maintained through observation, reporting, and routine maintenance of all electrical equipment. Most procedure rooms are now equipped with sufficient electrical outlets to prevent overloading the system, and through the installation of ceiling columns for gas, vacuum, and electrical outlets, the danger of tripping over cords or hoses has been mostly eliminated as a danger to the staff working in the rooms. Although an isolated power system is no longer required, some surgical suites have a system referenced to a common ground, thereby reducing the hazard of shock or burns from electrical current flowing through the body to the ground. An alarm should notify personnel when this system detects a fault or leakage. To determine the cause of the leakage, disconnect one electrical device at a time until the alarm is silenced.

All electrical equipment, new or used, should be routinely checked by qualified personnel and certified as safe to use according to national, state, and local safety codes. Equipment that fails to function at 100 percent efficiency should be taken out of service immediately, reported, and removed for repair or replacement as required. Several regulatory and voluntary agencies are concerned with safety within the hospital and the surgical suite. These agencies include the Occupational Safety and Health Administration (OSHA); Environmental Protection Agency (EPA); National Fire Protection Agency (NFPA); National Safety Code (NSC); The National Institute for Occupational Safety and Health (NIOSH); and The Centers for Disease Control (CDC), just to name a few. Questions and/or concerns for safety of patients and personnel should be directed to the hospital biomedical department or to these agencies directly.

Communication Systems, Internal and External

Since each procedure room becomes a separate entity within the suite during the surgical procedure, an effective, reliable means of communication must be established to maintain a safe environment. The system chosen should be capable of separating routine calls from those requiring immediate attention or assistance. In addition, the nursing core desk should have a direct communication link to each procedure room and ancillary area within the suite. Intercoms, telephones, or both provide a means of communication within and outside the suite, and all personnel should be taught how to use the system effectively and efficiently.

Self-assessment Exercise 2

Directions: Complete the following exercises. The answers are given at the end of this module.

1. List three important concepts that should be considered when designing a surgical suite.

2. The surgical suite is divided into three areas. Name them.

3. Each of the above areas are restricted to specific activities/equipment/supplies. Briefly describe each.

4. Four common surgical suite designs are in use today. Name them and give a brief description of each.

5. Name the five environmental factors important to patient safety in a procedure room.

6. List three factors associated with traffic control within the surgical suite.

INFECTION CONTROL: PRINCIPLES AND PRACTICES

Operating Room Attire

All persons who enter the semirestricted and restricted areas of the surgical suite should wear surgical attire intended for use within the surgical suite.[5]

OR attire is an important factor in controlling the potential spread of infection to the surgical patient and to the population outside the protected area. By restricting the clothing worn within the suite, the first barrier to infection has been established, and it is an essential component for the maintenance of an aseptic environment.

The Scrub Suit

In accordance with the AORN recommended guidelines, the scrub suit should be made of a lint-free, flame-resistant fabric that meets or exceeds the National Fire Prevention Association (NFPA) standards for proper fabric construction.

The scrub suit top should have short sleeves, and be tucked into the pants to prevent accidental contamination during movement within the restricted area. When donning the scrub attire, care should be taken to avoid contacting the floor with the pants or bottom of the dress.

Scrub attire should be changed daily or when it becomes soiled or wet. Scrub suits can be either cloth or paper fabric, as long as the fabric meets the minimum standards as previously stated. Reuseable surgical attire should be "Laundered in a laundry facility approved and monitored by the practice setting. . . . Laundering at home is not recommended."[6] Name tags and protective eye wear are included as part of proper OR attire, and circulating nurses and anesthesia personnel should wear jackets to prevent shedding from bare arms. Jackets should be closed to prevent

excess air movement, and removed prior to performing any aseptic procedure, for example, the surgical skin prep, thus avoiding possible contamination of the sterile field.

Headgear

Head and facial hair, including sideburns, should be covered when in the semirestricted and restricted areas.[7]

The scrub cap or hood must be clean and lint-free, and made of a fabric that meets or exceeds the NFPA standards. The headgear should be donned before the scrub attire to prevent fallout from the hair collecting on the scrub attire. The headgear should be discarded before leaving the surgical suite, and a new one applied prior to reentry into the semirestricted area.

Protective Barriers

Protective barriers should be made available to reduce the risk of exposure to potentially infective materials.[8]

Protective barriers include gloves (sterile and nonsterile), eye wear (goggles or shield masks), shoe covers or calf-high boots, and liquid-resistant aprons whenever the individual is exposed to blood or potentially infectious materials/solutions.

The Question of Shoe Covers

Shoes worn during the surgical procedure have a chance of becoming soiled by solutions, blood, and organic debris, and it is extremely difficult to clean contaminated shoes properly. Therefore, shoe covers, or "booties," should be worn over shoes by all personnel whether they are directly or indirectly involved with patient care areas, and changed as needed to prevent tracking of contaminants throughout the suite. Shoe covers should be removed before leaving the suite, and new ones applied prior to reentry into the semirestricted area. Be aware, however, some experts consider shoe covers an added, unnecessary expense.

Surgical Masks

All persons entering restricted areas of the surgical suite should wear a mask when there are open sterile items and equipment present.[9]

Since large numbers of potentially pathogenic microorganisms reside in the respiratory tract, a high-filtration mask, covering both the nose and mouth, should be worn at all times while in the procedure rooms or substerile and scrub areas.

Guidelines for the Proper Use of Masks

1. Masks must be changed between each procedure, if it becomes moist or wet, or both.
2. While wearing a mask, conversation should be kept to a minimum to prevent moisture build-up.
3. Masks should be removed by the strings and properly discarded before leaving the procedure room.
4. Masks are *never* worn outside the surgical suite.
5. Masks are either *on* or *off*. They should not be left dangling around the neck or placed in a pocket for future use.
6. Masks should fit snugly around the nose and chin, and should be tied securely to prevent accidental slipping during a procedure.

Surgical attire should be worn only within the surgical suite, but if it becomes necessary to leave the suite in OR attire, a cover gown may be worn over the scrub attire. Changing the scrub attire upon reentry into the surgical suite is governed by the institution's policies and procedures for OR attire.

To Cover or Not to Cover . . .

In 1993, AORN suggested that a "single-use cover gown should be worn over surgical attire when leaving the surgical suite."[10]

Today, because of cost-containment management and several research studies conducted concerning the value of cover gowns, hospitals have decided to create their own policies and procedures concerning the use of cover gowns. Alternative suggestions range from using a cover gown only when leaving the physical confines of the hospital, to not using a cover gown and changing scrubs on return to the OR, to not using cover gowns while in the hospital (lunch, breaks, and so on) and not changing scrub attire. Whatever the decision, a well-delineated policy, standardized throughout the institution, regarding cover gowns should be established, written, and enforced without exception. The recommendations for this policy should be made in collaboration with the infection control department of the institution.

Additional Recommendations

Wearing jewelry, such as rings, watches, and necklaces, is not recommended since they can harbor bacteria. Earrings should be small (i.e., stud earrings) and must be totally contained within the cap or hood.

Fingernails should be short, free from polish that has chipped, and maintained in good condition. As to artificial nails, they could harbor microorganisms or a fungus could develop due to frequent hand washing. Artificial nails are not recommended for personnel working in semirestricted or restricted areas.[11]

In addition, the Occupational Safety and Health Administration (OSHA) requires that all members of the staff use protective eye wear if the individual does not use corrective glasses. Contact lenses do not provide adequate protection for the eyes; therefore, protective eye wear is required for those individuals, including anesthesia personnel.

By adhering to these recommended practices for proper OR attire, the staff member can effectively assist in controlling and containing potential contaminants within the surgical suite, thus protecting the patient, visitors, themselves, and their coworkers from infection or accidental cross-contamination outside the protected area.

ENVIRONMENTAL SANITATION

Patients should be provided with a safe, clean environment, free from dust and organic debris.[12]

Effective environmental sanitation programs must be established to reduce the possibility of cross-contamination, which may lead to surgical wound infections, as well as the protection of personnel within and without the surgical suite.

The basis for such a program is the concept of universal precautions, which states that *all patients should be considered potentially contaminated* and therefore treated exactly alike regardless of the procedure being performed.

Although the environment cannot be sterilized, appropriate cleaning and disinfection procedures can reduce the possibility of transmitting pathogens, thus maintaining an aseptic environment. Environmental sanitation practices are performed by all members of the staff who are present in the suite before, during, and after a surgical procedure, and require constant observation to maintain a safe, therapeutic environment.

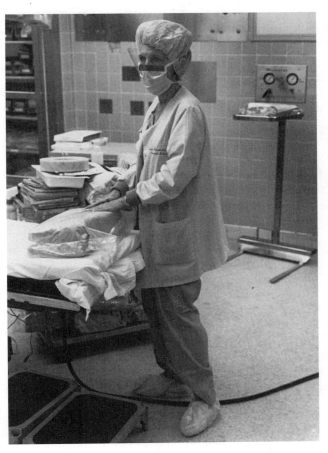

OR attire—clean scrub suit and mask with eye protector, cap, and shoe covers

Careful attention is given to the preparation of a procedure room by the surgical team, and the principles of containment and control become of primary importance to all personnel associated with the surgical procedure. Methods used to accomplish this goal should include:

1. Containment in clear plastic bags of soiled sponges during the procedure.
2. Double-bagging all soiled linen and disposable items before their removal at the conclusion of the procedure.
3. Immediate cleaning with an effective disinfectant solution of spills and debris from floors and walls.
4. Removing soiled shoe covers before leaving the procedure room, thus eliminating the "tracking" effect within the suite.

In addition to these recommendations, specific procedures should be used before and after each surgery and before the first case of the day. These are referred to as *preliminary, interim,* and *terminal cleaning* proce-

dures. In addition, a weekly and/or monthly cleaning program should be established by environmental services personnel.

Preliminary Cleaning

Proper preparation of the procedure room before the first case is essential to an effective surgical outcome. It is the responsibility of the scrub and circulating nurses to see that everything is ready prior to the acceptance of a patient.

To avoid unnecessary clutter, furniture and equipment not expressly required for the procedure should be removed. Before bringing in the selected surgical supplies for the case, horizontal surfaces should be damp-dusted with a hospital-approved disinfectant solution. Damp-dusting reduces viable microbial contamination from air and other sources by 90 to 99 percent. Adequate containers, properly lined, should be available and placed well away from the sterile field to avoid possible contamination during the set-up phase.

During the procedure, all efforts must be made to contain and confine the contaminated items. If an instrument falls to the floor, and requires immediate sterilization, the item should be washed first to reduce the number of contaminated microorganisms on the instrument.

At the conclusion of the case, gross soil and debris should be removed from the instruments if necessary, and the tray covered and taken to the appropriate area for decontamination and reprocessing.

If a case cart system is used, all reusable items and equipment are placed inside the cart. The cart is closed and taken to the decontamination area. The cart should be emptied and then washed with disinfectant solution or cleaned in an automatic steam cart washer system before it is restocked with items for the next procedure.

Interim Cleaning

All items that have come in contact with the patient or sterile field should be considered contaminated. Disposable items should be disposed of according to regulations. Reusable items should be processed according to institutional policy.[13]

Interim cleaning of the procedure room is performed at the end of each case, using an established protocol. Wet vacuuming is the method of choice for cleaning the floors since it is more effective than manual cleaning methods. If the wet-mop method is used, the mop head and disinfectant solution *must* be changed after each case and properly disposed of according to hospital policy. Adequate time must be allowed for proper disinfection and set-up of the procedure room.

Environmental services personnel, working within the suite to assist the surgical team, must be thoroughly knowledgeable about aseptic technique and proper methods used during the interim cleaning process, and should be supervised during the procedure to ensure maximum efficiency. With a well-coordinated team effort, turnover time between procedures can be accomplished in an average of 15 to 20 minutes.

Terminal Cleaning

At the conclusion of the day's schedule, operating (procedure) rooms, scrub/utility areas, corridors, furnishings, and equipment should be terminally cleaned.[14]

At the end of the day, or after use of a room is finished for the day, a more stringent and rigorous cleaning procedure is performed, usually by environmental services personnel with the assistance of the surgical staff.

All furniture is thoroughly cleaned with an appropriate disinfectant. Casters and wheels should be cleaned, and debris, such as suture strands, removed. Horizontal surfaces should be cleaned; ceiling and wall fixtures and tracks are cleaned on all surfaces. Floors are flooded after the furniture has been removed, and a thorough wet vacuuming is performed along with spot removal from the walls as needed. Once the floor is dry, the furniture is replaced and clean linen is placed on the OR table.

The cabinets in the room should be restocked with sterile supplies, with the assistive personnel being careful to rotate the stock of "in-hospital" sterilized items to reduce the risk of using "out-dated" sterile supplies. Avoidance of overstocking shelves will assist in easy retrieval of the items when needed.

Weekly and/or Monthly Cleaning

All areas and equipment in the surgical practice setting should be cleaned according to an established rou-

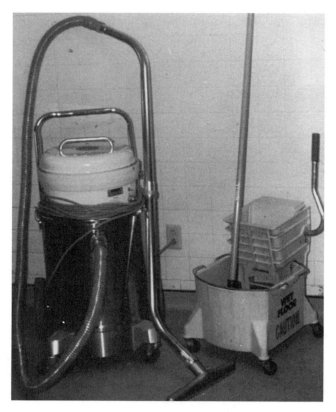

Environmental cleaning equipment—wet vac system, mop and bucket

tine.[15] In addition to the routine daily cleaning procedures, a weekly and/or monthly cleaning program, set up with environmental services personnel, should be established in the surgical suite. It should include thorough cleaning of ceilings, walls, floors, air-conditioning grills, sterilizers, and solution dispensers. Kick buckets should be washed and sterilized, and the cleaning equipment routinely used should be disassembled and disinfected.

Self-assessment Exercise 3

Directions: Complete the following exercises. The answers are given at the end of this module.

1. Environmental control in the surgical suite is based on the principles of _____ and _____.

2. Describe the proper OR attire for the following areas:
    a) Semirestricted area
    b) Restricted area
    c) Outside the surgical suite

3. Equipment should be damp-dusted before entering the semirestricted area.

    True   False

4. Clean supplies need not be separated from sterile supplies inside the surgical suite.

    True   False

5. Terminal cleaning is performed after each surgical procedure.

    True   False

6. The recommended temperature within the surgical suite is between _____ and _____, with the humidity maintained between _____ and _____.

7. Discuss the reason(s) for keeping the door closed during a surgical procedure.

8. Protective eye wear is part of proper OR attire for all personnel.

    True   False

9. Describe the proper method for terminal cleaning of a procedure room.

UNIT 2

Organizational Structure: The Team Concept

One of the best ways in which to develop a supportive climate, is to foster a feeling of group cohesiveness.

—E. J. Sullivan and P. J. Decker

Surgery is a complex field that requires a coordinated, well-directed team effort. There are three basic objectives of surgical patient care, and each team member plays a vital role in achieving these objectives:[16]

1. The delivery of a physiologically and psychologically prepared patient for the planned surgical experience.
2. The safe, efficient, and therapeutic alleviation of the patient's problem based on sound scientific knowledge and proficiency in technique.
3. The careful guidance of the patient's immediate postoperative care in order to minimize the possibility of future problems or complications.

These objectives are partially met in the clinical unit during the preoperative phase, and in the PACU immediately following surgery. But it is during the intraoperative phase that the surgical team provides much of the care necessary to meet the stated objectives of surgical patient care successfully.

The surgical team, usually consisting of the surgeon, his or her assistant, the scrub nurse/technician, the circulating nurse, and the anesthesiologist/anesthesia clinician (nurse anesthetist) must coordinate their efforts if the surgical experience is to be successful and therapeutic. Although each team member has specific duties and responsibilities, one member cannot function efficiently without the assistance and support of the others.

THE DEPARTMENT OF SURGERY

Administrative Structure

The OR Supervisor/Nurse Manager is responsible for the clinical aspects of the surgical suite in addition to its day-to-day management, including the delegation, planning, staffing, and directing of nursing activities occurring in the area. Additional nursing management personnel include, but are not limited to:

1. Head nurse
2. Assistant head nurses (speciality coordinators)
3. Clinical nurse specialist (education/management)
4. Team leaders

The position titles and responsibilities will vary with each institution and hospital, depending on its size and organizational structure (Fig. 2-5), but the goal is the same:

To render quality patient care during all three phases of surgical intervention.

Administrative Practices

Any successful organization or department relies on the orderly arrangement and efficient execution of patient care activities. In surgery, due to its critical nature, a team effort is essential to maintain quality patient care. The contribution of each person is like one level of a building. The AORN Standards and Recommended Practices[17] provides the interior design of the structure, while the Standards of Administrative Practices: OR[18] provides the framework of the structure. The quality and strength of each level is vital to the successful completion of the original objective.

These administrative standards are intended to serve as guidelines for the development of a successful program that will provide efficiency while promoting professional perioperative nursing care through research, education, and effective management skills.

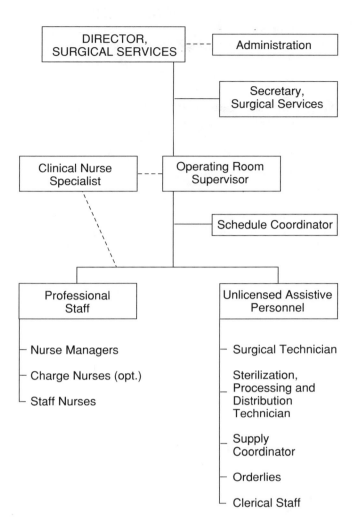

Fig. 2-5. Organizational chart—Department of surgery (Courtesy of Broward General Medical Centre, Ft. Lauderdale, FL, 1990.)

FUNCTIONS OF THE SURGICAL TEAM

Each person involved with the surgical patient has a vital role in the overall quality of care rendered. The implementation of efficient surgical intervention requires team work by all members, whether they are involved directly or indirectly with patient care. This team work requires vigilance, intelligent cooperation, and a readiness to assist whenever and wherever needed. The surgical team is divided into the sterile members (those who scrub, gown, and glove) and the non-sterile members. Satisfactory service in the operating room becomes a reality when all staff members within the department know their job and perform it efficiently and professionally.

Let's look at each position to gain a better understanding of the team concept.

AORN Standards: Administrative Practices, 1995

I   A philosophy, purpose, and objectives shall be formulated to guide OR services.

II An organizational plan for the OR shall be developed and communicated.

III A registered nurse shall be authorized with administrative accountability and responsibility for the OR services.

IV The registered nurse administrator shall be accountable and responsible for developing mechanisms that assure optimal patient care.

V   The OR management team shall develop and manage the budget for OR services.

VI The OR service shall have written standards of nursing practice.

VII The OR services shall have written policies and procedures that serve as operational guidelines.

VIII The OR management team shall be responsible for establishing staffing requirements, selecting personnel, and planning for appropriate utilization of human resources.

IX Staff development programs shall be provided for OR personnel.

X   A safe OR environment shall be established, controlled, and consistently monitored.

XI The OR management team shall promote the discovery and integration of new knowledge by encouraging development and use of nursing research.

XII The OR staff shall maintain appropriate documentation related to OR activities.

XIII The OR management team shall recognize a professional responsibility to promote, provide, and participate in a learning environment for students in health-care disciplines.

XIV There shall be a quality assurance program for OR services.

Source: AORN. Standards and recommended practices. Denver: The Association, 1995. Pp. 99–105.

The Surgeon
A physician who has specialized in the practice of surgery. Major responsibilities include, but are not limited to:

- performance of the operative procedure according to the needs of the patient
- the primary decision maker regarding surgical technique to use during the procedure (instruments, sutures, etc.)
- may assist with positioning and prepping the patient or may delegate this task to other members of the team

The First Assistant to the Surgeon
- May be a resident, intern, physician's assistant, or a perioperative nurse
- Assists with retracting, hemostasis, suturing, and any other tasks requested by the surgeon to facilitate speed while maintaining quality during the procedure

The Anesthesiologist
- A physician who specializes in the administration and monitoring of anesthesia while maintaining the overall well-being of the patient
- A non-sterile member of the surgical team

The Nurse Anesthetist (Anesthesia Clinician)
- The nurse anesthetist or anesthesia clinician is an advanced registered nurse practitioner who after additional training and certification in anesthesia (the Certified Registered Nurse Anesthetist [CRNA]) may administer and monitor the anesthesia using the anesthesiologist as a consultant if necessary
- A non-sterile member of the surgical team

The Scrub Assistant
- May be either a nurse or a surgical technician
- Responsible for assisting the surgeon and assistant with instrumentation, set-ups, suture presentation, sponges, and so on, while maintaining the sterility of the surgical field through aseptic practices

Key elements for successful implementation of this role is based on knowledge of anatomy and the sequence of the surgical procedure, to facilitate and anticipate the needs of the surgeon and the assistant.

The Circulating Nurse
- Must be a registered nurse who, after additional education and training, is specialized in perioperative nursing practice
- A non-sterile member of the surgical team
- Responsible and accountable for all activities occurring during a surgical procedure, including, but not limited to, the management of personnel, equipment, supplies, and the environment during a surgical procedure, and managing the flow of information to and from the surgical team members scrubbed at the field
- Patient advocate, teacher, researcher, manager, leader, and role model
- May be responsible for monitoring the patient during local procedures if a second perioperative nurse is not available

Unlicensed Assistive Personnel (UAP)
In addition to the above team members, UAP play a vital role in the day-to-day operation of the surgical suite. These positions include, but are not limited to:

- nursing aides
- patient care aides
- orderlies
- anesthesia technicians

Although these individuals are involved with direct patient care activities, they function in an "assistive role to the registered professional nurse. . . ."[19]

The surgical suite may also have ancillary personnel such as instrument room technicians (SPD technicians), clerical personnel and environmental services personnel, who although they do not have patient contact, are responsible, under the supervision of a professional (perioperative) nurse, for maintaining an aseptic environment and processing surgical supplies and equipment according to established criteria.

NURSING MANAGEMENT

> Effective leadership/management involves a sound educational process.
> —*L. M. Douglas, 1994*

A Conceptual Overview

Management, or supervision, can be described as the process of getting work done with and by others proficiently and within given constraints, such as budget or available human resources.

In surgery, as in any other area of nursing practice, all nurses are leaders and managers of patient care to some degree; either in an appointed role or in one the individual has assumed.

Nursing, as a decision-making, process-oriented profession, has required leadership/management skills from the beginning, in order to accomplish specific goals with the help of others.

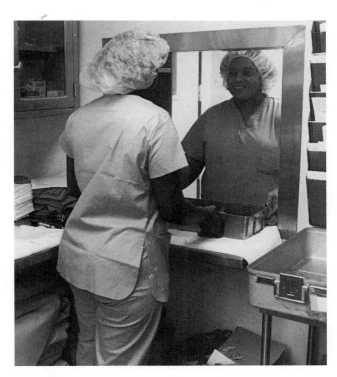

SPD technicians provide a vital service to the department of surgical services

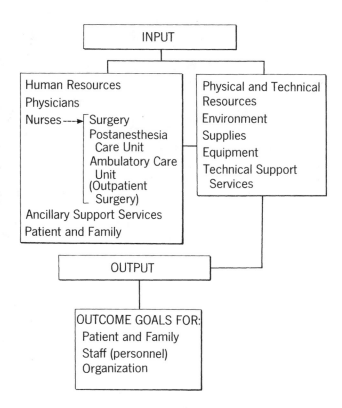

Fig. 2-6. Managing resources through input and output (Adapted from Douglas, LM. *The Effective Nurse/Manager* [3rd ed.]. St. Louis: CV Mosby, 1995.)

Role Definitions

Leader

Leadership is the effective use of skills that can influence or motivate others to perform to their fullest potential.

The leadership process influences the actions of a person or group to attain stated desired goals. It is dependent upon effective interpersonal skills, mutual respect, and mutually satisfying action and/or results for both the leader and the follower.

Leadership can occur in two distinct forms:

1. *Informal leadership* in which a person or team member is chosen by a group, but who is not specifically designated and who lacks formal authority, yet still influences group decision-making processes
2. *Formal leadership* in which a person who is by virtue of education and preparation appointed to the position and is given official authority to act and make decisions in the name of the organization or department

Manager

Management, or supervision, is described as the ability to get things done, making use of human, technical,

and physical resources, while providing guidance and directing people toward the organization's goals.

The management process consists of accomplishing organizational objectives through four distinct, yet integrated, functions: (1) planning, (2) organizing, (3) directing, and (4) controlling human, physical, and technical resources.

Management is a series of inputs and outputs: inputs occur through the use of human, physical, and technical resources, while outputs are the realization of specific goals (Fig. 2-6).

Leadership is usually a prerequisite to effective management: management requires a more global responsibility, while leadership is recognized as the "change-factor," assisting management in achieving stated goals.

Leadership and Management: Similarities and Differences

Although similar, leadership and management are different, not only in their official status but also in their overall effect.

The leader, whether formal or informal, can command power and authority only as long as there are followers, and may or may not have the ability to be an effective manager.

The perioperative nurse, by virtue of his or her educational preparation, is the natural "leader" within the surgical environment, and therefore must project a positive role model for others to follow.

Managers, on the other hand, have the power and authority to command action from individuals, owing to their position within the organization, but they may or may not be effective leaders if they lack the ability to achieve their goals due to a weak interrelationship with the group.

To be successful, one has to blend the qualities of both the leader and the manager, so that the followers continue to be influenced by them, by choice. This concept is applicable not only in business, but can be applied to perioperative nursing practice.

While leadership is an art, management is a science, deriving its basis from educational preparation consisting of sociologic and technical skills. Each can enhance the other in daily practice.

Sullivan and Decker (1995) describe management as having six basic yet essential responsibilities:

1. *Planning* Short- and long-term objectives and goals for a specific area or group of people within that area that are designed to complement the institution's philosophy and meet the needs of the individuals working within the department
2. *Staffing* To select the appropriate staff members to meet the goals and objectives stated, and to place them in appropriate positions so that implementation is effective
3. *Organizing* The effective use of human and material resources to achieve maximum efficiency to accomplish the stated goals and objectives
4. *Directing* Involves leadership and motivation so that the selected personnel can accomplish the institutional/department objectives
5. *Controlling* Relies on the use of criteria or standards of performance and the corrective actions needed when personnel deviate from the acceptable standards, policies, or regulations of the institution and/or department
6. *Decision-making* Relies on the ability to identify problems and search for alternative solutions to correct the problem

Factors Affecting the Nurse Manager

Six common factors can ultimately affect the nurse manager's effectiveness.[20]

A. Institutional structure
    Authority and power (where and how much)
    Centralization versus decentralization concepts
    Recruitment and selection system
    Reward system/clinical ladders
B. Social structure
    Role conflicts
    Organizational climate
    Philosophy
C. Staffing
    Group process/cohesiveness
    Motivation
    Change factors
D. Tasks/technology
    Personnel requirements
    Work environment
    Educational support
E. Organizational objectives
    Realistic
    Dynamic
    Participation in research
F. Environmental factors
    Economic climate
    Legal restraints
    Physical layout and design

The transition from a clinical role to a managerial role calls for learning and practicing a new set of skills. Nurses are not prepared for management during their initial educational preparation, so they must learn the necessary skills for effective leadership/management roles as they pursue higher education.

In the day-to-day practice of nursing, perioperative nurses are required to use management skills as they provide quality patient care during the surgical experience. This type of management is based on decision-making processes, which can determine the right approach to manage safely and effectively the patient and the environment.

Management and Leadership Styles

There are many theories and styles of management, some that are effective and others that may not always be successful, depending on their application. A new manager and/or leader should be familiar with the essential elements of each style, and decide which style is comfortable and yet still produces the best results. By the same token, experienced managers need to reassess their own management styles occasionally to evaluate the effectiveness of their current management practices and/or modify the style as needed. Such reassessment is necessary to accomplish the overall goals and objectives of the department and/or the organization.

According to Douglas (1995) there are four management styles, each with its own individual strengths and weaknesses.

Authoritarian/Autocratic Style

Managers who use the authoritarian style make all decisions *alone*, never involving others in the process. This usually results in lack of group support or respect for the position or the manager.

Such managers usually exhibit a low opinion of the workers, and feel that they (the worker) must be controlled to accomplish requested tasks.

Many situations require this style of management owing to the nature of the task required or requested, but it should not be the only style used if the manager is seeking to establish a cohesive, satisfied group.

Democratic/Consultative Style

The democratic style is also know as *participative* management, and emphasizes team work, open communication, and group dynamics. By using this style, the leader or manager becomes people-oriented rather than task-oriented. There is a mutual responsiveness to meeting group goals, and the manager/leader serves as a consultant when decisions affecting the group need to be made.

Permissive Style

Also known as "laissez-faire" managers, permissive managers usually have no established goals, and do not lead. They *assume* that the staff is self-motivated and that the job will be done with or without direction or control. This is directly opposite to the autocratic style of management, and can be highly effective, but only when used with motivated professional groups. It is rarely successful when the institution, or top management, believes in a highly structured, controlled management style.

Multicratic Style

In the multicratic management style, the positive aspects of the traditional styles just mentioned are combined to produce a flexible approach to management.

Since operating room nursing is a team effort, the perioperative nurse manager and/or leaders need to have an understanding of group dynamics, develop effective communication skills and interpersonal relationships, and be able to apply this knowledge to develop a supportive climate that fosters group cohesiveness and positive change.

ROLE ASSESSMENT: AN ADMINISTRATOR'S PERCEPTION

Now that we have discussed the concepts and components of effective management, let's get to the heart of the matter, since this is where management starts: in the heart.

Management is working *with* people, not having people work *for* you.

Think of management as building relationships with people, since management is people-oriented, whether it involves encouraging growth of key personnel or managing patient care. It is people working *with* people for the good of the organization and/or the improvement of nursing practice and patient care standards.

In many ways, the ability to manage people is a gift that, when cultivated through education and practice, becomes an effective tool that can motivate people to accomplish specific outcomes.

Many times, just a person's presence suggests he or she is a manager, by his or her manner of communication, actions, or reactions to and with people. These people possess a quality known as *charisma*; such people usually accomplish what they need to with the help of other people.

Desired Characteristics in an Administrator (Manager)

Many successful managers possess certain characteristics that enable them to be effective, including

1. Being able to make decisions
2. Being able to praise honestly and sincerely
3. Being able to think independently
4. Looking at the global picture before making decisions
5. Listening to and hearing what people are saying
6. Delegating and allowing those delegated to do the job and grow at the same time
7. Being self-motivated, dynamic, and willing to take constructive criticism, in order to grow

And, the most important of all,

8. Being honest, sincerely concerned, and caring about the people working with you on your team.

A manager (administrator) is there to facilitate learning and growth for the staff and ultimately for the organization. For the process to be successful, however, open lines of communication and an open-door policy must be in force. If the manager (administrator) is inaccessible or unapproachable, the group cohesiveness will break down, which can result only in failure to accomplish the goals that were originally established by your organization and/or your staff.

The Dichotomy of Administration/Management

An effective administrator needs to be a people-oriented person first, and an administrator second. The person-to-person aspect of managers in today's healthcare setting demands more than knowledge about being a manager, it demands a sixth sense about dealing effectively with people.

Although nurses routinely make management-type decisions involving the quality of patient care, not everyone is management (administrative) material, and here lies the dichotomy.

All nurses manage patient care, but not all nurses should be managers. There is absolutely nothing wrong with this, since nursing, as a profession, requires a *team* effort of both clinicians and managers to deliver effectively quality patient care.

Although theories and styles can and should be learned, the individual must decide which aspect of nursing accomplishes his or her individual goals and objectives, and being the best clinician in a specific area or setting is just as important as being a successful manager.

Perioperative nursing is no exception. The nurse must manage the clinical activities for a specific procedure using the clinical skills and independent thinking required to provide a safe, therapeutic environment for the surgical patient.

By the same comparison, the staff nurse working on the medical/surgical floor, or any other area within the institution, is the heart of the organization, while the manager, if successful, can assist in developing that staff nurse to his or her full potential, since without the staff nurse, management, regardless of the style used, cannot be successful. Management, therefore, revolves around *people.*

Impacts of Cost-Effective Administration/Management

One aspect, not yet introduced in this unit, is budgeting responsibilities; that is, the allocation of funds for specific needs of the department.

A budget helps control the organization or department, and because of its specialty and complexity, budgets will not be discussed in this chapter, except to speak about cost-effectiveness as it relates to training and education of the staff, and its impact on the organization as a whole.

The Perioperative Nursing Educator

Unfortunately, when budget cuts are requested, the first or second position to be eliminated is the *educator,* since that position is not usually perceived as being directly involved with patient care, nor does it generate revenue for the department. However, this assumption is what can cause the majority of unforeseen problems, for without education, a direct link to cost-effective and proficient management is in jeopardy, especially in surgery.

It is the successful administrator who recognizes the need for continuing quality education. Through this process the staff not only knows what to do, but more importantly, how to do it effectively and safely.

A dynamic education program in surgery can save the department and organization unnecessary expenses in the areas of:

- Recruitment and retention of staff
- Efficiently managing highly technical equipment
- Producing patient and physician satisfaction
- Maintaining an awareness of new technologies and maintenance of quality patient care as required by accrediting bodies

But most important, education can promote enhancement of professionalism through an on-going learning process, whether self-motivated or directed through formalized educational programs. It is impossible to be effective in any department, especially surgery, without continuing and effective educational support.

The educator or clinical nurse specialist is an important component of the management team, and is essential in maintaining quality patient care in a rapidly changing and highly technical environment. In institutions that promote education, management will be more successful and efficient. If not, it should become the job, of the administrator/manager, to promote education by stressing its contribution to the organization and the staff.

The administrator serves as the official representative of an assigned division or department, and is primarily responsible for planning, directing, coordinating, implementing, controlling, evaluating, and improving the quality of patient care. Whoever fills that position is expected to use current theories and acquired skills to enhance the department and ultimately the organization.

The Importance of Advanced Nursing Education

Most staff nurses have had little educational or practical experience in management positions. By being self-motivated, people-oriented, and having a commitment to the organization, selected nurses are likely to become well respected, and can become successful managers through formal educational programs.

Nurses in all areas of patient care must learn how to use both knowledge and people skills to manage effectively all aspects of their professional nursing practice.

Effective administration requires advanced nursing education in order to advance the management of perioperative nursing practice.

Self-assessment Exercise 4

Directions: Complete the following exercises. The answers are given at the end of this module.

1. State, in your own words, the three basic objectives of surgical patient care.

2. List the primary role functions of the
   a. Circulating nurse
   b. Scrub nurse/surgical technician
   c. CRNA
   d. Surgeon/first assistant

3. List the six responsibilities of management.

4. Compare the four leadership/management styles, and state the differences of each.

5. Assessment of personal characteristics is a reliable tool for determining the potential of a leader/manager.

                True   False

References

1. AORN. Standards and recommended practices. Denver: The Association, 1995. Pp. 141–144.
2. Ibid, pp. 283–284.
3. Department of Health and Rehabilitative Services. Hospital Licensure, Vol. 5, Washington, DC: 1986:854–855.
4. Ibid, p. 856.
5. Op. cit., p. 141.
6. AORN, 1995, p. 141.
7. Ibid, p. 142.
8. Ibid, p. 144.
9. Ibid, p. 143.
10. Ibid, p. 105.
11. Ibid, p. 143.
12. Ibid, p. 249.
13. Ibid, p. 250.
14. Ibid, p. 251.
15. Ibid, p. 252.
16. LeMatrie G, Finnegan J. The patient in surgery: A guide for nurses. 4th ed. Philadelphia: WB Saunders, 1980:34.
17. AORN 1995, op cit.
18. AORN. Standards of administrative practices: OR. Denver: The Association, 1995. Pp. 99–105.
19. American Nurses Association. Registered professional nurses and the unlicensed assistive personnel. Washington, DC: The Association, 1992.
20. Sullivan EJ, Decker PJ. Effective management in nursing. Menlo Park, CA: Addison-Wesley, 1995.

3 Standards for Perioperative Nursing Practice

Development of Nursing Standards
What Is a Standard?
Standards of Clinical Practice
Standards of Professional Performance
Outcome Standards—Perioperative Nursing
Competency Statements

... Standards reflect the definitions, purpose, and framework ... in the perioperative setting.

—AORN—1995

In the past, employee efficiency and effectiveness were usually measured by the amount of work produced, the speed of performance, or both. Today, nursing productivity cannot be limited to these parameters since the number of cases or tasks performed cannot adequately reflect the quality of care provided by the individual.

When the product involves professional nursing services rendered to a patient, it becomes necessary to distinguish between quantity and quality, and that quality must include competency levels of performance.

DEVELOPMENT OF NURSING STANDARDS

For nursing professionals to determine competency levels, the profession must first establish, maintain, and improve where possible the standards of care, and these standards must serve as the minimum levels of acceptable performance by the professional and/or the organization.

As a professional body, nursing must guarantee the quality of its service to the public, and these standards are a commitment and an assurance that the highest quality of care will be provided to all patients in all health-care settings, as guaranteed by the Patient's Bill of Rights, American Hospital Association, 1985.

To evaluate the quality of care provided, the nursing profession has established Standards of Practice through the American Nurses Association (ANA), the professional body for all professional nurses in the country, and these standards serve as a guideline for peer evaluation, employee assessment, and self-evaluation of nursing practice according to the latest theories and technologic advances associated with the practice of professional nursing.

Since perioperative nursing is referred to as *the practice of professional nursing in the operating room*, it too needs standards that state the minimum performance competencies required for the implementation of quality patient care during the perioperative period.

WHAT IS A STANDARD?

A standard is described as a criterion used by general agreement to denote an acceptable level of practice or an established norm.[1]

Nursing practice standards are descriptive statements that reflect the nature of current nursing practice, current knowledge, and current quality of patient care. As such, they are a means for establishing accountability of nursing care rendered by the professional nurse.

Broad in scope, and relevant to today's technology, standards provide for the uniformity of perioperative nursing practice on a national level, and are modified or revised continually to accommodate changes in theory, skill, or knowledge of nursing practice during the perioperative period.

Because a standard is considered the minimum level of performance required, they must be achievable to meet competency levels.

Standards are derived from four acceptable sources:

1. *Opinion* of knowledgeable professionals
2. *Authority* national organizations/agencies
3. *Research* concurrent and descriptive
4. *Theory* scientific basis

Types of Standards

The nursing profession has three types of standards:

1. *Structural standards* These provide the framework for the system in which nursing care is delivered. Examples include the Joint Commission for Accreditation of Healthcare Organizations (JCAHO), ANA, and AORN Administrative Standards.
2. *Process standards* These are nursing-oriented and describe the activities and behaviors designed to

achieve patient-centered goals. Examples include the ANA Standards and Perioperative Nursing Standards, both based on the nursing process, which describe the correlation between the nursing process activities and the quality of patient care rendered.
3. *Outcome standards* These standards focus on what has happened to the patient as a direct result of nursing intervention. Examples include oncology outcome standards and patient outcome standards: perioperative nursing.

Why We Need Standards

Five major reasons define why standards are an important aspect of professional nursing practice.

1. *Communications* Communications provide for sharing a common language with nursing professionals, which can cross barriers between specialties.
2. *Research* The standards provide a framework for further investigation, so that current practices are no longer based on intuition or "word-of-mouth" but are derived from theory developed by authorities within the nursing profession.
3. *Legal implications* The nursing profession must be self-regulating to maintain credibility as a profession. The courts use the professional standards "as a yard stick to determine whether hospitals and health care professionals have provided quality patient care according to nationally acceptable standards."[2]
4. *Quality improvement* Standards can be used as the criteria for quality improvement studies, to assess the current levels of practice rendered by the health-care team, services provided by the organization, or both.

Types of Standards: Nursing and Perioperative Nursing

Structure	Process	Outcome
Administrative practice—AORN	Clinical practice standards—AORN	Patient outcome standards—AORN
JACHO standards	Professional performance standards—AORN	Patient outcome standards—ANA
Administrative standards—ANA	Quality improvement standards—AORN	Patient outcome standards—ASPAN
Administrative standards—ASPAN	Job descriptions	
	Procedures	
	Guidelines	
	Protocols	
	Standards of care	

5. *Professional accountability* Standards set guidelines for nursing practice, providing a uniform basis for collecting and reviewing individual and departmental performance in conjunction with an established quality assurance program and/or performance appraisal system.

Standards for Perioperative Nursing

These standards, originally written in 1975, establish a basic model with which to measure the quality of perioperative nursing practice. Today, they have a new name and a new format, but the goal and purpose are the same:

To provide quality patient care to those undergoing surgical intervention.

By establishing these standards, the profession puts its obligation to quality patient care into daily practice. Through AORN, the professional body for perioperative nursing practice, the standards have created a tool with which to measure how the profession in general and individuals in particular are performing compared with acceptable levels of practice expected by their colleagues, society, and the patient entrusted to their care.

The revised standards have been grouped into two major categories:

1. **Standards of Clinical Practice**—describe how perioperative nurses utilize the nursing process for the delivery of patient care during the perioperative period.
2. **Standards of Professional Performance**—describe how the perioperative nurse combines several essential characteristics to the variety of role functions during the implementation of direct patient care.

STANDARDS OF CLINICAL PRACTICE

Standard I

Assessment

The primary goal of this standard is to obtain, systematically, as much information about the patient as possible through:

1. chart reviews
2. patient interview and observation
3. physical assessment

Clinical Practice Standards
I. Assessment The perioperative nurse collects patient health data.
II. Diagnosis The perioperative nurse analyzes the assessment data in determining diagnosis.
III. Outcome Identification The perioperative nurse identifies expected outcomes unique to the patient.
IV. Planning The perioperative nurse develops a plan of care that prescribes intervention to attain expected outcomes.
V. Implementation The perioperative nurse implements the interventions identified in the plan of care.
VI. Evaluation The perioperative nurse evaluates the patient's progress toward attainment of outcomes.

Source: AORN. Standards and recommended practices. Denver: The Association, 1995. Pp. 107–109.

---

4. conferences with other health-care providers involved with the patient
5. interviews with patient's family/significant others

Assessment Factors
1. Health data should include:
   a. current medical diagnosis and therapy
   b. individual's participation and expectations of proposed intervention
   c. previous responses to illness, hospitalization, and surgery
   d. psychosocial information as it relates to the individual's habits and social work roles
   e. understanding of the surgical procedure and signed informed consent
   f. psychological behaviors, for example, anxiety, coping, etc.
2. Health data are collected by appropriate methods
3. Health data collection is complete

When the nurse has satisfied these criterion or assessment factors, the data collection expected by Standard I is complete.

Standards of Professional Performance

I. Quality of Care
The perioperative nurse systematically evaluates the quality and appropriateness of nursing practice.

II. Performance Appraisal
The perioperative nurse evaluates his or her practice in context with professional practice standards and relevant statutes and regulations.

III. Education
The perioperative nurse acquires and maintains current knowledge in nursing practice.

IV. Collegiality
The perioperative nurse contributes to the professional growth of peers, colleagues, and others.

V. Ethics
The perioperative nurse's decisions and actions on behalf of patients are determined in an ethical manner.

VI. Collaboration
The perioperative nurse collaborates with the patient, significant others, health care providers, and others providing care.

VII. Research
The perioperative nurse uses research findings in practice.

VIII. Resource Use
The perioperative nurse considers factors related to safety, effectiveness, efficiency, environmental concerns, and costs in planning and delivering patient care.

Source: AORN. Standards and recommended practices. Denver: The Association, 1995. Pp. 111–113.

Standard II

Diagnosis

A nursing diagnosis is a concise statement that identifies clinical judgment about an individual, family, or community response to actual or potential health care problems/life processes. Nursing diagnoses provide the basis for selection of nursing interventions in order to achieve outcomes for which the nurse is accountable.[3] The information is derived from the nursing assessment data collected, and forms the basis for the plan of care created for that individual patient.

The term "diagnosis" is defined as a concise technical description of facts to determine the cause, nature, or manifestation of a condition, situation, or problem, and the decision or opinion resulting from such an examination and analysis of data.[4]

The goal of a nursing diagnosis is management of the nursing care problems, and is a major component of the nursing process.

Assessment Factors

a. the nursing diagnosis is based on identifiable data determined by continuous analysis and interpretation of the data

b. health status deviations are determined by comparing the identified data to established norms and/or the patient's previous condition

c. nursing diagnosis is consistent with current scientific theory

Standard III

Outcome Identification

The goals of perioperative nursing intervention are stated as desired or expected patient outcomes—what the nurse wants to observe, hear, or see as a direct result of nursing actions.

Patient outcome statements should be brief and concisely stated in measurable terms. Each outcome should include specific criteria for measuring the success or failure of the intervention. Outcomes should be attainable, considering the individuality of the patient, the nature of the surgery, and the resources available for the patient, family, and significant others.

In many instances, there is a tendency to focus on the nurse's goals rather than the patient's. Outcomes should always be related to the patient and the planned nursing intervention.

Assessment Factors

a. patient outcomes are derived from the nursing diagnoses statements, and are prioritized according to the individual needs of the patient

b. patient outcomes are stated in measurable terms of observable actions or reactions

c. patient outcomes are formulated through input from the patient, family, and health care providers

d. patient outcomes are realistic, determined by the patient's present and potential physical capabilities and behavioral patterns

e. patient outcomes are obtainable through available human and material resources

f. patient outcomes are achievable within an identified period of time

Standard IV

Planning

Developing a plan of care is an intellectual process requiring the perioperative nurse to have knowledge and skills specific to patient care in surgery.

The department should have a care plan form consistent with other nursing service areas, or the perioperative plan should be incorporated into the care plan used throughout the hospital, and should be documented in writing somewhere in the patient's record or on the nursing care plan form.

Assessment Factors

a. the plan of care includes setting priorities for appropriate actions
b. the plan includes a logical sequence of events and actions to attain the stated goals
c. the plan is based on current scientific knowledge
d. the plan incorporates available and appropriate human and material resources
e. the plan is realistic and can be implemented
f. the plan is developed with, and communicated to, the patient and other appropriate personnel and family
g. the plan specifies what nursing actions are performed and when, where, and by whom
h. the plan reflects preoperative assessment
i. the plan includes, but is not limited to:
preoperative teaching
verification of all documents
adherence to principles of asepsis, positioning, safety, monitoring, psychological and physiologic support, communication methods, and documentation of nursing activities performed

Standard V

Implementation

As the perioperative nurse begins to implement the plan of care, he or she draws on intellectual skills involving decision-making, observation, judgment, critical thinking and interpersonal relationships, in addition to manual dexterity, technical skill performance, and application of nursing knowledge.

While the plan is being implemented, additional data are being collected, and the original goals are being revised as necessary.

It is during this phase that *documentation* of all nursing activities performed becomes a major aspect, both legally and professionally, since the written record will serve as a communication tool for the nurses resuming postoperative care of the patient.

Assessment Factors

a. nursing actions are consistent with the plan of care and provide continuity during all three phases of surgical intervention
b. nursing actions are performed with safety, skill, and efficiency, and reflect the individualism of the patient
c. nursing activities are documented on appropriate forms

Standard VI

Evaluation

The term "evaluation" refers to the appraisal of the quality of care and the results of nursing intervention.

Actual measurements of goal attainment can be a formal or informal process. Making notations on the care plan, describing achievements, or developing an evaluation tool such as a Postoperative Interview Sheet are methods that can be used to determine to what extent the patient outcome goals have been accomplished.

Assessment Factors

a. current data about the individual are recorded and used to measure progress toward the goals
b. all parties involved assist in the evaluation process, including patient and family

The reevaluation (reassessment) of the client, appropriate nursing diagnoses, of goals, and changes or modifications reformation of the care plan should be a continuous ongoing process.

As the perioperative nurse cares for the patient, new information is continuously being gathered that effects the original goals and plan of care.

Based on this new information, or patient problems, the perioperative nurse must re-examine the original goals and determine if they are still pertinent, realistic, and obtainable.

When patient outcomes or goals have been restated, the plan of care needs to be modified and followed through with appropriate nursing actions, and the cycle begins again, and will continue until the patient no longer requires nursing intervention.

Assessment Factors

a. reassessment is directed by goal achievement and/or new data
b. the care plan is modified to meet the changes in conditions or needs of the patient

STANDARDS OF PROFESSIONAL PERFORMANCE

Originally drafted in 1993, the Standards of Professional Performance focus on how the nurse performs his or her various roles during the perioperative period. These standards depict the characteristics every professional nurse should ascribe to, and reflect a collaborative statement between the American Nurses Association (ANA) "Standards of Professional Performance" and AORN. (See P. 36.)

If the perioperative nurse can incorporate the Standards of Clinical Practice and Professional Performance into daily activities, he or she will have met all the expected professional obligations, resulting in a higher caliber of patient care during the perioperative period. The extent to which these perioperative standards can be implemented depends on the individual's commitment to quality patient care.

OUTCOME STANDARDS— PERIOPERATIVE NURSING

Originally drafted in 1984, the goal to provide nurses practicing in the OR with guidelines for providing the highest quality of patient care has not changed in today's complexity of perioperative nursing practice.

Used as a tool to measure the extent to which quality patient care has been achieved, the following Standards can assist the perioperative nurse during the Evaluation and Reassessment Phases of the process.

COMPETENCY STATEMENTS

Throughout this chapter we have used the term "competency" as a basis of quality patient care. Competency is described as the ability to practice a skill with safety and efficiency, and usually is a result of continual application of knowledge and skill.[5]

During the initial phase of exploration into the perioperative nurse's role, the nurse is in the *entry* level of practice, acquiring new skills and knowledge relating to patient care during the perioperative period. This phase usually lasts 6 months, and its completion is based on the nurse's ability to safely function independently as a perioperative nurse.

The next level, beginning at 6 months and continuing for approximately 2 years, is referred to as the "competency phase" of practice. It is characterized by an increase in knowledge and skills that reflect the total aspect of perioperative nursing practice.

To assist the nurse in determining whether this level has been achieved, the AORN has researched and developed the Competency Statements for Perioperative

---

> ### Patient Outcome Standards—Perioperative Nursing
>
> **Standard I**
> The patient demonstrates knowledge of the physiologic and psychological responses to surgical intervention.
>
> **Standard II**
> The patient is free from infection.
>
> **Standard III**
> The patient's skin integrity is maintained.
>
> **Standard IV**
> The patient is free from injury related to positioning extraneous objects or chemical, physical, and electrical hazards.
>
> **Standard V**
> The patient's fluid and electrolyte balance is maintained.
>
> **Standard VI**
> The patient participates in the rehabilitation process.
>
> *Source:* AORN. Standards and recommended practice. Denver: The Association, 1995. Pp. 125–126.

Nursing Practice, applicable to nurses working in surgery for 6 months or longer (see Fig. 1-1 for a continuum model).

Using the nursing process format and the Standards of Perioperative Nursing Practice as the framework, the competency statements can be directly correlated with current technology and implementation of patient care activities.

The statements are written in measurable terms, clearly redefining the need for qualified registered nurses performing specialized tasks for the patient undergoing surgical intervention.

Additionally, the perioperative nurse can use the competency statements as a self-assessment tool and as a study guide for the Certification Examination in Perioperative Nursing Practice (CNOR).

Assessment Phase
1. Competency to assess the physiologic health status of the patient.
2. Competency to assess the psychosocial health status of the patient, family, or both.
3. Competency to formulate nursing diagnoses based on health status data.

Planning Phase
4. Competency to establish patient goals based on the nursing diagnoses.

5. Competency to develop a care plan that prescribes nursing actions to achieve patient goals.

Implementation Phase
6. Competency to implement nursing actions in transferring the patient according to prescribed plan.
7. Competency to participate in patient/family teaching.
8. Competency to create and maintain a sterile field.
9. Competency to provide proper equipment and supplies based on patient/team needs.
10. Competency to perform sponge, sharp, and instrument counts at proper intervals.
11. Competency to administer drugs and solutions as prescribed.
12. Competency to physiologically monitor patients during surgery.
13. Competency to monitor and control the environment.
14. Competency to respect patient's rights.

Evaluation Phase
15. Competency to perform nursing actions that demonstrate accountability.

16. Competency to evaluate patient outcomes.
17. Competency to measure effectiveness of nursing care.
18. Competency to continually reassess all components of patient care based on new data.[6]

By continually using the standards of practice, outcome standards, and competency statements as a guide, the perioperative nurse practicing in today's ORs can assure the delivery of quality patient care during all three phases of surgical intervention.

Perioperative nursing practice is a concept that has become a reality for nurses caring for patients during the perioperative period. Through continuing education, research, and commitment to this specialty, perioperative nursing will continue to develop as it strives toward providing even more comprehensive nursing care to patients undergoing surgical intervention.

The assurance of this goal is the responsibility of every nurse practicing today, since perioperative nurses are *Specialists in Caring*.

Self-assessment Exercise 5

Directions: Complete the following exercises. The answers are found at the end of the Module.

1. Give one example of each type of professional standard:
   a) Structural
   b) Process
   c) Outcome

2. Describe one nursing activity related to each of the
   a) Standards of Clinical Practice
   b) Standards of Professional Performance

3. Outcome Standards are used to measure the effectiveness of nursing care rendered to the patient

   True   False

4. Competency Statements describe minimal levels of practice for the beginning practitioner

   True   False

5. Competency Statements use the *Nursing Process* format, and serve as a self-assessment tool for acceptable levels of practice.

   True   False

6. Identify and describe the framework for Perioperative Nursing Practice.

References

1. Kelly LU, Joel LA. Dimensions of professional nursing. 7th ed. New York: Macmillan Publishing Co., 1995.
2. Fiesta J. The law and liability: A guide for nurses. New York: John Wiley & Sons, 1983.
3. North American Nursing Diagnosis Association. NANDA's working definition of nursing diagnosis. St. Louis: In press.
4. Miller BF, Keane CB. Encyclopedia and dictionary of medicine, nursing and allied health. 2nd ed. Philadelphia: W.B. Saunders Co., 1980.
5. AORN. Standards and recommended practices. Denver: The Association, 1995. Pp. 76–84.
6. Ibid, Pp. 125–126.

Questions for Review for Module I

Complete the following questions by indicating the correct response. Answers are given at the end of the module.

1. Perioperative nursing practice involves the professional registered nurse caring for the patient during
   1. the preoperative phase
   2. the intraoperative phase
   3. the postoperative phase
   4. the admission procedure for surgery
      a. 1, 2, 4
      b. 1, 2, 3
      c. 2 only
      d. all of the above

2. The primary purpose of the AORN during its early years was to
   a. create standards of practice
   b. write policy and procedure for surgery
   c. establish a separate group for OR nurses
   d. gain national attention for nurses in surgery

3. According to the three-zone concept of surgical suite design, the dressing rooms are located in the
   a. restricted area
   b. clean area
   c. semirestricted area
   d. nonrestricted area

4. When preparing a procedure room for the first case of the day, the perioperative nurse notices the room humidity level to be 70 percent. The *first* action should be to
   a. open the sterile supplies and call plant engineering to report the humidity level
   b. notify plant engineering of the problem before opening the sterile supplies
   c. adjust the thermostat to make the room colder
   d. do nothing since this reading is within acceptable limits

5. Traffic flow in and out of a procedure room should be kept to a minimum to
   1. decrease microbial count
   2. reduce noise level
   3. increase team concentration

4. maintain positive pressure within the room
   a. 1 and 2
   b. 3 and 4
   c. 1, 3, 4
   d. all of the above

6. OR floors should be flooded with _____ and _____ at the end of each _____ as part of terminal cleaning procedures.
   a. germicidal solution; mopped; case
   b. detergent germicide; wet-vacuumed; case
   c. germicidal solution; wet-vacuumed; day
   d. detergent solution; mopped; day

7. Following a preoperative visit, the perioperative nurse creates a nursing diagnosis to
   a. identify the patient's needs and to define actions to meet those needs
   b. follow a specific surgeon's orders
   c. document the level and progress of nursing care
   d. alert the OR team of specific instruments needed for the case

8. The Standards of Perioperative Nursing Practice, first adopted in 1978, can be used as a guide for
   a. basic competency statements
   b. patient outcome standards
   c. policy and procedure manuals
   d. all of the above

9. The most common hazard associated with electricity in a procedure room is
   a. fire
   b. burns
   c. electric shock
   d. all of the above

10. Personnel entering the semirestricted area of the surgical suite are required to wear
    a. clean scrub suit; mask
    b. clean scrub suit; cap; mask
    c. clean scrub suit; cap; shoe covers
    d. clean scrub suit; cap

Glossary

Accountability: the process of being answerable to one's self, the profession, and the institution providing patient care

Basic Competencies: the knowledge and skills needed to perform safely and effectively the role of the perioperative nurse as defined in the AORN Standards of Practice in the competency phase of the continuum

Criterion: a means for judgment; standard or attributes with which to judge a condition or establish a diagnosis

Intraoperative Phase: the time beginning with the induction of anesthesia and ending with the admission of the patient to the postanesthesia care unit

Operating Room Nurse: a registered nurse who assumes the perioperative role (*see* Perioperative Nursing Practice)

Outcome Standards: standards used to determine intended or realistic expectations of the patient's problem within a specific time frame

Perioperative Nursing Practice: nursing activities performed by the professional registered nurse during the three phases of surgical intervention: preoperative, intraoperative, and postoperative

Perioperative Period: the time beginning with the decision to undergo surgery and ending with the termination of required nursing intervention and evaluation of care rendered

Preoperative Phase: the time beginning with the patient's decision to have surgery and ending at the time of the induction of anesthesia

Procedure Room: the environment in which the patient's surgical procedure is performed (*syn:* Operating Room)

Postoperative Phase: the time beginning with the admission of the patient to the postoperative unit and ending with the follow-up visit and/or discharge of the patient

Surgical Service: the department, involving all services related to the care and management of the surgical patient, including support and ancillary areas for the preoperative and postoperative periods

Surgical Suite: the cluster of rooms and support areas where surgical treatment is managed and/or performed

Surgical Team: personnel performing direct patient care during a surgical procedure in both the sterile and nonsterile positions

Bibliography for Module I

Association of Operating Room Nurses. *AORN Standards and Recommended Practices.* Denver, CO: The Association, 1995.

American Hospital Association. Statement on Patient's Bill of Rights. AHA House of Delegates. Chicago, 1973.

Atkinson LJ, Kohn ML. *Berry and Kohn's Introduction to Operating Room Technique,* 6th ed. New York: McGraw-Hill, 1978.

Crooks B. *Operating Room Technique for the Surgical Team.* Boston: Little, Brown, 1979.

Douglas LM. *The Effective Nurse Leader/Manager,* 3rd ed. St. Louis: Mosby, 1988.

Department of Health and Rehabilitative Services. *Hospital Licensure V.* 5, Washington, DC, 1986.

Driscol J. *Preserving the Legacy: AORN 1949–1989.* Denver, CO: Association of Operating Room Nurses, 1989.

Fairchild SS. Critical Elements: A Workbook for Perioperative Nursing Practice. Unpublished manuscript, 1987.

Fiesta J. *The Law and Liability: A Guide for Nurses.* New York: John Wiley & Sons, 1983.

Gordon M. *Nursing Diagnosis: Process and Application,* 2nd ed. New York: McGraw-Hill, 1987.

Groah L. *Operating Room Nursing: The Perioperative Role.* Reston, VA: Reston Publishers, 1983.

Gruendemann B. *The Surgical Patient: Behavioral Concepts for the Operating Room Nurse.* St. Louis: Mosby, 1974.

Hoeller ML. *Surgical Technology: Basis for Clinical Practice,* 3rd ed. New York: McMillan, 1994.

Kneedler J, Dodge G. *Perioperative Patient Care: The Nursing Perspective,* 3rd ed. Boston: Jones and Bartlett Publishers, 1993.

Kneedler JA. *MILS Series: The Nursing Process Series.* No. 6. Denver, CO: AORN, 1979. P. 28.

La Matrie G, Finnegan J. *The Patient in Surgery: A Guide for Nurses,* 5th ed. Philadelphia: Saunders, 1980.

Meeker M, Rothrock J. *Alexander's Care of the Patient in Surgery,* 9th ed. St. Louis: Mosby, 1991.

Miller BF, Keane CB. *Encyclopedia and Dictionary of Medicine, Nursing and Allied Health,* 2nd ed. Philadelphia: Saunders, 1980.

Seifert PC, Grandusky RJ. Nursing diagnosis: Their use in developing care plans. *AORN Journal* 51 (April 1990): 1008–1021.

Sullivan EJ, Decker PJ. *Effective Management in Nursing,* 4th ed. Menlo Park, CA: Addison-Wesley, 1994.

Tabor's Cyclopedic Medical Dictionary, 17th ed. Philadelphia: FA Davis, 1994.

Answers for Module I

Self-assessment Exercise 1

1. Incorporates the role of the professional nurse during all three phases of surgical intervention; is patient-oriented rather than task-oriented.
2. True
3. True
4. True
5. Patient; task

Self-assessment Exercise 2

1. Efficiency; flexibility; safety
2. Nonrestricted; semirestricted; restricted
3. Nonrestricted: available to outside personnel; requires no restricted activities
   Semirestricted: not accessible to outside traffic; connects inside corridors and supply areas to procedure rooms; supplies from outside cannot enter unless properly prepared or decontaminated
   Restricted: not accessible to outside traffic; area involves preparation of surgical team and actual performance of surgical procedure
4. 1. Central corridor: small surgical suite; all rooms open to one common corridor
   2. Double corridor: work area in the center, with procedure rooms on either side; can be open at one end (U shape) or closed. Most common shape; easy to access all areas
   3. Inner core/outer core: sterile/clean areas located in the center with outer core providing entry and ancillary support areas not requiring strict isolation; reserved for large areas devoted to surgical suite
   4. Cluster/pod/modular: procedure rooms attached to sterile supply core within a surgical suite; allows for easy expansion without interruption of existing services
5. Size of room; temperature and humidity; ventilation and air quality; electrical safety; communication
6. Separation of sterile, clean, and dirty supplies; well-delineated traffic patterns; recognition of specific areas and restrictions of traffic and activities within the areas

Self-assessment Exercise 3

1. Contain and control
2. a. Clean scrub attire; cap; shoe covers
   b. Clean scrub attire; cap, shoe covers, mask
   c. Cover gown over scrub attire (closed in front); cap, mask, and shoe covers removed
3. True
4. False: Clean must always be separated from sterile and dirty to avoid cross-contamination

5. False: Interim cleaning is performed after each procedure
6. 68°F to 76°F (20°C–22°C); 50 to 55 percent
7. To maintain the efficiency of the filtering system within each room, including 10 percent positive pressure, which forces old air out
8. True
9. All furniture is moved and the floor is cleaned from wall-to-wall; all furniture is cleaned and shelves are restocked with sterile items

Self-assessment Exercise 4

1. (Concepts should include, but not be limited to)
   Preparation of patients both physically and psychologically; use of scientific knowledge to alleviate existing problems; effective postoperative management, etc.
2. a. Circulating nurse: a registered nurse who is responsible for controlling and directing activities in a procedure room during a surgical procedure. The nonsterile member of the surgical team.
   b. Scrub nurse/technician: a sterile member of the surgical team responsible for assisting the surgeon and assistant with sterile supplies, equipment, and instrumentation.
   c. CRNA: a registered nurse who specializes in the monitoring and administration of anesthesia under the direction of an anesthesiologist.
   d. Surgeon: the physician responsible for the implementation of the surgical procedure.
3. Planning; staffing; organizing; directing; controlling; decision-making
4. Authoritarian: total control; no group dynamics; task-oriented
   Democratic: emphasis on team work and group dynamics; goal-oriented
   Permissive: nonleading; non–goal oriented
   Multicratic: combination of directed-group dynamics; people-oriented
5. False: Personal characteristics should not be considered as a reliable indicator

Self-assessment Exercise 5

1. Structural: JCAHO, State Nurse Practice Act, AORN
   Process—AORN; AACN, ANA
   Outcome—AORN; Oncology Nursing; AORN
2. Standards: Clinical Practice
   Assessment
   Nursing diagnosis
   Outcome identification
   Planning
   Evaluation
   Reassessment

Standards: Professional Performance
  Quality of care
  Performance appraisal
  Education
  Collegiality
  Ethics
  Collaboration
  Research
  Resource use
3. True
4. False: They describe expected activities for a nurse who has worked in surgery for 6 months or longer

5. True
6. Framework: Nursing process format during all three phases of surgical intervention that are reflected in the Perioperative Nursing Standards of Practice

Questions for Review

1. B
2. C
3. D
4. B
5. D

6. C
7. A
8. D
9. D
10. C

MODULE II

Biophysical Sciences

Chapter Outline

Content Overview

The correlation between biophysical sciences and the care of the surgical patient are inseparable during the perioperative period, since one forms the basic foundation for the other.

This module reviews the basic sciences and introduces new concepts related to the tasks performed by the surgical team during the three phases of surgical intervention.

Module Objectives

Upon completion of this module, you will be able to:

1. Review the principles of microbiology and epidemiology and describe the relationship between the surgical patient and the environment.
2. Discuss the wound healing process as it relates to the surgical patient.
3. Discuss the actions and nursing implications associated with specific pharmaceutical agents used during the perioperative period.
4. Describe the major factors and nursing considerations related to maintaining intravascular homeostasis during the three phases of surgical intervention.

4 Microbiology and the Surgical Patient

Humans and Microbes
Microbiology and Surgical Sepsis
The Early Years of Surgery
Principles of Microbiology
Bacteriology: General Concepts
Pathogen versus Nonpathogen
The Infectious Process
Infection Control: Principles and Nursing Implications
Physiology of Wound Healing
Types of Wounds
Methods of Surgical Wound Healing
Phases of First Intention Healing
Factors Influencing Normal Wound Healing
Complications of Wound Healing
Monitoring Postoperative Surgical Wound Infections
Centers for Disease Control Classification of Surgical Wounds

UNIT 1

Principles of Microbiology

HUMANS AND MICROBES

Many microorganisms inhabit the human body. Usually these microorganisms are harmless and in some cases may be beneficial. Occasionally, they invade the tissues and cause disease.

When microbes live together or in close association with each other, it is called *symbiosis*. In another arrangement, one organism benefits without causing harm or benefit to the other. This is known as *commensalism*. In *parasitism*, one organism (the parasite) de-

rives benefit from the association at the expense of the other (the host), usually resulting in disease.

Microorganisms that normally inhabit the skin and mucosa in a symbiotic relationship are referred to as *normal* or *resident flora*. Under some circumstances, such as a compromised defense system, resident flora may invade the tissues and multiply, causing tissue damage or infection, or serving as an entry for disease.

To understand the world of microorganisms, it is necessary to explore the general concepts associated with the fields of microbiology and bacteriology.

MICROBIOLOGY AND SURGICAL SEPSIS

The modern surgeon takes for granted aseptic technique and antisepsis, and fully expects the incision to heal cleanly and by first intention. This healthy situation was not always so before our understanding of the causes of wound infection and the preventive measures we use today.

The practice of medical and surgical asepsis dates back to the ancient Hebrews. Very specific laws relating to sanitation, purification, and isolation of individuals with infections are interspersed with laws relating to morality and obedience to God throughout the books of the Old Testament. It appears that throughout recorded history, humans have valued health and practiced some form of purification to protect themselves from infection.

Hippocrates, the father of scientific medicine, reportedly cleansed his hands before operating and boiled the water he used to irrigate the wound.[1] This action suggests his recognition of the importance of destroying or removing the germs or causative factors associated with wound infections.

Three centuries later, the Roman physician Marcus Trentures Varro stated "small creatures, invisible to the eye, fill the atmosphere and breathed through the nose could cause dangerous disease."[2] This germ theory was not validated until the seventeenth century and the invention of the microscope by the Dutch scientist Anton Van Leeuwenhoek.

THE EARLY YEARS OF SURGERY

In its infancy, the practice of surgery was discouraging and distressing, and was used only as a last resort for dying and terminally ill patients. In the early nineteenth century, the complications of sepsis were so common they were considered a "normal" consequence of surgery. According to early beliefs, when purulent drainage occurred from the incision, it signaled the evacuation of an abscess and the beginning of clinical improvement.[3] In some instances, nearly 80 percent of all clean wounds developed sepsis, and the mortality from limb amputations was even greater.

High on the list of problems associated with sepsis was puerperal fever. The mortality rates from postpartum uterine sepsis reached epidemic proportions throughout Europe's hospitals between the 1820s and 1830s. This was due to poor or nonexistent handwashing between examination of each patient.

Since there was no practice of aseptic technique, surgeons would operate in an open theater, dressed in Prince Albert lab coats, using no gloves, gowns, or masks. Strange as it may seem, a bloody lab coat became a status symbol, that of a successful, busy surgeon. The use of clean sheets or a clean environment, according to the surgeon, had little effect on the transmission of germs. Sepsis was the result of only the patient's lack of stamina for the procedure.

Great strides toward scientific methods relating to aseptic technique were made in the later nineteenth century. For example, in 1847, Semmelweis instituted the practice of handwashing before examining his maternity patients, reintroducing the ancient theory of purification by water, and thus reducing the potential of infections and puerperal fever.[4] Eighteen years later, in 1865, Lord Joseph Lister proposed that germs should be prevented from entering the surgical wound; hence, the Listerian technique was introduced, and Lister become known as the Father of Antiseptic Surgery.

In addition to the improvements already mentioned, other scientists were working toward revising the practice of surgery based on further germ theory research, including the spread of disease, and their contributions opened the door for the epidemiologic concepts that are used today in both surgery and general medicine.

It is obvious that surgery had a strange beginning, but it is easy to understand why, when you consider previous methods and techniques, surgical treatment has been considered a science only during the past 150 years. Today, microbiology and epidemiology have vital roles in providing a safe, therapeutic environment for the surgical patient, through the practice of aseptic technique.

PRINCIPLES OF MICROBIOLOGY

Microbiology is the science that studies submicroscopic life forms that cannot be seen by the naked eye.

The human species coexists with a large number of microorganisms, which are generally classified into seven major groups that are either plant or animal:

1. Algae — Plant
2. Protozoa — Animal
3. Yeasts — Plant (fungi)
4. Molds — Plant (fungi)
5. Bacteria — Animal
6. Rickettsiae — Animal
7. Viruses — Classified according to the host they dominate

Although a wide variety of microorganisms can cause infection, infection from bacteria and viruses is the primary concern for the surgical patient.

BACTERIOLOGY: GENERAL CONCEPTS

Bacteria are single-celled organisms that range in size from 1 to 10 microns in length and from 0.2 to 1 micron in width. Bacteria are classified according to (1) shape, or morphology, (2) spore-forming capability, (3) biochemical and physiologic characteristics, (4) staining properties, and (5) *pathogenicity*, or ability to cause disease.

Morphology (Shape)

Bacterial cells exist in three distinct shapes: (1) spherical (round), (2) cylindrical (rod), and (3) spiral or helical.

Spherical bacteria are called *cocci* (singular: coccus) and the cylindrical are known as *bacilli* (singular: bacillus). Helical cells may be curved like a comma, as in a *vibrio*, or may form several curves, as in the spiral or *spirilla* (singular: spirillum) or *spirochete.* Some short, thick, oval-shaped bacilli are referred to as coccobacilli (Fig. 4-1).

Cell Structure

In common with other cells, bacterial cells have a cell membrane that encloses the cytoplasm. In addition, most bacterial cells have a cell wall that surrounds the cell membrane. Most bacteria have a rigid cell wall that maintains its shape, but some, such as the spirochete or spirilla, have a flexible cell wall.

Some bacteria have an outermost layer called a *capsule*. The capsule is a loose-fitting gelatinous structure composed of either a polysaccharide or polypeptide substance, and it is this capsule that is associated with the pathogenic capabilities of the bacteria (Fig. 4-2).

Sporulation

Under certain conditions, some bacteria, especially species of bacilli, undergo a process called *sporulation*. In this process, a vegetative cell forms within it a round or oval slime layer that is surrounded by a capsule. As

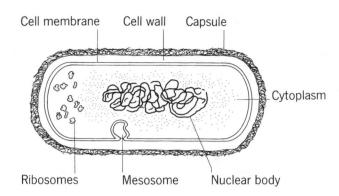

Fig. 4-2. Cell structure

the rest of the cell degenerates, only the spore remains. These are usually resistant to a variety of conditions that would kill vegetative cells, such as freezing and exposure to chemicals, heat, or radiation. When conditions are right, the spore germinates again and produces another vegetative cell. In essence, then, a *spore* is a dormant phase in the lifecycle of a bacterial cell.

Growth and Reproduction

Bacteria multiply by a process called *binary fission*, in which one cell divides to produce two primary cells. However, as with human growth and development, conditions must be favorable for the cell to mature. Bacterial growth is influenced by both nutritional and physical factors.

Nutritional Factors

Although a bacterium's nutritional requirements may vary, in general the materials necessary for the synthesis of cell components and for the production of energy must be available. Some bacteria feed off living tissue, while others feed off dead or devitalized tissue.

Some organisms, called *heterotrophic*, use organic substances as a source of carbon, while the *autotrophic* organisms obtain their energy from the sun or by metabolizing inorganic compounds, such as hydrogen, ammonia, nitrites, or hydrogen sulfide.

Physical Factors

1. *Suitable temperature* The optimum temperature for most bacteria is between 15°C and 50°C (59°F to 122°F). The pathogenic bacteria are adapted to grow in the human body, and grow best at temperatures between 35°C and 40°C (95°F and 104°F).
2. *Suitable moisture* Most bacteria can grow in a variety of solutions, since the cell wall prevents the cell from rupturing in a hypotonic medium. If bac-

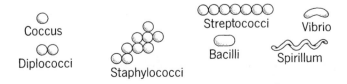

Fig. 4-1. Morphology of bacteria

terial cells are placed in a solution that is too hypertonic, however, water is drawn out of the cell by osmosis and growth is inhibited. Some bacteria can live in dried pus, sputum, mucus, or feces for long periods.

3. *Suitable pH* Most bacteria can tolerate a pH range from 5 (acid) to 8 (base), but grow best in a neutral pH (7). If the pH changes, cell growth and metabolism can be greatly decreased.
4. *Suitable atmosphere* Bacteria vary in their oxygen requirement, reflecting differences in the metabolic process used to generate energy. There are three types of bacteria with different oxygen requirements:
   a. Strict aerobes—these bacteria *must* have oxygen for growth (*obligate aerobes*)
   b. Strict anaerobes—to these bacteria, oxygen is toxic, so these organisms grow only in the absence of oxygen (*obligate anaerobes*)
   c. Facultative—these bacteria can grow with or without oxygen, although they grow faster when oxygen is available.

Energy Metabolism

Bacteria respond to the environment around them as well as to the chemical activity within the cell. This chemical activity is called *metabolism*. Metabolism allows the cell to produce energy required to perform specific tasks.

Metabolism occurs in two stages:

1. *Catabolism* the breaking down of the cell
2. *Anabolism* the building up of substances needed for growth and development

These two processes are essential to all cell growth and reproductive functions.

PATHOGEN VERSUS NONPATHOGEN

Microorganisms, especially bacteria, are commonly classified according to their ability to cause disease.

Pathogenicity is the ability of microorganisms to cause disease, while other microorganisms live in harmony (*commensalism*) with the body or even at times help to fight disease. The latter relationship is referred to as a nonpathogenic existence.

Some pathogenic microorganisms exist only as a parasite in the human body (*host*). Others exist as free-living organisms or exist in a mutualistic arrangement, neither helping nor hurting the host, though they are capable of causing infections if the natural body defenses are compromised.

Nosocomial infections, those that are hospital-acquired, are commonly caused by a pathogenic organism, so it is referred to as an *opportunistic pathogen.*

Another important procedure that further classifies bacteria is Gram's stain, used to differentiate bacterial cells into positive and negative categories.

In this staining procedure, bacteria are stained with crystal violet, treated with strong iodine solution, decolorized with ethanol or ethanol-acetone, and counterstained with a contrasting dye. Those retaining the stain are gram positive, and those losing the stain but staining with the counterstain are gram negative.

Gram-Positive/Gram-Negative Microorganisms

Gram-Positive Cocci

Members of the staphylococci and streptococci groups are the most common gram-positive cocci. They can be further divided by their sporulation capabilities. These bacteria are non–spore forming and are facultative. Staphylococci form a "grape-like" cluster, while streptococci resemble a short or long chain. Staphylococci are specifically associated with infections of the skin and intestinal tract. Streptococci are further classified into three groups according to their behavior when cultured on a blood-agar plate: α-hemolytic streptococci, β-hemolytic streptococci, and γ-hemolytic streptococci (nonpathogenic).

Gram-Negative Cocci

The clinically important gram-negative cocci are *Neisseria gonorrhoeae* and *N. meningitidis*. These are non–spore forming diplococci that cannot survive for long outside the human body. *N. gonorrhoeae* causes the venereal disease gonorrhea, while *N. meningitidis* causes meningitis and septicemia in a susceptible host.

Gram-Negative Enteric Bacilli

Gram-negative enteric bacilli are non–spore forming rods that are facultative anaerobes. Some of them are pathogenic, while others, such as the resident flora found in the intestinal tract, are not normally pathogenic but can become so under certain circumstances; for example, contamination of a surgical wound. Examples include, but are not limited to *Escherichia coli*, *Salmonella*, *Shigella*, *Pseudomonas*, and some species of *Proteus*.

Gram-Positive Non–Spore Forming Bacilli

Two important genera of gram-positive non–spore forming bacilli are *Corynebacterium* and *Lactobacilli*,

Table 4-1 Bacteria Reference Chart

Bacteria	Classification	Location
Staphylococcus (S. aureus)	Gram positive, facultative	Hair, skin, nasopharynx
Enteric bacilli	Gram negative, facultative, non–spore forming	Large intestines, perineum
Streptococcus	Gram positive, facultative, non–spore forming	Nose, oropharynx
Tuberculi bacillus (Mycobacterium tuberculosis)	Gram positive, aerobic, acid fast	Respiratory tract
Pseudomonas	Gram negative bacilli, facultative, non–spore forming	Intestinal tract, skin
Serratia	Gram negative bacilli, aerobic, non–spore forming	Respiratory tract, intestinal tract
Clostridium	Gram positive bacilli, anaerobic, spore forming	Soil, dust, feces

Anagram: S-E-S-T-P-S-C

which cause diphtheria and dental caries, respectively. Although neither directly affects the surgical patient, their presence could postpone surgery until the infection is under control.

Gram-Positive Spore Forming Bacilli

Bacillus and *Clostridium* are two major groups of gram-positive spore forming bacilli. *Bacillus anthracis,* a facultative anaerobe, can cause acute infectious disease in sheep, cattle, and horses. Humans contract the disease via contact with animal hair, hides, or waste, causing anthrax.

Clostridium are anaerobic spore forming rods commonly found in soil and the intestinal tract, and frequently found in wound infections. Several are pathogenic in humans, being the primary causative agents for gas gangrene (*C. perfringens*), while other strains cause such diseases as tetanus (*C. tetani*) and food poisoning (*C. botulinum*).

Gram-Negative Aerobic Coccobacilli

Gram-negative aerobic coccobacilli are non–spore forming organisms that are capable of forming capsules. Several species of *Haemophilus* are resident flora of the upper respiratory tract; the most common is *H. influenzae.* Encapsulated strains of this species are primarily pathogens that cause meningitis in younger children, and can also cause pneumonia, bronchitis, otitis media, and epiglottis, while nonencapsulated strains commonly cause secondary infections of the upper respiratory tract.

To remember the most common causes of surgical wound infections, the following anagram may be useful:

Search Every Source To Provide Safe Care

Table 4-1 will help identify these microorganisms, using the first initial of their name.

Self-assessment Exercise 1

Directions: Complete the following exercises. The answers are given at the end of this module.

For each of the bacteria listed, state the type/group and its classification (sporulation; oxygenation, etc.).

1. *STAPHYLOCOCCI*
    Type/Group: _____
    Classification: _____

2. *STREPTOCOCCI*
    Type/Group: _____
    Classification: _____

3. *CLOSTRIDIUM PERFRINGENS*
    Type/Group: _____
    Classification: _____

4. The two groups (tests) that can further divide the bacterial classifications are _____ and _____.

5. Illustrate the shapes for the following bacteria:
    1. *Streptococci*   4. *Staphylococci*
    2. *Diplococci*   5. *Spirillum*
    3. *Bacilli*

6. Disease producing microorganisms are called _____ and are the main source of _____ (hospital-acquired) infections.

7. Match the bacteria (left column) with their proper description/definition (right column):

    a. *Pseudomonas*   1. ___ Acid-fast bacillus
    b. *Escherichia coli* 2. ___ Gram-positive
                               bacteria; grape-
                               like cluster
    c. *Mycobacteria*   3. ___ Chain-like cluster
    d. Spore   4. ___ Water-loving
                               bacteria
    e. *Staphylococci*   5. ___ Gram-negative
                               rod
    f. *Streptococci*   6. ___ Resistant; hard
                               shell form of bac-
                               teria

8. List the five factors essential for the growth and reproduction of bacteria. State the preventive measures *YOU* could take to prevent contamination.
    1.
    2.
    3.
    4.
    5.

UNIT 2

Epidemiology and Infection Control

Epidemiology is the study of the relationships of various factors that determine the frequency and distribution of diseases or specific causes of infection.

THE INFECTIOUS PROCESS

Host–Microbe Interaction

The mere presence of microorganisms in or on the body does not signify disease. As discussed in Unit 1 of this chapter, many microorganisms inhabit the body surface and lumen of the intestinal tract as resident flora, never causing disease or harm to the host. But when a microorganism is allowed to invade tissues and multiply, it can become capable of causing infection or disease and stimulating a host response.

The infection may or may not be accompanied by overt symptoms of the disease. A local infection, for example, is usually restricted to a specific anatomic site, causing only an inflammatory response to that site. A systemic or generalized infection can occur as the result of microorganisms and their products spreading throughout the body.

An initial infection, caused by one kind of microorganism, is called a *primary infection,* while the *secondary infection* usually involves a second microorganism entering the system and can result in a more toxic form of infection, making it harder to arrest or destroy.

When a tissue becomes damaged, either by injury or disease, the initial stage of acute inflammation occurs, causing vascular and cellular changes. This acute inflammation will persist as long as the tissue damage occurs. Bacteria are the most common cause of injury to the surgical patient; therefore, every effort must be made to prevent this injurious substance from entering the surgical wound.

Sources of Infection

Infections caused by microorganisms that are considered part of the normal resident flora are said to be *endogenous.* An endogenous infection occurs when the normal balance between the organism and the human host is upset owing to impaired defenses, or when the organism is introduced into a part of the body where it does not normally occur, for example, *Escherichia coli* from the intestinal tract into the urinary tract.

Infections caused by microorganisms that are not part of the normal resident flora are said to be *exogenous.* These infections are usually acquired through personnel or hospital environments, and are referred to as *nosocomial infections* caused by opportunistic pathogens. Exogenous infectious agents can be transmitted by a variety of causes, either directly or indirectly.

Most nosocomial infections occurring during the postoperative period (endogenous or exogenous) appear to result from contamination acquired in the operating room, not only because the patient is compromised by illness, but also because the natural defense system, mainly the skin and mucous membranes, has been violated.

Transmission of Infection

Two methods of contact can result in contamination and postoperative wound infection in the surgical patient.

1. *Direct contact:* close association between an infected person and a susceptible host through blood, sputum, or mucous membrane.
2. *Indirect contact:* contact between a susceptible person and infectious material derived from an infectious host or contaminated source, such as skin, air, instruments, or dust particles.

Entry of Microorganisms

To gain entry into the body, microorganisms must penetrate natural barriers, such as the skin, the mucous membranes lining the respiratory, gastrointestinal, and urologic tracts, or the conjunctivae (Fig. 4-3).

These barriers constitute the body's first line of defense against microbial invasion. When these barriers are intact, the microorganisms establish themselves on the body's surface and wait to gain entry.

If the surgical patient is compromised before surgery, either by treatments or diagnostic procedures performed during the preoperative phase, the intraoperative phase can pose the greatest hazard to the patient, since the skin and mucous membranes are no longer intact or the system has been weakened.

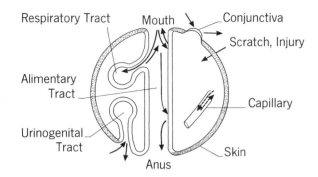

Fig. 4-3. Microbial entry (Adapted from Muir, BL. *Pathophysiology: Introduction to Disease.* New York: John Wiley and Sons, 1980. P. 515.)

Once pathogenic microorganisms have entered the body, they may establish a local infection at the site of entry or may disseminate throughout the body and establish themselves at sites remote from the site of entry (Fig. 4-4).

Whether or not the invading microorganisms establish an infection at the site of entry or at another location depends on the growth requirements of the organism, the local tissue environment, the strength of the host, and the ability of the microorganism to overcome the host defenses.

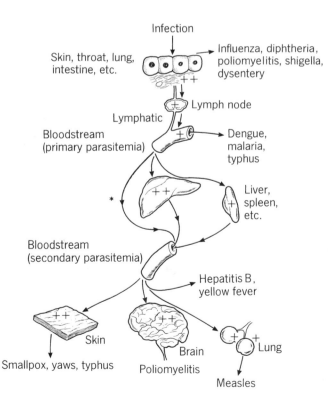

Fig. 4-4. Spread of infection (Adapted from Muir, BL. *Pathophysiology: Introduction to Disease.* New York: John Wiley and Sons, 1980. P. 524.)

The Immune Response

Resistance to infection involves the ability of the immune system to not only recognize a substance as foreign to the body (e.g., non-self), but also to initiate mechanisms to destroy and eliminate the substance. The exact mechanism by which the immune system distinguishes between pathogenic and nonpathogenic invaders or self and non-self is not understood. It appears that exposure of the immune system to circulating and tissue substances during fetal development results in a state of immunologic tolerance to these substances. In other words, the body recognizes these substances as *self* and does not normally initiate an immune response against them.

The Inflammatory–Reparative Response

Inflammation is the local response of tissue to damage, whether by injury or pathogenic microorganisms. Many agents can cause tissue damage, which starts an inflammatory reaction. This response proceeds through several stages, until the tissue has been healed. These stages are commonly described as the *acute inflammation, demolition,* and *restoration* stages (Fig. 4-5).

Clinical signs and symptoms of this process consist of redness, swelling, warmth, pain, and limitation of movement, and are present immediately following any invasive procedure in which the natural defense system has been compromised.

INFECTION CONTROL: PRINCIPLES AND NURSING IMPLICATIONS

According to the AORN Patient Outcome Standards, protecting the patient from infection is a primary goal. Therefore, it becomes the responsibility of all persons rendering care to the patient during the perioperative period.

Since the majority of infections can be acquired in the OR, most preventive measures should be directed toward three primary areas: (1) the preparation of the surgical patient, (2) technical and aseptic practice of the surgical team, and (3) the maintenance of the surgical environment.

Preoperative Preparation of the Patient

Measures aimed at preventing microbial contamination of the wound begin before the operation, by treating active infections and improving the general health

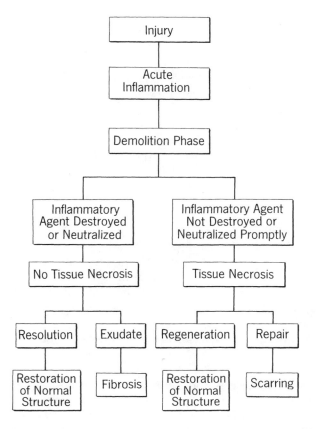

Fig. 4-5. Inflammatory–reparative pathways (Adapted from Muir, BL. *Pathophysiology: Introduction to Disease.* New York: John Wiley and Sons, 1980. P. 123.)

of the patient to reduce the risk of postoperative infections.

Other preoperative measures include keeping the preoperative stay as short as possible; avoiding hair removal, or, if necessary, removing the hair with clippers or depilatories rather than a razor; and proper antimicrobial preparation of the skin. This preparation may include a shower using an antimicrobial agent (e.g., Betadine) the night before and the morning of surgery, in addition to the surgical skin preparation performed immediately before the start of the procedure.

Intraoperative Aseptic Technique

Contamination from the surgical team is another potential source of infection, usually related to direct contact from hands or from shedding skin or mucous membranes.

The use of a surgical hand scrub with an effective antimicrobial agent prior to the application of sterile gloves should assist in retarding bacterial growth, and

corrective action should be taken immediately if this barrier is compromised in any way before or during the surgical procedure.

According to recent studies conducted by the Centers for Disease Control (CDC), the most important factor in preventing wound infections is operative technique.[5]

Poor technique can result in the contamination of the operative wound, causing an extension of the anesthesia time, and unnecessary injury to surrounding tissue, which can result in necrosis and delayed healing. Any of these conditions can result in postoperative wound infections, since the patient's natural defense system has been compromised.

Maintenance of the Surgical Environment

Air is also a potential source of microorganisms that can contaminate the surgical wound.

Air inside the OR is often contaminated with microorganisms that can be attached to airborne particles (dust, lint, respiratory droplets) that could be potential pathogens.

A large number of airborne particles are directly related to the number of persons in the OR (procedure), to the OR doors remaining open and personnel talking near or in the procedure room and to traffic patterns within the surgical suite. Failure to adhere to proper OR attire in the semirestricted and restricted areas of the suite may also account for potential problems, and must be addressed through rigid adherence to policies and procedures for all persons entering these areas.

Movement or activity in the OR can be decreased by keeping the procedure room doors closed and by limiting the number of persons in the procedure room and adjacent corridors. This can be accomplished through the implementation of strict traffic control procedures and policies, as suggested by the AORN Recommended Practices for Traffic Control.

In the modern, well-managed surgical suite, the risk of infection related to the physical environment is not as great as the human factor. This does not, however, reduce the need for constant vigilance on the part of all personnel, since the environment must be maintained to render safe, aseptic patient care.

Principles of Universal Precautions

While there are several means of transferring pathogenic microorganisms during the perioperative period, exposure to blood and body fluids presents the greatest threat to personnel working in the surgical suite.

In 1987, in response to the needs of persons working in "high-risk" areas, the CDC established the Universal Precautions concept for health-care workers, designed to protect personnel from unknown exposure from the patient or the environment.

Through the implementation of the Universal Precautions, the need for isolation of specific cases and the special cleaning procedures associated with these cases is no longer applicable. *All procedures and/or patients are potentially contaminated;* therefore, they are treated alike.

The CDC stated that "since medical history and examination cannot identify all patients who are potentially infected with blood-borne pathogens, specific precautions should be used with *ALL* patients, thereby reducing the risk of possible exposure to its minimum."[6] Accordingly, the CDC recommended that health-care workers could reduce the risk of contamination and exposure by adhering to the following guidelines[7]:

1. All health-care workers should routinely use appropriate barrier protection to prevent skin and mucous membrane exposure when contact with blood or other body fluids of ANY patient is anticipated.

   Gloves, masks, and protective eyewear or face shields should be worn during all surgical procedures and when handling soiled supplies or instruments during or after a procedure to prevent exposure of mucous membranes.

2. Hands and other skin surfaces should be washed immediately and thoroughly if contaminated with blood or other body fluids.

   Although gloves are worn by all personnel during a surgical procedure, handwashing after the removal of gloves should become a routine practice for both scrub and nonsterile personnel working in a procedure room.

3. Health-care workers should take all necessary precautions to protect against injuries caused by needles, scalpels, and other sharp instruments or devices during procedures; when cleaning used instruments; and when handling sharp instruments after a procedure.

   Needles should never be recapped or bent after use. Suture needles and sharps should be contained in a puncture-resistant container, and sealed for proper disposal according to recommended practices and established protocols. Sharp instruments should be placed in a tray in such a way that their points are not exposed, to avoid injury to persons working with the trays.

   During the procedure, care must be taken when handling suture needles to ensure that no one receives an injury by placing the needle on a needle holder and passing it with the point down.

4. Health-care workers who have exudate lesions or weeping dermatitis should refrain from all direct patient care and from handling patient care equipment until the condition resolves.

   Minor breaks in the skin, especially on the hands of the scrub nurse, should restrict scrubbing activities until the break has healed. Circulating nurses should wear sterile gloves if a skin lesion is present, and should cover the lesion with a protective covering when working in a procedure room.

The above guidelines can assist in reducing the risk of contamination, and have been adapted by the Occupational Safety and Health Administration (OSHA) to maintain a safe working environment.

Additionally, the CDC and OSHA recommend that aspirated or drainage material never be allowed to come in contact with the health-care worker, either during the aspiration process or following the procedure. Therefore, use of an efficient suctioning system is imperative during surgery, with extreme caution used during its disposition following the procedure.

When dealing with soiled sponges, towels, or disposable supplies, the principle of *Contain and Control* must be used by all personnel both during and after the procedure.

The perioperative nurse, along with the other staff members, must insist that the surgical suite be maintained at the safest possible level to avoid possible injury or harm to staff or the patient, and immediately correct situations that could cause contamination or harm.

Epidemiologic Monitoring Program

Through a surveillance technique initiated by the CDC that monitors postoperative infections, the surgeon and the nurse-epidemiologist can monitor those patients who are more likely to develop postoperative infections and those who, owing to the nature of their surgery, should be least likely. This technique establishes a criteria for monitoring the surgical infection rates and taking appropriate steps to reduce the incidence of these infections. This system is referred to as the *CDC Classification of Surgical Wounds* (see Unit 3 of this chapter) and is used throughout the country as a quality assurance measure for all surgical patients.

Managing the Postoperative Patient

In the postoperative period, the risk of wound infection can be reduced by proper techniques when handling

CDC Recommendations for Prevention of Surgical Wound Infections

Preoperative Phase

1. Medical treatment of active infections including the prophylactic administration of antibiotics as recommended by established protocols
2. Reducing preoperative hospital stay (same-day surgery)
3. Avoiding hair removal or removal when necessary by the use of clippers or depilatories, rather than a razor
4. Antimicrobial bath/shower the evening before surgery and the morning of surgery
5. Preoperative hand scrub using acceptable antimicrobial solution and technique

Intraoperative Phase

1. Strict adherence to aseptic technique
2. Proper surgical skin preparation
3. Usage of effective barrier materials to establish the sterile field
4. Proper environmental control within the surgical suite
5. Proper OR attire in the semirestricted and the restricted areas of the surgical suite
6. Proper operative techniques; that is, preventing possible contamination or perforation; prolonged operative time; and careful tissue handling
7. Classification and documentation of all surgical procedures/patients

Postoperative Phase

1. Aseptic dressing changes
2. Proper handwashing between patients/treatments
3. Discontinuance of antibiotic therapy unless the condition merits treatment
4. Protection of patients from other infected patients or personnel
5. Routine postoperative surveillance of all surgical patients
6. Quality assurance programs and periodic audits of patient care, including preventive measures for preventing wound infections

By following the recommendations given, all members of the health-care team involved with the surgical patient during the perioperative period can strive toward the optimal patient outcome: an infection-free surgical experience.

Source: Modified from Centers for Disease Control. Guidelines for prevention of surgical wound infections Today's OR nurse 8:38, 1987.

the wound, proper and frequent handwashing, and by the use of closed wound-drainage systems when indicated.

If a drain is used, having it enter through an adjacent, separate stab wound rather than the incision will, according to some physicians, lessen the chance of infection, since the incision site is not directly involved.

When changing a dressing, strict aseptic technique must be used by all personnel working with the postoperative patient, including proper handwashing before and after the procedure. This will reduce the risks of contamination during the critical stages of wound healing and cross-contamination from or to other patients.

A patient's intrinsic susceptibility to infection is also an important factor in determining the risk of postoperative wound infections. Patients with preexisting diseases or conditions pose a greater risk than those who begin the surgical experience in optimal health. If the patient has a preexisting disease, postponement of elective surgery and/or the initiation of corrective treatment may help reduce the potential risk factors, thus protecting the surgical patient from infection.

In other words, infection control is the responsibility of all health care workers.

The above box cites the CDC's recommendations for preventing surgical wound infections, encompassing all three phases of surgical intervention.

Self-assessment Exercise 2

Directions: Complete the following exercises. The answers are given at the end of this module.

There are two major sources from which microorganisms can be transferred to the operative site. Describe the preventive measures that could be taken to avoid their invasion of the patient/suite.

1. PERSONNEL/PATIENT
    a. Skin—Preventive Measures:

    _____

    b. Blood/Body Fluids—Preventive Measures:

    _____

    c. Respiratory Tract—Preventive Measures:

    _____

    d. GI Tract—Preventive Measures:

    _____

2. ENVIRONMENTAL FACTORS
    a. Circulating Air—Preventive Measures:

    _____

    b. Linens/Instruments/Supplies—Preventive Measures:

    _____

    c. OR Sanitation (within the suite)—Preventive Measures:

    _____

    d. Personal Hygiene—Preventive Measures:

    _____

UNIT 3

Principles of Wound Healing

The medical definition of wound healing is described as a "process which restores the structure and function of injured or diseased tissue." This process includes four aspects: (1) blood clotting, (2) tissue mending, (3) scarring, and (4) bone healing.[8]

PHYSIOLOGY OF WOUND HEALING

The body is extremely efficient in its ability to recover from trauma. In fact, a surgical wound begins to heal as soon as the surgeon makes the initial incision.

The acute inflammatory response, discussed earlier, occurs immediately after tissue damage and begins its cycle as the smaller blood vessels in the area of the injury constrict, followed by vasoconstriction, thereby supplying the injured site with nutrients needed to accomplish the healing process.

In the pathologic context, the lost or destroyed tissue is replaced by living tissue and the healing process begins.

TYPES OF WOUNDS

There are two types of wounds. The first involves possible tissue loss, and is known as the *open wound*, while the second are those without tissue loss, known as *closed wounds*.

The loss or destruction of tissue can occur in several ways:

1. By traumatic excision (accidental or surgical)
2. By chemical or physical agents (burns, ischemia)
3. By severe inflammation resulting in tissue necrosis

Replacement of lost tissue can be accomplished by repair or regeneration.

Repair is the replacement of lost tissue with granulation tissue that matures to form a fibrous connective tissue scar. Although it does not restore function, it fills the anatomic defect and restores tissue integrity.

Regeneration is the replacement of lost tissue with tissue of the same type, through multiplication of undamaged cells that replace those that were damaged. When regeneration occurs, normal function is usually restored.

If both restoration and repair occur, the basic framework of the tissue will survive, producing a tissue mass that will be completely restored.

METHODS OF SURGICAL WOUND HEALING

The *open wound* heals in three distinct ways, depending on the variables present during the healing cycle.

Primary Union (First Intention)

First intention wound healing occurs with incised or sutured wounds with no tissue loss, or minimum tissue loss without "dead space."

This is the *ideal* wound, since no contamination has occurred, and it results in a cosmetic effect similar to the normal skin surface. The edges are approximated, resulting in a "hairline scar."

Granulation (Second Intention)

Granulation occurs when wounds experience tissue loss, preventing the approximation of edges and thereby forcing the wound to heal with granulation tissue, which is finally covered by epithelial cells. The cause may be infection or necrosis of tissue, and it produces a wider and deeper scar.

Delayed Primary Closure (Third Intention)

Third intention healing uses a combination of first and second intention healing, and occurs when a wound is left open to heal. After 4 to 6 days, the granulation tissue covers the surface of the wound, at which time it is sutured closed (delayed closure).

This procedure is used when there is a high risk of infection or the need for drainage, but because the wound must be left open, this technique can result in additional complications during the postoperative period.

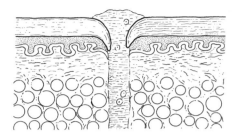

Fig. 4-6. Substrate phase—healing phase lasts about 4 days after wounding (Adapted from Stroumtos, O. [ed.]. *Perspectives on Sutures*. Davis and Geck, Co., Pearl River, NY: American Cyanamid Co., 1978.)

PHASES OF FIRST INTENTION HEALING

The normal wound healing process, when no complications or barriers are interposed to prevent the normal course of events, occurs in three phases.

Phase 1: Substrate Phase (Inflammatory or Lag)

Time: at the time of injury, lasting 4 to 6 postoperative days.

Condition of the Wound: extremely delicate; held together by fibrin bands from blood clots and plasma. Color appears a pinkish-red due to "proud flesh" (Fig. 4-6).

Abnormal State: a prolonged inflammatory state can delay formation of new tissue, resulting in retarded development of wound strength. Dehiscence is likely to occur during this time.

Phase 2: Proliferative Phase (Fibroplasia/Healing)

Time: begins at the third or fourth postoperative day, and continues for approximately 2 weeks.

Condition of the Wound: new cells form and actual repair of tissue takes place. Epithelial cells move along the cut edges to the base of the fibrin clot, forming capillaries and lymphatics. The wound still appears reddish-pink owing to increased blood flow and the delivery of oxygen and nutrients to the new granulation tissue (Fig. 4-7).

Abnormal State: if the wound is not approximated uniformly, or if dead space is present, the scar will be wide and irregular since the skin will grow over the unapproximated edges.

Phase 3: Maturation Phase (Remodeling)

Time: may last as long as 2 years from the date of initial healing.

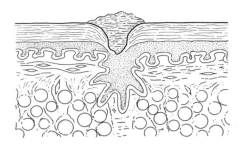

Fig. 4-7. Proliferative phase—epithelialization, wound contraction, and connective tissue repair occur from about the fifth to the twentieth postoperative days (Adapted from Stroumtos, O. [ed.]. *Perspectives on Sutures*. Davis and Geck, Co., Pearl River, NY: American Cyanamid Co., 1978.)

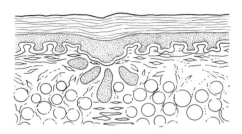

Fig. 4-8. Remodeling phase—phase may continue for many months before the wound regains maximum tensile strength (Adapted from Stroumtos, O. [ed.]. *Perspectives on Sutures*. Davis and Geck, Co., Pearl River, NY: American Cyanamid Co., 1978.)

Condition of the Wound: regains at least 80 percent of its original strength. The increase in strength is due largely to reconstruction of collagen fibers. This network is usually adequate to withstand normal activity around the fourth postoperative week. The suture line continues to contract, and the pink color fades to flesh tone. Although it is now stronger, it will never achieve the full strength of uninjured tissue (Fig. 4-8).

Abnormal State: if an infection is present, closure does not occur, and the wound may require debridement and/or possible reclosure at a later date. If abnormal strain occurs during this time, an incisional hernia may develop.

The entire wound healing process might be likened to the demolition and reconstruction of a building: the removal of debris occurs at the same time as the production of new materials and building configuration.

FACTORS INFLUENCING NORMAL WOUND HEALING

The general health status of an individual, as well as local factors and intraoperative considerations, can influence the process of wound healing.

General Factors

Nutrition

Nutrition is an important factor in the total healing process. *Protein* deficiencies impair the formation of granulation tissue and collagen, which can decrease wound strength. Sufficient amounts of *amino acids* necessary for wound healing are usually available from a well-balanced diet and from mobilization and breakdown of tissue protein.

Vitamin C (ascorbic acid) is necessary for the formation of collagen, and deficiencies can add to the delay of wound healing and decrease strength. Adequate *calcium* and *vitamin D* are necessary for the healing of fractures, since vitamin D is required for calcification of bone.

Cell Oxygenation

Adequate oxygen is critical for wound healing. Anemia would be expected to interfere with wound healing because it impairs oxygen transport in the blood.

Age

Age can influence wound healing, since it is generally believed that healing is better and faster in the young than in the elderly. Impaired healing in the elderly is most often associated with inadequate circulation due to atherosclerosis, or the presence of coexisting diseases.

Chemical Imbalances

Fluid and electrolyte imbalances can delay wound healing since these components and the ultimate affect of the acid-base status of the patient will delay the effectiveness of the lag phase.

Drugs, such as steroids, chemotherapeutic agents, and abused substances, including alcohol and tobacco, can affect the production of collagen and protein synthesis, directly affecting the total healing process.

General Physical Condition

Patients with preexisting or coexisting diseases are more prone to wound infections due to a compromise in the body's immune response.

Specific diseases, such as uremia, uncontrolled diabetes, malignancies, respiratory dysfunction, or the effects of radiation therapy make the wound more vulnerable to disruption and/or infection, resulting in an abnormal healing process.

Smoking has an impact on wound healing, since it can reduce the amount of functional hemoglobin by 10 to 15 percent. The result is a prolonged or abnormal healing process.

Obese patients are also at risk, since fatty tissue is relatively avascular and is therefore prone to microbial contamination and general weakening.

Local Factors

Adequate Circulation

An adequate blood supply is probably the most critical factor in wound healing. Oxygen and nutrients are brought to the injured site via the circulatory system. Therefore, anything that impairs blood flow to the area will interfere with the healing process.

Inflammation

Although healing begins shortly after injury, while the acute inflammatory phase is in progress, repair or regeneration cannot be completed until the acute inflammation subsides and debris is removed from the wound.

Any factor that incites inflammation, such as the presence of infection or foreign bodies, will delay healing. Sutures, for example, must be chosen carefully and handled with precision, because they are foreign substances. Too many sutures or one that is not absorbing properly can interfere with healing. Some sutures can form keloids, stones, or other disruptive factors.

Hemorrhage

Excessive bleeding into the wound not only stimulates inflammation but requires repair before healing can begin. Both inflammation and hemorrhage can delay the healing process, posing additional risks to the patient.

Immobilization

In the treatment of fractures, immobilization of the wound is crucial. It may also promote healing of soft tissue wounds, especially if they are large or deep, since movement may separate the wound edges and disrupt the fragile granulation tissue, which can cause excessive bleeding.

Stress

Stress, which in some instances produces a chemical imbalance, can be a major factor in the wound healing process. Acute stress apparently does not interfere with wound healing, but chronic stress may retard healing and decrease wound strength.

Intraoperative Factors

Improper Tissue Handling

Rough handling of tissue can damage the fibers and delay the healing process. Tissue should be handled with minimal trauma to preserve whatever is naturally available to assist in the healing process.

Previous Surgery

Previous surgery that produced scar tissue or adhesions can slow down the healing process, since circulation may not be adequate in that area. Following a lysis of adhesions, the wound may be weak, resulting in a delay of the healing process.

Suturing and Wound Closure Materials

Too many sutures or the wrong type for a specific area can interfere with the healing process.

Patients may react adversely to suture material, which can set up an inflammatory response due largely to irritation to tissue, similar to when the body tries to reject foreign bodies as a defense mechanism. Synthetic monofilament suture material causes less reaction than braided suture material, and has proven to be less reactive than that made of natural substances. Surgical gut and nonabsorbable sutures, especially those made of silk or cotton, are often associated with inflammation or irritation, resulting in a delayed healing process.

For this reason, if an infection is present at the time of surgery, the surgeon will request a synthetic suture rather than one made from natural fibers.

Recently, the use of internal staples has become a popular replacement for sutures, since they are generally nonreactive, thus minimizing the risk of irritation. Additionally, they can aid in the reduction of operative time, and possibly decrease the extensive handling of tissues.

Exogenous Factors

Maintaining an aseptic environment is paramount in preventing exogenous contamination of the surgical wound.

The perioperative nurse must ensure the sterility of the instruments and supplies and proper preparation of the surgical site, and monitor all activities and personnel involved with the procedure to maintain a safe, therapeutic environment.

COMPLICATIONS OF WOUND HEALING

Even with the best technique and precise nursing care during the perioperative period, some patients may experience complications involving the surgical wound.

The greatest concern during the first 2 to 5 postoperative days is wound disruption causing either dehiscence or evisceration.

Additionally, incisional hernias, fistulas and sinuses, and keloids are complications that may be encountered during the postoperative period.

Wound Dehiscence or Evisceration

Wound dehiscence is the partial or total separation of the wound. It occurs most often during the lag phase of the healing process, while the wound is still in a delicate condition.

Total dehiscence, usually involving an abdominal incision, results in *evisceration,* or protrusion of the viscera through the incisional line. When this occurs, a true surgical emergency exists, requiring immediate action by the nurse caring for the patient.

Incisional Hernias

Incisional hernias result from incomplete wound dehiscence in which the skin remains intact. Incisional hernias can occur as late as 2 to 3 months postoperatively, and occur most frequently in lower abdominal incisions. Incisional hernias can lead to bowel obstructions, which must be surgically corrected.

Fistulas and Sinuses

Fistulas and *sinuses* usually occur during the second phase of normal healing (fibroplasia phase). A fistula is a tract between two epithelium-lined surfaces, open at both ends. This type of complication is usually associated with head and neck, bowel, or genitourinary surgery, and results in drainage that is not expected from the anatomic area.

A sinus, on the other hand, is open at only one end, producing an abnormal sinus tract. This usually requires drainage and closure, but only after the inflammation has subsided.

Keloids

Changes in the metabolism of collagen during the healing process may result in the development of *keloid* scars, producing a dense, fibrous tissue around the outside of the original incision. These scars can be revised; however, the condition can reappear again with each new incision or manipulation of the incisional site.

Self-assessment Exercise 3

Directions: Complete the following exercises. The answers are given at the end of this module.

1. Number the following descriptions of normal wound healing (1. Lag Phase; 2. Maturation Phase; 3. Healing Phase) in their proper sequence:

   a) _____ 14 to 21 days; strengthening by collagen fiber formation

   b) _____ 4 to 6 days; delicate condition with proud flesh, held together by fibrin clots

   c) _____ 4 to 14 days; rapid build-up of fibroblasts; approximation of edges with connective tissue

2. The normal phases of wound healing occur only with

   _____

3. Describe the look of the scar in second intention healing.

   _____

4. Dehiscence differs from evisceration because it

   _____

MONITORING POSTOPERATIVE SURGICAL WOUND INFECTIONS

Many factors can influence the acquisition of a postsurgical wound infection, but basically an infection requires the interaction of three potential causes:

1. The patient's intrinsic resistance (susceptibility of the host).
2. A source of the microorganisms (environmental or personnel).
3. A means of transmission (entry into the system).

Some of these causes may include air, various hospital personnel (carriers), equipment, food, heating/cooling systems, and other patients, in addition to the sources discussed earlier in this chapter.

While all hospital areas pose some degree of risk to the patient of acquiring an infection, surgical patients are the highest risk population within the institution, and therefore require constant monitoring to avoid possible complications.

Surgical wound infections are the second most frequent cause of nosocomial infections and are an important reason for the increase of morbidity, mortality, and increasing hospital-stay costs.

CENTERS FOR DISEASE CONTROL CLASSIFICATION OF SURGICAL WOUNDS

Surgical wound infections are divided into two types:

1. Those confined to the incisional wound.
2. Those involving structures adjacent to the wound

that were entered or exposed during the surgical procedure.

To track infections involving the surgical patient, and to learn how they may have occurred or how to prevent their reoccurrence, the CDC established a classification system for surgical wounds based on the risk factor of possible postoperative infections occurring due to the nature of the surgical procedure. There are four categories, or *classes,* of surgical wounds, each with a specific criterion for placement:

1. Class I Clean wounds
2. Class II Clean-contaminated wounds
3. Class III Contaminated wounds
4. Class IV Dirty (infected) wounds

The following descriptions can assist in classifying a wound, and are used throughout the country to describe a specific type of surgical procedure and its risk factor.[9]

Class I Clean Wounds

Definition: Uninfected operative wounds in which no inflammation is encountered, and the respiratory, alimentary, genital, or uninfected urinary tracts are not entered. Additionally, clean wounds are elective surgery, with primary closure and, if necessary, drained with a closed drainage device.

Operative incisional wounds that follow nonpenetrating (blunt) trauma should be included in this class, if all other criteria have been met.

Risk Factor: 1 to 5 percent risk of postoperative infection.

Examples: include, but are not limited to, eye surgery, hernia repairs, breast surgery, neurosurgery (nontraumatic), cardiac or peripheral vascular surgeries.

Class II Clean-contaminated Wounds

Definition: Operative wounds in which the respiratory, alimentary, genital or urinary tract is entered under controlled conditions and without unusual contamination. Specifically, operations involving the biliary tract, appendix, vagina, and oropharynx are included provided there is no evidence of infection or no major break in aseptic technique is encountered.

Risk Factor: 3 to 11 percent risk of postoperative infection.

Examples: include, but are not limited to, gastrectomy, cholecystectomy (without spillage), elective appendectomy, cysto or cysto-TUR (negative urine cultures), total abdominal hysterectomy (TAH), dilation and curettage, "C" sections and tonsillectomy (noninfected at time of surgery).

Class III Contaminated Wounds

Definition: Surgery that involves open, fresh, traumatic wounds, or with major breaks in sterile technique or with gross spillage from the GI tract, and incisions in which acute, nonpurulent inflammation is encountered.

Risk Factor: 10 to 17 percent risk of postoperative infection.

Examples: include, but are not limited to, rectal surgery, laparotomy (significant spillage), traumatic wounds (e.g., gunshot, stab wounds [nonperforation of visceral]) or acute inflammation of any organ without frank pus present (e.g., acute appendicitis or cholecystitis, compound fractures).

Class IV Dirty (Infected) Wounds

Definition: Old traumatic wounds with retained devitalized tissue, and wounds that involve existing clinical infection or perforated viscera and/or delayed primary closure wounds. This classification suggests an infectious process was present prior to surgery.

Risk Factor: greater than 27 percent risk of postoperative infection.

Examples: include, but are not limited to, debridement, incision and drainage, total evisceration, perforated viscera, amputations, or positive preoperative blood cultures.

It is important to remember, when deciding what classification the surgical procedure belongs in, that coexisting diseases do not influence the classification, only preexisting infectious processes that may be present at the time of surgery.

Placing a surgical procedure in its proper category is an important responsibility of the perioperative nurse, since it will help the epidemiology department and the surgeons effectively monitor and care for the postoperative patient.

Self-assessment Exercise 4

Directions: *Complete the following exercises. The answers are given at the end of this module.*

1. List four physical conditions that if present could increase the patient's risk of developing a postoperative wound infection.

   1. _____

   2. _____

   3. _____

   4. _____

2. No special cleaning procedures are performed following a septic case. Why? _____

   _____

3. The circulating air in a procedure room is a potential source of contamination, owing to dust particles.

4. Soiled sponges should be handled only with _____ and/or _____.

5. For each of the following wound classifications, state one procedure that correlates with its description.

   Class I Clean _____

   Class II Clean-contaminated _____

   Class III Contaminated _____

   Class IV Dirty (infected) _____

6. A patient scheduled for an inguinal hernia repair has been diagnosed with AIDS. The classification for this procedure would be Class II.

   True   False

References

1. Zimmerman LM, Veith I. Great ideas in the history of surgery. New York: Dover Publishing, 1987. P. 21.
2. Groah LK. Operating room nursing: The perioperative role. Reston, VA: Reston Publishing, 1983. P. 136.
3. Cartwright F. The development of modern surgery. New York: Thomas Crowell, 1968. P. 48.
4. Ibid, p. 50.
5. Centers for Disease Control. Guidelines for prevention of surgical wound infections. Atlanta, GA: U.S. Department of Health and Human Services, 1987.
6. Centers for Disease Control. Morbid mortal weekly report Aug. (Suppl.), 1988: MMWR.
7. Ibid.
8. Miller BF, Keane CB. Encyclopedia and dictionary of medicine, nursing and allied health. 3rd ed. Philadelphia: WB Saunders, 1983. P. 441.
9. American College of Surgeons. Committee on control of surgical infections. Manual on control of infections in surgical patients. 2nd ed. Philadelphia: JB Lippincott, 1984.

5 Surgical Pharmacology

Systems of Measurement
Administering Intravenous Solutions
Calculating Intravenous Flow Rates
Preparation and Administration Guidelines
Categories of Drugs

UNIT 1

Basic Calculations

An important part of the perioperative nurse's role is the preparation and administration of pharmacologic agents during the perioperative period.

To provide the patient with the exact amount of a drug as ordered by the surgeon, the perioperative nurse must be able to perform simple calculations in order to deliver to the surgical team the correct amount of a drug, under sterile conditions.

This unit reviews the basic mathematical principles as they relate to the safe preparation and administration of drugs and drugs in solution that are commonly used at the sterile field.

SYSTEMS OF MEASUREMENT

The three systems of measurement commonly associated with the administration of medications are the metric, apothecary, and household systems.

The metric and household systems measure weight, volume, and length, while the apothecary system measures weight and volume.

The metric system is most commonly used in surgery since most of the agents are prepared in this format.

The Apothecary System

The apothecary system, an old English form of measurement, is being replaced by the metric system, although it is still used by some physicians and hospitals.

The terms *dram* and *ounce* are usually expressed in lowercase Roman numerals, but their values are being replaced by their metric equivalency for standardization of weights and measures, as European countries have already accomplished.

The Household System

Household measures, the least accurate system, are used only when it is impractical to calculate and measure doses, or when teaching a patient how to take his or her prescribed medication once he or she leaves the hospital.

Since household utensils from each manufacturer may differ in measurement, the American Standards Institute has established national standards to assist in dispensing drugs or solutions requiring the use of household measurements. Examples include:

60 drops = 1 teaspoon
1 teaspoon = 1 fluid dram = 4 or 5 milliliters
1 pint = 16 ounces = 473 milliliters
8 fluid ounces = 1 glassful = approx. 237 mL

The Metric System

The metric system, invented by the French in the late eighteenth century, is also called the *decimal* system. It is used primarily because of its accuracy, and is the only system used in the U.S. Pharmacopeia, the official listing for drugs.

The metric system is very logically organized and flexible. The basis of measurement was chosen as a quarter of the Earth's circumference measured across the poles. One ten-millionth of the distance was accepted as the standard unit of linear measurement—the distance from the Equator to the North Pole—and this distance was divided by 10,000 and chosen as the unit of length: a *meter*.[1] Calculations within the system are based on divisors and multiples of units of 10.

Units of Measure: Metric

Units of measurement include volume of fluids (*liter; L*); weight of solids (*gram; g*); and measures of length (*meter; m*).

Subdivisions of metric units include *deci, centi, milli,* and *deca, hecto,* and *kilo.* Units of weight are expressed in grams (*g*), milligrams (*mg*), kilograms (*kg*), and micrograms (*μg*), while units of capacity are expressed in liters (*L*) and milliliters (*mL* [formerly *cc*]). Distance is expressed in meters (*m*) and millimeters (*mm*).

Review of Frequently Used Equivalencies

The following lists represent the common equivalencies between one system and another.

METRIC		DECIMAL
	0	hundred thousandths
	0	ten thousandths
kilo	0	thousands
hecto	0	hundredths
deca	0	tenths
meter, liter, gram	0	units
deci	0	tenths
centi	0	hundredths
milli	0	thousands
	0	ten thousandths
	0	hundred thousandths
	0	millionths

Weights

APOTHECARIES	METRIC
60 grains (gr) = 1 dram (dr)	60–65 mg = 1 gr
8 drams = 1 ounce	4 g = 1 dr
12 ounces = 1 pound	30–32 g = 1 oz
	370–375 g = 1 lb
	0.37–0.375 kg = 1 lb
gr 1/60 = 1 mg	1000 μg = 1 mg
gr 15–16 = 1 gm	1000 mg = 1 gm
2.2 lb = 1 kg	1000 g = 1 kg

Volume

APOTHECARIES	METRIC
1 minim (m) = 1 gtt =	0.06 mL
15–16 minims =	1 mL
60 minims = 1 fl oz	4 mL = 1 fl dr
8 fl dr = 1 fl oz	30 mL = 1 fl oz
16 fl oz = 1 pint	500 mL = 1 pt
	500 mL = 0.5 L
2 pt = 1 quart	1000 mL = 1 qt
	1000 mL = 1 L
4 qt = 1 gallon	4000 mL = 1 gallon
	4000 mL = 4 L

(heparin) 10 mg = 1000 units (U)

Common Conversion Formulas

In most instances, the drug requested will be supplied by the pharmaceutical company in a unit of measure that does not require conversion or calculation to another system. However, the perioperative nurse will occasionally have to perform calculations to determine the correct dosage; therefore, the rules of conversion from one system to another must be used.

NOTE: Whenever you make a conversion, it is easiest to convert the unit of measure ordered to the unit of measure on hand.

Some of the more common conversion formulas are listed on the following pages.

To change minims to milliliters: Divide by 15
To change milliliters to minims: Multiply by 15
To change milligrams to grains: Divide by 60
To change grains to milligrams: Multiply by 60
To change pounds to kilograms: Divide pounds by 2.2 kilograms
To change kilograms to pounds: Multiply kilograms by 2.2 pounds

To change grams to milligrams: Multiply grams by 1000 *or* move decimal point three places to the **right**

To change milligrams to grams: Divide milligrams by 1000 *or* move decimal point three places to the **left**

To change liters to milliliters: Multiply liters by 1000 *or* move decimal point three places to the **right**

To change milliliters to liters: Divide milliliters by 1000 *or* move decimal point three places to the **left**

NOTE: 1 mL and 1 cc are equivalent. The abbreviation mL is used here.

Self-assessment Exercise 5

Directions: *Complete the following exercises. Answers are given at the end of this module.*

1. Convert the following:

    a. 0.5 g = _____ mg

    b. 30 mg = _____ gr

    c. 500 mg = _____ gr

    d. 2000 mg = _____ g

    e. 10 mg = _____ units (heparin)

2. Compute the following:

    a. A vial of MS is labeled gr 1/4 = 1 mL. How many minims would you give for gr 1/2?

    b. Atropine 0.3 mg is ordered. On hand you have gr 1/150 per mL. How many minims would you give? _____

    c. A drug contains 2 mL = 1 g. The surgeon orders 250 mg in irrigation. How many mL of medication would you prepare?

    _____

ADMINISTERING INTRAVENOUS SOLUTIONS

All surgical patients will have a preoperative intravenous (IV) line started, and in some instances, especially during a local procedure, the perioperative nurse will be responsible for monitoring the infusion rate.

Intravenous administration sets are constructed to deliver a specific number of drops per milliliter. This is referred to as the *drop factor* and can be found on the outside of the IV administration package. For example:

Baxter-Travenol	10 gtt/mL
Abbott	15 gtt/mL
McGaw	13 gtt/mL
Cutter	20 gtt/mL
minidrip (all)	60 gtt/mL
infusion pumps	mL/HR

CALCULATING INTRAVENOUS FLOW RATES

The following formulas can help determine the correct flow rate, and are calculated according to the number of drops (gtt) delivered per unit of time by the IV solution set:

1. To determine the mL/hr rate:
Divide the total volume to be infused by the total number of hours.

EXAMPLE: 1000 mL D_5W q8h = 125 mL/hr

2. To determine the drops-per-minute rate (gtt/min):

$$gtt/min = \frac{total\ IV\ volume \times gtt/mL\ (drop\ factor)}{total\ time\ (in\ min)}$$

EXAMPLE: 1000 mL D_5W q8h =
    15 gtt/mL = 31 gtt/min
    10 gtt/mL = 21 gtt/min
    60 gtt/mL = 125 gtt/min

3. Short-cut formulas (10 or 15 gtt/min):

    a. determine the mL/hr rate

    b. divide the mL/hr rate by 6 (10 gtt/mL) or 4 (15 gtt/mL)

    c. The answer is the gtt/min rate

4. For minidrip: Drops per minute = mL/hr.

Self-assessment Exercise 6

Directions: Complete the following exercises. The answers are given at the end of this module.

1. Calculate how many drops/min for 1000 mL to be given over 8 hours with a tubing that delivers 10 gtt/mL.

2. Infuse 2000 mL of fluid over 24 hours (drop factor = 15).

   a. How many gtt/min? _____

   b. How many mL/hr? _____

3. Infuse 500 mL in 8 hours using a minidrip IV tubing.

   a. How many drops/min? _____

   b. How many mL/hr? _____

UNIT 2
Drugs Used in Surgery

Drugs used in surgery include those that are

- administered parenterally
- administered topically
- administered in irrigation solution
- introduced into a hollow organ or duct for diagnostic purposes

PREPARATION AND ADMINISTRATION GUIDELINES

Reconstituted powders or liquid medications are delivered to the scrub nurse/technician by the circulating nurse. The contents may be transferred via a sterile syringe or by pouring vial contents into an appropriate receptacle according to acceptable institutional policy. In either case, the procedure for accepting or preparing a drug requires the use of strict aseptic technique.

As with any drug, the nurse must:

- Know the allergies of the patient.
- Know the proper reconstitution and preparation procedures, using the manufacturer's recommendations and/or the institutional policies.
- Know the proper dosage, routes of administration, and possible complications and side effects of each drug administered.
- Check with the manufacturer's recommendations for storing a drug to maintain the drug's maximum effectiveness.
- Confirm the drug type and dosage requested before administration to the sterile field (both the scrub and circulator must do this). The drug should be checked for color and consistency, and if a change has been noticed, the product should not be used.
- Label each agent or agent in solution with the name and amount on the container/syringe after administration to the sterile field.
- Use a sterile "decanting spout" when delivering solutions from an IV bag (e.g., Heparinized saline) to the sterile field, to avoid contamination of the field.
- Document on the intraoperative record all drugs/solutions administered to the sterile field.

As an added precaution, neither the circulating nurse nor the scrub nurse/technician can permit familiarity with a bottle shape or size, label, or color to interfere with the proper checking procedures. Poor technique and disregard for safety may result in injury to or adverse reaction by the patient. Drug allergies (food allergies) should be reexamined before administration of all substances used during the perioperative period.

CATEGORIES OF DRUGS

Pharmacologic agents are commonly placed into categories according to their similarities in action and/or their physiologic effect when introduced into the system.

As with any medication, the nurse should have knowledge of the actions, methods of administration, and nursing considerations associated with each drug.

Unlike other medications administered by the nurse, administration of these agents does not require a written physician's order, since it is considered standard protocol during the intraoperative period, based on the physician preference card and/or a verbal order from the surgeon during surgery.

The following monograph describes the ten categories of drugs commonly administered in the OR:

1. Antimicrobial (antiinfective, antibiotic)
2. Anticoagulants
3. Hemostatic agents
4. Oxytocics
5. Steroids (antiinflammatory)
6. Diagnostic imaging agents
7. Dyes
8. Diuretics
9. CNS agents
10. Emergency protocol drugs

Monograph of Common Drugs Used in Surgery

Category: Antimicrobial (Antiinfective; Antibiotic)
General Description:
Chemical agents that eliminate living organisms pathogenic to the host (patient). The methods for classifying these agents include:

- Mechanism of action—inhibition of protein synthesis, activity on the cell membrane, alteration of the nucleic acid metabolism.
- Spectrum of activity—gram positive or gram negative.
- Similarity in chemical structure—penicillins; cephalosporins; aminoglycosides; sulfonamides.
- Source—living organisms; chemical synthesis.

Selection is based on the organism's sensitivity, patient variations, and the relative toxicity of the proposed agent.

EXAMPLES: include, but are not limited to:

- penicillins (e.g., ampicillin)
- cephalosporins (e.g., cefazolin sodium [Ancef])
- aminoglycosides (e.g., neomycin sulfate; gentamycin sulfate [Garamycin])
- sulfonamides (e.g., gantrisin)
- others (e.g., bacitracin, chloromycetin, vancomycin, tetracycline)

Administration Method:
  in saline irrigation solution
Nursing Considerations for Surgery:

- Although cephalosporins may be used for patients allergic to penicillin, some patients may show sensitivity and subsequently develop allergies to this group.
- All drugs in irrigation solution in the sterile field must be labeled to avoid confusion with plain solutions.
- All agents used in irrigation must be documented on the intraoperative record.

Category: Anticoagulants
General Description:
  Anticoagulants are given to prolong the time it takes the blood to clot by preventing the conversion of fibrinogen to fibrin. In addition, they are used to prevent the occurrence of clot enlargement or fragmentation (thromboembolism).

EXAMPLE:

- heparin (generic, liquaemin sodium)

Administration Method:
  IV (administered by anesthesiologist) or in irrigation solution (Heparinized saline solution)
Nursing Considerations for Surgery:

- It is clinically safer and far more accurate to measure the dose in units than in milligrams.

- Intravenous heparin must be administered via an infusion pump.
- Heparin should be administered in an isotonic sodium chloride solution (IV), not a sodium chloride irrigation solution.
- Heparin is available in units/mL; available either as Bovine or Porcine. Check with physician as to proper dosage.
- Document irrigation solution on intraoperative record.

Category: Hemostatic Agents
General Description:
  Hemostatic agents reduce capillary bleeding and arrest blood flow, thereby assisting in blood clotting during surgery.

EXAMPLES:

- absorbable gelatin sponge (e.g., Gelfoam)
- microfibrillar collagen (e.g., Avitine)
- oxidized cellulose (e.g., Surgicel; Oxycel)
- topical thrombin
- systemic hemostatic/Amicar

Administration Method:
  placed topically on the bleeding surface to absorb blood and reduce bleeding; sprayed directly on area
Nursing Considerations for Surgery:

- Topical thrombin is reconstituted before use, and is generally used with an absorbable gelatin sponge (Gelfoam) for greater absorbancy. It can also be used in spray form.
- Amicar must be reconstituted, and is given IV
- Absorbable gelatin sponges do not have to be removed; however, the oxidized cellulose should be removed after hemostasis has been accomplished.
- Microfibrillar collagen (Avitine) is applied directly to the bleeding area in dry-powdered form, but will adhere to wet gloves, instruments, or tissue surfaces. Handle with smooth, dry forceps.

Category: Oxytocics
Oxytocics are normally found in the posterior pituitary gland and stimulate smooth muscle of the uterus during childbirth, thereby forcing the uterus to contract and thus decreasing bleeding after a cesaraen section.

EXAMPLES:

- oxytocin (Pitocin)
- methergine

Administration Method:
  added to IV (by anesthesiologist)
Nursing Considerations for Surgery:

- Store at temperatures below 25°C (77°F); avoid freezing.
- Oxtocics can have an antidiuretic effect; monitor intake and output.
- They are usually administered after delivery of the placenta.
- Use cautiously in patients with a history of cervical or uterine surgery and in primigravida women over 35 years of age.
- Rotate bottle gently to distribute drug in solution.
- Do not use ampules with discolored solution.
- IV methergine is used for emergencies only.

Category: Steroids (Antiinflammatory)
General Description:
Corticosteroids are hormones produced naturally by the adrenal cortex. They are used in surgery to reduce inflammation and possible postoperative swelling.

EXAMPLES: include, but are not limited to:

- dexamethasone (Decadron)
- dexamethasone (Hexadrol)
- hydrocortisone sodium succinate (Solu-Cortef)
- methylprednisolone sodium succinate (Solu-Medrol)
- methylprednisolone acetate (Depo-Medrol)
- hydrocortisone (Aristocort)
- trimethasone (Kenalog)

Administration Method:
administered parenterally to the affected site by the surgeon
Nursing Considerations for Surgery:

- Reconstitute according to manufacturer's recommendations.
- Agitate to dissolve particles prior to delivery.
- Label syringe on back table to avoid accidental usage.
- Provide scrub nurse/technician with a 19g needle for withdrawal and a 23g to 27g needle for injection (surgeon's preference).
- Hydrocortisone (Solu-Cortef) should be given deep IM.
- Carefully check label for recommended route of administration.
- Document medication on intraoperative record.

Category: Diagnostic Imaging Agents
General Description:
Contrast imaging agents are also known as *radiopaque media.* They allow radiologic visualization of internal structures during operative procedures, such as intraoperative cholangiograms, cystoretrogrades, and so on.

Depending on its structure, the contrast media may be instilled directly into a duct or organ and may or may not be diluted with normal saline. Therefore, check with the surgeon for administration preferences.

EXAMPLES: include, but are not limited to:

- Renografin (cholangiography, hysterosalpingography)
- Cystografin, Cysto-Conray (cystourethrography)
- Hypaque
- Hyskon

Administration Method:
direct instillation into duct or organ via tube or special catheter
Nursing Considerations for Surgery:

- Although the incidence of iodine hypersensitivity related to contrast media is low, preoperative assessment of problems associated with previous x-ray procedures should be reported immediately.
- Be prepared to treat any adverse reactions (usually with Benadryl) when using contrast media.
- The surgeon is responsible for instillation of the agent during the x-ray procedure.
- Label all syringes and check with surgeon as to dilution strength if requested or required.
- Document agent on intraoperative record.

Category: Dyes
General Description:
Solutions used to stain or mark a specific surface or area. Most solutions for skin marking have been replaced by sterile ''marking pens''; however, dyes can also be used to color solutions or to test the patency of specific organs.

EXAMPLES: include, but are not limited to:

- methylene blue
- indigo carmine

Administration Methods:

- added to solution
- administered directly into structure
- used as a topical marker on skin

Nursing Considerations for Surgery:

- No adverse effects have been reported
- May be diluted per surgeon's preference

- Rinse container immediately after use as it may cause permanent discoloration.
- If instilled internally, document use on intraoperative record.

Category: Diuretics
General Description:

Diuretics reduce the body's total volume of water and salt by increasing their urinary excretion. This occurs mainly because diuretics impair sodium chloride reabsorption in the renal tubules. Additionally, diuretics can increase the osmotic pressure, inhibiting tubular reabsorption of water and electrolytes, thus reducing retention of water and possible reduction of swelling in traumatized areas, for example, the brain.

EXAMPLES: include, but not limited to:

- furosemide (Lasix)
- mannitol (Osmitrol)

Administration Method:

IV (by anesthesiologist)
Nursing Considerations for Surgery:

- Lasix should be given over 1 to 2 minutes.
- Monitor serum potassium levels. Make note of patients on digitalis.
- Mannitol solution often crystalizes, especially at low temperatures. Therefore, store it in a solution-warming cabinet.
- Do not use solution with undissolved crystals.
- Hemodynamic monitoring equipment should be available (e.g., central venous pressure catheter, Foley catheter with urimeter).

Category: Central Nervous System Agents
General Description:

CNS agents are those that affect the body's response to stimuli, coordination of activity, and level of consciousness. This category includes agents such as analgesics, tranquilizers, anticonvulsants, and anesthetic agents (see Chap. 6).

All these agents can alter the patient's perception of pain or well-being, and must be used with extreme caution since unfavorable interactions and/or reactions are often encountered.

EXAMPLES:
1. Analgesics: bind with opiate receptors at many sites in the CNS, altering both pain and the emotional response to pain. Examples include, but are not limited to:

- fentanyl and fentanyl derivatives (Sublimaze); (Alfenta); (Sufenta)
- morphine sulfate
- Meperidine (Demerol)
- codeine
- Hydromorphone (Dilaudid)

NOTE: In high doses, narcotic analgesics can be further classified as anesthetic agents, and are administered by the anesthesiologist and/or CRNA, not the perioperative nurse.

2. Tranquilizers: reduce anxiety without inducing sleep. Most tranquilizers have muscle-relaxant and anticonvulsive properties, and closely resemble sedative-hypnotics in pharmacologic properties. Examples include, but are not limited to:

- diazepam (Valium)
- midazolam (Versed)
- droperidol (Inapsine)

Administration Method: IV
Nursing Considerations for Surgery:

- Know the institutional policies for administration protocols before administering these agents.
- During a local procedure, document all patient responses every 15 minutes or more often as needed.
- Keep antagonist agents available when administering these agents.

Chapter 6 contains further discussion specific to anesthetic agents, narcotics, and tranquilizers.

Category: Emergency Protocol Drugs
General Description:
This category includes:

- cardiac stimulants (e.g., epinephrine)
- vasoconstrictors (e.g., levophed)
- vasodilators (e.g., nipride)
- cardiotonics (e.g., digitalis)
- antiarrhythmics (e.g., lidocaine)

Nursing Considerations for Surgery:
The perioperative nurse should be prepared, through annual Basic Life Support review, to handle correctly the common drugs used during emergency situations, including dosages, administration routes, and indications for use.

By following the current American Heart Association protocol for Advanced Cardiac Life Support (ACLS), the perioperative nurse can deliver comprehensive emergency care and assist as necessary in the preparation and administration of emergency drugs and solutions.

Supplemental Drugs and Solutions

In addition to the previous categories, the surgical patient may receive additional drugs and solutions to maintain hemostasis during the perioperative period. These agents include:

1. Volume expanders, to increase circulating fluid volume. (Examples include hespan, albumin, and hetastarch.)
2. Blood and blood components, to restore cell volume. (Examples include fresh-frozen plasma, washed packed cells, whole blood, cryoprecipitate, and factor VIII.)
3. IV solutions, with or without electrolytes. (Examples include D_5W, D_5LR, Lactate ringer's.)

Self-assessment Exercise 7

Directions: Complete the following exercises. The answers are given at the end of this module.

1. Match the description in Column A with the category in Column B.

   COLUMN A

   a. kills or inhibits the growth of microorganisms
   b. promotes blood clotting
   c. reduces tissue swelling and inflammation
   d. radiopaque; visualizes internal structures
   e. prolongs blood clotting
   f. draws fluid out of tissues
   g. changes perception; reduces pain
   h. increases blood volume
   i. causes contraction and constriction
   j. first line drugs for cardiac arrhythmias

   COLUMN B

   1. _____ Diuretics
   2. _____ Contrast media
   3. _____ Oxytocics
   4. _____ Steroids
   5. _____ Antimicrobials
   6. _____ CNS agents
   7. _____ Anticoagulants
   8. _____ Hemostatics
   9. _____ Emergency drugs
   10. _____ Volume expander

2. Parenteral administration includes IM and IV.

   True   False

3. Internal irrigation usually requires the use of 0.9% NaCl.

   True   False

4. Contrast media is usually prepared as a mixture of the agent and normal saline.

   True   False

5. Fentanyl is the generic name for _____.

Reference

1. Nurse's Reference Library, Drugs. Springhouse, PA: *Nursing* 90: 58, 60, 1990.

6

Anesthesia and Perioperative Nursing Implications

Alfredo Ferrari

Three events have had a great impact on modern surgery: *hemostasis*, the control of bleeding; *antisepsis*, the control of infection; and *anesthesia*, the ability to control pain.

HISTORICAL OVERVIEW OF ANESTHESIA

The ability to deaden or relieve pain sensations has been in existence since biblical times, although most of the methods used during its early years were associated with mysticism and the administration of potions and topical agents containing plant substances that were capable of anesthetizing a specific area.

Anesthesia in Ancient Cultures

Anesthesia is based on changes produced due to chemical substances, and relies on pharmacodynamics, toxicology, and pharmaceutical chemistry as it relates to the human body.

The ancient Hebrews used wine and mandrake root (mandragora) to cause a loss of pain during circumcisions and surgical procedures performed during that time.[1]

The Egyptian pharmacopeia was vast in its remedies and medicines used to deaden pain. Medicines were administered by temple priests and physicians, and were available in many different forms, from salves to potions taken internally.

It is well known that substances derived from the opium poppy were in use during the second millennium B.C., and drugs such as *hyoscyammas* and *scopolamine*, both related to the mandrake root, probably were used along with potent mixtures of wine and secret herbal substances.[2]

The ancient Greeks, including Hippocrates, used the juice of the opium poppy and hyoscyammas for anesthesia and the relief of pain caused by disease.

In ancient China, wine, drugs, and acupuncture were used to deaden pain, although according to ancient writings a proper Chinese attitude toward pain was to bear it without a sign of emotion.

Pain management in pre-Columbus America used plants that not only deadened pain, but also had a profound psychic effect, and these were frequently used both in religious ceremonies and to control pain.[3]

Today, skillful specialists administering anesthesia have a variety of methods and techniques to choose from, depending on the individual patient's needs, the surgeon's preference, and the proposed surgical procedure.

DEVELOPMENT OF MODERN ANESTHESIA

In the early years of medicine and surgery, the anesthetic techniques of hypnosis, alcohol intoxication, or the ingestion of herbal concoctions were acceptable methods for controlling pain. The gastrointestinal tract remained the only avenue for anesthesia administration until the inhalation of vapors became an alternative approach, and the intravenous method for administering drugs became a reality.

With the techniques of anesthetic administration more or less divided between physicians and chemists, the use of *inhalation, intravenous,* or *regional* techniques or a combination of the three, became more readily available. All three methods began to emerge during the Middle Ages, although they were not widely practiced for fear of reprisals from the church and the medical community.

Inhalation Anesthesia

Around 1540, a Swiss physician is said to have sweetened the feed of chickens with a substance known as oil of vitrol, formally named *aether*, which became the diethyl ether that would be inhaled by most surgical patients over the next 100 years. The effect that was discovered was amazing: one of profound sleep, but the chickens "awakened without harm."[4]

Regional Anesthesia

Cocaine and local agents had a much different beginning. The coca leaf was believed to be an Incan gift from the god Manco Capac to relieve the daily suffering of his people, especially during childbirth.

By the time the Conquistadors arrived in South America in the sixteenth century, the lower-class peasants and slaves were paid for their work in coca leaves, which were formed into a ball containing guanco and cornstarch, and chewed to produce a euphoric effect, thereby generating a greater output of labor for the Spanish builders who were busy erecting great monuments and cities for their countrymen.

There is substantial documentation of simple surgical procedures being performed while the patient was under the influence of cocaine, thereby proving it had a powerful anesthetic effect. Also, when the substance was topically applied to an injured area, the site became desensitized to pain, producing local anesthesia.[5]

Intravenous Anesthesia

In 1628, following William Harvey's studies concerning the circulation system and how it nourished the organs of the body, Sir Christopher Wren and Daniel-Johnson Major began to experiment with the idea of injecting medications into the bloodstream to deaden pain throughout the system.

Wren is credited with administering the first opiate solution intravenously via needle and syringe in 1657. Although the patient died because of an overdose, a new era in pain management was developing.

As the intravenous method became more widely accepted for administering other medications, it was not much later that this pain-management method was used during surgical procedures, although still technically "shunned" by the church as an "unholy" act.

THE IMPACT OF ANESTHESIA ON SURGERY

Although operations have been performed for centuries, they were generally associated with superficial problems such as fractures, amputations, or the removal of cataracts or bladder stones. Even as surgery was progressing, it was very slow compared with medicine, largely due to a lack of effective pain control during the procedure and by devastating postoperative infections. Both of these obstacles were substantially reduced by the discovery of anesthesia and the proof that germs caused infection and thus must not be allowed to enter an open wound.

Superficial surgery could be performed with the aid of alcohol, opiates, and mandragora, but abdominal procedures would not be feasible until the patient could be put deeply to sleep yet safely enough to permit unhurried operative maneuvers and ability to reawaken.

As anatomic knowledge and surgical techniques improved, the search for safer methods to prevent pain became more pressing. By 1831, three basic inhalation agents—ether, nitrous oxide, and chloroform—had been discovered, but no successful medical application of their pain-relieving properties had yet been made.[6]

In 1846, W.T.G. Morton finally showed the worth of nitrous oxide during a tooth extraction. From that demonstration, great strides were made in the use of anesthesia for a variety of surgical, obstetric, and diagnostic procedures.[7]

THE CREATION OF A SPECIALTY

In 1902, physicians began to specialize in anesthesia. Nurses, however, have been administering anesthesia for over 100 years. In addition, the American Association of Nurse Anesthetists identified Sr. Mary Bernard (in 1877) as the first nurse anesthetist in the United States.

In 1937, the American Board of Anesthesiology was created to certify those physicians wishing to practice anesthesiology. In 1986, this board was made responsible for proposing recommendations to expand the existing educational preparation for anesthesiologists by including a 4-year clinical program following the completion of a generic medical education.[8] Today, anesthesiology is a mature speciality, but its limits have not yet been clearly defined.

PHASES OF ANESTHESIA PRACTICE

Anesthesia consists of making the patient insensitive to pain in a specific area of the body or the body as a whole. The objectives of anesthesia are (1) to produce analgesia, (2) to produce amnesia, (3) to induce muscle relaxation, and (4) to provide control of the autonomic nervous system reflexes.

Anesthesia, like perioperative nursing practice, can be related to the three phases of surgical intervention: *preoperative, intraoperative,* and *postoperative management.*

PREOPERATIVE PHASE

The preoperative phase revolves around the assessment and preparation of the patient for surgery.

Preparation for Anesthesia

According to the recommendations from the Joint Commission on Accreditation of Health Care Organizations, all patients receiving anesthesia (general, regional, or local with monitored anesthesia care) should undergo an evaluation and assessment by an anesthesia practitioner before the administration of anesthesia. Past and present medical history should be reviewed with attention focused on prior surgical experiences and the physiologic alterations induced by disease. The ability to tolerate the adverse effects of anesthesia and surgery depends largely on the normality of respiration and circulation and the homeostatic functions of the liver, kidneys, and endocrine and central nervous systems.

A formal evaluation program should be established, consisting of an interview, a systems review, and a record of important data that can be used later as a guide for an individualized anesthesia program, depending on the needs of the patient (Fig. 6-1).

If special diagnostic procedures and tests are needed, they should be carried out as soon as possible so that the results are on the chart before the scheduled surgery date, in order to perform a comprehensive assessment of the patient's physical status.

Once the preliminaries are over, the patient should be told of the plan for anesthesia, including the methods proposed so that the patient can make an intelligent decision. At that point, an informed consent should be signed and witnessed.

Although from a medicolegal point of view the anesthesia summary is more meaningful than a signed anesthesia consent, most institutions will insist on both in order to protect the patient and the anesthesia practitioner administering the anesthesia therapy (Fig. 6-2).

AMERICAN SOCIETY OF ANESTHESIOLOGY CLASSIFICATION SYSTEM

For the purpose of providing appropriate anesthesia, a classification of the patient's physical status was adapted by the American Society of Anesthesiology (ASA) in 1963,[9] and is used to determine the risk factors based on the current health status of the patient. Included in this evaluation are the presence of coexisting diseases and the type of surgery (emergency or elective) to be performed.

As part of the preoperative evaluation, the anesthesia practitioner will place the patient into one of the following classifications, according to the physiologic description of the patient.

	No	Yes	AIRWAY ASSESSMENT:	PERTINENT LABORATORY:
Have you had or still have:				$H/_H$ Plat
High Blood Pressure			Neck:	
M.I. Date:			Teeth Condition:	SMA
Chest Pain, Angina:			Natural	ECG
Murmur:			Dentures	CXR
Arrhythmia:			Bridge	Others:
Asthma:			Caps	
Bronchitis:			Risks Explained:	
C.O.P.D./Emphysema:				
Recent Cold:			MEDICATIONS:	
Rhinitis/Postnasal Drip:				
Back/Disc Disease:				
Paresthesia/Pain Down Legs:				
Spine Deformity:				
Seizures:				
C.V.A.:			ASA NPO at: ANESTHETIC PLAN	
T.I.A.:			COMMENTS:	
Diabetes:				
Bleeding Problems:				
Sickle Cell Disease/Trait:				
Obstetrical Pregnant				
Other Problems:				
Renal System:				
Jaundice. Hepatitis				
Other:				

Date of Surgery: _____ Procedure: _____ O.R. No.: _____
Allergies: _____ Age: Wt.: Ht.: Race: Language: _____
Previous Anesthesia: No/Yes Type _____ Problems: _____

SMOKES: No Yes
ALCOHOL: Heavy / Social / None
DRUGS: No Yes

PREANESTHESIA MEDICATION:

DATE: _____ TIME: _____

Signature _____

Fig. 6-1. Preoperative evaluation, record (Adapted from Broward General Medical Center, Department of Anesthesia, Ft. Lauderdale, FL)

Classification: Class 1
Description:
The patient has no organic, physiologic, biochemical, or psychiatric disturbances. The pathologic process for which the operation is to be performed is localized and does not entail a systematic disturbance.
Examples include, but are not limited to:
hernia repairs, uterine fibroids, dysmenorrhea

Classification: Class 2
Description:
Mild-to-moderate systemic disturbance caused either by the condition to be treated surgically or by another pathophysiologic process. The extremes of age (neonate or adult between 80 and 90 years old) may be added to this classification, even though no discernible systemic disease is present. Extreme obesity and chronic bronchitis may be included in this category.
Examples include, but are not limited to:
nonlimiting or slightly limiting organic heart disease, mild diabetes, essential hypertension, anemia.

Classification: Class 3
Description:
Severe systemic disturbance/disease from whatever cause even though it may not be possible to define the degree or disability with finality.

GENERAL MEDICAL CENTER

CONSENT FOR ANESTHESIA

Patient's Name: _____   Date: _____

I am to have an operation soon and request that an anesthetic be administered for the operation. I understand that there are various forms of anesthesia that can be used, such as general anestheisa (intravenous or inhalation agent), spinal anesthesia (such as saddle block), nerve block anesthesia, local anesthesia, or a combination of the above. The choice and any medically acceptable alternatives have been discussed with me by the anesthesia practitioner. I hereby consent to the administration of anesthesia by the following method(s):

_____

Since I realize that it is possible that, for whatever reason, the above type of anesthesia might not be effective for me, I hereby also consent to alternative means of anesthesia as may be determined by the anesthesia practitioner under the circumstances of my condition and situation.

I understand that although modern anesthesia is relatively safe and uneventful, unexpected reactions and complications may occur and these can vary between patients whose medical conditions appear otherwise similar. I realize that my complete medical history, particularly as to allergic reactions in the past, is extremely significant and I have fully advised the anesthesia practitioner of everything that I know in this regard.

Risks and hazards which are recognized by anesthesia practitioners as substantial and which can occur regardless of the experience, care and skill of the anesthesia practitioner include, but are not limited to, broken teeth, allergic reactions, pneumonia, phlebitis (inflammation and infection of the veins), nerve injury or paralysis, damage to or failure of the heart, liver, kidneys, and/or the brain, and death. If I am pregnant, the above risks may also affect the fetus. In most cases these risks and hazards are rare. I realize that the anesthesia practitioner will do the best to protect me from such risks and hazards, but no guarantee as to the outcome of any anesthtic can be made.

I understand that the anesthesia practitioners in the hospital practice as a group or as individuals, that because of a variety of circumstances which can occur in any operating room, that another anesthesiologist or certified registered nurse anesthetist under the supervision of an anesthesiologist, may actually administer all or part of my anesthetic. I accept these circumstances without reservation.

I have fully read this Consent and I understand and agree with all its terms. I have been able to discuss the proposed anesthesia with the anesthsia practitioner and any questions that I have had have been answered to my satisfaction.

_____   _____
            Witness to Patient Signature Only   Patient or Guardian

                                                _____
                                                          Interviewing Anesthesia Practitioner

Fig. 6-2. Anesthesia consent form (Adapted from Broward General Medical Center, Department of Anesthesia, Ft. Lauderdale, FL, 1993)

Examples include, but are not limited to:
severely limiting organic heart disease, severe diabetes with vascular complications, moderate to severe pulmonary insufficiency, angina or old myocardial infarction (MI).

Classification: Class 4
Description:
Severe systemic disorders that are already life-threatening, not always correctable by surgery or operation planned.

Examples include, but are not limited to:
marked signs of cardiac insufficiency, persistent (unstable) angina, active myocarditis, advanced pulmonary, hepatic, renal, or endocrine insufficiency.

Classification: Class 5
Description:
The moribund patient who has little chance of survival but is submitted to surgery in desperation. The patient may require surgery as a resuscitative measure, with little or no anesthesia.

Examples include, but are not limited to:

leaking or ruptured abdominal aortic aneurysm, cerebral trauma with increasing intracranial pressure, comatose patient requiring a tracheostomy, massive pulmonary embolism.

Classification: Class 6 (1990)
Description:

A patient declared legally dead according to state statutes and definition, whose organs are being removed for donor preparation.

Status: E (Emergency)
Description:

Any patient in one of the classes previously listed who is operated on as an emergency. The letter *E* is placed beside the numerical class, reflecting that this patient is considered a poor risk and/or is in poor physical condition, with minimal evaluation performed owing to the acuity of the situation (for example: 1E; 2E).

Perioperative Nursing Implications

As part of the perioperative nursing assessment, this classification system can serve as a guide to assist the nurse in anticipating unusual events that may occur as a direct result of anesthesia and/or the surgical procedure.

By reviewing the preoperative evaluation, and by becoming familiar with the classification system, the perioperative nurse and the surgical team can be prepared to use greater safeguards to care effectively for the patient undergoing surgery.

Self-assessment Exercise 8

Direction: Complete the following exercises. The answers are given at the end of this module.

1. _____ was the first inhalation agent associated with general anesthesia.

2. The first *local* anesthetic agent, which came from the coca leaf, was called _____.

3. List the four major objectives of anesthesia.

4. Describe the purpose of the preoperative anesthesia evaluation.

5. According to the ASA Classification System, a healthy 7-year-old child with acute appendicitis would be considered a __. (Class number)

Preoperative Medications

In addition to the preoperative assessment and evaluation, ordering preoperative medications is an essential component of this phase.

Preoperative medications are given to (1) reduce preoperative anxiety, (2) decrease secretions in the mouth and respiratory tract, (3) reduce reflux irritability, (4) relieve pain, and (5) lower the body's metabolism so that less anesthetic agent is required.

Selection of Preoperative Medications

The selection of preoperative medications is made by the anesthesia practitioner, based on the preoperative assessment of the patient, including the patient's physical and emotional status, age, weight, past medical history (including medication history), and demands of the proposed surgical procedure.

When choosing a preoperative medication, the anesthesia practitioner tries to avoid causing disturbances in the cardiorespiratory system, while providing both physical and emotional support and comfort.

Pharmacologic Agents and Physiologic Effects

Preoperative medications are usually derived from five categories, depending on the physical and psychological needs of the patient, and may include:

1. *Sedative-hypnotics* to promote relaxation and rest, and to stabilize the blood pressure and pulse (used less frequently today than several years ago)
2. *Anticholinergics* to decrease secretions in the mouth and tracheobronchial system
3. *Narcotics* to promote relaxation, enhance the effect of the anesthetics, and to control pain
4. *Antianxiety* to produce relaxation and reduce anxiety
5. *Antiemetics* to inhibit nausea and vomiting

The following pages describe some of the more commonly used preoperative medications, their desired effects, and possible adverse patient responses.

COMMON PREOPERATIVE MEDICATIONS

Sedative-Hypnotics
Medication: pentobarbital sodium (Nembutal)
Desired Effects: reduces anxiety and promotes sleep
Adverse Effects: may cause confusion in the elderly; no analgesia actions

Anticholinergics
Medication: atropine sulfate (Atropine)
Desired Effects: decreases secretions; helps prevent laryngospasms; prevents anesthesia-induced bradycardia
Adverse Effects: excessive dry mouth; tachycardia; blurred vision; restlessness; confusion; possible urinary retention, temperature elevations
Medication: glycopyrrolate (Robinul)
Desired Effects: Same as atropine (secretions decrease rapidly)—five to six times more potent than atropine sulfate
Adverse Effects: same as atropine sulfate; does not cross the blood–brain barrier, so CNS effects are usually absent; long-lasting dry mouth (good for outpatient surgery)
Medication: scopolamine (Hyoscine)
Desired Effects: same as atropine sulfate with additional amnesic effect
Adverse Effects: same as atropine sulfate can produce CNS depression and bradycardia. More profound CNS effects are due to ease of agent crossing blood–brain barrier—more likelihood of confusion, disorientation.

Narcotics
Medication: meperidine hydrochloride, synthetic (Demerol)
Desired Effects: analgesia with sedation and mild euphoria; rapid onset with short duration
Adverse Effects: CNS disturbances; potent myocardial depressant; hypotension; syncope; bradycardia; nausea/vomiting; pupillary constriction
Medication: Morphine sulfate (Generic)
Desired Effects: analgesia with sedation (peak analgesia within 50 to 90 minutes with intramuscular [IM] pain management up to 4 hours)
Adverse Effects: CNS disturbances; bradycardia; orthostatic hypotension; syncope; gastrointestinal (GI) disturbances
Medication: fentanyl citrate (Sublimaze)

Desired Effects: Same as morphine sulfate, but action is faster and less prolonged
Adverse Effects: 75 to 125 times more potent than morphine sulfate; if given rapid IV push, it can produce "frozen chest," circulatory depression, and cardiac arrest. (When given with other analgesics or CNS depressants on board, use ¼ to ½ usual dose.)
NOTE:
Medication: fentanyl citrate and droperidol (Innovar)
Desired Effects: General calmness with euphoria; analgesia (fentanyl); antiemetic/tranquilizer (droperidol)
Adverse Effects: Respiratory depression; hypotension; muscle rigidity; occasional dysphoria (outer tranquility with inner anxiety)

Antianxiety/antiemetics
Medication: hydroxyzine (Vistaril)
Desired Effects: reduces anxiety, with antiemetic property; mild skeletal muscle effect
Adverse Effects: drowsiness; dry mouth; headache; dizziness (can only be given PO or IM)
Medication: droperidol (Inapsine)
Desired Effects: reduces anxiety with antiemetic effects
Adverse Effects: orthostatic hypotension; tachycardia; drowsiness; mental depression; severe depression of blood pressure following administration of parenteral analgesics; and, despite the appearance of tranquility, calmness with severe inner irritability can occur (very long acting)
Medication: diazepam (Valium)
Desired Effects: provides sedation and amnesia in 40 to 50 percent of patients; reduces anxiety and apprehension
Adverse Effects: respiratory depression; excessive drowsiness (long-acting effect postinjection can last up to 2 to 4 hours, with half-life remaining in the system 3 to 8 days); no analgesic effect; mild to moderate amnesia
Medication: midazolam hydrochloride (Versed)
Desired Effects: short-acting depressant with clinical action similar to diazepam with fewer adverse effects; potent amnesiac
Adverse Effects: three times more potent than diazepam; potent respiratory depressant; laryngospasm; cardiac changes (ventricular)

Antiemetics
Medication: metoclopramide (Reglan)
Desired Effects: increases gastric motility with increase in lower esophageal sphincter tone; helps prevent nausea and vomiting
Adverse Effects: restlessness; headache; dizziness; sedation (use cautiously with anticholinergics and narcotics—can antagonize effects of these agents)

Nursing Implications: Preoperative Medications

Most patients do not understand the purpose of the preoperative medication and tend to think that the shot they receive should "put them out"; so they arrive in the preoperative holding area anxious because they are still awake, thinking the medication is not working properly. With proper education concerning the purpose of the medication, the patient will arrive relaxed, which will assist in the administration of the actual anesthetic agents and adjunctive agents used during surgery. Advise patient that medication may be given before leaving for the preoperative holding area or may be given while in the surgical holding area.

If a preoperative oral or IM injection is not given in the unit following the initiation of an IV line, the medication may be given via IV push while the patient is in the holding area, depending on the patient's immediate needs.

In addition, an extremely effective method that nurses can use to reduce anxiety is an attitude of caring. A nurse who understands the patient's feelings, and provides both physiologic and emotional support during the preoperative period can make all the difference in the world.

When planning nursing intervention for the surgical patient, the responses to the preoperative medication should be considered and the patient continually monitored for possible adverse side effects while waiting to be transported to the procedure room.

Signs and symptoms of adverse reactions could include vomiting, hypotension, cardiac changes, and changes in sensorium to a greater degree than expected. All responses should be reported immediately to the anesthesia practitioner for intervention and correction as necessary, with corresponding documentation of the events.

Self-assessment Exercise 9

Directions: Complete the following exercises. The answers are given at the end of this module.

1. _____ and _____ are examples of anticholinergic agents.
2. List three major reasons for prescribing preoperative medications.

3. The single most important cause of preoperative anxiety in the otherwise well-balanced patient is the _____.
4. Using your answer to No. 3, identify three supportive nursing interventions that may be helpful in reducing patient anxiety during the preoperative period.

INTRAOPERATIVE PHASE

The focus of the intraoperative phase is to produce anesthesia, which requires the use of drugs and techniques that abolish the sensations of pain, achieve adequate muscle relaxation, produce amnesia, and control the autonomic nervous system. These agents include

- Inhalation agents—gases or volatile liquids that produce general anesthesia
- Intravenous agents—agents that produce anesthesia in large doses through sedative–hypnotic–analgesic actions
- Local anesthetics—agents that block nerve conduction in a specific area

Anesthesia Methods and Techniques

Anesthesia methods fall into two general categories: *general* and *regional*.[10]

General anesthesia is described as a state of analgesia and complete loss of consciousness as a direct result of anesthesia agents, with conservation of the regulative (autonomic nervous system [ANS]) functions. *Regional anesthesia* is described as causing insensibility to pain owing to the interruption of sensory nerve conduction via a nerve block, field block, or by topical application to skin or mucous membranes.

General Anesthesia

There are two methods used, either alone or together, to produce general anesthesia. These are *inhalation,* in which gases are administered into the systemic circulation through the alveolar membranes of the lungs, with diffusion to the pulmonary circulation and finally to the brain; and *intravenous,* in which agents are adminis-

tered as a bolus or continuous drip infusion directly into the systemic circulation. The IV technique can be used primarily as an induction agent, for relaxation, analgesia, and/or sleep.

Balanced Anesthesia

Balanced anesthesia is a term used to describe anesthesia methods that combine a muscle relaxant, a hypnotic-sedative, a narcotic, and inhalation agent, which when combined produce a state similar to that produced by a general anesthetic agent.

Phases of General Anesthesia and Nursing Activities

General anesthesia is accomplished in phases, and each phase requires specific nursing activities to successfully facilitate effective, safe anesthesia.

Phase 1: Preinduction Phase

Scope: Begins when the patient enters the induction room or the procedure room and is placed on the operating table, and ends before the induction of anesthesia.

Nursing Activities: Nursing actions revolve around the safety and comfort of the patient, and include proper positioning of the patient on the table, padding of the pressure points, and applying safety straps as needed. The perioperative nurse must be available to assist anesthesia personnel and to provide emotional support to the patient during the preliminary preparations. Additionally, the nurse must be sure that the anesthesia practitioner's suction is readily available and in proper working condition before the start of this phase. Other perioperative assistance will be dictated by procedures at individual hospital or operative centers.

Phase 2: Induction/Intubation

Scope: Begins with the introduction of anesthetic agents, and ends with securing the airway, which may include intubation of the trachea.

Nursing Activities: This phase is considered to be the most dangerous for the patient; therefore, all precautions must be taken to ensure the patient's safety.

The atmosphere must be calm and quiet; devoid of any extraneous noise that could result in uncontrolled patient movement or reflexes during the induction period. The perioperative nurse should remain beside the patient, assisting anesthesia personnel with the induction/intubation procedure, including the performance of the Sellick maneuver (cricoid pressure) as needed, while all other activities and movement have been stopped.

It is only after successful intubation and stabilization, and with permission of anesthesia personnel, that the patient can be transferred to the procedure room or repositioned as necessary and the surgical prep can be performed. (If a radio is on in the procedure room, the volume should be turned down as hearing is acute during this phase.)

NOTE: At no time during the induction phase should the circulating nurse leave the room, since she or he may be the only person available to assist anesthesia personnel should a complication arise.

Phase 3: Maintenance

Scope: Begins when stabilization has been accomplished and ends prior to the start of the reversal process, toward the end of the surgical procedure.

Nursing Activities: Perioperative nursing activities may differ in each institution during this phase, but usually consist of helping monitor urinary output and blood loss; arranging for various lab tests as requested; and obtaining additional drugs, solutions, and/or supplies. By remaining alert to any unforeseen events, and assisting anesthesia personnel during the procedure as necessary, the team will be able to maintain a safe, therapeutic environment.

It is important to remember that you, as the circulating nurse, are the only nonscrubbed member of the team who can assist anesthesia personnel if an emergent situation arises, so if you must leave the room to get urgent supplies, notify anesthesia personnel you are leaving, and return as quickly as possible.

Never leave the room for an extended period of time without another nurse to replace you while you are gone.

Phase 4: Reversal/Extubation

Scope: Begins somewhat before the closure of the operative wound and ends immediately before transporting the patient to the postanesthesia care unit or designated postanesthesia area.

Nursing Activities: As with Phase 2, the extubation phase is a dangerous time for the patient, since physiologic changes could trigger unexpected events, such as laryngospasm, vomiting, slow spontaneous respirations, or uncontrolled reflex movement.

Some patients can emerge from anesthesia with wild, uncontrolled movements that could cause harm if not handled gently, while others emerge smoothly, without difficulty. The perioperative nurse must constantly be aware of the patient's status and be prepared to assist anesthesia personnel to prevent unnecessary injury.

If special equipment is needed during the immediate postanesthesia period, arrangements should be made by the perioperative nurse before transport, and the recovery room nurses alerted to these special needs.

Additionally, the perioperative nurse should *always* accompany the patient with anesthesia personnel to the postanesthesia care unit (PACU), since the perioperative nursing role has not ended until the patient is transferred to another professional nurse and a report of nursing activities during the intraoperative phase has been given to the nurse who will continue the patient's postoperative care.

Stages of Anesthesia: Classic Characteristics and Nursing Implications

According to Arthur E. Guedel (1920),[11] **unpremedicated inhalation** anesthesia has four classic stages, which can be seen with ether. Although each stage is not seen today because of the use of ancillary intravenous agents, the responses to each stage may still be present, though not as obvious as in earlier practice. As a historical teaching aid, the classic stages of anesthesia will be reviewed (Fig. 6-3).

Stage I: Relaxation (Amnesia/Analgesia)

Scope: From the beginning of anesthesia to the loss of consciousness. Pain sensation is not completely lost, but reaction to pain has been altered.

Patient Reaction/Biologic Response:

- feelings of drowsiness and dizziness
- hearing becomes exaggerated
- may appear inebriated
- pain sensation is decreased

Nursing Implications:

1. Close the OR doors to reduce extraneous noises.
2. Confirm proper positioning, including all safety factors.

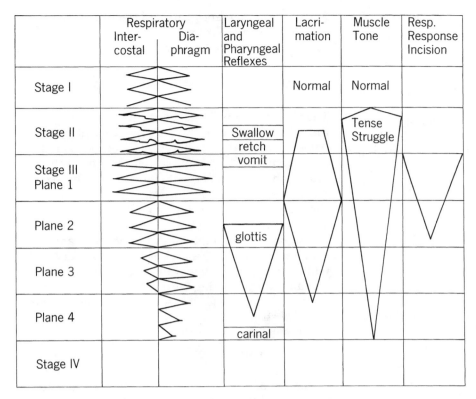

| | Respiratory | | Laryngeal and Pharyngeal Reflexes | Lacri-mation | Muscle Tone | Resp. Response Incision |
	Inter-costal	Dia-phragm				
Stage I				Normal	Normal	
Stage II			Swallow retch vomit		Tense Struggle	
Stage III Plane 1						
Plane 2			glottis			
Plane 3						
Plane 4			carinal			
Stage IV						

Fig. 6-3. Classic stages of general anesthesia (Adapted from Gillespie, NA. *Anesth Analg* 22: 275, 1943. Cited in Dripps, RD, Eckenhoff, JE, and Vandam, LD. *Introduction to Anesthesia.* [6th ed.] Philadelphia: WB Saunders, 1987. P. 233.)

3. Verify anesthesia suction is available and working correctly.
4. Reduce talking, unnecessary movement, and noise to only what is absolutely necessary.
5. Remain at the head of the OR table; assist the anesthesia clinician, and provide the patient with emotional support.

Stage II: Delirium/Excitement
Scope: From the loss of consciousness to the onset of respiratory depression and loss of lid reflexes.

Patient Reaction/Biologic Response:

- irregular respirations
- loss of consciousness
- loss of lid reflexes
- increased muscle tone and involuntary motor response
- sensitive to external stimuli (can be startled)

Considered an extremely dangerous stage that could result in laryngospasms, vomiting, aspiration, arrhythmias, and myoclonic movement.
NOTE: Short-acting sedative-hypnotics (barbiturates,

ketamine, versed, narcotics, propofol) reduce time related to Stages I and II.

Nursing Implications:

1. Avoid any type of extraneous stimulation.
2. Lightly restrain extremities to avoid injury.
3. Remain at the head of the table to assist anesthesia personnel as needed (e.g., cricoid pressure, etc.).
4. Remain alert for any emergency situations that could arise.

Stage III: Surgical Anesthesia
Scope: From the regular pattern of respirations to the total paralysis of intercostal muscles and cessation of voluntary ventilation.

This stage can be further divided into four planes ranging from light anesthesia through excessively deep anesthesia.

Plane 1: Light Anesthesia

- loss of lid reflexes; pupils are smaller
- patterns of normal breathing visible
- vomiting/gag reflex gradually disappearing

- respiratory rate and depth may increase
- eye movement may still be present

Plane 2: Medium Anesthesia (surgery could begin)

- ventilations are more regular, but tidal volume has decreased
- loss of eye movement; pupils in midline, concentrically fixed
- vocal cord reflex (which could result in laryngospasms) begins to disappear
- decreased muscle tone as anesthesia deepens

Plane 3: Deep Surgical Anesthesia

- begins with decreased intercostal muscle movement
- only diaphragmatic activity remains
- increased muscle relaxation

NOTE: These stages will be seen in reverse order during the emergence or reversal stage.
Plane 4: Deeper Anesthesia

- begins with intercostal paralysis and progresses to complete cessation of spontaneous ventilation
- if allowed to go deeper, circulatory system failure is imminent
- pupils no longer react to light

Nursing Implications:

1. Be available to assist anesthesia personnel as necessary.
2. Validate with anesthesia appropriate time to reposition and prep.
3. Recheck patient positioning and reaffirm safety precautions.

Stage IV: Danger
Scope: From the time of cessation of ventilation to failure of the circulation, caused by high levels of anesthesia in the CNS. Accidentally reached; not desirable.
Patient Reaction/Biologic Response:

- medullary paralysis; cardiac/respiratory collapse
- pupils fixed and dilated
- pulse rapid and thready
- ventilation ceases, coma develops
- circulatory and respiratory arrest

Nursing Implications:

1. Be prepared to assist in emergency resuscitation measures (CPR).

2. Obtain emergency cart and defibrillator.
3. Remain in the room at all times.
4. Document all events and therapies as they occur.

Sequence for Inhalation Anesthesia

The patient is usually given oxygen via a mask before the administration of the anesthesia agent. When the patient is relaxed, after the administration of an induction agent and/or a muscle relaxant, the anesthesia practitioner will hyperventilate with oxygen securing the airway, which may include intubation of the trachea. The tube will be attached to the breathing circuit and the maintenance stage begins.

On completion of the surgical procedure, and before extubation, the anesthesia clinician will hyperventilate with 100 percent oxygen, then remove the tube and continue administering the oxygen with the mask until the patient is stable for transport with no signs of ventilatory obstruction.

Inhalation Anesthesia Agents

Inhalation anesthesia agents are categorized into two types: those that are gaseous, and those that are volatile.

Gaseous Agents—Include Cyclopropane and Nitrous Oxide

Cyclopropane, one of the first inhalation agents (no longer in use), is a colorless, sweet-smelling, flammable, explosive gas. It is considered a very potent anesthesia agent, characterized by rapid induction and emergence. Cyclopropane can cause respiratory depression and cardiac arrhythmias owing to its potency and ability to sensitize the myocardium.

Nitrous oxide, on the other hand, is a colorless, odorless, nonexplosive gas that has been referred to as a "carrier of gases."

Nitrous oxide was first discovered by Joseph Priestly in 1772, yet its ability to relieve pain was not recorded until decades later. Nitrous oxide is rarely used alone since it is a weak inhalation agent, but when combined with other agents and oxygen, N_2O serves as a potentiator for other inhalation agents. High-concentration nitrous oxide can produce hypoxia; therefore, caution is always used when administering this agent.

Volatile Agents

Volatile agents are liquids that are easily vaporized and produce anesthesia when inhaled. Volatile agents include ether, trichloroethylene, chloroform, halo-

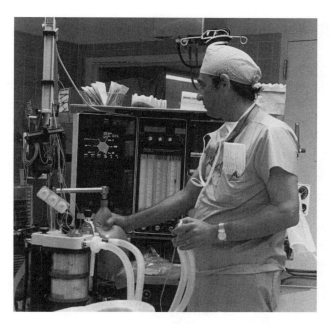

The anesthesia machine is checked by an anesthesia practitioner before use

thane, enflurane, methoxyflurane, isoflurane, and desflurane, the last five of which are halogenated compounds.

All these agents require a special vaporizer for administration. Since some agents (especially ether) are flammable and explosive, and since some cannot be used with carbon dioxide absorbers (trichloroethylene), they are no longer in use in centers other than teaching centers. The last five inhalation agents are used to varying degrees, depending on the medical condition of the patient, as well as other factors.

MONOGRAPH OF INHALATION AGENTS

Pioneer Agents

Trichloroethane (Chloroform)

Trichloroethane is one of the original inhalation agents. It is considered the most potent of all inhalation agents and is very difficult to control.

Trichloroethane is nonflammable and colorless with a somewhat pungent odor and sweet taste. It produces a rapid, yet pleasant induction, but frequently causes cardiac arrhythmias that result in myocardial depression, and causes severe hepatic disorders.

Trichloroethane was used during the Civil War and early surgeries, but because of its potency and difficulty in safe administration, it was eventually replaced by ether.

Ether (diethyl ether)

Ether is another of the original inhalation agents, and is found today only in major teaching hospital labs, to illustrate the "classic stages" of anesthesia. Ether was safe since the range between therapeutic and dangerous doses was large; in addition, it produced profound skeletal muscle relaxation.

Ether, however, has its drawbacks. It is highly explosive and flammable, and has properties that cause long induction and long emergence, with increased nausea and vomiting and irritation to the skin, mucous membranes, lungs, and kidneys.

Because it is inherently safe, ether is still used in some Third World countries, although it has been removed from American hospitals owing to its dangerous explosive properties.

Ether and trichloromethane are considered "pioneer" anesthetic agents, and although they are no longer permitted in ORs today, the eventual discovery of all other inhalation agents developed from early experiments with these substances.

Modern Inhalation Agents

Halothane (Fluothane)

Halothane is one of the first halogenated hydrocarbon compounds developed—producing a rapid, smooth induction. It is nonflammable, nonexplosive, and very potent. The speed of emergence is intermediate; it is therefore used in conjunction with nitrous oxide and muscle relaxants.

Halothane can cause cardiopulmonary depression, and ventricular fibrillation can be seen when it is administered with epinephrine. It seldom causes nausea and vomiting and is nonirritating to mucous membranes. It is an excellent bronchodilator, but patients may be subject to decreased blood pressure owing to depression of the myocardium and peripheral blood vessel dilation.

Halothane is contraindicated in patients with liver disease, since it is suspected of being hepatotoxic.

"Shivering" is common during the recovery phase, due to either vasodilation or neurogenic responses.

Halothane is considered one of the "trigger" agents associated with malignant hyperthermia; because of this, and because it may be hepatotoxic, most anesthesia practitioners avoid using halothane on adults or patients requiring long or multiple procedures. It is important to note, however, that this agent is used extensively for the inhalation induction of children.

Methoxyflurane (Penthrane)

Methoxyflurane is a potent agent that provides a slow induction and emergence with some nausea and vomiting.

Although methoxyflurane has superb analgesic properties and excellent muscle relaxation, and provides good anesthesia in low doses, it is nephrotoxic and may have adverse renal effects, especially when used with certain antibiotics (tetracycline, gentamycin, tobramycin, and kanamycin). CNS depressants, including alcohol, potentiate its effects and prolong postoperative drowsiness and analgesia.

Methoxyflurane is contraindicated in patients with renal or liver disease, and because of this and other factors, it is not widely available in the United States.

Enflurane (Ethrane)

Enflurane, like halothane, is a colorless, nonflammable agent, producing pleasant and rapid induction and emergence.

Enflurane is rapid-acting, and induces good muscle relaxation, and good analgesia with very little nausea and vomiting. However, enflurane depresses respiration and lowers blood pressure proportionally to the amount administered, although with minimal alteration in cardiac rate or rhythm.

Enflurane also produces a moderate blockade to surgical stress related to the release of adrenal hormones.

Enflurane is thought to be free of hepatic or renal toxicity, but is contraindicated in patients with seizures, head injuries, and certain obstetrical conditions.

Since it produces some muscle relaxation, it is often used with intraabdominal surgery. Like halothane, enflurane can produce postoperative shivering.

Isoflurane (Forane)

Isoflurane is a nonflammable, nonexplosive clear liquid.

Although it is an isomer of enflurane (Ethrane), its vapors have a strong odor, which may account for the respiratory irritation it can produce. Isoflurane is a potent respiratory depressant, but it does not produce cardiovascular instability, although it tends to cause mild sinus tachycardia.

Isoflurane provides slow induction due to its respiratory tract irritation and rapid emergence, with a low incidence of nausea or vomiting. Additionally, it does not stimulate excessive secretions, nor has there been evidence of renal or hepatic toxicity, owing to the minimal metabolism of the agent.

Isoflurane is an excellent choice for neurosurgical procedures. It has excellent cardiovascular stability and has no deleterious hepatic, renal or CNS effects.

Postoperatively, emergence is rapid, but shivering may be seen with isoflurane, although to a lesser extent than with ethotoin.

Desflurane (Suprane)

Desflurane is a halogenated ether similar to isoflurane. It is a liquid with an extremely low boiling point and requires a special electronically heated, pressurized vaporizer for delivery of stable, accurate inspired concentration.

This relatively new agent is a good smooth muscle relaxant causing bronchodilatation and decreased arteriolar muscle tone. It may cause an early increase in intracranial pressure, does not sensitize the heart to catecholamines, does not cause coronary artery vasodilation, as does isoflurane, and has a direct muscle-relaxant effect. Very rapid changes in depth of anesthesia are possible due to its low tissue solubility. Elimination is via the lungs, liver, and kidneys.

Sevoflurane (Sevoflurane)

Sevoflurane is also a halogenated ether and is a liquid but, unlike desflurane, does not require a specially heated, pressurized vaporizer for delivery.

This agent is a relatively good muscle relaxant and, similar to Desflurane, causes increased cerebral blood flow and increased intracranial pressure. Very rapid changes in anesthetic levels are possible due to low blood solubility. It is irritating to the bronchial mucosa (although not as much as is Desflurane) and so is seldom used for inhalation induction. It does not cause arrhythmias in the presence of infected Epinephrine. Elimination is via the lungs and liver.

Anesthesia Safety Measures

During the administration of any inhalation agents, a scavenging method for waste anesthetics and carbon dioxide must be used to avoid unnecessary exposure to health-care personnel. A chemical absorber containing granules of the hydroxides of sodium, calcium, or barium absorb moisture and carbon dioxide from the exhaled gases. As the granules become saturated with the carbon dioxide, and the absorbent substance becomes exhausted, the granules change color; therefore, the absorber must be monitored and changed as needed. Excess anesthetic gases are evacuated to the outside atmosphere by scavenging systems.

Additionally, the breathing circuits, masks, endotracheal (or nasotracheal) tubes, and reservoir bags are all disposable, providing a clean circuit for each patient, thus avoiding potential cross-contamination or unwarranted mixtures of inhalation agents.

Intravenous Anesthesia Agents

Intravenous medications are frequently used to supplement the inhalation technique, and thus provide a safe, reversible state of anesthesia.

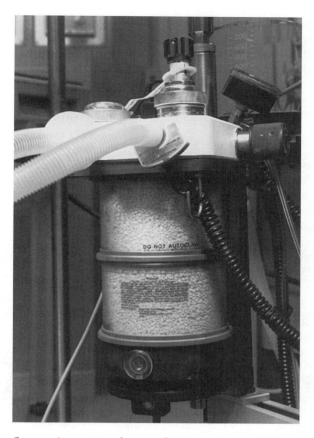

Scavenging system for anesthesia waste materials

Unlike inhalation agents, which can be "blownoff" through ventilation of the lungs with oxygen, intravenous drugs must be metabolized and/or excreted by the kidneys. Their elimination is essentially independent of respiratory function.

Intravenous agents can be administered by bolus dose or by continuous drip infusion, depending on the effect desired.

Three categories of intravenous drugs are associated with general anesthesia:

1. *Barbiturates* and others act directly in the CNS, producing an effect ranging from mild sedation to sleep
2. *Narcotics* render the patient pain-free and, in some cases, produce a euphoric state
3. *Muscle relaxants* provide total relaxation of skeletal muscles, resulting in reduced tissue trauma (this cannot be accomplished by other intravenous agents)

In addition, tranquilizers, neuroleptanalgesics, and phencyclidines are used to supplement the inhalation technique, each producing specific effects not available with other agents.

Some agents, such as narcotics, can be totally reversed (antagonized), while others can be only partially reversed; and this factor can play a part in the choice of intravenous agent to be administered.

MONOGRAPH OF COMMON INTRAVENOUS AGENTS

Barbiturates and Others

Thiopental Sodium—NSP (Pentothal)

Thiopental sodium is an ultra–short-acting barbiturate, usually administered via bolus injection, that produces rapid induction and emergence with decreased emergence delirium. The dosage is based on the kilogram (kg) weight of the patient, and his or her pathophysiologic status and psychological need.

Respiratory and cardiac depression are frequent occurrences, so preparation for ventilator support must be completed before administration. Thiopental sodium must be used with caution in patients with severe cardiac disease, myxedema, and neuromuscular disorders, and is absolutely contraindicated in a rare disorder of metabolism called *porphyria*.

Thiopental sodium is excellent for "rapid-sequence" inductions, when the patient requires emergency surgery, and/or has a full stomach.

There is not an agent currently available that is an antagonist to thiopental sodium; it can produce a "shivering" effect, prolonged somnolence, arrhythmias, laryngospasm, bronchospasms, and severe cardiovascular depression.

Methohexital Sodium (Brevital) and Thiamylal (Surital)

Like thiopental sodium, both methohexital sodium and thiamylal are short-acting barbiturates, administered by bolus injection, with the dose based on the kilogram weight of the patient.

Methohexital sodium is frequently used as an anesthetic agent before electroconvulsive therapy (ECT), oral surgery, gynecologic and urologic examinations, or closed reductions of fractures, whereas thiamylal sodium is mainly used in conjunction with general anesthesia.

Both methohexital sodium and thiamylal can produce side effects similar to thiopental sodium; in addition, they can cause muscular twitching, headache, excessive salivation, and acute allergic reactions. For this reason, methohexital sodium is infrequently used with general anesthesia techniques.

Similar precautions used with thiopental sodium

must be used before the administration of these agents, and, like thiopental sodium, neither is reversible.

Others

Ketamine HCl (Ketalar)

Ketamine is a phencyclidine derivative of use for induction of hypovolemic or hypotensive patients. It has been associated with emergent phenomena, some very pleasant, others very unpleasant. These emergent reactions can be eliminated by the concomitant use of either Valium or Versed injection.

Since this agent produces no pharyngeal relaxation, airway patency is well-maintained, but no oropharyngeal procedures are usually performed. Intra- and postoperative emergent surroundings should be free of loud noises or noisy activity.

Propofol (Diprivan)

Known familiarly as "milk of amnesia" for its anesthetic qualities, and as "dream cream" because of its ability to induce erotic dreams during emergence, propofol is a potent, ultra short-acting agent used both for induction and maintenance. It is particularly appreciated by surgeons because most patients awake with a clear sensorium, unlike those given barbiturates.

If administered rapidly, or undiluted into smaller veins, severe pain may result at the site of injection, so it is usually preceded with IV narcotics and IV lidocaine to decrease awareness and to desensitize the vein.

Propofol has no analgesic properties, and is not approved for use in pregnant women.

Opioid Analgesics

As previously discussed, opioids can be used both as a preoperative medication and as adjunct therapy during local, regional, or general anesthesia.

Commonly used opioids are meperidine HCl, morphine sulfate, fentanyl, alfentanil, sufentanil, and codeine (codeine is discussed in the section on Topical Anesthesia Agents).

The respiratory and cardiovascular depressive effects of opioids are well known, and these agents are most often given by bolus injection. However they could be given via infusion drip, under certain conditions or procedures such as open-heart surgery.

Because all opioid analgesics are derived from basically the same substance or synthetic derivatives, their basic characteristics are very similar:

- produce potent analgesia
- fast-acting, with prolonged analgesic effect
- reversible with a opioid antagonist (naloxone)

- possibility of accompanying nausea and vomiting
- must be administered slowly to avoid severe cardiopulmonary depression
- do not necessarily render unconsciousness

There are, however, some differences that should be mentioned.

Meperidine Hydrochloride (Demerol)

- Reversal agent is naloxone (Narcan)
- Meperidine hydrochloride acts within 10 to 15 minutes of injection, and is therefore slower than the other agents.
- When given IV, meperidine hydrochloride should be diluted and given slowly; it can cause hypotension, bradycardia, and respiratory depression.
- Spasmolytic compared with ms

Morphine Sulfate

- Reversal agent is naloxone (Narcan)
- Is known to cause respiratory depression as a side effect.
- Morphine sulfate has little adverse effect on blood pressure, cardiac rate, or cardiac output; it acts within 5 to 7 minutes of injection and is usually the drug of choice when dealing with cardiac patients due to its cardiovascular stability.
- The pharmacology of morphine sulfate provides a reference base for narcotics.
- Spasmogenic as compared to meperidine hydrochloride

Fentanyl (Sublimaze)

- Fentanyl is 75 to 125 times more potent than morphine sulfate, and more rapid in action (1- to 2-minute onset); therefore, smaller dosages are recommended to achieve the same effect.
- Rapid injection of fentanyl can result in a "frozen chest" syndrome, which can be reversed with a muscle relaxant such as anectine.
- Fentanyl is shorter in duration than morphine sulfate (20–40 minutes), and is therefore an ideal agent for patients undergoing ambulatory surgery.
- Nonanesthesia personnel who administer fentanyl, such as during a local procedure with IV sedation, should refer to hospital policy for administration guidelines, since it can produce cardiorespiratory complications.
- Reversal agent is naloxone (Narcan)

Alfentanil (Alfenta) and Sufentanil (Sufenta)

- Alfentanil and sufentanil are derivatives of fentanyl.

- Both are similar to fentanyl in action, yet differ in potency and duration of action.
- Like fentanyl, both can be used alone for short-duration procedures in bolus dosages, or for procedures lasting over 45 minutes via the continuous infusion method.
- Sufentanil citrate is 5 to 7 times more potent than fentanyl, while alfentanil hydrochloride is one third to one quarter as potent. Sufentanil citrate produces a remarkably stable cardiovascular state. Alfentanil hydrochloride is ultra–short acting and so is used for very short procedures or given by continuous IV infusion for slightly longer procedures.
- When these agents are administered, ventilatory maintenance should be constantly available; therefore, these modern synthetic narcotics can be administered only by qualified anesthesia personnel familiar with artificial ventilation and maintenance techniques.
- Reversal agent is naloxone (Narcan)

Tranquilizers

Valium, Versed, and Inapsine were previously mentioned as preoperative agents, but they too can be used as adjunct agents for general, regional, or local anesthesia.

Droperidol (Inapsine)

- Droperidol potentiates both narcotics and barbiturates, with an onset of 10 minutes and a duration of 2 to 4 hours, to a maximum of 12 hours depending on the dosage and patient reaction.
- It possesses strong antiemetic and antipsychotic properties, and can be mixed with fentanyl (Innovar) or given separately with other narcotics. Droperidol can produce hypotension and tachycardia.

Diazepam (Valium)

- Diazepam can produce antegrade amnesia in 40 to 50 percent of patients, with good relaxation effects that last 8 to 12 hours after injection.
- Diazepam cannot be *mixed* with other agents, but can be given at the same time. Ventilation must be monitored, since it is a potent respiratory depressant.
- Reversal agent is flumazenil (Romazicon)

Midazolam Hydrochloride (Versed)

- Midazolam hydrochloride is one of the newer of the tranquilizers. It has a minimal residual effect, yet in smaller doses provides potent antegrade amnesia in 70 to 80 percent of patients, without the adverse side effects of diazepam. It is three times more potent than diazepam.
- Midazolam hydrochloride is water soluble; therefore, it is easily diluted in the circulation, metabolized, and excreted.
- Reversal agent is flumazenil (Romazicon)

Muscle Relaxants (Anesthesia Adjuncts)

Neuromuscular relaxants, as they are often called, are used to provide muscle relaxation during surgery and/or to facilitate the passage of an endotracheal tube.

These agents work on the striated muscles of the body by interfering with acetylcholine binding at the motor-end plate where the nerve fiber connects with the muscle fiber.

Although they have excellent therapeutic properties, special problems do exist with these agents:

- Mycin interaction (neomycin, streptomycin) tends to prolong the action of neuromuscular blocking agents
- Hypothermic states increase the duration of action
- Bradycardia due to neostigmine/atropine reversal techniques is not uncommon
- Depolarizing agents cannot be lessened (reversed); therefore, they must be used cautiously

Muscle relaxants are subdivided into two groups: depolarizing and nondepolarizing, based on their specific actions and properties.

Depolarizing Muscle Relaxants

Depolarizing muscle relaxants mimic acetylcholine by binding with the motor-end plate receptors to cause prolonged depolarization. Thus, the muscle remains relaxed, and repolarization is very slow. The onset of action is rapid (within 1 minute), with a short duration (3 to 5 minutes).

Depolarizing muscle relaxants can be very useful in the treatment of profound laryngospasm; in reversing frozen chest syndrome, or assisting ventilatory management with insertion of an endotracheal tube, both inside and outside the surgical area.

Succinylcholine (Anectine or Quelicin) is a rapid-acting agent (within 1 minute) with a short duration of action (3 to 10 minutes) depending on the amount given. It is frequently administered before intubation, and can be given either by bolus injection or continuous drip infusion when longer periods of muscle relaxation are required.

Succinylcholine is rapidly metabolized, and is the drug of choice to reverse "frozen chest syndrome," which can occur if fentanyl is given too quickly.

The disadvantages of succinylcholine include bradycardia, a transient rise in intraocular pressure, and increased intragastric pressure. It can also cause muscle fasciculations, and postoperative myalgia. Succinylcholine requires refrigeration.

Succinylcholine is contraindicated in recent CVAs, crush injuries, patients with recent burns, muscle trauma, or neuromuscular disorders, and is thought to be the major IV triggering agent for malignant hyperthermia, *especially* when used with halothane.

NOTE: Since succinylcholine is colorless and clear, the IV solution should be colored to differentiate it from a standard IV, thus avoiding accidental administration during a procedure. (Use several drops of indigo carmine or methylene blue.)

Nondepolarizing Muscle Relaxants

These agents, unlike the depolarizing agents, occupy acetylcholine receptor sites and block the depolarizing action of acetylcholine at the neuromuscular junction. However, they do not cause depolarization, and are therefore referred to as *competitive* neuromuscular blocking agents.

They have a slower onset of action than depolarizing agents, and a significantly longer duration (20–60 minutes). These agents are administered via bolus or continuous IV infusion, and can be reversed by neostigmine, physostigmine, pyridostigmine, or edrophonium by allowing the acetylcholine to accumulate at the neuromuscular junction. (Atropine or glycopyrolate are used to decrease vagal stimulation before reversal.)

Examples include tubocurarine, pancuronium bromide, gallamine triethiodide, vercuronium bromide, and atracurium besylate.

Curare (d-Tubocurarine; tubocurarine; dTc) Curare is the oldest of the muscle relaxants, discovered originally by the South American Indians, who used a similar compound at the end of their arrows when hunting for food to paralyze their catch prior to the kill.

The onset time is 3 to 5 minutes, with its peak action occurring within 30 minutes and its duration lasting up to 60 minutes.

Curare, when given too rapidly, frequently causes histamine release, with symptoms of tachycardia, hypotension, and bronchospasm, leading to cardiac arrhythmias.

Curare is potentiated by several anesthetic agents, including fluothane, methoxyflurane, and enflurane, and by some antibiotics, and is not widely used in today's anesthesia practice.

Curare is contraindicated in patients with crush injuries or fresh spinal cord injuries.

Reversal agents include neostigmine, pyridostigmine (Regonol), or edrophonium (Tensilon).

Pancuronium Bromide (Pavulon) Pancuronium bromide is longer acting than curare, and is approximately 5 times as potent. Pancuronium bromide is administered by bolus injection or continuous infusion.

Pavulon can increase heart rate and arterial pressure, and is therefore not recommended for patients with cardiac or hypertensive disorders. Additionally, pancuronium bromide can cause residual muscle weakness, and should be used cautiously in elderly or debilitated patients and in the presence of renal or hepatic impairment or neuromuscular disorders. Pancuronium bromide is excellent for procedures of long duration.

Reversal agents include neostigmine, pyridostigmine, and edrophonium.

Gallamine Triethiodide (Flaxedil) Gallamine triethiodide has a slightly shorter duration of action than the other muscle relaxants, and is synthetically produced. It is less potent than dTc (one fifth) and its duration is 25 percent shorter.

Gallamine triethiodide can frequently affect the vagus nerve causing tachycardia and slight hypotension, but does not produce bronchospasms.

Gallamine triethiodide is contraindicated in patients with hypersensitivity to iodides or impaired renal function and patients in shock. Gallamine triethiodide should be used with caution in elderly and debilitated patients. Additionally, electrolyte imbalance can potentiate neuromuscular effects.

Gallamine triethiodide needs to be protected from light, and only fresh solutions should be used. It should *not* be mixed with meperidine HCl, and should be given slowly (over 30–90 seconds) as with all nondepolarizing relaxants that are histamine releasers. It is rarely used in today's anesthesia practice.

Vecuronium Bromide (Norcuron) Vecuronium bromide is an intermediate duration muscle relaxant, about one third more potent than pancuronium bromide, with a shorter neuromuscular blocking effect.

There are no known contraindications, but prolonged recovery has been seen in patients with hepatic disease and conditions associated with acute circulatory disorders.

Vecuronium bromide must be reconstituted and protected from light. After reconstitution, the drug should be refrigerated; it should be used within 8 hours, or discarded.

Reversal agents include pyridostigmine and neostigmine.

Atracurium Besylate (Tracrium) One of the newer muscle relaxants, atracurium besylate has a faster recovery time (8–10 minutes for complete reversal). Rapid administration or overdosage of atracurium besylate can produce a histamine-like reaction, which can cause flushing; hypotension; bradycardia; tachycardia; and vasodilation when administered too fast.

Atracurium besylate requires refrigeration, and fresh solution should be used each time the agent is administered.

Atracurium besylate is unique in one way: it is broken down (physically) and spontaneously as long as the patient maintains normal temperature and pH (Hofmann elimination). Therefore it is useful in the presence of liver and/or kidney disease.

Reversal agents include neostigmine and physostigmine.

Safety Considerations

The safe use of neuromuscular blocking agents requires the establishment of an effective airway, either by oral airway and mask, or by endotracheal intubation, along with controlled, monitored ventilation.

For anesthesia to be safe, the anesthesia practitioner/CRNA must carefully monitor the patient's physiologic status and be prepared to correct any adverse effects caused by the agent(s) being used. Muscle relaxation can be evaluated by using a nerve stimulator placed between the ulnar nerve at the elbow or wrist, which can determine the presence or absence of contractions or diminished strength of the hand muscles.

In addition to evaluating the muscle relaxation, the saturation of oxygen within the red blood cells can be monitored with a pulse oximeter, and because of its accuracy, is now considered the standard of care for all patients receiving anesthesia or IV sedation not only in surgery but in any area where the patient's physiologic status has been compromised.

COMPLICATIONS OF GENERAL ANESTHESIA

The most common complications of general anesthesia that may lead to severe disability or death are aspiration pneumonitis, failure to ventilate adequately, and malignant hyperthermia.

Malignant hyperthermia syndrome (MHS) has been described as a complication that can occur in one out of 15,000 children and one out of 50,000 adults, without warning or preexisting symptoms.

First identified in 1960, MHS is a potentially fatal hypermetabolic, genetically transmitted syndrome. It may also be induced by currently used inhalation agents, particularly halothane, and can be triggered by injection of the depolarizing muscle relaxant succinylcholine. The crisis, however, is not limited to the surgical setting exclusively, nor to the administration of an-

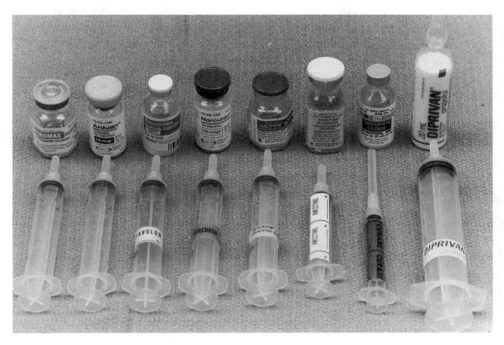

Common IV agents

esthesia agents. It has been seen occasionally in the emergency department following severe trauma or shock producing elevated stress levels.

Etiologic Considerations

Malignant hyperthermia syndrome is a dominantly inherited trait, but it remains dormant until one of the triggering agents or circumstances activates the self-propagating crisis. It can be seen in young men with some types of muscle deformity or abnormality, and is most often associated with circumstances producing anxiety, stress, or trauma or in persons who pursue strenuous exercises on a routine basis. Malignant hyperthermia syndrome is also reported to be higher in children with strabismus. Patients with occult myopathies of any type, and not necessarily related to malignant hyperthermia, or to the use of succinylcholine, may develop these potentially and rapidly disastrous anesthetic events.[12]

Physiologically, the patient apparently has a defect in the reticuloendothelial system of the muscle cell, allowing the anesthetic to trigger a sudden rise of calcium within the muscle cell. This increased calcium then sets off a series of biochemical reactions that lead to an increased metabolic rate, transforming the energy of the contracted muscle into heat (*hyperthermia*).

Malignant hyperthermia syndrome, if untreated or not treated fast enough, has a 50 to 80 percent mortality rate, but this has improved through education about immediate treatment and the ability to prescreen (with a muscle biopsy) individuals with familial histories or previous complications with anesthesia.

Signs and Symptoms

The most consistent early symptom is tachycardia, usually sudden and unexplained, with a sudden increase in end-tidal carbon dioxide, followed by tachypnea, and occasionally, even if the patient is partially paralyzed, spontaneous respirations.

Other signs include unstable blood pressure; arrhythmias; dark blood at the surgical field; cyanosis and mottling of the skin; profuse sweating; fasciculations and/or rigidity; metabolic/respiratory acidosis; elevation of serum potassium and creatine phosphokinase, and a sudden rise in temperature (1°F every 15 minutes) to as high as 108°F or more.

Emergency Treatment

Each institution should have its own written protocol for treating a malignant hyperthermia crisis, which should include the following actions:

1. Stop the surgery and anesthesia immediately.
2. Change the anesthesia breathing circuits, and hyperventilate with 100 percent oxygen.
3. Administer dantrolene sodium (Dantrium) IV, starting with 1 mg/kg up to a maximum cumulative dose of 10 mg/kg via rapid infusion. If arrhythmias are present, follow standard protocol.

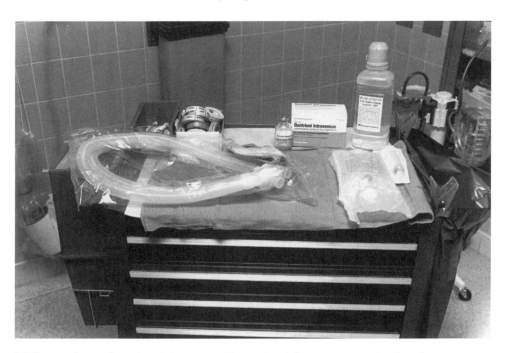

Malignant hyperthermia crisis cart—self-contained for prompt retrieval and usage

4. Initiate cooling:
    - Iced saline solution (not Ringer's lactate) IV
    - Surface cooling via hypothermia blanket or ice packs or immersion in an ice bath
    - If necessary, extracorporeal perfusion (femoral to femoral) may be needed to reduce fever, then warm until normothermia is regained.
    - Gastric or rectal lavage
5. Monitor all hemodynamic indicators: urinary output, arterial pressure, central venous pressure and arterial blood gas readings. Maintain urinary output of at least 2 mL/kg per hour with mannitol and/or furosemide (Lasix) if needed.
6. Once the patient is stable, transfer him or her to the ICU for 24 to 48 hours of observation, follow-up monitoring, and postcrisis treatment.

PERIOPERATIVE NURSING CONSIDERATIONS

General Nursing Considerations

Although an MHS crisis is not a common occurrence, it is always prudent to prepare for one in advance to avoid wasting precious time.

Each surgical suite should have an emergency MHS crisis cart available, stocked with the necessary drugs, supplies, and solutions according to the written protocol created by the department of anesthesia.

A sheet with specific assignments should be kept on the cart, and each person or group of persons in the suite should be familiar with the standard operating procedure during a crisis.

If preoperative evaluations reveal an unusual anesthesia history, all precautions should be taken prior to the start of the procedure, including the availability of iced saline solutions; dantrolene sodium (unmixed), and additional drugs and supplies as directed by protocol.

During the crisis, additional RN's will be needed to assist with the preparation of the drugs and solutions, since 36 vials or more of dantrolene sodium may have to be reconstituted, depending on the kilogram weight of the patient.

Postcrisis Follow-Up

Although 80 percent of MHS crises occur in surgery, the patient should be closely monitored for the next 72 hours, since the mortality rate from latent crisis is still high.

A comprehensive scenario of all events should be documented as part of the patient's record, and the attending physician (if not the surgeon) should be informed, to continue follow-up therapy.

Fast, comprehensive nursing actions, coupled with a *team effort*, can be the factor that prevents MHS from becoming a life-threatening situation.

Self-assessment Exercise 10

Directions: Complete the following exercises. The answers are given at the end of this module.

1. List the five factors that influence the type of anesthesia a patient receives.

2. Differentiate between general and regional anesthesia in their overall patient responses.

3. Why is it important for an anesthesia machine to have a scavenging system in perfect working condition?

4. Describe the technique used when performing a Sellick maneuver, and its purpose.

5. Succinylcholine (Anectine), Atracurium Besylate (Tracrium), Tubocurarine (Curare), Pancuronium Bromide (Pavulon), Vecuronium Bromide (Norcuron) are neuromuscular blockers. Name the one that is a depolarizing agent.

_____

6. Identify at least three supportive nursing measures that may be helpful in reducing a patient's anxiety level prior to the induction of anesthesia.

7. MHS can be triggered by volatile anesthesia agents, but the onset is more abrupt with:

   a. nitrous oxide
   b. succinylcholine
   c. halothane
   d. pancuronium bromide

8. Once the diagnosis of MHS is made, vigorous treatment must be immediately instituted, including:

   a. termination of anesthesia and the procedure
   b. hyperventilation with 100 percent oxygen
   c. administration of dantrolene sodium
   d. all of the above

9. MHS can be diagnosed preoperatively with muscle biopsy studies.

   True   False

10. A sudden rise in temperature is an early warning sign of MHS requiring immediate action.

    True   False

11. Once the crisis is past, additional monitoring is not necessary.

    True   False

REGIONAL ANESTHESIA: TECHNIQUES AND AGENTS

Regional anesthesia has been described as a temporary interruption of the transmission of nerve impulses to and from a specific area or region.

When using this technique, the patient does not lose consciousness, but motor function may be affected, depending on the extent of the anesthetized field, the level of injection, and the penetration capabilities of the agent.

Regional anesthesia was first introduced in Germany in 1898 by August Bier, followed by Matas in America and Tuffie in France,[13] as an alternative to general anesthesia.

The major agent being used at that time was procaine hydrochloride (Novocaine), replacing cocaine, whose addictiveness, toxicity, and short duration of action were apparent.

Today, regional anesthesia has several advantages, including less systemic disturbance to body function; the infeasibility of general anesthesia owing to recent ingestion of food; the presence of cardiac and/or pulmonary dysfunctions; or when surgery is superficial or general anesthesia is not required.

Regional Anesthesia Techniques

Several techniques are used with regional anesthesia, and the choice depends on the type and duration of surgery; the preference of the anesthesia practitioner and surgeon; and the patient's preference when feasible.

Topical anesthesia: the anesthetic agent is applied directly to the skin and mucous membranes, which readily absorb the agent; therefore, it acts rapidly.

Local anesthesia (infiltration): used for minor and superficial procedures in which the agent is injected into a specific area. If the presence of an anesthesia practitioner is required during the procedure, the technique is referred to as *local with MAC* (monitored anesthesia care).

Nerve block: a technique in which the anesthetic agent is injected into and around a nerve or a nerve group that supplies sensation to a small area of the body. Major blocks involve multiple nerves or a *plexus,* while minor blocks involve a single nerve.

Intravenous block (Bier block): involves the intravenous injection of a local agent and the use of an occlusion tourniquet. The occlusion tourniquet prevents infiltration of the anesthetic agent beyond the ex-

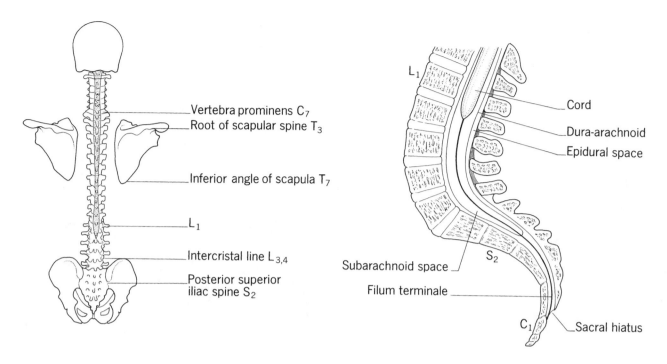

Fig. 6-4. Anatomy of the spinal column

tremity, thus preventing absorption into the general circulation.

Bier blocks are used most often for procedures involving the arm, wrist, hand, and the lower extremity.

Spinal and Epidural Anesthesia

Although spinal and epidural techniques have many similarities in physiologic effects, the two methods have definite differences.

A review of the anatomy involving the selected areas may help to better understand these differences and to differentiate the two methods.

Anatomic Review   The spinal column and its ancillary structures consist of the following (Fig. 6-4):

1. Vertebral column—consisting of 33 vertebrae: seven cervical; 12 thoracic; five lumbar, and four sacral. The column is surrounded by at least five strong ligaments.
2. The spinal cord—extends from the medulla oblongata about 18 in. (or two thirds of the way) down the spinal column, to approximately the lumbar area (L_1 or L_2).
3. The spinal cord is encased in three layers:
    a. Dura mater—a tough, fibrous sheath outside (surrounding) the cord.
    b. Arachnoid/subarachnoid space—a cobweb-like structure, which contains the circulating

cerebrospinal fluid (CSF); lies between pia and dura mater.
    c. Pia mater—the layer immediately on top of the spinal cord.
4. Spinal nerves—31 symmetrical pairs of nerves that exit from the intervertebral foramina: eight cervical, 12 thoracic, five lumbar, and one sacral. It is these nerves that are selectively blocked during spinal and epidural anesthesia.
5. Dermatomes—Segmental distribution of opinal nerves (Fig. 6-5).

Spinal Anesthesia Techniques

Spinal anesthesia occurs when the anesthetic agent is injected into the CSF within the subarachnoid space. Spinal anesthesia is also known as a *subarachnoid block* (SAB).

The injection is performed through one of the interspaces between lumbar disk 2 (L_2) and the sacrum (S_1); the level of anesthesia depends mainly on the amount of the anesthetic injected, the position of the patient, and the level of the interspace used for the spinal (Fig. 6-6).

Spinal anesthesia can be divided into three levels: low, mid, and high spinals. Low spinals (saddle or caudal blocks) are primarily used for surgeries involving the perineal or rectal areas. Mid spinals (below the level of the umbilicus—T_{10}) can be used for hernia repairs or appendectomies, while the high spinal (reaches the nipple line—T_4) can be used for surgeries such as cesarean sections.

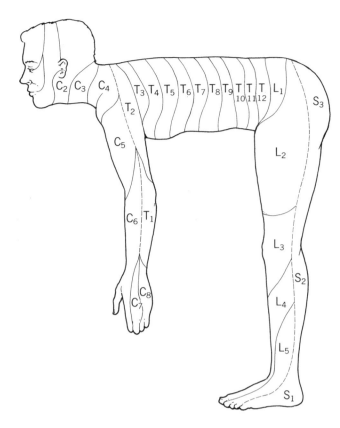

Fig. 6-5. Dermatomes of the body

Spinal anesthesia produces excellent analgesia and relaxation for abdominal and pelvic procedures, and is administered, most commonly, via a one-time bolus injection through a small-gauge needle; a smaller gauge needle is used to reduce the size of the hole in the dura matter.

The level of analgesia depends on the following factors:

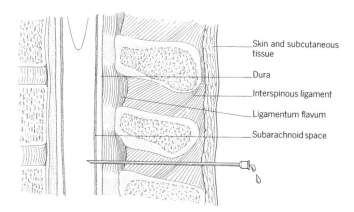

Fig. 6-6. Insertion of spinal needle

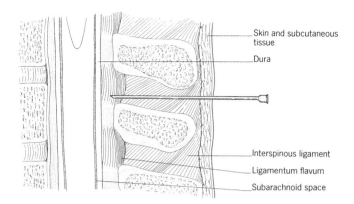

Fig. 6-7. Needle placement for epidural anesthesia

1. dose and concentration of agent used
2. volume of agent used
3. specific gravity of the solution
4. CSF pressure
5. positioning of the patient during and immediately after the injection

The most common position for spinal anesthesia is sitting or lateral decubitus (knee to chest) with the back curled outward.

Epidural (Peridural) Anesthesia Technique

Epidural anesthesia, commonly associated with obstetric surgery, involves the injection of an anesthetic agent into the epidural space, the area outside the dura mater, but inside the spinal column (Fig. 6-7).

Epidural anesthesia can be administered via bolus injection or through a small, thin catheter, and can be used for anorectal, vaginal, and perineal procedures, as well as higher, intraabdominal procedures.

Patient positioning for epidural anesthesia is similar to spinal positioning. When a catheter is used, it must be securely taped to avoid migration of the catheter.

Because the anesthetic agent does not enter the spinal cord, greater quantities of the agent must be used with the epidural technique.

Possible Complications and Corrective Actions

Although spinal and epidural anesthesia produce excellent analgesia and relaxation, the perioperative nurse should be prepared to assist anesthesia personnel if complications occur either during or after injection of the local agent.

Hypotension

The most common adverse effect of spinal/epidural anesthesia is hypotension due to the anesthetic agent and vasodilation that can occur peripherally, reducing the venous blood return to the heart.

Treatment begins before the anesthetic agent is administered. This includes fluid loading to increase the circulatory volume, administration of oxygen, and proper positioning. After the agent is administered, the above measures are employed, as well as the use of vasopressors.

Total Spinal Anesthesia

Another, more critical adverse effect is a condition referred to as *total spinal,* which occurs when the anesthetic level is too high, depressing the respiratory and cardiac systems.

Treatment involves respiratory assistance and cardiovascular support. This condition reverses itself, however, as the agent is absorbed and metabolized within the body.

Nausea and Vomiting

Nausea and vomiting are not uncommon during the injection sequence. They may be due to the agent, hypotension, abrupt position change, apprehension, or all of these factors.

Treatment consists of administration of oxygen, antiemetics, fluid loading, and vasopressors.

Urinary Retention

Urinary retention is caused by an anesthetic-induced decrease in bladder tone; it may occur intraoperatively and postoperatively.

Treatment is to monitor urinary output, increase fluid volume, and administer appropriate diuretics according to severity.

Paralysis and/or Muscle Weakness in Legs or Feet

Peripheral paralysis is caused by a decrease in neuromuscular sensation, sometimes to a dangerous level. It is very rare, occurring in only 1 of 1000 to 2000 blocks.

Treatment consists of careful and continuous assessment of the patient and immediately reporting any untoward reactions to the anesthesia practitioner for corrective action.

Postspinal Headache

A postspinal headache is due to intraspinal CSF pressure changes or leaks in the dura.

Cerebrospinal fluid pressure causes stress on the nerves between the cranium and the brain. Postspinal headaches, not seen with epidural techniques, can occur immediately or 24 to 48 hours after injection; the treatment usually consists of bedrest, increased fluid intake, sedation, and, in severe cases, a blood patch graft to seal the hole (5–10 mL of the patient's blood via an epidural injection).

Backache

Tenderness at the level of the block may last for a few weeks after spinal anesthesia.

Epidural anesthesia has fewer adverse effects than spinal anesthesia, but occasionally urinary retention, pruritus, nausea, respiratory depression, and pronounced orthostatic hypotensive episodes can occur.

PERIOPERATIVE NURSING MANAGEMENT

The prevention of possible complications can be accomplished through specific nursing activities when working with patients receiving spinal or epidural anesthesia. These should include, but not be limited to:

1. Assisting anesthesia personnel in obtaining and maintaining optimum positioning during and after injection. Since the sensory system has been compromised, protection of all areas of lost sensation from pressure or improper body alignment is essential.
2. Moving the patient slowly when changing his or her position.
3. Maintaining sterile technique during the procedure.
4. Assessing the security of the catheter by anchoring it to prevent its possible migration.
5. Reporting any return of feelings expressed by the patient.

The success of spinal and epidural anesthesia techniques requires patient cooperation. Providing emotional support and reassurance during the procedure, answering questions, and remaining close to the patient will in most instances reduce the patient's anxiety level and produce a successful result.

Regional Anesthetic Agents

Regional anesthetic agents fall into two primary groups, amides and esters, based on their chemical composition and actions (Table 6-1).

Amides are organic substances that are primarily metabolized in the liver and excreted in the urine. Examples of amides include marcaine, carbocaine, and duranest.

Ester derivatives are metabolized rapidly and almost completely by plasma cholinesterase. The remaining drug is then metabolized by the liver and ex-

Table 6-1   A Summary of Local Anesthetic Agents

Generic Name	Trade Name	Type of Agent	Concentration	Maximum[a] Dose Rate (mg/kg)	Upper Limit Maximum Total Dose[b] (mg)	Onset/Duration
Procaine	Novocain	Ester	2–4%	10	1000	Slow/30 min
Chloroprocaine	Nesacaine	Ester	1–2%	10	1000	Fast/1 hr
					800	
Tetracaine	Pontocaine	Ester	0.1–0.25%	1	200	Slow/2–3 hr
					100	
Lidocaine	Xylocaine	Amide	1–2%	6	500	Fast/1–2 hr
					300	
Prilocaine	Citanest	Amide	1–2%	8	600	Moderate/2–3 hr
Mepivacaine	Carbocaine	Amide	1–2%	6	500	Fast/2–3 hr
					300	
Bupivacaine	Marcaine	Amide	0.5%	2	225	Slow/5–7 hr
					175	
Etidocaine	Duranest	Amide	0.5–1%	4	400	Fast/4–6 hr
					300	

[a] Indicates maximum dose rate with epinephrine; reduce by 25% if epinephrine is not used.
[b] Top figure indicates maximum dose total with epinephrine, the bottom indicates maximum dose total without epinephrine.
Adapted from Davidson HC. A Practice of Anesthesia. Chicago, IL: Yearbook Medical Publishers, Inc., 1984; Lebowitz P, Newberg L, Gillette M. Clinical Anesthesia of the Massachusetts General Hospital. Boston: Little, Brown, 1992; Snow JC. Manual of Anesthesia. Boston: Little, Brown, 1983.

creted in the urine. Examples of esters include Nesacaine, metycaine, procaine, pontocaine, and cocaine (the first local anesthetic agent).

Only a few of these agents are used routinely during regional anesthesia, and the choice largely depends on the type of regional technique to be used and the choice of the anesthesia practitioner based on the surgical procedure and its anticipated length.

Mechanism of Action

Local anesthetics block depolarization by interfering with sodium movement into the nerve cell, prevention generation and conduction of the nerve impulses.

Epinephrine Additive

It is not uncommon to administer an agent that contains epinephrine; therefore, most commercially prepared agents come both without epinephrine and with epinephrine (1:100,000 or 1:200,000).

Epinephrine serves two purposes:

1. It produces vasoconstriction, thus aiding in the control in bleeding.
2. It prolongs (slows) absorption of the drug, so the duration of action is longer.

Epinephrine has specific problems, however, that

should be anticipated: such as local irritation and dermatitis, tachycardia, palpitations, restlessness, or feelings of anxiety.

In large doses, signs of epinephrine overdose may include convulsions, severe hypertension, respiratory depression, and anaphylactic reactions.

Absorption varies according to dose, site of injection, and vasodilation produced by the drug. Epinephrine combined with a local anesthetic decreases absorption.

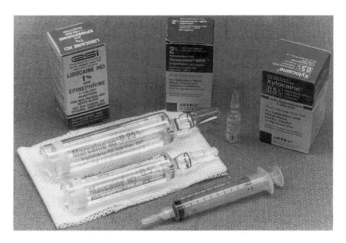

Local anesthesia agents

Self-assessment Exercise 11

Directions: Complete the following exercises. Answers are given at the end of this module.

1. A regional anesthesia technique especially useful in labor and delivery is:
   a. epidural
   b. spinal
   c. nerve block
   d. intravenous block

2. In spinal anesthesia (circle correct answer[s]):
   a. injection is made at L_2 to L_3 or above
   b. levels of anesthesia are influenced by position following injection
   c. the anesthetic agent may be Xylocaine
   d. an adverse reaction may include respiratory depression

   e. a headache 24 to 48 hours after epidural anesthesia is not uncommon

3. Identify two appropriate patient positions associated with spinal and epidural anesthesia.

4. Describe four nursing interventions that could reduce patient anxiety and/or maintain patient dignity when regional anesthesia is used and the patient is awake.

5. Spinal anesthesia may result in sudden hypotension.

   True   False

LOCAL ANESTHESIA AND INTRAVENOUS CONSCIOUS SEDATION

The increase of diagnostic procedures and surgical procedures continues to challenge perioperative nurses in today's practice setting. The combination of local anesthesia with IV conscious sedation with opioids and sedatives is seen more frequently in today's practice than ever before. With the increasing number of these procedures, perioperative nurses utilizing this technique need to be aware of the safe practices related to the administration of these agents, and the monitoring responsibilities for those patients using local anesthesia with IV conscious sedation.

In an effort to provide safe guidelines for practice, AORN has created two recommended practices related to this area: 1) monitoring the patient receiving IV conscious sedation, and 2) monitoring patients receiving local anesthesia (see Boxes on pp. 104, 105).

Managing Intravenous Conscious Sedation Agents

Opioid analgesics and *sedatives* are the medications routinely administered to provide IV conscious sedation. Because scope of practice limitations almost always preclude nurses (except CRNAs) from administering any anesthetics, IV conscious sedation, administered by the perioperative nurse, is limited to those agents classified as analgesics and sedatives (tranquilizers).

Perioperative nurses administering these agents must be familiar with dosage requirements, onset, and duration of actions. During conscious sedation, special

consideration must also be given to drug interactions and precautions. Additionally, knowledge of titration techniques with prescribed ranges is necessary to attain the desired effect with a minimum of medication to reduce the potential for adverse effects.

Opioid Analgesics

An analgesic agent is one that has the capability to change both pain perception and the reaction of the patient to pain. Opioid analgesics are usually understood to include natural and semisynthetic alkaloid derivatives from opium as well as their synthetic surrogates with actions that mimic those of morphine.[14]

Frequently used opioid analgesics include morphine sulfate, meperidine hydrochloride, and fentanyl. With these agents, analgesia can usually be produced without disturbing other CNS function such as protective reflexes or breathing.

The most serious adverse effect of opioids is *respiratory depression,* which can progress to apnea and may suddenly and unexpectedly occur in arousable, responsive patients. If apnea is not promptly treated, it can result in cardiac arrest.

It is important for the perioperative nurse to remember that the effects—including adverse effects—of any opioid may be potentiated when given in combination with sedatives, as is generally done with IV conscious sedation. Hypovolemic states may also cause opioid effects to become more pronounced.

Sedatives

An effective sedative agent (formally known as tranquilizers) should reduce anxiety and exert a calming effect with little or no effect on motor or mental functions.[15] Combined with analgesics, sedatives reduce anxiety and to some degree, produce short-term amnesia. Agents frequently used include those that belong to the *benzodiazepine* family, specifically, diazepam and midazolam.

Diazepam (Valium) has been found to act on parts of the limbic system (thalamus and hypothalamus) inducing a calming effect. Each patient reacts differently to diazepam, but amnesia has been most pronounced when sedation is produced.

Clinical sedation is usually recognized by heavy, slurred speech and nystagmus preceding the onset of sleep. These two signs are often used as the end point when titrating doses. Common adverse effects include venous thrombosis, phlebitis, local irritation, confusion, drowsiness, hypotension, and apnea.

Midazolam (Versed) is a short-acting sedative about three times more potent than diazepam. Midazolam is considered by some anesthesia practitioners as superior to diazepam for sedation and amnesia due to its rapid onset of actions. Because it is rapidly metabolized, midazolam is quickly excreted, resulting in a shorter duration of action. Additionally, unlike diazepam, midazolam does not cause venous irritation nor produce the ''hang-over''-like effect that may be present with diazepam.

Due to the natural aging process, reduced doses of all benzodiazepines and longer postoperative evaluation are indicated for patients over 60 or whenever other CNS depressants are used. The elderly and chronically ill patient is also at risk for hypoventilation and apnea, especially in the presence of COPD or compromised renal function.

Reversal Agents

Naloxone hydrochloride (Narcan), a narcotic antagonist, and flumazenil (Romazicon), a benzodiazepine antagonist, are the currently available reversal agents. These agents can enhance the safety of conscious sedation and may be used as needed, depending on institutional policy and clinical judgment.

AORN Recommended Practice—Intravenous Conscious Sedation

The following recommended practices can provide a guideline for the perioperative nurse administering IV conscious sedation agents.

Managing Complications

When monitoring a patient during IV conscious sedation, the goal of the perioperative nurse is to maintain

---

Monitoring Patients Receiving IV Conscious Sedation

I. The nurse should know the goals and objectives of IV conscious sedation.

II. Each patient receiving IV conscious sedation should be assessed physiologically and psychologically before the procedure.

III. Each patient receiving IV conscious sedation should be monitored for reaction to drugs and for physiologic and psychological changes.

IV. The nurse monitoring the patient should have a working knowledge of resuscitation equipment and the function and use of monitoring equipment and should be able to interpret the data obtained.

V. Documentation on the patient record during the administration of IV conscious sedation should reflect evidence of continued assessment, diagnosis, outcome identification, planning, implementation, and evaluation of patient care.

VI. Patient's receiving IV conscious sedation should be monitored postprocedure, receive written discharge instructions, and meet specified criteria before discharge.

VII. Policies and procedures on monitoring the patient receiving IV conscious sedation should be written, reviewed annually, and readily available within the practice setting.

Source: AORN. Standards and recommended practices for perioperative nursing. Denver: The Association, 1995. Pp. 205–209.

---

the patient in a relaxed, arousable, cooperative state with intact protective reflexes.

Overdosage or adverse effects in either the procedure, stress, or the medication may occur at anytime. Therefore, the patient's vital signs, blood pressure, and oxygen saturation must be assessed and documented at least every 5 minutes.

Should adverse reactions or complications occur, the perioperative nurse should initiate the appropriate supportive measures, which may include establishing and maintaining a patent airway, ventilatory support via mask and ambu, and CPR if indicated. Nursing-initiated measures for hypotension may include administration of appropriate IV fluids (directed by the surgeon), leg elevation, and use of vasopressors, nalox-

---

Monitoring the Patient Receiving Local Anesthesia

I.   All patients receiving local anesthesia should be monitored by a perioperative nurse for reaction to drugs and for physiologic and behavioral changes.

II. The perioperative nurse should have the knowledge, skill, and ability to use and interpret the data from monitoring equipment.

III. Documentation on the patient record during the administration of local anesthesia should reflect evidence of continuous assessment, planning, implementation, and evaluation of patient care.

IV. Policies and procedures for monitoring the patient receiving local anesthesia should be written, reviewed annually, revised as necessary and readily available within the practice setting.

Source: AORN. Standards and recommended practices for perioperative nursing. Denver: The Association, 1995. Pp. 217–218.

---

one or flumazentil as directed. All patient responses and interventions should be documented and reported to the surgeon. Additionally, an anesthesia practitioner may be needed to assist in managing the duration of the incident and/or case.

PERIOPERATIVE NURSING CONSIDERATIONS

According to AORN, the following recommended practices are considered the minimal standards of care for the patient undergoing surgery with local anesthesia.

Nursing Management

The establishment of standardized protocols for the management of local anesthesia procedures ensures quality nursing care for the patient and provides the necessary legal guidelines for the perioperative nurse, according to hospital and department approval and the Nurse Practice Act governing that practice (Fig. 6-8).

Often times nurses tend to assume that less preparation is needed for the surgical patient who is receiving local anesthesia. However, this assumption is not only

inaccurate, but is in direct opposition to the realities of the situation.

In addition to the preparation of instruments and supplies required for the case, the perioperative nurse who cares for the patient must meet the psychological and physiologic needs before, during, and after the procedure, apply sound nursing judgment based on a knowledge of the biophysical sciences, and perform accurate assessment techniques in addition to precise documentation of the patient's responses and the care provided.

Protocols should be written to define ongoing care and precise management of nursing interventions and to provide concrete direction for all staff involved with a specific aspect of care. Protocols for management of the patient receiving local anesthesia, therefore, should include, but not be limited to:

- Patient selection criteria
- Extent and responsibility for monitoring
- Method of recording patient data
- Frequency of documentation of physiologic data obtained
- Medications that may be administered by the perioperative nurse
- Discharge criteria

As mentioned previously, local anesthesia falls under the category of regional anesthesia, and is used when it is desirable to block the neuromuscular conduction system in a small, specified area, without affecting adjacent structures.

Local infiltration, or "field block," can be used for a wide variety of cases ranging from oral surgery to furnishing a field block surrounding a hernia or the incision and drainage of an abscess. In this technique, the subcutaneous branches of the appropriate sensory nerves are anesthetized by the injection of a local anesthetic agent. When the agents are combined with epinephrine, the effect of the agent is prolonged, in addition to aiding in the control of bleeding due to vasoconstriction.

In addition to the local agent administered at the field, the patient may also receive an IV sedative to minimize the fear and anxiety associated with being "awake" during the procedure, in addition to minimizing the discomfort that may occur from the procedure.

To provide a safe environment for the patient, the perioperative nurse must be knowledgeable about how these agents work together, or alone, and be prepared to counteract their adverse effects in a safe and effective manner (Table 6-2).

Most local anesthetics begin to act in less than 15 minutes after application or infiltration, but the duration of their action varies with each agent.

Department of Nursing Services

DIVISION: Surgical Services
UNIT: Surgery

STANDARD OF CARE STATEMENTS ON
PATIENTS WITH: __Local Anesthesia__

OUTCOME STANDARDS	Date Met & R.N. Int.
1. Patient will demonstrate physiologic stability in all body systems within 4 hours.	
2. The patient will utilize the sequence of events pertaining to surgical experience.	
3. The patient will demonstrate and participate in self-care management activities.	

SUBJECT HEADINGS / POTENTIAL CARE PROBLEMS	Initiated Date	R.N	NURSING INTERVENTIONS	Discontinued Date	R.N.
PRE-OPERATIVE PHASE					
Knowledge deficit, lack of specific information relating to surgical experience.			Provide explanations regarding sequence of events during the peri-operative period. -Encourage patient to verbalize questions and concerns. -Remain with patient to provide support. -Provide non-verbal support thru touch.		
Potential altered sensory perception related to pre-op meds			Protect patient during transport & moving. Assess status prior to administration of next med dose. -Encourage patient to verbalize discomforts. -Discuss with patient availability of pain medication.		
INTRA-OPERATIVE PHASE					
Possible discomfort related to required positioning and length of surgical procedure.			Position patient anatomically with appropriate support & flex table slightly at knees to reduce strain on back muscles. Place pillow beneath knees and pad all boney prominences.		
Potential loss of dignity related to excessive exposure & lack of personal care.			A. Limit exposure of patient only to required area for surgical procedure. B. Call patient by name. C. Only permit team members in the room. D. Maintain quiet & professional atmosphere.		
Possible adverse reactions to local anesthetic agent related to sensitivity or overdose.			A. Check chart for allergies. B. Obtain base line vital signs. C. Monitor all physiologic aspects as directed by protocol. D. Communicate any changes to surgeon.		
Potential for injury related to: Burns (chemical or electrical) Foreign Objects Nosocomial Infection			A. Place electrosurgical ground pad as close to incision site as possible with total skin contact around periphery. B. When prepping, place towels along patient's sides to prevent pooling of solutions. C. Perform sponge, needle, & instrument counts according to protocol. D. Ensure compliance with principles of asepsis.		
POST-OPERATIVE PHASE					
Potential lack of continuity of patient care related to returning patient to primary nurse/inpatient unit.			A. Inform primary care nurse of procedure performed & physiological data during procedure. -Patient's response. -Fluids & medications administered -VS pre,intra, & post procedure. -Presence of drains.		
Potential alteration in comfort related to pain at incisional site.			A. Review post-op pain management with patient & family. B. Instruct patient how to most benefit from paid medication. -When -How		

Fig. 6-8. Protocol for local anesthesia management (Modified from Broward General Medical Center, Department of Surgical and Anesthesia Services, Ft. Lauderdale, FL)

Table 6-2   Treatment of Problems with Local Anesthesia

Problems	Signs and Symptoms	Treatment

Allergic reaction	Initial signs: rash, redness of skin, itchiness, hives, and swelling. Later signs: bronchoconstriction, asthmatic breathing, hypotension, and syncope	1. Ensure airway patency
		2. Administer
		  a. Oxygen
		  b. Diphenhydramine 50 mg IV
		  c. IV fluids for hypotension
		  d. Vasopressors
		  e. Bronchodilators

Reaction to epinephrine	Headache, increased heart rate, increased blood pressure, palpitations, apprehension, sweating, tremors	1. Ensure airway patency 2. Administer oxygen 3. Continue to monitor for potential cardiovascular problems

Toxic overdose	Initial signs: numb tongue, blurred vision, tinnitus, dizziness, drowsiness, confusion. Later signs: loss of consciousness, tonic-clonic convulsions, CNS depression, respiratory depression, respiratory arrest	1. Ensure airway patency
		2. Administer
		  a. Oxygen
		  b. Diazepam 50 mg IV
		  c. Succinylcholine 0.1–0.2 mg/kg IV followed by intubation

The dosage and choice of agent will vary according to the procedure, the level of anesthesia needed, tissue vascularity, patient responses, and surgeon's preference, but the nurse monitoring the patient should be aware of these variables to render safe care.

Physiologic Monitoring

By definition, physiologic monitoring consists of the continual observation of the patient's vital signs, including blood pressure (B/P), pulse (rate and rhythm), and respiratory rate; oxygen saturation; skin condition and color; and any changes in the patient's physical or behavioral status.

The patient must be constantly monitored during the procedure, and documentation of this monitoring must be specific as to frequency and methods used.

Effective physiologic monitoring cannot be performed without baseline information to use as a guide; therefore, the nurse should obtain, through interview and observation, all pertinent data regarding the patient's past or present medical history, including allergies; history of hypertension; physical limitations (which could affect positioning); and emotional status.

An IV line should be started preoperatively, or be readily available, according to hospital policy, and the information recorded on the appropriate form.

On entry into the OR, and following the positioning of the patient on the OR table, the perioperative nurse should apply the electrocardiograph leads and blood pressure cuff, explaining the procedure to the patient to relieve the "fear of the unknown." Initial baseline data should be recorded, which will serve as a reference point throughout the procedure. Additionally, oxygen via nasal cannula may be started, and a pulse oximeter should be used to monitor oxygen saturation levels.

Emergency equipment and medications should be in the room or be available for immediate use, according to established protocols.

Assessment and recording of the physiologic status should continue at least every 5 to 15 minutes during the procedure, depending on hospital protocol, and before and after each dose of medication. Any significant changes, either in vital signs, cardiac rhythm or sensorium should be reported to the surgeon immediately for appropriate corrective action.

Documentation of the physiologic status should flow throughout the record, with special notations of when medications are administered and the amount given. This critical documentation should reflect the patient's responses to the drugs, and can serve as a reference in the event that complications develop during the procedure (Fig. 6-9).

Additional Nursing Management Recommendations

In addition to physiologic monitoring, the establishment and maintenance of IV solutions, and medication administration, the perioperative nurse is responsible for the assessment, planning, implementation, and evaluation of nursing care throughout the perioperative period, including the environmental management and psychological support.

Creating a Therapeutic Environment

The atmosphere of the procedure room plays an important part in contributing to the patient's comfort during a local procedure.

Soft music tends to relax the awake patient, while rock or jazz tends to excite and sometimes disturb the patient and possibly the surgical team. In fact, music may be the only familiar experience the patients encounter during their brief visit to the surgical suite. Maintaining a natural environment, talking to the patient, and allowing the patient to express his or her feelings and needs should be encouraged, since levels of pain tolerance are somewhat higher when concentration is shifted to other areas.

It is equally important, however, that a nonprofessional, carefree environment should be avoided, to maintain the patient's confidence in not only the surgeon, but also the nursing team. Careful planning and consideration, coupled with sound nursing judgment, are the best guidelines for creating and maintaining a safe, therapeutic environment.

Providing Patient Comfort

Many times the patient receiving local anesthesia will be on the OR table for several hours. By providing physical comfort during the procedure, anxiety and pain levels can be reduced, resulting in the need for less medication through a few simple comfort measures.

For example, a flotation mattress (egg crate) should be placed on the operating table, under the sheet, to provide padding for bony areas of the back and hips. Another measure involves positioning the patient in proper body alignment, with the elimination of ridges caused by sheets or gowns. Extremity pads should be used on elbows and heels, especially if the patient is to be in the supine position, with a small pillow under the lower back, and, if it does not interfere with the patient's airway, a small pillow under the head should be available. Finally, warm blankets can reduce the chill factor, since these patients will be more acutely aware of a temperature drop than patients totally anesthetized.

An explanation to the patient about limitations in movement during the procedure is always recommended. The patient should be informed that a slight shift in position is permissible as long as the surgeon approves and the change does not interfere with the surgery or the positioning of the sterile drapes.

If the patient requires oxygen administration during the procedure, a brief explanation of the nasal cannula and its purpose is in order, since the patient may interpret this therapy as a sign of an impending problem. Nasal cannulae, which incorporate monitoring of end tidal carbon dioxide levels ($ETCO_2$), are desirable to monitor ventilation.

Controlling Extraneous Noise and Traffic

For all local cases, a sign posted on the OR door stating "This Patient is Awake" or something similar should be used, and the staff should be cautioned to avoid extraneous noise outside the room.

Because the patient is awake, use of the intercom should be restricted, and if pathology is needed for a diagnostic examination of tissue specimens, a notation on the requisition stating that the patient is awake can eliminate any misinterpretation of the information heard by the patient.

The provision of comfort measures and the maintenance of the patient's safety is the primary responsibility of the perioperative nurse, in addition to monitoring physiologic responses to the surgery and the medications. For this reason, two nurses should be assigned to local cases; one to serve in the circulating capacity and one to provide the monitoring and nursing care activities required to make the surgical experiences as pleasant as possible.

Documenting Perioperative Nursing Care

As with any surgical procedure, documentation is the legal responsibility of the perioperative nurse. Documentation during a local anesthesia case not only requires the nurse to record the surgical aspects of the case (e.g., intraoperative nurses record), but also requires that the monitoring of physiologic and psychological status, and the appropriate nursing care and patient responses to that care, be accurately described.

In some institutions, the use of a narrative nurse's note serves as the local anesthesia record, in addition to the operative record required for all operative procedures. In other hospitals, a local anesthesia record (see Fig. 6-9) has been created for the documentation of this information, and like the narrative note, is used in addition to the operative record. This record, then, becomes a substitute for the anesthesia record. It has been further recommended that since anesthesia personnel are not monitoring this patient, the anesthesia record should not be used by the perioperative nurse for documentation during a local procedure.

As the perioperative nurses' responsibilities and tasks increase, so too does the need for detailed documentation. As the patient advocate and the professional nurse caring for the patient, the perioperative nurse must share the responsibility with the surgical team for maintaining a safe, therapeutic environment

Table 6-3 **Intravenous Sedation Monograph**

Agent	Classification	Recommended Dosage	Nursing Implications
Diazepam (Valium)	Tranquilizer, anticonvulsant	2–10 mg (0.4–2.0 mL) given in 1-mL increments	1. Do not mix with any solution 2. Inject close to site of infusion cannula 3. Reduce dose in debilitated or elderly patients 4. Do not give if respirations are less than 12/min 5. Contraindicated in patients with acute narrow-angled glaucoma 6. Slow absorption rate; effect can last for several days 7. When used with narcotic, reduce dose 8. Reversible
Meperidine (Demerol)	Narcotic analgesic (synthetic)	10–50 mg diluted (100 mg diluted with 20 mL of sterile water yields concentration of 5 mg/mL)	1. Consult with physician if respirations are below 12/min before giving the next dose 2. When given with tranquilizers, reduce dose by 25–50% 3. Administer slowly over 1 min 4. Reversible with Narcan
Morphine sulfate	Narcotic analgesic (opiate derivative)	2.5–10 mg (g $\frac{1}{16}$–$\frac{1}{6}$) diluted (10 mg diluted with 10 mL of NS yields a concentration of 1 mg/mL)	1. Do not give if respirations are less than 12/min 2. Contraindicated in patients with COPD and debilitated, elderly patients 3. Onset immediate with duration lasting 4–6 hr 4. Reversible with Narcan
Midazolam (Versed)	Tranquilizer, sedative	1–5 mg diluted, slow IVP (5 mg in 5 mL NS or D$_5$W yields concentration of 1 mg/mL)	1. Three times more potent than Valium; therefore, give $\frac{1}{4}$–$\frac{1}{2}$ Valium dose 2. Do not give if respirations are less than 12/min 3. Rapid onset with duration of 2–6 hr 4. Potentiated by narcotics and CNS depressants; Reversible 5. Optimum level usually indicated by slurring of speech

Key: COPD = chronic obstructive pulmonary disease; IVP = intravenous push; NS = normal saline (0.9% NaCl).

during any surgical procedure, but most importantly during a local anesthesia procedure.

Postprocedural Follow-Up

The preoperative interview offers the perioperative nurse the opportunity to individualize the care planned for the patient undergoing surgical intervention; the effectiveness of this care is evaluated during the postoperative phase of surgical intervention.

Unlike general anesthesia patients, who are transported to the postanesthesia care unit for immediate monitoring and assessment, the local anesthesia patient usually returns to the designated postprocedural area (Ambulatory Surgery Unit or Patient Care Unit)

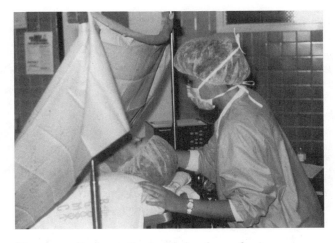

Nurse monitoring patient with local anesthesia

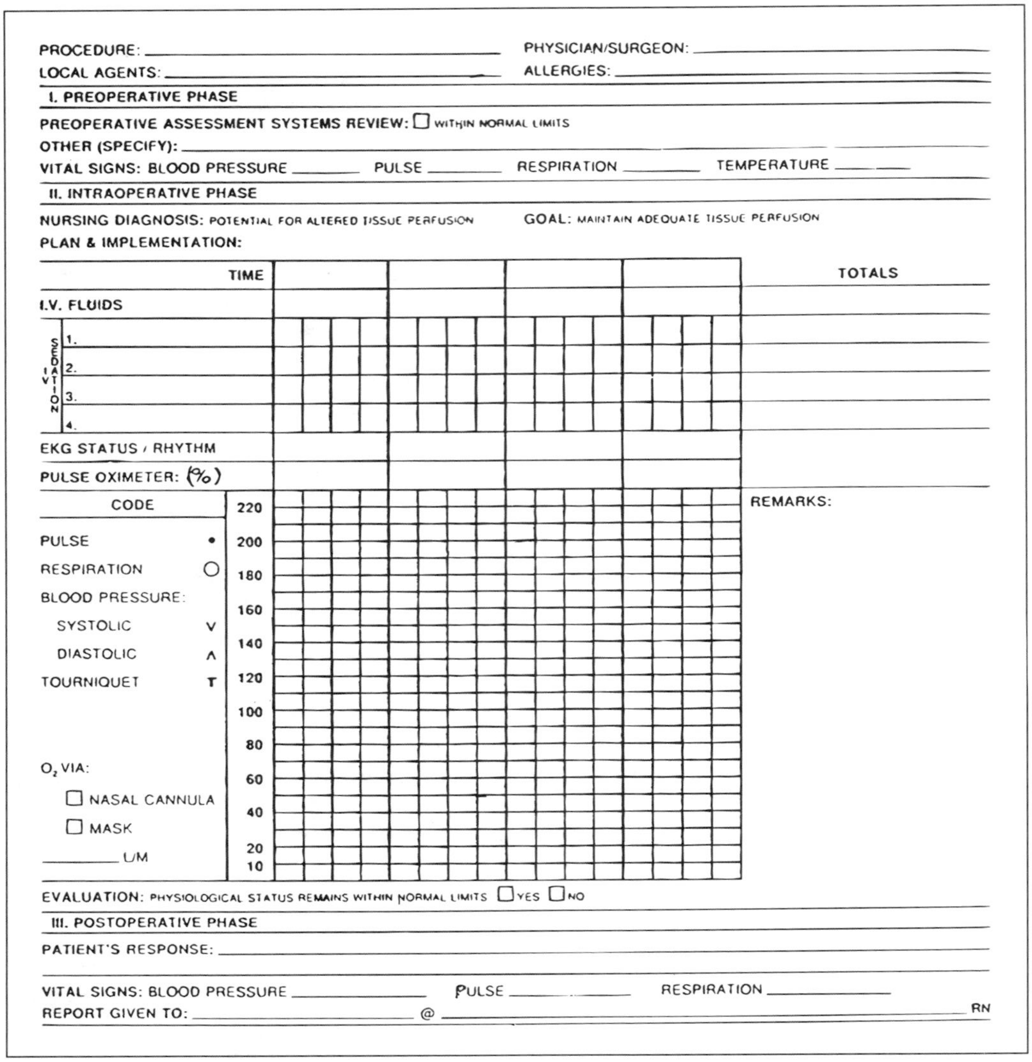

PROCEDURE: ______ PHYSICIAN/SURGEON: ______
LOCAL AGENTS: ______ ALLERGIES: ______

I. PREOPERATIVE PHASE

PREOPERATIVE ASSESSMENT SYSTEMS REVIEW: ☐ WITHIN NORMAL LIMITS
OTHER (SPECIFY): ______
VITAL SIGNS: BLOOD PRESSURE ______ PULSE ______ RESPIRATION ______ TEMPERATURE ______

II. INTRAOPERATIVE PHASE

NURSING DIAGNOSIS: POTENTIAL FOR ALTERED TISSUE PERFUSION GOAL: MAINTAIN ADEQUATE TISSUE PERFUSION
PLAN & IMPLEMENTATION:

TIME					TOTALS
I.V. FLUIDS					
SEDATION 1.					
2.					
3.					
4.					
EKG STATUS / RHYTHM					
PULSE OXIMETER: (%)					

CODE: PULSE •; RESPIRATION ○; BLOOD PRESSURE: SYSTOLIC V; DIASTOLIC Λ; TOURNIQUET T

Scale: 220, 200, 180, 160, 140, 120, 100, 80, 60, 40, 20, 10

REMARKS:

O_2 VIA: ☐ NASAL CANNULA ☐ MASK ______ L/M

EVALUATION: PHYSIOLOGICAL STATUS REMAINS WITHIN NORMAL LIMITS ☐ YES ☐ NO

III. POSTOPERATIVE PHASE

PATIENT'S RESPONSE: ______

VITAL SIGNS: BLOOD PRESSURE ______ PULSE ______ RESPIRATION ______
REPORT GIVEN TO: ______ @ ______ RN

Fig. 6-9. Local anesthesia monitoring record (Courtesy of North Broward Hospital District, Department of Surgical Services, Ft. Lauderdale, FL)

for follow-up monitoring, which must continue to maintain the patient's safety.

Psychological stress, in conjunction with the administration of medications and the trauma of surgery, makes postoperative management of the local anesthesia patient as important as the preoperative and intraoperative phases of surgical intervention.

The main objective of postoperative care is to facilitate the rapid, safe, and comfortable recovery of the patient's normal functions. Therefore, a safe rule of practice dictates that patients receiving IV sedation be returned to the PACU for a minimal period of time before being transferred to the designated postoperative area.

If the patient received only the local agent, without IV sedation, transfer to the PACU area may not be necessary, depending on the policies of the hospital and the postoperative condition of the patient.

In either situation, the perioperative nurse's responsibility for patient care does not end in surgery, but continues until an accurate report of the patient's status has been given and documented to provide continuity of care.

For patients who are returning home the same day as surgery, the perioperative nurse should accompany the patient to the Ambulatory Care Unit, where a verbal report can be given to the nurse assigned to the patient, and the patient can relax and recover from the surgical procedure prior to returning home. Additionally, any postoperative instructions can be given to both the patient and family, with explanations as necessary.

It is hard to differentiate the care given to the patient receiving local anesthesia from the care given to the general anesthesia patient, since both types of patient have the same basic supportive needs, anxieties and concerns. Patients under local anesthesia, however, are awake and acutely aware of all that is happening around them, which requires additional planning by the surgical team.

The perioperative nurse must always provide optimum patient care to ensure that the surgical experience is as pleasant and nontraumatic as possible, while maintaining a safe, therapeutic surgical environment.

Self-assessment Exercise 12

Directions: Complete the following exercises. Answers are given at the end of this module.

1. List the signs and symptoms associated with a toxic overdose of a local anesthetic.

2. Describe the nursing activities for care of the patient receiving local anesthesia during the preoperative period.

3. Headache, increased heart rate, and increased blood pressure are signs and symptoms usually associated with the administration of

    _____

4. A tranquilizing agent, used during a local anesthesia case and administered by the perioperative nurse, would be:
    a. meperidine hydrochloride
    b. fentanyl
    c. midazolam hydrochloride
    d. ketamine

5. The recommended interval for monitoring vital signs for a patient receiving local anesthesia is

    _____

References

1. Lyons AS, Petrucelli B. Medicine: an illustrated history. New York: Harry N. Abrams, 1978. P. 135.
2. Ibid, p. 137.
3. Ibid, p. 139.
4. Dripps RD, et al. Introduction to anesthesia, 7th ed. Philadelphia: WB Saunders, 1988. P. 4.
5. Miller RD, ed. Anesthesia, Vol. I. 2nd ed. New York: Churchill-Livingstone, 1986. P. 8.
6. Ibid, p. 15.
7. Ibid, p. 17.
8. Ibid, p. 19.
9. American Society of Anesthesiology. ASA classification of surgical patients. Chicago, IL: The Association, 1991.
10. Dripps RD, op. cit. Pp. 17–18.
11. Dripps RD, op. cit. Pp. 196–197.
12. Miller RD. P. 1086.
13. Miller RD, op. cit. P. 10.
14. Katzung, B. Basic and clinical pharmacology 15th ed. Norwalk, CT, 1992. P. 42.
15. Ibid, p. 306.

Intravascular Homeostasis and Hemodynamics

James Mulchay

Intravascular Homeostasis
Body Fluids
Solutes and Electrolytes
Hemodynamic Monitoring

Surgical procedures impose a variety of stressors on the patient, both psychologically and physiologically. Among those that require constant monitoring are body fluids, electrolytes, and acid–base disturbances.

Most patients facing elective operative procedures have oral intake withheld during the 8 to 12 hours preceding surgery, resulting in unreplaced solute and water loss. In view of this preoperative loss, the monitoring and restoration of normal fluid balance becomes the primary concern of the anesthesia clinician, since this deficit can ultimately affect all body systems and directly or indirectly affect the outcome of the surgical procedure.

INTRAVASCULAR HOMEOSTASIS

Both fluid and electrolyte balance are part of a larger homeostatic process. The internal and external factors that attempt to keep the body in a state of equilibrium (*homeostasis*) are connected through the *circulatory, gastrointestinal (GI), pulmonary,* and *renal (urinary)* systems. Because of this connection, if the external exchange processes are not properly regulated, the internal balance cannot be maintained within normal limits and will require outside intervention to correct the imbalanced state.

Achieving internal balance requires the steady-state exchange of energy, solutes, and water between body fluid compartments: exchanges between plasma and interstitial fluid (ISF), and exchanges between ISF and the intracellular fluid (ICF).

All the essential exchanges occur in the microcirculatory bed (the capillaries and venules) which then transport their substances to their designated locations.

BODY FLUIDS

Functions of Body Fluids

The body fluids of an adult consist of approximately 70 percent water and solutes which serve two major functions:

1. They transport nutrients to cells and remove waste from cells.
2. They provide a medium in which chemical reactions can occur.

Body fluids serve as a universal solvent to create solutions of various substances. In a diseased state, an overproduction or underproduction of any substance disrupts this balance, which can prolong the recovery phase and ultimately the total hospitalization time.

The body maintains homeostasis through the movement of liquids and solutes from one compartment to another (a process called *diffusion*), allowing the fluids to nourish and maintain all the cells and tissues of the body.

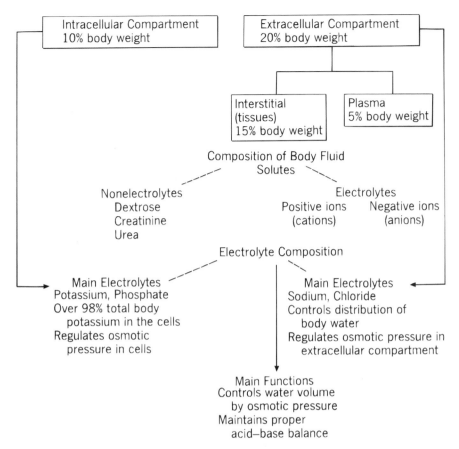

Fig. 7-1. Fluid compartments and composition (Adapted from Travenol Labs, Inc. Fundamentals of Body Water and Electrolyte. Deerfield, IL, 1974.)

Measurement of Fluid Status

Osmolar imbalances involve disturbances in osmolarity and therefore in water distribution in fluid compartments in the body. Water always moves from an area of lesser solute concentration to an area of greater solute concentration until both are equal.

A clinical measure of osmolarity in the body is the measurement of the solute sodium in the serum. An elevated serum sodium level indicates *hyperosmolarity* (water-deficit syndrome) and conversely, a lowered serum sodium level indicates *hypoosmolarity* (water-excess syndrome).

Additionally, measurement of intravascular fluid status can be accomplished by the *hematocrit* level, which is a volume percentage of red blood cells and other solids (WBC, platelets, and so on) in whole blood, determined by centrifuging the blood sample to separate the cellular elements from the plasma. The test results indicate the ratio of cell volume to plasma volume, differentiating *hypovolemia* and *hypervolemia*.

For example, a hematocrit (Hct) level of 40 percent signifies that 40 percent of the total blood volume is cell and 60 percent is plasma (fluid).

Fluid Compartments

The body is divided into two major fluid compartments (Fig. 7-1):

1. Intracellular (ICF)—found within the cell
2. Extracellular (ECF)—contained outside the cell

Intracellular Fluid

The ICF is the largest compartment, accounting for 50 percent of total body weight (Fig. 7-2).

Because of the larger muscle mass in males, the percentage of total body weight that is ICF is somewhat greater than that in females. In a newborn infant, the proportion is approximately three fifths intracellular and two fifths extracellular. This ratio changes and reaches adult levels by the time the infant is about 30 months old.

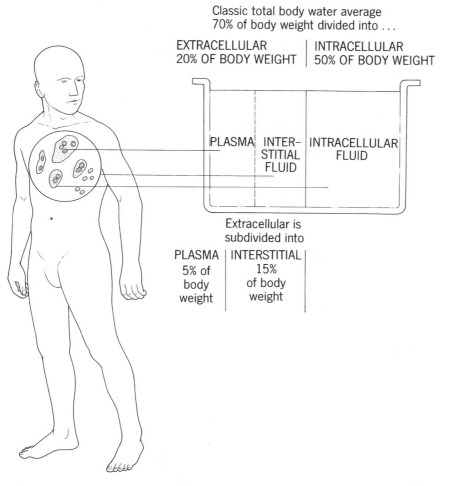

Fig. 7-2. Fluid spaces/compartments within the body (Adapted from Travenol Labs, Inc. Fundamentals of Body Water and Electrolyte. Deerfield, IL, 1974.)

Extracellular Fluid

The extracellular fluid (ECF) accounts for 20 percent of total body weight, and is divided into two additional sections:

1. *Interstitial fluid* contained in the spaces between the cells (15 percent).
2. *Intravascular fluid* contained within the blood vessels; that is, plasma (5 percent).

There is one additional fluid compartment, the *transcellular compartment*, which some scientists classify as part of the ICF. It includes the fluid found in joints, peritoneal and pleural cavities, the cerebrospinal fluid, fluid in the chambers of the eye, and secretions of the gastrointestinal system. Analysis of this system may assist the anesthesia clinician in tracing lost electrolytes and prescribing proper replacement therapy.

Fluid and Electrolyte Disturbances

Fluid and electrolyte imbalances occurring in an ill patient are serious complications that can threaten life. The correction of these imbalances is vital. Knowledge of the endocrine responses to stressors assists the perioperative nurse and anesthesia practitioner to achieve a better understanding of imbalances and problems associated with them.

Endocrine Response to Stress

The endocrine controls are affected by stress. At times, stress from preoperative apprehension triggers an undesirable endocrine response, making it necessary to postpone an operation.

Apprehension, pain, and duration and severity of trauma give rise to surgical stressors and cause an increased endocrine response during the first 2 to 5 days after surgery.

Because these stress reactions are normal, correction is often unnecessary and correction may in fact be harmful, yet the patient must be monitored for unforeseen complications.

Two major endocrine controls directly affected by stress are the *pituitary gland* and the *adrenal gland.*

The posterior pituitary controls quantitative secretions of antidiuretic hormone (ADH), while the anterior pituitary controls secretions of adrenocorticotropic hormone (ACTH). The latter stimulates the adrenal gland, producing an increase of mineralocorticoids (aldosterone) and glucocorticoids (hydrocortisone). The adrenal medulla secretes vasopressors (epinephrine and norepinephrine) to help maintain blood pressure.

A direct physiologic effect is produced when stress increases the secretions of these various hormones. When the posterior pituitary increases ADH secretions, antidiuresis is produced, thus helping maintain blood volume. When the anterior pituitary increases ACTH secretions, the adrenal gland is stimulated to increase the secretion of aldosterone and hydrocortisone. These two adrenal hormones help maintain blood volume by (1) causing the kidneys to retain sodium and chloride, resulting in water retention, and (2) promoting the excretion of potassium. There is also a shift between the intracellular-extracellular space, the direction of which depends on the relative osmolarity of each space and the presence of ADH.

Hydrocortisone also promotes the breakdown of proteins to provide the necessary amino acids for healing in addition to stimulating the conversion of protein and fat to glucose for energy production during the stressful period (Fig. 7-3).

Therapeutic Considerations

Abnormalities of body fluids and electrolyte metabolism present certain therapeutic problems.

When the mechanisms normally regulating fluid volume, electrolyte composition, and osmolarity are impaired, therapy becomes complicated. An understanding of these metabolic abnormalities enables the nurses and physicians caring for the patient during the perioperative period to manage the patient with greater efficiency.

Regulation of Body Fluids

Certain organs assist in the maintenance of body fluid and electrolyte balance.

The lungs and skin are important monitors, but the kidneys are the main body fluid regulators. They con-

trol the ECF compartment by regulating concentration of particles (osmolarity), volume of ECF, blood volume, and blood pH.

In addition, the GI tract, heart, blood vessels, pituitary gland, adrenal glands, and parathyroid glands are part of this fluid and electrolyte regulation mechanism.

Types of Body Fluids

Fluids within the body are *isotonic*—that is, the concentration of dissolved particles (tonicity) is equal to that of the intracellular fluid in a dynamic and constantly changing state.

When an isotonic solution (IV or irrigation) is used, it causes no net movement of water across the cell membrane, thus maintaining the osmotic pressure within the cell. Because this pressure remains the same, the cell does not change in size (Ex. 0.45 NS). However, when external fluids (i.e., *hypertonic* or *hypotonic* fluids) are introduced, changes can occur that can cause an imbalanced state.

Hypertonic Fluids

Hypertonic fluids are those with a greater tonicity than that of the intracellular fluid. When this type of solution is infused into the body, water will rush out of the cell, causing the cell to shrink *(crenation).* Examples include D_5LR; $D_{10}W$, or 3% saline solutions. Dehydration can also produce the same effect.

Hypotonic Fluids

Hypotonic fluid has less tonicity than the intracellular fluid, and when water surrounds the cell, the water will diffuse into the cell, causing the cell to swell to the point of bursting *(hemolysis).* Inappropriate use of IV or irrigation solutions, or severe electrolyte loss, as in severe diarrhea with tap water replacement, will cause the body to become hypotonic. Examples include 0.45 NS or 2.5% dextrose in water.

Fluid Imbalances

Fluid imbalances are presented in Table 7-1.

Hypovolemia

Description
Low fluid volume in ECF compartment

Possible Causes
- decreased water intake
- excessive vomiting/diarrhea

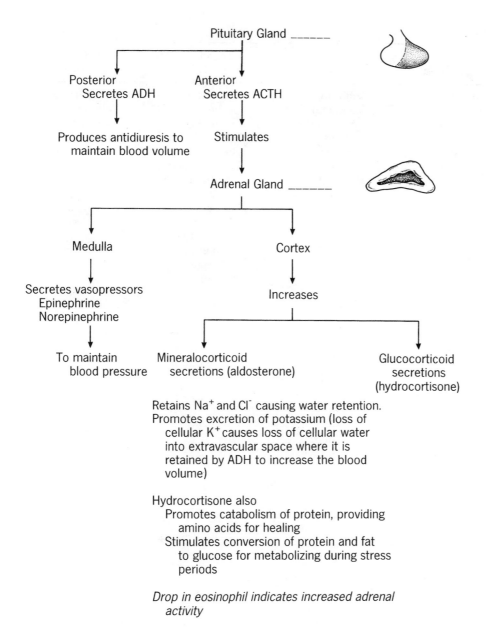

Fig. 7-3. Endocrine response to stress (Adapted from Bullock, B., and Rosendahl, P. *Pathophysiology: Adaptation and Alteration in Function.* [3rd ed.]. Philadelphia: Lippincott, 1984.)

- systematic infection leading to an increase in body temperature
- fistulous drainage
- intestinal obstruction
- burns; salt water drowning
- bleeding
- increased ADH

Laboratory Findings

Increased Hct, hemoglobin (Hgb), and red blood cells (RBCs)

Serum: hypertonic (specific gravity [SG] increased)

Decreased cardiac output

Decreased central venous pressure (CVP); pulmonary artery pressure (PAP)

Chlorides: absent from urine (if renal function is normal)

Signs and Symptoms
- dry skin and mucous membranes
- oliguria/anuria
- increased temperature
- decreased blood pressure (BP)
- increased heart rate

Table 7-1   Summary of Fluid Imbalance

Substance	Function	Gains	Losses	Effects of Too Little	Effects of Too Much
Water	Medium of body fluids Allows chemical changes Regulates body temperature Lubricant	Ingested H$_2$O Ingested food Tube feedings Parenteral fluids Rectal feedings Oxidation of food	Vomiting Ventilation Wound exudate Suction Perspiration Internal pooling Paracentesis Thoracentesis Colitis Urine Interstitial pooling	Concentrated urine Oliguria Thirst Fever Increased serum sodium Circulatory failure Flushed dry skin Poor skin turgor Increased Hct, blood urea nitrogen, creatinine	Dilute urine Polyuria Headache Confusion Nausea, vomiting Weakness Muscle cramps Muscle twitching Convulsions Decreased sodium concentration in serum and Hct Increased intracranial pressure

Therapy
- provide both water and electrolytes to compensate for loss
- insert a CVP line to prevent overload during replacement therapy

Hypervolemia

Description
High fluid volume in the ECF compartment

Possible Causes
- congestive heart failure
- excessive ACTH therapy
- excessive ingestion or infusion of sodium chloride
- renal disease (portal hypertension/chronic kidney disease)
- acute respiratory failure/fluid shift
- "near" drowning

Laboratory Findings
decreased Hct, Hgb, and RBCs
Serum: hypotonic
decreased cardiac output
increased osmolarity
increased CVP; PAP

Signs and Symptoms
- pitting edema
- moist rales in lungs
- puffy eyelids
- dyspnea
- bounding pulse
- increased BP

Therapy
- remove excess sodium and water from plasma through diuretic therapy
- reduce sodium chloride intake

Self-assessment Exercise 13

Directions: Complete the following exercises. Answers are given at the end of this module.

1. The body fluid compartments consist of the

   _____ located within the cell, and the

   _____ located outside the cell.

2. Interstitial fluid is located within the

   _____ compartment, and accounts for

   _____ of total body water.

3. When body fluid has a concentration of dissolved

particles equal to that of the intracellular fluid, it is referred to as a *hypotonic state.*

True   False

4. An example of a *hypertonic* fluid would be

   _____. What would this do to the cell?

   _____

5. Body fluids are called the *universal solvent.*

True   False

SOLUTES AND ELECTROLYTES

Two types of solutes can be found in body fluids:
1. *Nonelectrolytes* molecules that do not break down when placed in water (e.g., glucose, urea, creatine)
2. *Electrolytes* molecules that split into charged particles *(ions)* when placed in water. Some molecules develop a positive charge *(cations)*, while the others develop a negative charge *(anions)* (e.g., Sodium [Na^+], Potassium [K^+], Calcium [Ca^{++}], Chloride [Cl^-]).

Electrolytes are related to four fundamental physiologic functions: (1) water distribution and maintenance, (2) osmotic pressure regulation, (3) neuromuscular irritability, and (4) acid–base balance.

Normal Electrolyte Distribution

In each fluid compartment, various electrolytes balance each other to achieve neutrality, but when a disease condition or trauma (such as surgery) occurs, the fluid, electrolyte, and acid–base regulation is disturbed, creating an imbalanced state.

Since surgical patients are under a great deal of stress, which can produce physiologic and metabolic changes, the electrolyte status of the patient becomes an important assessment tool during the perioperative period.

The normal plasma concentration of electrolytes is 154 cations and 154 anions, measured in milliequivalents (mEq) per liter (Fig. 7-4).

Carbonic acid plays a major role, since it represents the combination of carbon dioxide and water.

The cations Na^+, K^+, Ca^{++}, and Mg^{++}, unite with the anion bicarbonate to form base bicarbonate, and as long as the ratio of 1 mEq of carbonic acid to 20 mEq of base bicarbonate is maintained, the hydrogen ion (pH) remains neutral.

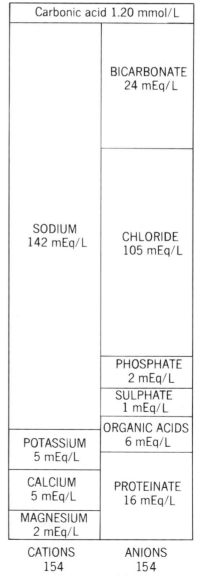

Fig. 7-4. Electrolyte distribution in extracellular fluids

Table 7-2   Electrolyte Profiles

Substance	Function	Gains	Losses	Effects of Too Little	Effects of Too Much
Sodium (Na$^+$)	Osmotic pressure Muscle and nerve irritability (aldosterone)	Ingestion of high Na$^+$ foods Parenteral solutions Decreased intake of H$_2$O	Diuretics Decreased intake of Na$^+$ Perspiration Gastric suction Intestinal suction Increased intake of H$_2$O	Hypotension Nausea, vomiting Diarrhea Anxiety Abdominal cramps Anuria	Dry, sticky mucous membranes Intense thirst Fever Oliguria/anuria Agitation, restlessness Convulsions
Potassium (K$^+$)	Intracellular fluid balance Regulates heart rhythm Muscle and nerve irritability Cholesterol and protein metabolism	Leakage from cells into vascular bed following trauma Oral ingestion Renal disease Metabolic acidosis Addison's disease	Decreased K$^+$ intake Diarrhea Diuretics GI surgery Perspiration Fever Wound exudate Metabolic alkalosis	Apathy, lethargy Muscle weakness Nausea Tachycardia Cardiac/ respiratory failure EKG changes	Muscle weakness Nausea Colic Diarrhea EKG changes Oliguria/anuria
Calcium (Ca^{++})	Muscle contraction Regulates heart rhythm Nerve irritability Blood clotting Growth (parathyroid hormone)	Milk intake Parathyroid dysfunction Vitamin D intake	Diarrhea Wound exudate Pancreatitis Burns Massive transfusion	Tingling, numbness Tetany Muscle cramps Convulsions Pathologic fractures Softening of bones	Relaxed muscles Flank pain/ kidney stones Cardiac arrest Nausea, vomiting Stupor, coma
Magnesium (Mg^{++})	Activates enzyme system Nerve irritability Utilization of K$^+$, protein, calcium	Renal disease Administration of magnesium supplements Dialysis Addison's hyperparathy- roidism	Alcoholism Liver disease Gastric suction Diabetes Renal disease Diuresis	Tremor-tetany Athetoid movements Convulsions Confusion Hallucinations Tachycardia Hypertension	Lethargy, coma Respiratory problems Death Decreased deep tendon reflexes Dysrhythmias
Chloride (Cl$^-$)	Osmotic pressure Acid-base balance Ion transport	Obtained through sodium chloride (table salt)	Prolonged vomiting Gastric suctioning	Metabolic alkalosis	
Phosphorus (PO$_4^=$)	Building of bones, teeth Buffer system Transport of fatty acids Metabolism of fats and carbohydrates (parathyroid hormone)	Obtained through practically all foods	TPN therapy which does not contain phosphates	Poor mineralization of bones Rickets Lethargy; abnormal respiratory patterns	Tetany, hypocalcemia
Bicarbonate (HCO$_3^-$)	Acid–base balance	GI suction with loss of chloride ions Ingestion of baking soda Administration of ACTH	Renal disease Diabetic acidosis Infection Salicylate intoxication Ketogenic diet	Metabolic acidosis Deep rapid breathing Weakness Disorientation Coma	Hypertonicity of muscles Tetany Depressed respiration Metabolic alkalosis

If the electrolyte value changes, so too does the acid–base value of the plasma change, creating an acidotic or alkalotic state, depending on the changes in the system.

Primary Electrolytes for the Surgical Patient

Whenever tissue is injured or invaded by foreign organisms, a complex set of processes begin to protect the organism from imbalance, including the regulation of electrolytes and fluids in the major body compartments (Table 7-2).

Following surgical trauma, there is a period when capillary permeability is increased, and during this period fluid and electrolytes escape from the vascular space and produce edema and electrolyte imbalances. Several liters can be lost into the ISF, especially with extensive surgical procedures.

Sodium, potassium, chloride, calcium, and bicarbonate are the major electrolytes involved with the stress of surgery and the administration of anesthetic agents.

Sodium (Na⁺)

Sodium is the major extracellular cation comprising more than 90 percent of the total cation concentration. Sodium balance is integrated with regulation of extracellular fluid volume.

Normal Range
135 to 145 mEq/L.

Physiologic Functions:
- Body fluid control associated with hormonal secretion of ADH
- Conduction of nerve impulses and muscle contraction
- Because of its dominance in quantity, any appreciable changes in total cations represent a change in sodium
- When Na^+ is lost or retained, it is reciprocally accompanied by water and potassium

Major Disturbances
Hyponatremia
- ECF, concentration of Na^+ < 136 mEq/L
- Occurrence: reduced, normal, or expanded ECF volume, loss of Na^+ through the kidneys (renal disease, diuretics), adrenal insufficiency
Hypernatremia
- ECF concentration of Na^+ > 145 mEq/L
- Occurrence: loss of hypoosmotic fluid, infusion of fluids high in sodium, cellular dehydration, infu-

sion of $NaHCO_3$, renal loss, diabetes insipidus, stress

Potassium (K⁺)

Potassium is the major intracellular cation in the ICF fluid compartment. It is the only electrolyte with no mechanism of retention, so to maintain the potassium balance and consistent concentration levels in ECF, the excretion of potassium must be equal to the intake.

Normal Range
3.5 to 5.5 mEq/L

Physiologic Functions
- Plays a major role in regulating the excitability of nerve and muscle cell membranes
- Controls cellular osmotic pressure
- Activates enzyme reactions, and maintains special cell polarization/repolarization in cardiac muscle
- Reciprocal relationship between Na^+ and K^+ intake of large amounts of Na^+ results in an increased loss of K^+, and vice versa
- Entrance of K^+ into the cells depends on normal metabolism and glucose utilization

Major Disturbances
Hypokalemia
- Plasma K^+ concentration < 3.5 mEq/L
- Occurrence: increased cellular uptake, excessive renal excretion and gastrointestinal losses, acid–base imbalances, malnutrition
Hyperkalemia
- Plasma K^+ concentration > 5.5 mEq/L
- Occurrence: excessive intake of K^+, increased cell lysis, altered cellular uptake and decreased renal excretion (renal failure)

Calcium (Ca⁺⁺)

Calcium has many important functions in the body. Ninety-nine percent of it is found in bone. Calcium provides the major source for the development and maintenance of structure and function of the musculoskeletal system.

Normal Range
8.8 to 10.5 mg/100 mL Ca^{++} is the only electrolyte measured in milligrams; approximately half in ionized form. Calcium may also be measured in the mEq system, but milligram is more frequently used.

Physiologic Functions
- Maintains structure/function of cell membranes
- Involved as ionized Ca^{++} in normal clotting of blood

- Exerts a sedative effect on the nerve cells
- Vitamin D plays an important role in absorption of calcium (most intestinal absorption occurs in the duodenum and jejunum)
- Key role in activation of excitation–contraction coupling in muscles

Major Disturbances

Hypocalcemia
- Serum Ca^{++} concentration < 8 mg
- Occurrence: vitamin D deficiency, thyroid and parathyroid disease, acute pancreatitis, alkalosis (pH > 7.5), chelating agent infusion (citrate in whole blood to prevent coagulation)

Hypercalcemia
- Serum Ca^{++} concentration < 10.5 mg
- Occurrence: hyperparathyroidism, hyperthyroidism, adrenal insufficiency, neoplasia, excessive vitamin D intake, excessive Ca^{++} intake (antacids/bicarbonate)

Chloride (Cl^-)

Sodium and chloride are handled in a parallel fashion in the body, and tend to preserve osmotic pressure and water balance.

Normal Range
100 to 106 mEq/L

Physiologic Functions
- Major extracellular anion found in ISF and lymph
- Deficiency of either Cl^- or K^+ will lead to a deficit of the other
- Assists in maintaining fluid neutrality (both with osmotic pressure and body fluids)
- Aids in buffering action of O_2 and CO_2 exchange in the red blood cell and ion transport
- Aids in promotion of the chloride shift
- Involved in Na^+ reabsorption mechanism in the kidney to maintain osmolarity ("chloride pump")

Major Disturbances
Hypochloremia
- Serum chloride level < 100 mEq/L
- Occurrence: common component of metabolic alkalosis, prolonged vomiting/gastric suctioning

Hyperchloremia
- Serum chloride level > 105 mEq/L
- Occurrence: rare, but can occur in coma states, severe/uncorrected dehydration, hyperventilation, renal insufficiency, and overtreatment with NaCl solutions

Self-assessment Exercise 14

Directions: Complete the following exercises. Answers are given at the end of this module.

1. Electrolytes are electrically charged ions. A positively charged ion is called a(n) _____ and a negatively charged ion is a(n) _____.

2. The major cation found in the intracellular fluid compartments is _____, with a normal range between _____ and _____.

3. In controlling distribution of body fluids, the cation _____ plays a major role.

4. This cation provides the foundation for normal blood clotting at the capillary level:

    _____.

5. This cation is responsible for stimulating the polarizing/repolarization of cardiac muscle and is directly related to sodium: _____.

6. This anion is considered the major buffering agent for the system (_____). Its normal value in an arterial sample is _____.

Acid–Base Balance and Disturbances

For optimal functioning of the cells, metabolic processes maintain a steady balance between acids and bases. Arterial pH is an indirect measurement of the hydrogen ion (H^+) concentration, and is a reflection of the balance between carbon dioxide (CO_2), which is regulated by the lungs, and bicarbonate (HCO_3^-) a base buffer regulated by the kidneys.

During the perioperative period, values derived from blood gas analysis (ABG reports) become clear only when one has a thorough understanding of the physiology of the transport and movement of oxygen and carbon dioxide between the lungs and peripheral tissue.

As previously mentioned, a variety of stressors are working during the perioperative period, and these stressors produce metabolic changes that can be directly related to acid–base disturbances, in addition to fluid and electrolyte imbalances. This, coupled with the administration of anesthetic agents and the trauma of surgery, places the patient in a vicarious position which if not prevented and/or corrected could produce unfavorable results, even death.

The ABG report usually consists of the following components:

*   arterial oxygen tension—Pa_{O_2}
*   arterial carbon dioxide tension—Pa_{CO_2}
*   overall hydrogen ion concentration—pH
*   bicarbonate concentration—HCO_3^-
*   base excess—BE
*   oxygen saturation percentage—O_2 sat.

Normal Values of Arterial Blood

When analyzing arterial blood gas values, the following values are considered to be within normal range:

O_2 sat.	95 percent or greater
P_{O_2}	80–100 mm Hg
P_{CO_2}	35–45 mm Hg (dissolved CO_2 in blood)
pH	7.40 (7.35–7.45)
HCO_3^-	22–26 mEq/L
BE	−2 to +2

Physiology of Acid–Base Balance

Acid–base balance has a respiratory and a metabolic component. During normal metabolic processes, which primarily constitute aerobic metabolism, the body produces two forms of acids:

1. respiratory (volatile and carbonic) acids
2. metabolic acids

Carbon dioxide when combined with water forms carbonic acid (H_2CO_3). Carbonic acid is a volatile acid that is excreted by the lungs. Carbonic acid (CO_2 + H_2O) can also be produced by the combination of bicarbonate (HCO_3^-) with hydrogen ions (H^+), which are in a mass dynamic equilibrium (CO_2 + $H_2O \rightleftharpoons H^+$ + HCO_3^-).

The other acids, termed *metabolic acids,* are of a larger molecular size and normally are derived from intermediate metabolism of amino acids, fats, and carbohydrates. In addition, there are inorganic phosphoric and sulfuric acids, which are all excreted by the kidneys.

In the absence of adequate tissue oxygenation, lactic acid cannot be metabolized. Its quantity thus increases and the result is *metabolic acidosis.*

The oxygen content (carried by hemoglobin and dissolved in plasma), depends on the arterial oxygen tension (Pa_{O_2}) and the hemoglobin level.

If hypoxemia is present, it must be corrected, since a reduction of Pa_{O_2} can cause an acid–base abnormality.

Buffer System

A buffer system consists of a weak acid and the salt of that weak acid (or *base*). This innate defense system prevents marked changes in the acidity of the body.

The most important buffer system is the sodium bicarbonate and carbonic acid system, consisting of the salt of the weak acid ($NaHCO_3$) and a weak base (H_2CO_3), because it is regulated by the lungs and kidneys.

As oxygen is unloaded from the hemoglobin to the tissues, CO_2 is entering the circulation, and can be carried and buffered by the hemoglobin. Thus, an important function of hemoglobin is to act as a buffer, and it is considered the single most powerful buffer in plasma.

Hydrogen Ion Concentration

Hydrogen ion concentration is expressed as *pH.* It is an expression of the relationship between the base and the acid, normally 20 parts base to 1 part acid.

The normal pH is 7.40 (7.35–7.45). Thus, a pH less than 7.35 describes *acidosis,* while a pH in excess of 7.45 denotes *alkalosis;* a reflection of how well the buffer system is responding to change (Fig. 7-5).

In addition to pH, the other component essential for

the correct assessment of acid–base disturbance is the Pa_{CO_2}. The Pa_{CO_2} provides an important measure of the adequacy of the patient's ventilation. As ventilations increase, the Pa_{CO_2} decreases and conversely, as ventilations decrease, the Pa_{CO_2} increases.

Therefore, elevation of the carbon dioxide component (>45 mm Hg) is termed *hypercapnia* and constitutes *respiratory acidosis* (hypoventilation), while a decrease in carbon dioxide (<35 mm Hg) is termed *hypocapnia* and constitutes *respiratory alkalosis* (hyperventilation) (Table 7-3).

Base Excess

Base excess, another component of the ABG report, denotes the amount of strong base or acid per liter of blood, and is expressed as a negative or positive value.

General Assessment: Acidosis/Alkalosis

Acidotic State
- CNS depression
- decreased cell activity
- headache, lethargy, nausea and vomiting
- disorientation, coma, death

Alkalotic State
- CNS overexcitability
- fidgeting, twitching, tremors
- confusion, tetany
- convulsions, death
  (See Table 7-4, p. 126)

Interpreting Blood Gas Reports

In order to prescribe the correct therapy for acid–base imbalance, knowing how to interpret ABG reports is essential.

General Laboratory Values

Respiratory Acidosis
pH	<7.35
P_{CO_2}	>45 (increased P_{CO_2}, decreased respirations)
HCO_3^-	within normal limits (WNL)
BE	2.5

Metabolic Acidosis
pH	<7.35
P_{CO_2}	within normal limits (WNL) (respiratory system not primary)
HCO_3^-	<22 mEq/L
BE	negative (lost bicarbonate)

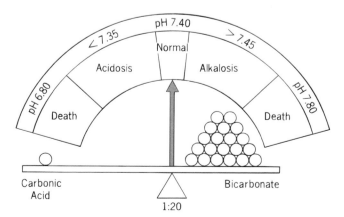

Fig. 7-5. Acid–base relationship

Table 7-3   Clinical Manifestations of Acid–Base Disturbances

Condition	CNS	Neuromuscular	Cardiac	Respiratory

Respiratory alkalosis	Vertigo
	Syncope
	Nervousness
	Seizures
	Decreased mentation
	Confusion
	Anxiety
		Paresthesia
		Muscle cramps
		Tetany
		Decreased
		  psychomotor
		  function
			Arrhythmia
			Hypotension
				Dyspnea
				Hypoventilation

Metabolic alkalosis	Seizures Belligerence Confusion Stupor Coma	Irritability Tetany	Dysrhythmia	Hypoventilation
Respiratory acidosis	Decreased mentation Apprehension Restlessness Drowsiness Disorientation Coma	Fatigue Muscle weakness Flapping tremors Uncoordination Reflexes	Tachycardia Cyanosis	Hyperventilation Dyspnea
Metabolic acidosis	Drowsiness Decreased mentation Confusion Coma Seizures	Fatigue	Hypotension Hypoxia Dysrhythmia	Kussmaul respirations

Respiratory Alkalosis

pH	>7.45
P_{CO_2}	<35 (decreased CO_2, increased respirations)
HCO_3^-	WNL
BE	2.5

Metabolic Alkalosis

pH	>7.45
P_{CO_2}	WNL (respiratory system not primary)
HCO_3^-	>26 mEq/L
BE	positive

Differentiating Acidosis from Alkalosis

Arterial blood gas values are reported to the surgical team, and corrections are made accordingly. But how do you interpret these values to determine whether the disturbance is respiratory or metabolic; acidosis or alkalosis?

These simple steps may make interpretation easier:

1. Determine whether the pH is acid (<7.35) or alkaline (>7.45)
2. Evaluate the respiratory component:
    if P_{CO_2} is greater than 45: acid
    if P_{CO_2} is less than 35: alkaline
3. Evaluate the metabolic component
    if HCO_3^- is less than 22: acid
    if HCO_3^- is greater than 26: alkaline

4. To diagnose, match term by the pH with the same term by either the P_{CO_2} or the HCO_3^-

EXAMPLE: pH 7.34 acid
P_{CO_2} 48 acid
HCO_3^- 25 WNL

Diagnosis: Respiratory Acidosis

The respiratory, cardiovascular, and urinary systems interact to maintain a homeostatic state, both in health and during illness. However, with proper intervention, these systems need not become imbalanced or can be corrected before a more serious consequence can develop during the perioperative period.

Perioperative Nursing Implications

Although the ultimate management of fluids and electrolytes and acid–base balance is part of the total anesthesia care, the perioperative nurse should have a working knowledge of the disturbances and how to prevent/correct them.

By carefully assessing the patient, the perioperative nurse can anticipate potential problems and therefore be of greater assistance to the anesthesia practitioner during the intraoperative period.

Table 7-4   Summary Sheet: Acidosis/Alkalosis

Condition	Definition	Probable Cause	Recognition	Laboratory Tests	Sample Lab Test: Uncompensated	Sample Lab Test: Compensated
Metabolic Acidosis	Excess of acid (H^+) and deficit of base (HCO_3^-)	Ketoacidosis, incomplete metabolism of fats (diabetes), renal acidosis, retention of inorganic phosphoric and sulfuric acids (renal failure), lactic acidosis, incomplete metabolism of CHO, (HCO_3^- deficit, diarrhea	Headache, nausea, vomiting, diarrhea, sensorium changes, tremoring, convulsions	pH < 7.35 Serum CO_2 < 22 mEq/L Pco_2 > 40 mm Hg if compensating Po_2 usually normal Serum K^+ elevated	pH 7.15 Pco_2 40 Po_2 88 (HCO_3^- 8 (HCO/H_2CO_3 ratio is 8:1)	pH 7.35 Pco_2 24 Po_2 88 HCO_3 8 (lungs "blow off" CO_2 by hyperventilation to decrease acids)
Respiratory Acidosis	Excess of acid (H_2CO_3) and elevated Pco_2	Hypoventilation: retention of CO_2 (i.e., COPD), muscular weakness	Decreased ventilation, sensorium changes, somnolence, semicomatose-comatose, tachycardia, arrhythmia	pH < 7.35 Serum CO_2 > 27 mEq/L if compensating Pco_2 > 40 mm Hg Po_2 usually normal or low Serum K^+ elevated	pH 7.15 Pco_2 60 Po_2 88 (HCO_3^- 24 ((HCO_3^-/H_2CO_3 ratio is 13:1)	pH 7.35 Pco_2 60 Po_2 88 (HCO_3^- 39 (kidneys hold HCO_3^- to neutralize H_2CO_3)
Metabolic Alkalosis	Deficit of H^+ and excess of base (HCO_3^-)	Gastric losses via vomiting, stomach tube, lavage, potent diuretics	Nausea, vomiting, diarrhea, sensorium changes, tremoring, convulsions	pH > 7.45 Serum CO_2 > 27 mEq/L Pco_2 > 40 if compensating Po_2 usually normal Serum K^+ decreased Serum chloride decreased	pH 7.52 Pco_2 40 Po_2 88 (HCO_3^- 36 ((HCO_3^-/H_2CO_3 ratio is 30:1)	pH 7.45 Pco_2 55 Po_2 88 (HCO_3^- 36 (lungs retain CO_2 by hypoventilation to increase acids)
Respiratory Alkalosis	Deficit of carbonic acid (H_2CO_3)	Hyperventilation from neurogenic cause, brain trauma, ventilators	Tachypnea, sensorium changes, numbness, tingling of hands and face	pH > 7.45 Serum CO_2 < 22 mEq/L if compensating Po_2 > 40 mm Hg Po_2 usually normal Serum K^+ decreased Urine alkaline	pH 7.52 Pco_2 24 Po_2 88 (HCO_3^- 24 (HCO_3^-/H_2CO_3 ratio is 40:1)	pH 7.45 Pco_2 24 Po_2 88 HCO_3^- 15 (kidneys excrete (HCO_3^- and retain H^+ ions)

Preoperative Assessment

1. Collection of data regarding:
   a. nutritional status
   b. GI, renal, cardiovascular, and respiratory systems
   c. general health
   d. current medications
2. Review of laboratory values, including CBC, electrolyte profiles, hematology studies, and ABG report
3. Assessment of psychologic status, coping mechanisms, support systems, and current therapies/treatments

Intraoperative Phase

Specific factors affecting the fluid, electrolyte, and acid–base balances include:

1. IV fluid administration of nonelectrolyte/electrolyte solutions
2. General anesthetic agents
   a. alter respiratory status and can predispose to cardiac arrhythmias related to retention of CO_2 and potassium loss
3. Regional anesthesia
   Spinal: possibly reduce urine volume output, creating hypervolemia (highly unlikely)
   Epidural: can increase urine volume output, sacrificing potassium and creating a hypovolemic state
4. Temperature control
   a. depression of heat-regulating mechanism can produce an increase in O_2 consumption and vasodilation and potentiate an acid–base disturbance
5. Positioning
   a. immobility causes body fluids to pool (shunt) and impair circulation, resulting in venous stasis and pressure in dependent positions

Monitoring Intraoperative Homeostatic Status

The following recommendations may help to prevent complications from hemodynamic disturbances:

1. Preoperative education to reduce stress levels
2. Proper positioning with supportive aids padding bony prominences; providing adequate support devices; maintaining near proper alignment
3. Use of pulse oximeter (measurement of O_2 saturation at tissue levels)
4. Hemodynamic monitoring for long or complicated cases, especially those involved with the cardiorespiratory systems
5. Accurate measurement of blood loss and urinary output during the procedure
6. Periodic measurement of intravascular status: Hct and Hgb; CBC; ABG; chemistry profiles

The perioperative nurse has an important role in performing functions that can assist the anesthesia practitioner in maintaining fluid, electrolyte, and acid–base balance; therefore, he or she should be able to:

1. Reduce stress through preoperative teaching programs and ongoing intraoperative supportive measures
2. Collaborate with anesthesia personnel by anticipating specific needs for the planned surgical procedure, and work as a team to provide quality patient care
3. Anticipate changes due to external and internal stressors and plan accordingly
4. Recognize imbalances and interventions needed to correct the disturbances
5. Accurately record patient's hemodynamic status (I & O; fluid/blood loss; amount of irrigation; etc.)

Self-assessment Exercise 15

Directions: Complete the following exercises. Answers are given at the end of this module.

1. The arterial blood analysis, representing the ventilatory component, is the _____.

2. pH is the measurement of _____ _____ .

3. ABG values and their normal ranges are:

   1. _____

   2. _____

   3. _____

   4. _____

5. _____

6. _____

4. The primary metabolic parameter in the ABG value is the _____.

5. Describe the ABG values of a patient experiencing respiratory acidosis. _____

6. _____ is usually seen as a result of over-mechanical ventilation.

HEMODYNAMIC MONITORING

Invasive hemodynamic monitoring is used primarily to (1) evaluate left and right ventricular function, (2) assess fluid volume status, and (3) evaluate cardiovascular therapies.

Changes in hemodynamic measurements always precede changes in the patient's clinical status, and early detection using hemodynamic monitoring can prevent critical conditions from developing.

Hemodynamic monitoring can be performed by noninvasive techniques, such as noninvasive blood pressure monitoring, measurement of intake and output, and so on, or by an invasive technique through the insertion of a catheter that measures values of hemodynamic status.

Although most patients may not need the invasive monitoring technique, the perioperative nurse must be aware of normal values and be able to recognize any abnormal values being presented by the patient during the perioperative period.

Components of a Pressure Monitoring System

Any pressure monitoring system will contain a *transducer*, an *amplifier*, and a *display monitor.*

The transducer changes the mechanical energy from a pressure wave into electrical energy. This electrical energy travels through a wire to the amplifier, which enlarges the amplitude of the electrical signal from the pressure wave, filters out extraneous interference, and then sends this signal to the display monitor.

In addition, all pressure monitoring systems need a specialized catheter and a pressurized IV solution bag usually containing a heparinized solution (normal saline or D_5W), a continuous flushing device, and a rigid pressure-resistant catheter tubing with a Luer-Lock connection.

Understanding Hemodynamic Physiology

To understand the meaning of hemodynamic measurements, an understanding of cardiac function is essential. One approach to this understanding relates to cardiac output and its components.

Cardiac output is the amount of blood pumped by the heart in 1 minute. It can be defined further as the product of *heart rate* and *stroke volume* (the amount of blood pumped per heart beat).

Stroke volume is influenced by contractility, afterload, and preload. *Contractility* is the ability of the myocardium to generate force and contract. *Afterload* is a combination of forces that tend to resist ejection of blood by the ventricles, while *preload* is defined as ventricular end-diastolic volume or pressure.

To simplify, an increase in end-diastolic volume increases the stretch of the myocardium muscle fibers, allowing the ventricles to eject a greater volume of blood.

Measuring Cardiac Performance

When invasive monitoring is indicated, the central venous pressure (CVP) and Swan–Ganz catheters pro-

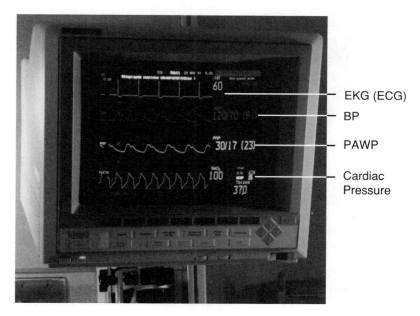

EKG (ECG)

BP

PAWP

Cardiac Pressure

Monitor screen displaying hemodynamic wave forms

vide the information needed about the physiologic status of the heart and vascular system.

Central venous pressure monitoring assesses fluid status and indicates pressure in the right atrium, which reflects right ventricular diastolic pressure. The normal CVP ranges from 5 to 10 cm of H_2O via manometer and 2 to 6 mm Hg via transducer when perfusion is adequate. If the patient became overhydrated, the CVP would rise and conversely, when there is a significant fluid loss, the CVP will fall. The CVP is measured from a catheter placed into the right atrium or superior vena cava (Fig. 7-6).

The Swan–Ganz catheter is a 4- or 5-lumen catheter, which can measure the pulmonary artery wedge pressure, left arterial pressure, and left ventricular end diastolic pressure, in addition to cardiac output and right-sided heart function (Fig. 7-6).

The catheter is inserted percutaneously into the internal jugular, subclavian, femoral, basilic, or brachial vein, and threaded toward the heart. As it passes through critical points, the monitor displays wave forms associated with each position so that the physician can determine exactly where the catheters is lying in relation to the pulmonary artery and ventricles (Fig. 7-7).

Normal Hemodynamic Values

Normal pressure readings include:

Pulmonary artery systolic	20–30 mm Hg
Pulmonary artery diastolic	<12 mm Hg
Mean pulmonary artery	<20 mm Hg
Pulmonary artery wedge pressure	4–12 mm Hg
Right atrium	2–6 mm Hg
Right ventricle	20–30 mm Hg (systolic)
	2–6 mm Hg (end diastolic)

Arterial Blood Pressure

Blood pressure can be monitored noninvasively (with a blood pressure cuff) or invasively via an arterial catheter inserted percutaneously into an artery (A-line).

Arterial wave forms consist of a systolic and diastolic component. Arterial pressure rises rapidly after the aortic valve opens during ventricular systole, and the wave form is usually in sync with the patient's ECG.

Pressure recorded in the peripheral arteries will have higher systolic and lower diastolic values than pressures recorded in the aortic arch. This change in systolic and diastolic pressures is caused by movement of blood through small elastic arteries, and because of the natural rise and fall of systolic and diastolic pressures, the mean pressure remains fairly constant regardless if the catheter is in a central or peripheral artery.

Hemodynamic Monitoring and Nursing Implications

One of the primary goals during surgery is careful and accurate assessment of the patient. Although hemodynamic monitoring is usually the responsibility of the anesthesia practitioner, the perioperative nurse should be aware of normal cardiac function and be able to

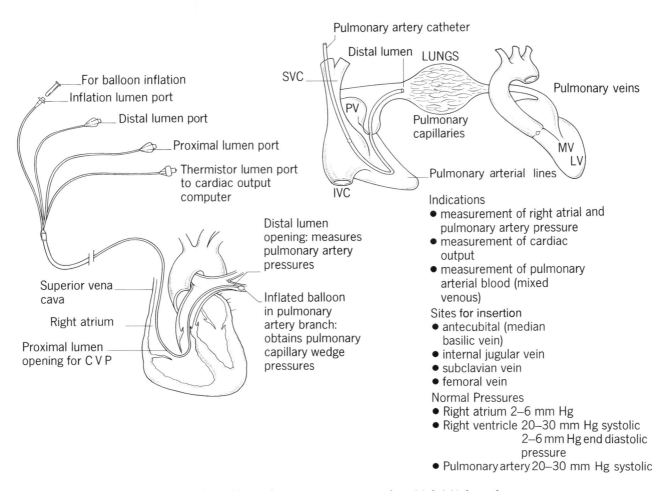

For balloon inflation
Inflation lumen port

Distal lumen port

Proximal lumen port

Thermistor lumen port
to cardiac output
computer

Superior vena
cava

Right atrium

Proximal lumen
opening for C V P

Distal lumen
opening: measures
pulmonary artery
pressures

Inflated balloon
in pulmonary
artery branch:
obtains pulmonary
capillary wedge
pressures

Pulmonary artery catheter

Distal lumen   LUNGS

SVC

PV

Pulmonary
capillaries

IVC

Pulmonary arterial lines

Pulmonary veins

MV
LV

Indications
● measurement of right atrial and
  pulmonary artery pressure
● measurement of cardiac
  output
● measurement of pulmonary
  arterial blood (mixed
  venous)

Sites for insertion
● antecubital (median
  basilic vein)
● internal jugular vein
● subclavian vein
● femoral vein

Normal Pressures
● Right atrium 2–6 mm Hg
● Right ventricle 20–30 mm Hg systolic
                 2–6 mm Hg end diastolic
                 pressure
● Pulmonary artery 20–30 mm Hg systolic

Fig. 7-6. Hemodynamic catheter (left) and hemodynamic monitoring valves (right) (Adapted from Datascope Corp. Teaching Materials for Principles of Hemodynamic Monitoring, Datascope Corp., Montvale, NJ.)

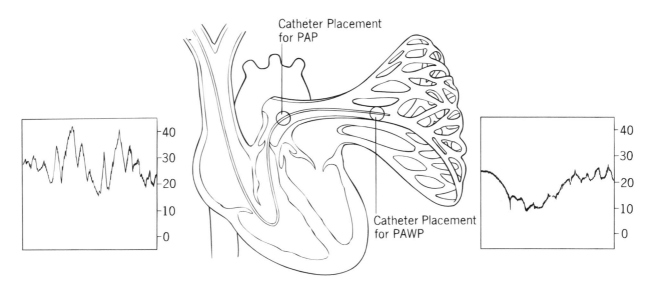

Catheter Placement
for PAP

Catheter Placement
for PAWP

Fig. 7-7. Catheter wave forms—hemodynamic monitoring

Table 7-5   Troubleshooting Monitoring Problems

Problem	Possible Causes	Action
Dampened arterial wave form resulting in abnormally low pressure readings	Catheter obstruction or clot at distal tip Air and/or leak in transducer and/or tubing Incorrect calibration or gain control	Flush line with Heparinized saline; check all connectors; recalibrate and check monitor settings; confirm appropriate transducer level
Arterial pressure tracing more than 20 mm Hg higher than cuff pressure	Catheter kinked or positioned against arterial wall Transducer not calibrated or zeroed correctly Transducer not at right atrial level	Check for kinks in tubing; reposition and splint arm/hand if needed; recalibrate and rezero
Pulmonary catheter will not "wedge" when balloon is inflated	Catheter has migrated out of position Insufficient air in balloon Balloon has ruptured	Assess location with x-ray/fluoroscopy and reposition; deflate and reinflate balloon slowly, if air placed in balloon is not recoverable, or if no resistance to inflation, catheter may require placement

recognize hemodynamic changes that accompany the physiologic stress associated with a disease state and/ or surgical intervention, to anticipate possible complications (see Table 7-6).

As with any therapy, invasive hemodynamic monitoring has definite advantages and disadvantages. Some of the advantages include:

- Earlier recognition of cardiogenic shock or disturbances in the fluid volume status
- Provision of accurate measurements of cardiac function for otherwise unstable patients or those undergoing extensive surgery
- Ability to detect minute changes in the physiologic status of the patient
- Provision of information as to the patient's response to drugs

Disadvantages might include:

- Risk of complications, such as bleeding, infection, vascular damage, or possibility of an embolism

- Need for proficiency in insertion techniques to prevent trauma and to monitor and interpret values
- Patient anxiety regarding the invasive technique and family anxiety seeing the multiple lines postoperatively without adequate explanation

Troubleshooting Possible Monitoring Problems

The perioperative nurse can assist in deciphering possible problems by understanding how the equipment functions (Table 7-5).

Hemodynamic monitoring offers a valuable tool for assessing and managing cardiac performance during the intraoperative period, and the perioperative nurse should be prepared to assist the physician or anesthesia practitioner during the insertion procedure in addition to recognizing the physiologic changes that may result through the use of invasive monitoring techniques (Table 7-6).

Table 7-6   Summary Chart: Hemodynamic Values and Clinical Problems

Etiology	Arterial Blood Pressure	Central Venous Pressure	Pulmonary Artery Pressures	Cardiac Index	Clinical Signs and Symptoms
Pulmonary congestion	Varies	Normal or increased	Increased, PAW > 18 mm Hg	Normal or decreased	Paroxysmal nocturnal dyspnea, shortness of breath, respiratory crackles found in dependent lung fields, dry hacking cough
Pulmonary edema	Normal or increased	Increased	Increased, PAW 25–30 mm Hg	Decreased	Frothy sputum, hemoptysis, dyspnea, orthopnea, diffuse rhonchi and crackles, S_3 and S_4 gallop
Cor pulmonale	Varies	Normal or increased	PAP normal or slightly increased, PAW normal PAW > 33/15 mm Hg PAEDP > PAW	Normal to decreased, increased	Chronic cough with sputum production, increasing dyspnea, pitting edema, occasionally ascites, distended neck veins, diffuse rhonchi and wheezes
Right ventricular dysfunction	Varies	Increased	PAP increased PAW low or normal	Decreased	Distended neck veins, ankle/leg edema, abdominal distention, nausea, sternal heave, increased numbers of premature atrial and ventricular beats, atrial fibrillation
Pulmonary embolus	Varies	Increased mean CVP > 6 mm Hg	PAW normal or low Mean PAP > 20 mm Hg PAEDP 5 mm Hg or more > PAW	Decreased, < 2.7 L/min/m²	Dry cough, pleuritic chest pain, hemoptysis, sudden dyspnea, apprehension, tachypnea, tachycardia
Acute mitral regurgitation	Decreased	Increased	Increased, large *v* waves in PAW	Decreased	Sudden onset of systolic murmur, heard best at cardiac apex; sudden onset of dyspnea and chest pain

(continued)

Table 7-6 (*continued*)

Etiology	Arterial Blood Pressure	Central Venous Pressure	Pulmonary Artery Pressures	Cardiac Index	Clinical Signs and Symptoms
Ventricular septal defect	Decreased	Increased	Increased	Decreased	Loud systolic murmur, sudden onset of dyspnea and chest pain
Myocardial ischemia	Normal or increased	Normal	PAW increased	Decreased	Angina pectoris, dyspnea
Hypovolemia	Normal or decreased	Normal or decreased	PAW decreased	Decreased	Postural hypotension, dry mucous membranes, lethargy, muscle cramps, elevated serum sodium
Increased SVR	Varies	Normal or increased	Increased	Decreased	Skin cool, pulses faint to palpation, audible blood pressure, significantly lower than direct blood pressure
Cardiac tamponade	Decreased	Increased	Increased CVP; PAEDP, PAW equalize	Decreased	Cyanotic discoloration of the neck, pulsus paradoxus, widened mediastinum present on X-ray
Left ventricular dysfunction	Decreased	Normal or increased	Increased	Decreased	Dyspnea, tachypnea, tachycardia, fatigue, crackles, S$_3$ gallop, distended neck veins
Cardiogenic shock	Decreased, systolic pressure below 90, or 30 mm Hg below normal	Increased or normal	PAW 15–30 mm Hg	Decreased < 2.0 L/ min/m^2	Dyspnea, tachypnea, cool, clammy skin, mental confusion, tachycardia, crackles, rhonchi, wheezes

Key: PAWP = pulmonary artery wedge pressure; PAP = pulmonary artery pressure; PAEDP = pulmonary artery end diastolic pressure; CVP = central venous pressure; SVR = systemic vascular resistance.
Source: Adapted from Datascope Corp. Teaching Materials for Principles of Hemodynamic Monitoring, Datascope Corp., Montvale, NJ.

Questions for Review for Module II

Directions: Complete the following questions. Answers are given at the end of this module.

1. An endogenous infection is acquired from organisms in the environment.

    True   False

2. Patients undergoing surgery are prone to infection. Four possible causes for this infection could include:
    1. Personnel
    2. Patient
    3. Instruments
    4. Environment
    5. Equipment/supplies
    6. Bacterial barriers
        a. 2, 3, 5, 6
        b. 1, 2, 4, 5
        c. 1, 3, 5, 6
        d. 3, 4, 5, 6

3. Certain factors or conditions can significantly influence the patient's risk for developing a postoperative wound infection. These include age, nutritional status, general health, and length of procedure.

    True   False

4. Antibiotic therapy eliminates the need for concern involving protecting the patient from infection during the perioperative period.

    True   False

5. A drop in blood pressure is a common side effect of:
    a. halothane
    b. enflurane
    c. isoflurane
    d. all of the above

6. Inhalation and intravenous agents may be used in combination to achieve general anesthesia.

    True   False

7. Cocaine is commonly used as a topical anesthetic agent in nasal surgery.

    True   False

8. Malignant hyperthermia is treated with which agent?
    a. dobutamine
    b. dopamine
    c. dantrolene
    d. adrenalin

9. Lactated Ringers is an example of a replacement IV solution. Fluid replacement therapy may be accomplished by administering what type of IV fluid?
    a. D_5W
    b. LR w/20 mEq KCL
    c. $D_{10}W$
    d. lactated ringers

10. Preoperatively, the patient is taking a diuretic. Which of the following electrolytes may be most affected?
    a. sodium
    b. potassium
    c. chloride
    d. magnesium

11. Body fluids are considered hypertonic.

    True   False

12. A possible cause of hypovolemia may include:
    a. excessive vomiting
    b. nasogastric suctioning
    c. intestinal obstruction
    d. all of the above

13. A CVP reading reflects venous tone and relative venous volume.

    True   False

14. The ABG report reveals the following values:
    pH 7.5; P_{CO_2} 33; P_{O_2} 45; O_2 Sat. 88
    Which of these values is within normal limits?
    a. O_2 Sat.
    b. P_{O_2}
    c. P_{CO_2}
    d. pH

15. A Swan–Ganz catheter is used to measure PAP and LVEDP.

    True   False

Glossary

Microbiology and Wound Healing

Adhesions: bands of fiber that hold two structures together that are normally separate

Aerobe: a microorganism that grows best in *free* oxygen
- *Facultative:* prefers an environment free of oxygen but can grow in the presence of oxygen
- *Obligatory:* grows *only* in the presence of free oxygen

Anaerobe: microorganism that grows best in the *absence* of oxygen
- *Facultative:* prefers an oxygen environment, but can grow without oxygen
- *Obligatory:* grows *only* in the absence of oxygen

Approximate: to bring tissue edges together

Bacilli (combining form): referring to bacteria having a form of straight or slightly bent rods

Bacteria: microscopic, unicellular organisms that reproduce by fission and do not contain photosynthetic pigments

CDC: Centers for Disease Control; branch of Department of Health and Human Services; watchdog for surveillance of nosocomial infections

Cocci: bacterium of spherical, round, or oval shape; singular or in groups

Collagen: fibrous, insoluble protein found in connective tissue

Cytoplasm: protoplasm within a bacteria cell, not including nucleus; site of major metabolic activities

Debridement: removal of necrotic or damaged tissue

Dehiscence: a bursting open of a wound; involving the abdominal cavity

Endogenous: produced or arising from within a cell or organism; concerning spore formation within the bacteria cell

Enzymes: compounds produced by living organisms to break down chemical reactions involved with metabolism; often named by adding *-ase* to substance (substrate)

Epidemiology: science concerned with defining and explaining the interrelationship of factors that determine disease frequency and distribution

Evisceration: protrusion of viscera through a cavity wall; usually abdominal contents resulting from wound dehiscence

Exogenous: originating outside an organ or part

Fibroblast: any cell or corpuscle from which connective tissue develops

First Intention Healing: ideal; a minimum of tissue destruction and close approximation of wound edges (syn: primary union)

Fungi: a division of plantlike organisms which includes molds and yeasts; lacking chlorophyll, they are dependent on parasitic/saprophytic existence; many forms are pathogenic to plants and animals

Gangrene: a necrosis or death of tissue due to deficient or absent blood supply

Granulation: fleshy projections formed on the surface of a gaping wound that is *not* healing by primary union

Gram Negative, Gram Positive: reactions of bacterial cells to a staining procedure; specifies characteristic of bacteria

Heterotrophic: requiring organic compounds as source of carbon and energy

Host organism: the organism from which a parasite obtains its nourishment

Infection (infectious process): the condition in which the body or a part of it is invaded by a pathogenic agent; local or systemic; capable of being transmitted with or without contact

Keloid: raised, firm, thickened scar; usually following traumatic injury

Microbes: unicellular forms of life, including bacteria, rickettsiae, viruses, fungi, and protozoa

Necrosis: death of areas of tissue or bone surrounded by healthy parts; due to insufficient blood supply

Nosocomial Infection: an infection acquired in a hospital or infirmary

Parasites: organisms that live off living tissues or other organisms

Proud Flesh: granulated raw tissue in a wound that shows no other sign of healing

Proteus: genus of gram-negative, variously shaped rods that inhabit intestinal tract; highly resistant to most antibiotics

Rickettsiae: small microorganisms usually occurring as intracellular bodies; cultivated outside host only in living tissues and embryonated chicken eggs

Saprophytes: organisms that live on dead plants and animals by breaking down chemical substances

Second Intention Healing: wound is left open to heal from inside toward the outer surface; edges are not capable of close approximation (syn: granulation healing)

Spirillium: spiral-shaped bacterial cells; belonging to the family *Pseudomonadaceae;* found in fresh water and salt water

Spores: inactive resting forms produced within protoplasm of certain bacilli; highly resistant to destruction by heat, cold, and chemicals; have been known to survive for decades

Staphylococcus aureus: spherical, gram-positive cocci; inhabit air, water, surfaces of the body, mucous membrane, and nasopharynx; cause suppuration of wounds, and with increase in antibiotic resistant strains can be responsible for grave systemic infections

Systemic: pertaining to the whole body rather than to one of its parts

Surgical Wound Infection: incisional and deep surgical wound infections

- *Incisional:* infection occurring at site within 30 days after surgery, involving the skin, subcutaneous tissue, or muscle located above fascial layer
- *Deep:* infection occurring within 30 days after surgery (no implant present) or within 1 year if implant is present, and infection appears related to surgery and invades tissue or spaces at or beneath fascial layer

Third Intention Healing: combination of first and second intention healing in that wound is left open and closed at a later time. Usually associated with gross infections *(syn: delayed primary union)*

Universal Precautions: management of all cases and patients using established criteria stating that all are potentially contaminated; includes usage of protective bacterial barriers and protection for eyes and mucous membranes of health-care personnel

Viruses: ultra-microscopic infectious agents, capable of passing through pores of most filters. Identified by host-range filtration and immunologic responses of infected animals; seen only with electron microscope. Major cause for concern in surgery: hepatitis and AIDS (blood and blood products)

Anesthesia

ASA: American Society of Anesthesiologists, which has a classification system based on the health status of individual scheduled for general, regional, or monitored anesthesia procedures

Analgesia: lessening of or creating insensibility to pain

Anesthesia: partial or complete loss of sensation, with or without loss of consciousness as a result of the administration of an anesthetic agent

Anesthetic: an agent that produces anesthesia; subdivided into general and regional, according to their actions

Anesthesia Clinician: a specially trained professional who specializes in the administration of anesthesia

Anticholinergic: an agent given for parasympathetic depression, resulting in decreased oral and tracheobronchial secretions

Balanced Anesthesia: anesthesia produced by administering a combination of two or more drugs/agents to provide a sufficient amount of muscle relaxation, analgesia, and sleep

Barbiturate: an agent given to promote sedation

Depolarizing Muscle Relaxant: an agent that produces a depolarization of the membrane at the motor end plate, causing a muscle contraction that is followed by a neuromuscular block

Dissociative Anesthetic Agent: a general anesthesia agent that produces a catatonic state by selectively interrupting associative pathways to the brain, in addition to providing analgesia and amnesia

Epidural Anesthesia: injection of anesthetic agent into the epidural space, blocking the transmission of nerve impulses to selective nerve fibers

Extubation: removal of an endotracheal tube

General Anesthesia: depression of the central nervous system, resulting in loss of consciousness, sensory perception, and motor function

Induction: the phase of general anesthesia from the beginning of administration of the anesthetic agent until loss of consciousness

Inhalation Technique: an anesthetic technique in which the agent enters the system via the lungs using a mask or indwelling tube in the nose or mouth and is carried into the bloodstream to the brain via the circulatory system. The agent is primarily removed by lung ventilation

Intubation: insertion of a tube directly into the trachea via the nose or mouth

Intravenous Block: local anesthesia obtained by injecting the anesthetic agent into a vein of a tourniquet-occluded extremity

Local Infiltration: injection of the anesthetic agent into subcutaneous tissue of the operative site

Narcotic Analgesia: an agent given to reduce pain sensation by altering perceptive and emotional responses to pain and providing sedation

Narcotic Antagonist: an agent that acts by blocking the effect of a narcotic

Neuroleptanalgesia: an agent that reduces motor activity, lessens anxiety, and produces profound tranquilization

Nondepolarizing Muscle Relaxant: an agent that blocks the action of acetylcholine at the neuromuscular junction, but does not cause depolarization at the motor end plate; therefore, fasciculations do not occur

Regional Anesthesia: a generic term referring to a technique that temporarily interrupts the transmission of nerve impulses to and from a specific area of region

Spinal Anesthesia: injection of an anesthetic agent into the cerebrospinal fluid in the subarachnoid space, blocking the transmission of nerve impulses to the nerve fibers *(syn: subarachnoid block [SAB])*

Topical Anesthesia: an agent applied directly to the skin and mucous membranes, affecting superficial nerve endings

Tranquilizer: an agent given for the purpose of sedation, reduction of anxiety, and potentiation of narcotics

Volatile Gases: liquids that are easily vaporized and, when inhaled, produce anesthesia

Homeostasis and Hemodynamics

Acid–base Balance: the maintenance of a normal balance between the acidity and alkalinity of body fluids within the extracellular and intracellular fluid compartments

Acidosis: an abnormal increase in hydrogen ion concentration in the body owing to an accumulation of an acid or the loss of a base

Alkalosis: an abnormal condition of body fluids characterized by a tendency toward an increased pH (excess base) or a deficiency of an acid

Anion: an ion that develops a negative charge when placed in solution

Cation: an ion that develops a positive charge when placed in solution

Central Venous Pressure (CVP): a measurement that directly reflects pressure within the right atrium, which ultimately reflects pressure within the right ventricle

Diffusion: a process in which ions and molecules move from an area of greater concentration to an area of lesser concentration in order to maintain equilibrium of particles within the area

Electrolyte: a molecule that when dissolved in solution dissociates into ions, thus becoming capable of conducting electricity

Extracellular Fluid (ECF): fluid that is situated or occurring outside a cell or cells

Hypotonic: having an osmotic pressure less than that of the solution with which it is being compared; less than body fluid

Hemodynamics: the study of the movement of blood through the cardiovascular network

Homeostasis: a tendency of biologic systems to maintain stability while continuously adjusting to internal and external changes *(adj. homeostatic mechanism)*

Hypertonic: having an osmotic pressure greater than the solution with which it is being compared; greater than body fluid

Interstitial Fluid (ISF): pertaining to fluid located between the cells or in the interspaces of the tissue

Intraarterial Blood Pressure (A-line): the use of a catheter in an artery, attached to a transducer, to provide continuous data via a display monitor and/or digital writeout or pressure meter

Intracellular Fluid (ICF): fluid within a cell or cells

Intravascular Fluid: fluid within a vessel or vessels

Isotonic Fluid: a solution having the same osmotic pressure as the solution with which it is being compared

Osmolarity: the concentration of the number of dissolved particles per unit of water in serum

Osmotic Pressure: the pressure exerted on a semipermeable membrane separating a solution from a solvent (membrane being impermeable to solvent)

pH: a scale representing the relative acidity or alkalinity of a solution. The numeric value indicates the hydrogen ion concentration in the solution compared to that of a standard solution

Plasma: the fluid portion of the blood, containing no cells, made up of water, electrolytes, proteins, glucose, fats, bilirubin, and gases; important in maintaining osmotic pressure

Swan–Ganz Catheter: a multilumen, balloon-tipped, flow-guided catheter used to monitor a patient's hemodynamic status by thermodilution techniques

Transcellular Fluid: smallest compartment of body fluids, consisting of fluid contained in joints, cavities, and CSF.

Bibliography for Module II

American College of Surgeons Committee on Control of Surgical Infections. Manual of Control of Infections in Surgical Patients. 2nd ed. Philadelphia: J. B. Lippincott, 1984.

American Heart Association. Textbook of Advanced Cardiac Life Support. Dallas: The Association, 1995.

Association of Operating Room Nurses. Standards and Recommended Practices for Perioperative Nursing Practice. Denver: The Association, 1995.

Barash RK, Cullen BF, Stoelting RK. Clinical Anesthesia. Philadelphia: J. B. Lippincott, 1989.

Barker WF, Howard JM, Culberton WR, et al. Postoperative Wound Infections: The Influence of the OR and Various Other Factors. Ann Surg, 1980.

Bocock EJ, Parker MJ. Microbiology for Nurses. Baltimore: Williams & Wilkins, 1982.

Brachman PS, Dan BB, Haley RW, Hostin TM. Nosocomial Surgical Infections: Incidence and Cost. Surg Clin North Am 1980; 60:15–25.

Bullock, B., Rosendahl P. Pathophysiology: Adaptation and Alteration in Function. Boston: Little Brown, 1984.

Burrows W. Textbook of Microbiology. 22nd ed. Philadelphia: W. B. Saunders, 1985.

Cartwright F. The Development of Modern Surgery. New York: Thomas Crowell, 1968.

Crowley LV. Introduction to Human Disease. 2nd ed. Boston: Jones and Bartlett, 1988.

Dripps RD, Eckenoff JE, Vandam LD. Introduction to Anesthesia: The Principles of Safe Practice. 7th ed. Philadelphia: W. B. Saunders, 1988.

Eckenhoff JE. Anesthesia from Colonial Times. Philadelphia: J. B. Lippincott, 1966.

Felver L. Understanding the Electrolyte Maze. Am J Nurs 80:1591–1595, 1980.

Felver L, Pendarvis JH. Electrolyte Imbalances: Intraoperative Risk Factors. AORN J 49:992–1005, 1989.

Gardner JS, Ed. CDC Definitions for nosocomial infections. Am J Infect Control 6. U.S. Department of Health and Human Services, Atlanta, 1988.

Gavoni LE, Hayes JE. Drugs and Nursing Implications. 6th ed. New York: Appleton-Century-Crofts, 1988.

Groah LK. Operating Room Nursing: The Perioperative Role. 2nd. ed. Reston, VA: Reston Publishing, 1992.

Guidelines for Prevention of Surgical Wound Infections. Atlanta, GA: Centers for Disease Control, 1985.

Halperin ML, Goldstein MB. Fluid, Electrolyte and Acid–Base Emergencies. Philadelphia: W. B. Saunders, 1988.

Katsung B. Basic and Clinical Pharmacology. 5th ed. Norwalk, CT: Appleton and Lange p. 42.

Keys JL. Fluid, Electrolyte and Acid–Base Regulation. Monterey, CA: Wadsworth Health Science Division, 1985.

Klein S. A Glossary of Anesthesia and Related Terminology. New York: Medical Examination Publishing, 1985.

Kneedler J, Dodge G. Perioperative Patient Care: The Nursing Perspective. 2nd ed. Boston: Blackwell Scientific, 1987.

Kozier B, Erb G. Fundamentals in Nursing. 3rd ed. Reading, MA: Addison-Wesley, 1987.

Miller BF, Keane CB. Encyclopedia and Dictionary of Medicine, Nursing and Allied Health. 3rd ed. Philadelphia: W. B. Saunders, 1983.

Miller RD, ed. Anesthesia, Vol. I. 3rd ed. New York: Churchill-Livingstone, 1990.

Centers for Disease Control MMW (Suppl. 37), Washington, DC. 1988.

Muir B. Pathophysiology: An Introduction to the Mechanism of Disease. New York: John Wiley and Sons, 1980.

Nentwich PF. Intravenous Therapy: A Comprehensive Application of Intravenous Therapy and Medication Administration. Boston: Jones and Bartlett, 1990.

Nurses Reference Library. Drugs. Springhouse, PA: NURSING 82, 1982.

Physician's Desk Reference. 43rd ed. Oradell, NJ: Medical Economics, 1989.

Stoelting RK, Miller RD. Basics of Anesthesia. 2nd ed. New York: Churchill-Livingstone, 1989.

Somerson SJ, Husted CW, Sicilia MR. Insights into Conscious Sedation Am J Nurs. 95:26–32, 1995.

Wardell SC, Bousard LB. Nursing Pharmacology: A Comprehensive Approach to Drug Therapy. Monterey, CA: Wadsworth Health Science Division, 1985.

Zimmerman LM, Veith I. Great Ideas in the History of Surgery. New York: Dover Publishing, 1987.

Answers for Module II

Self-assessment Exercise 1

1. Facultative cocci
   Gram positive; non–spore forming
2. Facultative cocci
   Gram positive; non–spore forming
3. Anaerobic bacilli
   Gram positive; spore forming
4. Gram positive and gram negative stain
5. For answers 1–5, see Figure 4-1, p. 49.
6. Pathogens; nosocomial
7. 1. C
   2. E
   3. F
   4. A
   5. B
   6. D
8. Suitable atmosphere; suitable temperature; suitable moisture; pH requirements; nutritional requirements

Self-assessment Exercise 2

I-A Skin
   Handwashing; surgical scrub; skin prep; *clipping* hair instead of shaving, and only when necessary
I-B Blood/body fluids
   Universal precautions; appropriate barrier protection; eye protection
I-C Respiratory tract
   Proper use of surgical mask by all team members; avoidance of direct patient care by team members with URI
I-D GI tract
   Proper bowel prep; hand washing; proper surgical technique

II-A Circulating air
   Damp-dusting all flat surfaces; limited talking/movement; OR door closed; proper ventilation and effective filtering system
II-B Linens/instruments/supplies
   Proper use of disposables; proper decontamination and sterilization methods; enforced traffic control for distribution of supplies (outside to inside)
II-C OR sanitation
   Enforced routine for interim/terminal cleaning; spot cleaning as required
II-D Personal hygiene
   Clean scrub attire; cleanliness; good personal hygiene practices

Self-assessment Exercise 3

1. a. 3
   b. 1
   c. 2
2. Primary union or first intention healing
3. Wide; heavier; healing from the inside out
4. Dehiscence—separation of wound edges
   Evisceration—protrusion of viscera through incisional line (total evisceration)

Self-assessment Exercise 4

1. 1. Poor nutritional status
   2. Age
   3. Chemical imbalance
   4. General physical condition
   5. Circulatory status

2. Universal precautions; all cases are treated as potentially contaminated; no special cleaning is required if sanitation practices meet required standards
3. True
4. Gloves and/or instrument (sponge stick)
5. 1. Hernia repair; breast bx.; primary open heart
   2. Hysterectomy; D&C; cholecystectomy; C-section
   3. Fx. Femur (trauma); gunshot/knife wound (not penetrating viscera); ruptured appendix
   4. I&D of old wound; total evisceration; amputation
6. False: the medical diagnosis does not change the risk factor for postoperative infection. The classification is directly related to the type of surgery being performed.

Self-assessment Exercise 5

1. a. 500 mg
   b. 8 minims
   c. 7.5 gr
   d. 2 gm
   e. 1000 U
2. a. 30 minims
   b. 12 minims
   c. 0.5 mL

Self-assessment Exercise 6

1. 20.8 (21) gtt/min
2. a. 20.8 (21) gtt/min
   b. 83.3 mL/hr
3. a. 62.5 (63) gtt/min
   b. 62.5 (63) mL/hr

Self-assessment Exercise 7

1. Matching
   1. F   6. G
   2. D   7. E
   3. I   8. B
   4. C   9. J
   5. A   10. H
2. True
3. True
4. True
5. Sublimaze

Self-assessment Exercise 8

1. Ether
2. Cocaine
3. a. produce analgesia
   b. promote amnesia
   c. induce muscle relaxation
   d. provide control of ANS reflexes
4. To establish a baseline of information in order to provide the correct anesthetic agents and methods based on individual needs and current health status
5. Class II

Self-assessment Exercise 9

1. a. age
   b. medical history

   c. current physical status
   d. nature of surgery
   e. expertise/preference of anesthesiologist
   f. previous anesthesia history
   g. surgeon/patient preference
2. Atropine; Robinul
3. a. facilitate induction
   b. alleviate anxiety
   c. decrease secretions
4. Fear of the unknown
5. Speak calmly; answer questions as best you can; provide assurance; explain activities being performed; touch (hold patient's hand)

Self-assessment Exercise 10

1. General anesthesia results in loss of consciousness, while regional anesthesia desensitizes a specific area without loss of consciousness
2. A scavenger system collects nitrous oxide so that it can be eliminated through the suction apparatus, and not released into the air, thus protecting OR personnel
3. Applying pressure on the cricoid cartilage posteriorly with thumb and forefinger
4. Anectine (Quelicin)
5. Remain at patient's side; speak calmly, explaining the procedure; maintain a quiet, relaxing atmosphere

Self-assessment Exercise 11

1. A
2. B, C, D
3. Sitting; lateral
4. Remain immediately available; provide verbal reassurance; limit patient exposure; restrict traffic flow and extraneous noise from the room
5. True

Self-assessment Exercise 12

1. Numbness of tongue; blurred vision; tinnitus; dizziness; drowsiness; confusion
2. Preoperative assessment and interview; establishing peripheral IV line; providing explanation of sequence of events; positioning; establishing a therapeutic environment
3. Epinephrine
4. C
5. 5 to 15 minutes, and before each dose of anesthetic and/or sedation agent

Self-assessment Exercise 13

1. Intracellular fluid; extracellular fluid
2. In the spaces between the cells; 15% of body weight
3. False: when particle distribution is equal, the fluid is *isotonic*
4. $D_{10}W$; D_5 0.45 NS; D_5LR
   Hypertonic solutions cause water to leave the cell and the cell shrinks (crenation)
5. False. Water is the "universal solvent."

Self-assessment Exercise 14

1. Cation; anion
2. Potassium; 3.5 to 5.5 mEq/L
3. Sodium
4. Calcium
5. Calcium
6. Bicarbonate; 22–26 mEq/L

Self-assessment Exercise 15

1. P_{O_2}
2. Concentration of hydrogen ions in solution
3. P_{O_2} 80–100 mm Hg
   P_{CO_2} 35–45 mm Hg
   pH 7.40 (7.35–7.45)
   HCO_3^- 22–26 mEq/L
   BE ± 2.5
   O_2 Sat. > 95 percent
4. HCO_3^- Bicarbonate
5. pH < 7.35
   P_{CO_2} > 45
   HCO_3^- WNL
   BE 2.5
6. Respiratory alkalosis

Questions for Review

1. False: *endogenous* infections are acquired from an organism *within* the body
2. B
3. True
4. False: as patient advocates, basic patient protection from harm (infection) cannot be disregarded
5. D
6. True
7. True
8. C
9. D
10. B
11. False: body fluids are *isotonic*
12. D
13. True
14. C
15. True

MODULE III Asepsis and the Surgical Environment

Chapter Outline

Content Overview

Surgery has advanced further in the past 100 years than in all the preceding years. The most important component of that advance is the ability to manipulate or operate on the human body without the fear of infection. The basis for this ability is a group of procedures known collectively as *aseptic technique*.

This module focuses on the specific tasks and clinical competencies for perioperative nursing practice, by describing the methods used to establish and maintain a safe, therapeutic surgical environment for the patient and personnel during the perioperative period.

Module Objectives

Upon completion of this module, you will be able to:

1. Discuss the current AORN recommended practices associated with an aseptic environment.
2. Identify the steps, procedures, and equipment required for establishing and maintaining a sterile field.
3. Describe the appropriate usage and care of the tools commonly used in surgery, including sutures, needles, and instruments.
4. Differentiate between the duties and responsibilities of the scrub and circulating roles, before, during, and after a surgical procedure.
5. Correlate the knowledge of aseptic principles with the implementation of the perioperative nurse's role during the perioperative period.

8 Operating Room Theory and Techniques

UNIT 1

Fundamentals of Asepsis

Whosoever touches the body of the afflicted man shall wash his garments and bathe in water . . . least their uncleanliness be the cause of their death.

—Leviticus 15

HISTORICAL OVERVIEW

The history of surgical asepsis is as old as civilization, as evidenced by the reference to cleanliness in the Old Testament. Regulations concerning personal hygiene showed an uncanny understanding of infection and how it was transmitted from one person to another without proper cleansing of the body or the mind. According to ancient writings, most primitive peoples, at one time in their history, regarded disease as the work of the *evil one* or *evil spirits*. Sickness also came from supernatural powers, along with the ability to rid the body of disease.

In the pre-Christian era, Hippocrates (460 B.C.) began to turn the art of healing away from the mystical rites of the priest-healers to an approach that everyone could understand and practice. In his teachings, he spoke of cleanliness to avoid infection when he stressed irrigating dirty wounds with wine or boiled water. Boiling water, as well as fire, was used often to clean instruments and prevent infection.[1]

In Babylon, the *Code of Hammurabi* established laws to mandate safe practices in surgery, including a penalty for surgeons whose patients suffered injury or infection as a result of their surgery. For example, if a patient lost an eye due to *faulty surgery*, including infection, the surgeon's eye was put out.[2]

Surgeons in ancient Egypt, with their vast knowledge of medicines, surgical procedures, and treatments, including the art of embalming, used herbs and drugs as an antiseptic, as well as the fumes of specially prepared incense to deodorize and disinfect the environment.

ANTISEPSIS/ANTISEPTIC

The origin of the word *antisepsis* is Greek, which, literally translated, means "against making rotten."[3] In scientific terms, antisepsis is described as a means of preventing sepsis (making rotten) by the destruction of microorganisms and infective matter.[4]

Antiseptic, stemming from the original Greek concept, was later described by Charles White (1728–1813) as any substance that inhibits the growth of bacteria, including heat, accomplished by boiling or burning or chemicals such as *chlorinated-lime solution*.[5] Louis Pasteur (1822–1895), a French chemist, developed his theories on germs and microorganisms, and in a lecture delivered at the *French Academy of Medicine*, explained his theory regarding the growth and reproduction requirements of microbes. He stated they could be found scattered on the surface of every object, particularly in hospitals. By removing these microbes through proper cleansing and application of heat, he could reduce their number on the surfaces, but they would still remain in the air. During this turbulent time, hospital deaths from infection were the rule, not the exception.

Pasteur pursued this theory on the drawing board, where he eventually conceived the first sterilizer that would be capable of destroying the microbes that might be harboring on instruments and supplies used in surgery. It was Robert Koch, however, in 1881, who would actually develop the first nonpressure flowing steam sterilizer.

Florence Nightingale (1820–1910), known as the pioneer of antiseptic principles, changed forever the role of the nurse related to protecting the patient from infection. Through her writings describing the deplorable conditions in British Army hospitals during the Crimea War, the correlation between cleanliness and recovery began to take on new meaning, and people were finally listening to her when she advocated clean sheets, clean gowns, and decent surroundings for all patients.[6] Through her efforts, housekeeping practices improved. Aseptic principles began to emerge, many of which are still practiced today.

Antiseptic Surgery

In England, based on the findings of Pasteur's experiments and the positive outcomes related to decreased infection rates, Lord Joseph Lister (1827–1912) began to identify the implications of this theory on postoperative surgical infections. Lister believed that if contamination by the air-borne particles could be prevented from entering the surgical wound, infection could be prevented. Lister, aware that *carbolic acid* was being used to destroy sewage odors, decided to try this agent as a soaking solution for his instruments and sponges and the cleaning of surfaces in the operating theater. Because of this experiment, and the reduction of infection in his patients, he insisted that these practices be carried out for every surgical case, even to the point of using a diluted solution to wash his hands and prepare the surgical incision site. Eventually, all members of his staff followed the same practices.

This *antiseptic* technique gave Joseph Lister the nickname "Father of Antiseptic Surgery," and the principles he established were the beginnings of the aseptic practices employed today.

Other concepts of aseptic technique were beginning to develop rapidly, now that it was proven that infection could be reduced drastically by following simple preventative measures:

- von Bergman (1880) advocated sterilization of surgical instruments, dry goods, and the cleaning of the surgeon's hands with bichloride of mercury
- Neuber (1881) was the first to use a cap and gown in the OR
- Bloodgood (1894) was the first to don sterile gloves, as did the members of his surgical team
- Mikulicz (1896) was the first to use a surgical mask

Surgical Technique Improves

In the field of surgical technique, William Halstead, an American surgeon teaching at Johns Hopkins Hospital in Baltimore, advocated proper procedures for tissue handling and wound closure, including the evacuation of debris, proper hemostasis, and prevention of *dead space* occurring during wound closure by careful approximation of the wound edges, thus reducing the risk of postoperative wound infections.

Surgery was finally becoming a positive alternative treatment, based on scientific principles and improvement in the general area of tissue handling and wound closure. Infections developing in clean wounds were becoming increasingly rare, thanks to the contributions of those pioneers in aseptic principles. Today it is reinforced by the development and appropriate use of chemotherapeutic agents, such as antibiotics, and a better understanding of aseptic technique.

SURGICAL CONSCIENCE

> With loyalty will I endeavor to aid the physician in his work, and devote myself to the welfare of those committed to my care. . . .
> —*Nightingale Pledge (1893)*

As a member of the health-care team, physicians, nurses, and para-professionals are entrusted with the safety and welfare of those who come to us for help or assistance. As a patient advocate, the perioperative nurse has, as one of his or her most important functions, the responsibility for monitoring and maintaining an aseptic environment during the perioperative period, thus preventing harm from befalling the patient.

Surgical conscience is that concept which allows for *no compromise in the principles of aseptic technique*, since anything less could increase the potential risk of infection, resulting in harm to the patient.

Developing a Surgical Conscience

A surgical conscience builds on the principles of asepsis, and is an act of mental discipline. It involves inspection and regulation of one's own practice, with particular attention to deviations from acceptable, safe practices, especially during the intraoperative phase of the surgical experience.

Surgical conscience does not only apply to the surgical team, but to all those directly involved with patient care. Surgical conscience demands the recognition and immediate action to correct improper practices observed during surgery by any member of the health-care team. This includes the ability to report one's own breaks in technique, so that corrective action may be taken, even if the person is not being observed.

Additionally, surgical conscience involves the ability to set aside personal preferences and prejudices in order to provide optimum patient care. Through continuous vigilance and evaluation of the patient, the environment, personnel, and equipment, we can reduce the possibility of complications that could rise out of complacency or lack of professional consideration for others.

When fully developed, surgical conscience can become a blend of several characteristics. Integrity, hon-

esty, and self-confidence, allow the individual to recognize the human trait of being fallible, requiring an alertness to wrongdoing and correcting it before it causes harm to another person. When rapport and mutual respect are established among the members of the health-care team, corrections will become constructive, not destructive, but it takes time for knowledge and practice to reach this level. In order to fully comprehend the concept of surgical conscience, ask yourself the following questions before the start of each procedure:

1. Is this the best set-up for this procedure?
2. Do I have everything that is logically necessary under existing conditions?
3. Do I understand what is required of me and how I can be of greatest assistance?
4. Have I done all I can do to provide a safe, therapeutic environment for my patient?
5. If I were the patient, what would I want the team/nurse to do for me to help reduce my fears and anxieties?

The *key* words involving surgical practice are *caring, discipline, vigilance, honesty,* and *integrity.* Surgical conscience, simply stated, is doing unto *others* (patient) *as you would have others* (health-care personnel) *do unto you.*

Florence Nightingale once summarized this concept, stating that the nurse must keep a "high sense of duty in her own mind, must aim at perfection and must be consistent always in herself."[7]

ASEPTIC TECHNIQUE: PRINCIPLES AND PRACTICES

The basis for all infection-free surgery is founded on the *principles of aseptic technique.* Every attempt must be made toward preventing the invasion of microorganisms into the surgical wound during the perioperative period.

Two methods are utilized which, if practiced with precision, can prevent serious complications to the already compromised surgical patient:

1. Aseptic Technique
2. Sterile Technique

Although they sound similar, they are very different in practice. *Aseptic technique* is a group of procedures which prevent contamination of microorganisms through the knowledge and principles of *contain and control. Sterile technique,* on the other hand, is a group of methods by which contamination of an item is prevented by maintaining the sterility of the item/area involved. Different, yet linked by their purpose of preventing contamination, both techniques, the supplies and equipment used, and the surgical environment can ultimately protect the patient from an unwarranted postoperative infection.

Aseptic technique is based on the premise that most infections are introduced into the body from outside (exogenous) sources. To avoid infection, it is necessary to ensure that any procedure performed on the body is done in such a way as to introduce no bacteria. The procedure must therefore be performed within a *sterile field* from which all living bacteria, including those initially present on the patient's skin, have been excluded. All instruments, sutures, and fluids must be sterile, that is, free of all living microorganisms, including spores. The surgical team member's hands must be cleansed of all bacteria, and they must be wearing a sterile gown, sterile gloves, and mask, or the procedure cannot be considered sterile.

The principles of aseptic technique are no less important when performing a procedure that does not require the strictness of the OR environment, but involves a break in the patient's skin or entering a sterile cavity, which renders the patient susceptible to invading microorganisms. Sepsis introduced through a venous cut down can kill just as surely as infection introduced at the operating table.

Principles of Aseptic Technique

Aseptic technique can be implemented in many different ways. While many may believe that some practices have become too ritualistic, or lack sufficient empirical research to support their implementation, the understanding of the basic principles remains an important aspect of safe perioperative nursing practice. Until empirical research demonstrates that any technique is not effective, these basic principles should remain in force and should be practiced by all members of the healthcare team.

By using the best theoretical knowledge available today to create and maintain a sterile field, perioperative nurses play a vital and significant role in *protecting the patient from infection*. The next few pages will outline the current AORN recommendations and principles for creating and maintaining an aseptic environment. These recommended practices stem from the original eight principles of asepsis derived from microbiology and epidemiologic concepts.

Principles of Asepsis

1. All items used within a sterile field must be sterile.
2. A sterile barrier that has been permeated must be considered contaminated.
3. The edges of a sterile container are considered unsterile once the package is opened.
4. Gowns are considered sterile in front, from shoulder to table level, and the sleeves to 2 inches above the elbow.
5. Tables are sterile at table level only.
6. Sterile persons and items touch only sterile areas; unsterile persons and items touch only unsterile areas.
7. Movement within or around a sterile field must not contaminate the field.
8. All items and areas of doubtful sterility are considered contaminated.

Recommended Practices— Aseptic Technique

The AORN recommended practices should be used as a guide for anyone who is present during the procedure, and is involved either directly or indirectly with patient care.[8] Additionally, they should be applied to any area where invasive procedures are being performed.

Recommended Practice I

Scrubbed persons should wear sterile gowns and gloves.

Nursing Implications The surgical team is divided into two groups: those who are directly working at the surgical field (sterile team), and those who are working around the sterile field (unsterile team).

All sterile team members perform a surgical scrub before entering the procedure room, in order to remove gross dirt from their hands and arms before applying their sterile gown and gloves (see Surgical Hand Scrub Procedure, p. 152). Since the scrubbed team members receive sterile equipment from the circulator (nonsterile member), and since sterile can only touch sterile, a bacterial barrier is needed between the person and the sterile item. That bacterial barrier is the sterile gown and gloves.

In order to maintain the sterile field, parameters of sterility for the gown have been established:

- the gown is considered sterile in front from chest to the level of the sterile field
- the sleeves are considered sterile from 2 inches above the elbow to the stockinette cuff, and therefore the cuff must be covered, at all times, by sterile gloves

The following areas are not considered sterile, for various monitoring reasons: the *neckline, shoulder areas, areas under the arms,* and the *back of the gown.*

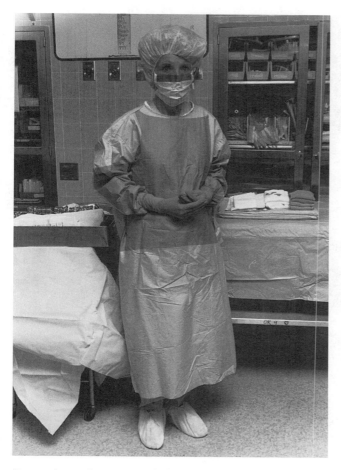

Person in sterile gown and gloves (note defined sterile area of gown)

In order to preserve the sterility of the gloved hands, they should be kept within the sterile boundary of the gown, and since the axillary region is not sterile, the arms should never be crossed with hands positioned into the axilla. Should either of these barriers be compromised, they must be discarded, and a new gown and/or gloves applied, depending on the nature of the break in technique.

Recommended Practice II

Sterile drapes should be used to establish a sterile field.

Nursing Implications Contamination of equipment and personnel is prevented by the placement of a bacterial barrier or sterile drape over an item located within the boundary of the sterile field. During surgery, the patient, once covered with the bacterial barrier, becomes the center of the sterile field. Specific pieces of furniture must be used to accommodate surgical instruments and supplies, and these surfaces must therefore be covered with a bacterial barrier before assembly and use by sterile members of the team.

Once the sterile field has been established, nonsterile persons must never reach over the draped areas, since this constitutes contamination of that area, requiring immediate corrective action to recreate the sterility of that item or field. The parameter for the sterile field is easily maintained, since only the top of the draped table and/or the patient is considered sterile. Anything below this level is unsterile, and must be treated as such by members of the sterile team.

In order to properly drape an unsterile surface with sterile drapes, the following guidelines should be practiced:

- Sterile persons drape an unsterile surface first toward themselves, protecting their gown and gloves at all times.
- When nonsterile persons drape an area, they do so away first, then toward them, avoiding reaching over a sterile field. (See Critical Element Task 9-3, p. 255.)

Should the drapes become permeated or moist, they must be considered contaminated and corrective action must be initiated to cover the area in question, or the drapes must be changed.

Recommended Practice III

All items used within a sterile field should be sterile.

Nursing Implications Under **no** circumstances can sterile and unsterile items/areas be mixed, since one contaminates the other. Some items used during surgery come presterilized from the manufacturer, for example, drapes, sponges, gowns, gloves, and so on, while others, such as instruments and trays, are sterilized in the hospital, either in the central processing area or in the OR.

Before opening or dispensing these items for sterile use, the integrity of the packaging and the assurance of sterility must be accounted for by those persons dispensing the item. This can be accomplished through several preparatory procedures:

- checking the outer wrapper or package to make sure there are no tears or holes
- confirming the items' sterility has not been compromised by handling
- inspecting to see that the items have gone through the proper sterilization process evidenced by the indicators on the outside of the package
- realizing that if sterility is doubted, the item is considered contaminated, and cannot be used

According to research findings, the sterility of a package is event-related, and not time-related; there-

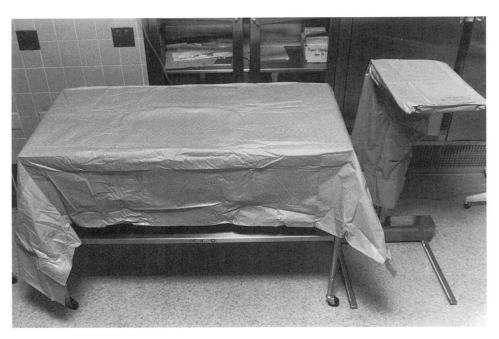

Bacterial barrier instrument table (left) and Mayo stand (right) draped with appropriate barriers

fore the item's sterility is dependent on the type of packaging material, handling, and storage conditions.[9]

For further discussion on sterilization processes and monitoring procedures, refer to Unit 2 in this chapter.

Recommended Practice IV

All items introduced onto a sterile field should be opened, dispensed, and transferred by methods that maintain sterility and integrity.

Nursing Implications The edges of a sterile container or wrapper cannot be considered sterile once the container or wrapper is opened. When opening a sterile item, a margin of safety must always be employed, that is, the hands of the unsterile person should be covered or protected from accidental contact with either the field or the scrubbed person during the transfer procedure. (See p. 149.)

When working with irrigation solution or fluid contained in a pour bottle, careful attention must be used to avoid "splash-back," and once the solution has been poured, the container cannot be recapped for future use, since its contents can no longer be considered sterile. The solution must be completely used, or the remaining fluid must be discarded.

When retrieving a sterile item from the autoclave, the circulating nurse cannot touch the item, and must present the item, maintaining its sterility, to the scrub nurse so that she can transfer it to the sterile field, without contamination. This can usually be accomplished by the use of a *flash pan* with a handle for retrieving items requiring emergency sterilization for immediate use. (See Critical Element Task 8-6, p. 188.)

Recommended Practice V

A sterile field should be constantly monitored and maintained.

Recommended Practice VI

All personnel moving within or around a sterile field should do so in a manner to maintain the integrity of the sterile field.

Nursing Implications The sterility of the supplies used during a surgical procedure can be affected by the events taking place within the room, and the length of time the items have not been used and/or exposed to the environment. Since contamination can accidently occur by any member of the team, the sterile field should be created as close to the time of the procedure as possible, and once created, be constantly monitored.

According to research findings, a sterile field should never be covered for use at a later time.[10] Covering and removal of the cover can cause contamination of the field. In order to monitor the field and maintain its integrity, the field should be in constant view, and you should therefore never turn your back on a sterile field.

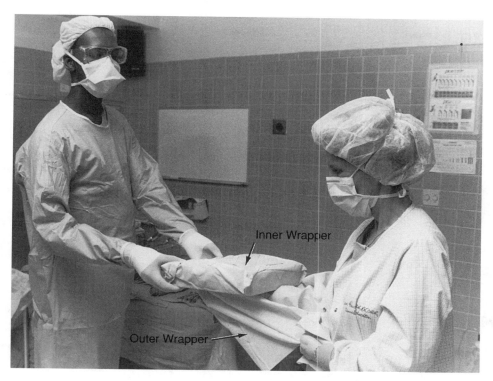

Square wrap—sterile item being dispensed to scrub nurse (notice position of hand)

Air currents can become a source of contamination, so that movement within or around a sterile field should be minimal to avoid contamination of the field. Sterile persons (in gown and gloves) should not wander in and out of the sterile area, or sit while in sterile attire, since the gown is considered contaminated below table level and may contaminate other parts of the gown and/or gloves. The only acceptable exception is when the entire procedure is performed in a sitting position. Persons in sterile gowns and gloves should not leave the procedure room or sterile area in gown and gloves (either during or after the procedure).

Since the patient is the center of the sterile field, scrubbed persons should not venture away from this area. Wandering around the room could cause contamination of the field. Scrubbed persons should not position themselves in an unsterile area of the procedure room. All of these actions constitute a break in technique, and must be avoided in order to protect the patient and maintain an aseptic environment.

Should scrubbed persons need to change positions, they should do so in a manner that maintains the sterility of their gown and gloves: face to face (sterile to sterile) or back to back (unsterile to unsterile).

In addition to the recommended practices for creating and maintaining a sterile field, there are other methods that can be employed to protect and maintain an aseptic environment. These include:

1. preventing moisture from contaminating a bacterial barrier
2. restricting talking in the room to a minimum
3. avoiding unsterile persons walking between two sterile fields (set-ups)
4. keeping unsterile persons a safe distance from the sterile field
5. keeping the OR doors shut during a procedure (recognizing that contamination by an intermediate source, such as air, moisture, or dust, can be minimized by reducing or eliminating the source)
6. monitoring for breaks in technique, if and when they occur, and taking immediate and appropriate steps to correct the break in technique

Maintaining an Aseptic Environment

The use of aseptic technique in controlling the operating room environment is guided by several principles and standards. There are many more factors, which are not included in this unit, and the perioperative nurse is encouraged continuously to review current literature concerning the principles and practices of aseptic technique.

Self-assessment Exercise 1

Directions: Complete the following exercises. The answers are located at the end of the module.

1. Define *aseptic technique*

2. Differentiate between aseptic practices and *sterile technique.*

3. The basis for implementation of aseptic technique begins with an understanding of _____.

4. List the five *AORN Recommended Practices for Basic Aseptic Technique*

    1. _____

    2. _____

3. _____

4. _____

5. _____

5. Describe how *you*, as the perioperative nurse, can help maintain an aseptic environment during the *intraoperative phase* of surgical intervention.

6. Maintaining the principles of aseptic technique is only necessary in the OR.

    True   False

IMPLEMENTING RECOMMENDED PRACTICES

As described in Chapter 2, environmental preparation of the surgical suite plays a major role in maintaining an aseptic atmosphere. Proper OR attire, traffic control, and environmental sanitation practices are all used to assure the continuing safety of the patient.

When working with sterile supplies and equipment during a surgical procedure, additional safeguards must be employed and sterility must be maintained.

The word "sterile" implies the destruction/removal of all microorganisms from an object or surface, including spores. In order for this definition to be accurate, specific preparatory procedures for both the team and the equipment must be completed before the start of the procedure.

Preparation of the Surgical Team

Since the skin cannot be sterilized, like inanimate objects, preparation of the surgical team requires a surgical hand scrub and the application of sterile gowns and gloves.

The Surgical Hand Scrub

Despite the fact that the surgical team's hands must be covered by sterile gloves, it is mandatory that a surgical hand scrub be performed, according to acceptable technique, before the beginning of each procedure (see Critical Task Element 8-1, p. 152.)

There are several reasons for this. Hands may carry pathogenic bacteria acquired from other sources within the environment. Gloves may become punctured or torn during the procedure, exposing the pa-

tient and the team to microbial contamination. By performing a surgical hand scrub, the skin is rendered *aseptically clean* in preparation for donning sterile attire.

The surgical hand scrub is a process that reduces the microbial count to as low as possible by mechanical washing. The scrub removes soil and transient organisms by a combination of friction and an antiseptic (antimicrobial) agent which reduces resident flora and deactivates microorganisms. The goals of the surgical scrub include (1) the removal of soil and transient microbes from the hands and forearms, (2) the reduction of the resident microbial count to as low a level as possible, and (3) the reduction of the potential rapid rebound growth of microbes.

Nursing Implications The surgical scrub is performed after proper preparation by the person performing the scrub. Skin and nails should be kept clean and in good condition. Fingernails should be short (not to reach be-

---

Recommended Practices for Surgical Scrub

1. All personnel should be in surgical attire before beginning the surgical hand scrub.
2. An effective antimicrobial surgical hand scrub agent approved by the facility's infection control committee should be used for all surgical hand scrubs.
3. The surgical hand scrub procedure should be standardized for all personnel according to institutional policy and procedure.

Source: AORN. Standards and recommended practices, Denver, CO: The Association, 1995, pp. 185–188.

yond the finger tips), and polish free. Artificial nails are not recommended because of their potential for harboring bacteria and fungal development under the nails. Jewelry, including watches, rings, and bracelets should not be worn. Hands should be inspected for breaks in the skin which could become an entry for microbial contamination. A clean scrub suit, a cap covering all hair, including facial hair, and a high filtration mask are required by all personnel performing the scrub procedure.

Antimicrobial Agents

Both the iodophors and chlorohexidine gluconates are commonly used for this purpose. They are prepared in combination with detergent to give a cleaning action along with the antibacterial action. Disposable, presterilized scrub brushes, impregnated with an antimicrobial agent, are available in most ORs. The choice of agent is dependent on effectiveness and personal preference (sensitivity) to the agent. Agents to be used for the surgical hand scrub should be standardized throughout the institution, and approved by the infection control department of the facility.

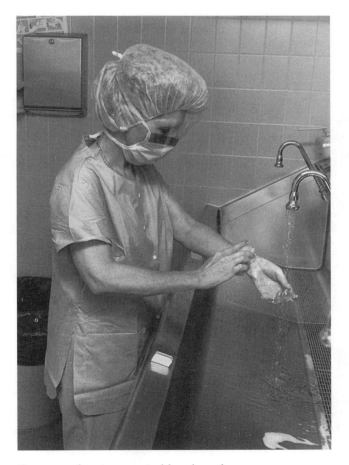

Person performing surgical hand scrub

Length of Scrub

According to the latest research, a 5-minute surgical scrub, covering hands and forearms, is adequate for removal of gross dirt and oils from the skin, as long as mechanical friction and antimicrobial action is present. Therefore all surgical scrubs are of 5-minute duration.

Donning Sterile Attire

Before scrubbed personnel can touch sterile supplies or the sterile field, they must put on sterile gowns and gloves to prevent microbial contamination on hands or clothing from being transferred to the sterile field and/or the patient's wound. Materials used as a bacterial barrier, such as gowns and drapes, may be an important link in the prevention of wound infection, and therefore the specifications for this material, whether disposable or nondisposable, must meet the recommended criteria established by AORN[11] in order to preserve an aseptic environment during a surgical or invasive procedure of any type.

Nursing Considerations   Materials should be resistant to penetration by either blood or other liquids used at the sterile field. The stockinette cuff is the most contaminated portion of the gown, since it absorbs moisture from the skin more rapidly than the gown fabric, and therefore must be covered at all times with sterile gloves. Materials should meet or exceed recommendations from the National Fire Protection Agency (NFPA) for flame retardation, be as lint-free as possible, and create and maintain an aseptic barrier when in use.

In some instances, due to the nature of the surgical procedure, extra protection gowns may be required (an additional layer of resistant material is added to the front of the gown and the sleeves) as an added precaution against penetration of copious amounts of fluids or contaminants, or both, during the procedure.

Recommended Practices: Protective Barrier Material

1. Surgical gowns and drapes should be made of material that minimizes the passage of microorganisms between nonsterile and sterile areas.
2. Gowns and drapes should be safe and comfortable for use in the practice setting.

Source: AORN. Standards and recommended practices, Denver, CO: The Association, 1995, Pp. 181–182.

CRITICAL ELEMENT
TASK 8-1

Procedure for Surgical Scrub

PURPOSE

To remove microbial organisms from hands and arms by both mechanical and chemical antisepsis

PREREQUISITE

Proper scrub attire, including mask

PROFICIENCY

One hundred percent accuracy at the time of performance

PROCEDURAL STEPS

Anatomic (Timed) Method: *(see diagram below)*

1. Assemble equipment and adjust water to a comfortable setting.
2. Wet hands and arms. If pre-washing with detergent from soap dispenser, lather hands and arms with soap and rinse.
3. Remove scrub brush from package, and using the nail cleaner provided, clean subungual spaces.
4. Squeeze brush under the water to dispense soap from the sponge.
5. Holding sponge perpendicular to finger tips, begin to scrub using back and forth motion. Scrub all four sides of each finger, including spaces in between.
6. Maintaining lather, scrub palm of hand and back of hand to the wrist, using circular motion.
7. Starting at the wrist, scrub to 2 inches above the elbow on all sides of the arm and wrist, rotating the arm from back to front.
8. Transfer sponge to the other hand and repeat steps 6 through 8, maintaining aseptic technique.

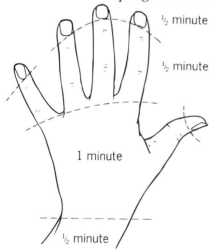

Timed method: 5-minute scrub

½ minute	fingers and nails
1½ minutes	palm and back of hand
½ minute	wrist to 2 in. above elbow

2½ minutes per extremity

Fig. A. Surgical hand scrub technique, anatomic scrub method

NOTE: Never go back over area already scrubbed.

9. Discard brush, and rinse hands and arms under the running water starting at finger tips and working toward elbows, keeping hand upright and elbows in a downward position.
10. Allow water to drip off elbows, maintaining proper position before entering the procedure room.

POINTS TO REMEMBER

1. Avoid "splashback" of water (scrub agent) on scrub suit.
2. Time interval: 5-minute scrub—2½ minutes for each extremity (see Fig. A).
3. Avoid unnecessary movement and talking during the scrub procedure.
4. Masks must be in place during the scrub procedure by all persons entering the scrub area.
5. If contact is made with unsterile surfaces during the scrub procedure, the entire scrub procedure must be started from the beginning.
6. Only those recommended antimicrobial solutions should be used during the surgical scrub.

Gowning and Gloving Procedures

Moisture remaining on the skin after the scrub procedure must be dried with a sterile towel before donning sterile gown and gloves. Therefore, the hand-drying process is part of the gowning procedure. (See Critical Element Task 8-2, Fig. A, p. 154.)

In order to preserve the sterility of the major sterile supplies opened before surgery, the gowning and gloving procedure should be performed close to the sterile field, but on a separate surface. This will help prevent the accidental contamination of the supplies during the procedure. (See Critical Element Task 8-2, Fig. B, p. 155.)

Sterile Gloves

Sterile gloves come presterilized and sized from the manufacturer. During the packaging of sterile gloves, provisions must be made for the scrubbed person to touch only the inner side of the glove cuff when donning the gloves. When opening the package, if a wide cuff is not available, discard the gloves and request another pair to avoid possible contamination during the gloving procedure.

Sterile gloves can be applied using two methods: the *open method* and the *closed method.* (See Critical Element Task 8-3, pp. 156–158.)

The closed glove method should be used any time you are initially applying sterile gown and gloves, while the open glove method should be used when gloving another team member or changing a glove during a procedure (self or team member), or when a sterile scrub or gown is not required (aseptic procedures).

Scrub persons, responsible for establishing and organizing the sterile field, are responsible for gowning and gloving with assistance from the circulating nurse (unassisted gowning and gloving), while the rest of the sterile team members will be assisted by the scrubbed person. (See Critical Element Task 8-4 pp. 159–161.)

Changing and Removing Sterile Gown and Gloves

Just as important as properly donning sterile attire is the procedure for changing gloves during a procedure and safe removal of contaminated gown and gloves. To protect the hands, the gown is removed first, followed by the gloves. Both are contained away from the scrub attire, and placed in the designated receptacle for contaminated disposable (or nondisposable) linen. (See Critical Task Element 8-5, p. 162.)

CRITICAL ELEMENT
TASK 8-2

Procedure for Application of Sterile Gown

PURPOSE

To provide assurance of maintaining a sterile field by covering those areas of the body and clothing with a sterile bacterial barrier

PREREQUISITE

Surgical hand scrub
Opening the sterile gown and glove package as designated in prescribed manner

PROFICIENCY

One hundred percent at the time of performance

PROCEDURAL STEPS

A. Drying Hands (see Fig. A)

1. Enter procedure room holding hands and arms away from the body at the appropriate height.
2. Approach the table where gown and gloves have been prepared, pick up the sterile towel touching only the sterile towel, and step back. Allow the towel to fall open.
3. Starting with one end of the towel, dry one hand and arm stopping 2 inches above the elbow.
4. Invert the towel, and with the other end, dry the other hand and arm.

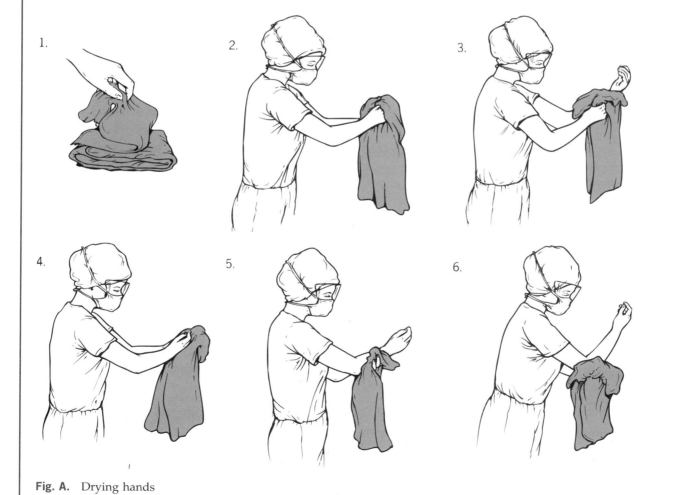

Fig. A.   Drying hands

NOTE: As you are drying the hand and arm, bend forward slightly to prevent any part of the towel from coming in contact with clothing.

   5.   When both hands and arms are dry, discard the towel.

B. Unassisted Gowning (see Fig. B)

   1.   Grasp the prefolded sterile gown by the neckline with both hands and step back from the table into an obstructed area.

   2.   Holding the folded gown with the inside toward you, locate the neckline of the gown, and holding the gown with both hands, allow the gown to unfold in front of you.

   3.   Holding the unfolded gown at shoulder level, push both hands and arms into the sleeves simultaneously.

NOTE: The circulating nurse will assist in bringing the gown over the shoulders by reaching inside the gown and closing and securing the gown at the waist and neckline. The hands should not be extended beyond the stockinette cuff.

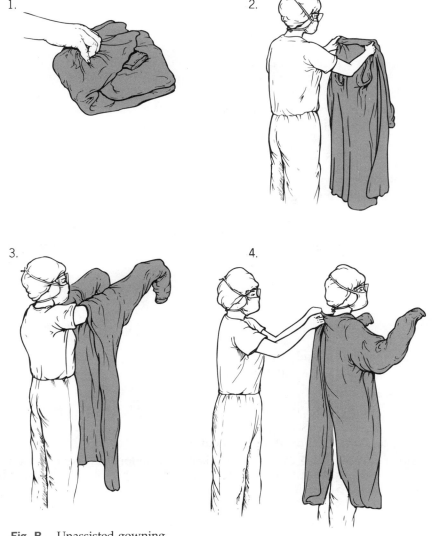

Fig. B.   Unassisted gowning

Procedure for Applying Sterile Gloves

PURPOSE

To provide a bacterial barrier over the hands, thus allowing contact with sterile items and protection from contaminants during the procedure

PREREQUISITE

A. Closed-gloved method: Surgical scrub and sterile gown

B. Open-glove method: None if sterile gown is not worn

PROFICIENCY

One hundred percent at time of performance

PROCEDURAL STEPS

A. Closed-glove method (see Fig. A)

1. Using the stockinette cuff of the glove as a "mitten," open the inside wrappers of the glove package, and with the left hand, lift the *right* glove off the wrapper by the cuff.
2. Extend the right forearm with palm upward. Place the palm of the glove against the palm of the protected hand *thumb-to-thumb* with *fingers pointing toward the elbow.*
3. Hold the cuff of the hand being gloved securely, and with the other protected hand, stretch the glove cuff over the end of the right sleeve and hand. (The cuff of the glove is now over the stockinette cuff of the gown, with the hand still inside the sleeve.)
4. Pull the glove on over extended right fingers until it completely covers the stockinette cuff.
5. Using the gloved hand, pick up the other glove from the package, and repeat steps 2 through 4.

B. Open-glove method (see Fig. B)

1. Open glove package by grasping the two center folds of the wrapper, and spreading them apart.
2. Lift the left glove up from the wrapper by the edge of the cuff using thumb and index finger of the right hand.
3. Slide the glove over the left hand, holding the cuff, and adjust each finger into its own slot.
4. Invert the gloved hand so that gloved fingers are touching the sterile glove and lift it off the wrapper.
5. Slide ungloved hand into glove and adjust fingers.
6. Adjust both gloves for comfort and covering of wrists.

POINTS TO REMEMBER

A. Gowning

1. When drying hands, do not go over areas already dried.
2. Avoid contact of towel with scrub suit by bending slightly at the waist during the drying procedure.
3. Use one end of the towel for each hand/arm.
4. When placing arms into gown, maintain proper level of arms and hands (*no higher than shoulders or lower than waist*).
5. For initial gowning and gloving, do not let hands go beyond cuff of gown.
6. When *removing a gown* at the end of the procedure, care must be taken to avoid touching contaminants on the gown. Therefore, it is removed inside out, pulling downward from the shoulders, toward the middle. (See Critical Element Task 8-5, Fig. B.)

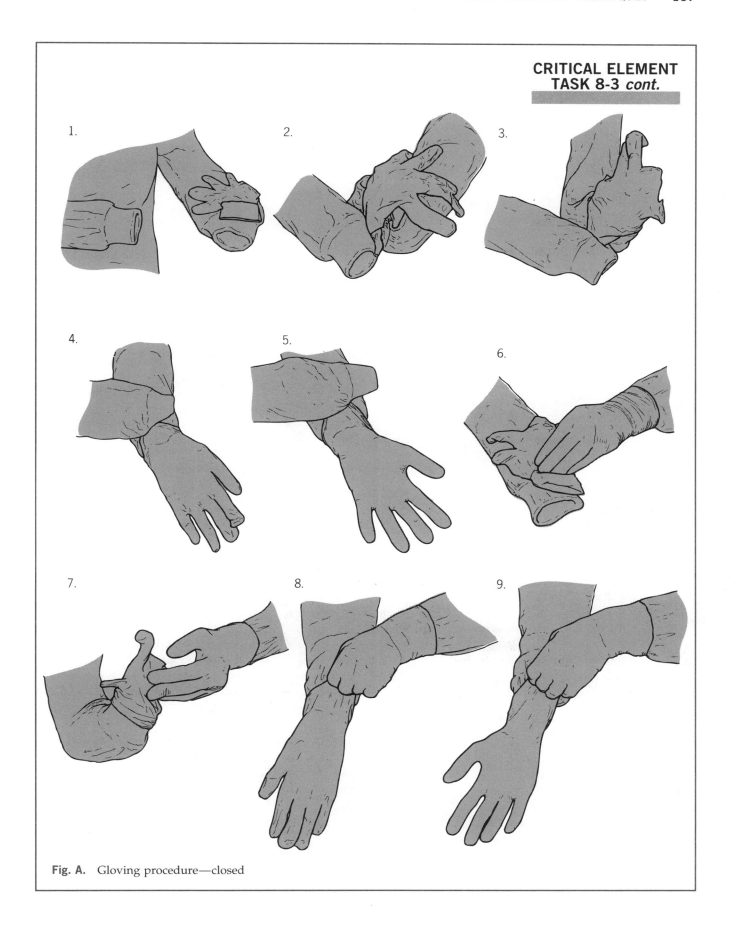

1.
2.
3.
4.
5.
6.
7.
8.
9.

Fig. A. Gloving procedure—closed

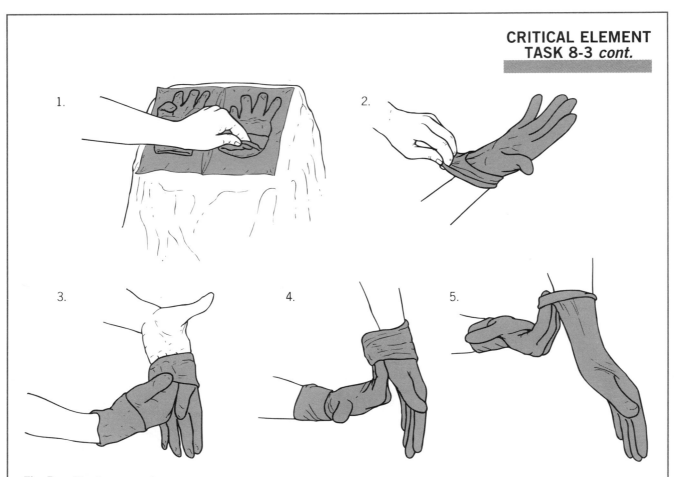

Fig. B. Gloving procedure—open

B. Gloving

1. Avoid contact of sterile gloves with ungloved hands during closed glove procedure.
2. For open glove, touch only the cuff of the glove with ungloved hand, and then only glove-to-glove for other hand.
3. For closed glove, never let the fingers extend beyond the stockinette cuff during the procedure. Contact with ungloved fingers constitutes contamination of the glove.
4. If contamination occurs during either procedure, both gown and gloves must be discarded and new gown and gloves must be used.
5. When removing gloves after a procedure is finished the gloves are removed *after* the gown is removed inside out, using glove-to-glove then skin-to-skin technique. (See Critical Element Task 8-3, Fig. B.)

Procedure for Gowning and Gloving Another Team Member (Assisted Gowning/Gloving)

PURPOSE

To assist another member of the sterile team in applying sterile gown and gloves before the start of a procedure

PREREQUISITE

Surgical hand scrub by team member
Procedure performed by person in sterile gown and gloves

PROFICIENCY

One hundred percent at time of performance

PROCEDURAL STEPS

A. Gowning Another Person (see Fig. A)

1. Open the sterile towel and lay it across the palm of the team member being gowned.
2. Unfold the gown carefully, holding at the neckband so that the inside of the gown faces the wearer.
3. Keeping gloved hands inside the gown shoulders, place the gown on the arms of the wearer, as he/she slips into the sleeves of the gown, and push up toward the shoulders.
4. Release the gown at shoulder height, and adjust the sleeves in preparation for assisted open gloving.

NOTE: The circulator will assist with the gowning procedure by pulling the gown onto the shoulders from the inside of the gown, securing the back of the gown by fasteners at the neck and waist from the inside.

B. Gloving Another Member (Open-glove method) (see Fig. B)

1. Pick up the *right* glove, grasping it firmly with fingers under the everted cuff, and present it so that the thumb and palm are facing the wearer. Announce the hand to be gloved.
2. Stretch the cuff sufficiently to allow hand access while protecting your gloved hand, and apply resistance while the wearer pushes hand into the glove.
3. Release the cuff.
4. Present the *left* glove in the same manner. The wearer will assist by stretching the cuff with his/her index finger of the gloved hand.
5. Apply resistance as needed; then release the cuff.
6. Offer a damp towel to remove powder from gloves, and discard towel after use.

POINTS TO REMEMBER

1. Protect your sterile gown and gloves during the gowning and gloving of another team member.
2. During gloving, do not let your hands fall below your waist when applying resistance.
3. If contamination occurs during either procedure, ask the circulator to assist in removing the gown and gloves, and repeat the gown and glove procedure.

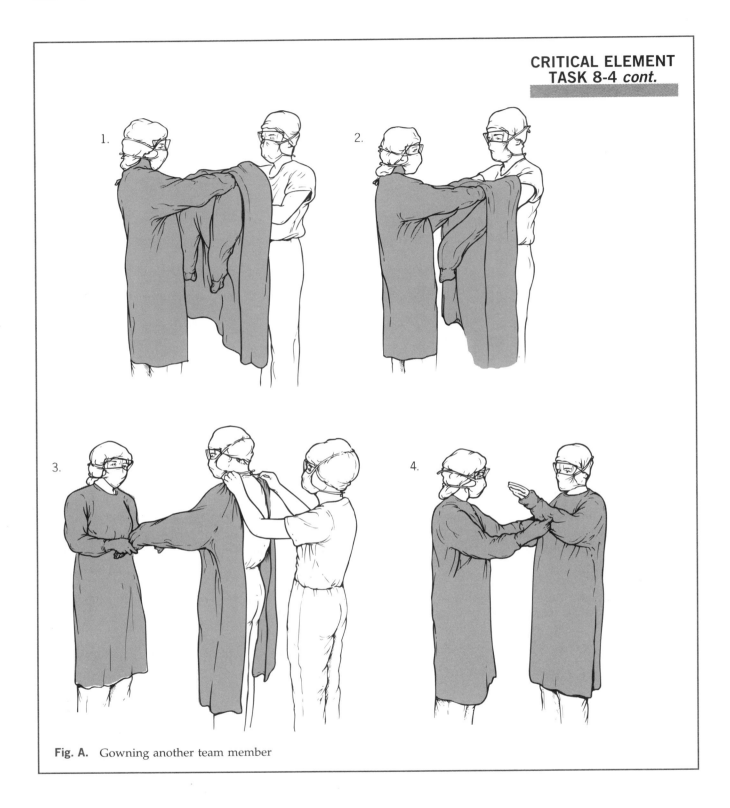

Fig. A. Gowning another team member

1.

2.

3.

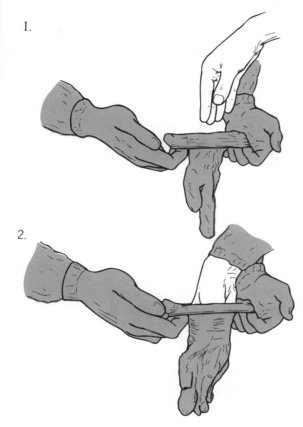
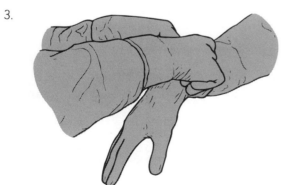

Fig. B. Gloving another team member

**CRITICAL ELEMENT
TASK 8-5**

Procedure for Changing Glove(s)
During a Procedure

PURPOSE

To remove contaminated glove(s) and replace with sterile glove(s) without interrupting the flow of surgery

PREREQUISITE

Prior application of sterile gown and gloves

PROFICIENCY

One hundred percent at time of performance

PROCEDURAL STEPS

A. Self

1. Holding contaminated glove away from the sterile field, ask the circulator to remove glove in the following manner:
   a. circulator grasps outside of glove, at palm, and pulls glove off
   b. scrubbed person holds onto the sleeve of gown, thereby preventing stockinette cuff from riding over hand

NOTE: Circulator should be wearing gloves during this procedure to protect uncovered hands from contacting contaminants.

2. Using the open-glove method, re-apply sterile glove to exposed hand.
3. Wipe off glove with damp cloth and discard cloth.

B. Team Member

1. Follow step 1 for removal of soiled glove.
2. Using the open-glove method, follow the procedure for Gloving Another Team Member (p. 159), and re-apply sterile glove(s) accordingly.
3. Offer damp towel to wipe off glove(s), then discard towel.

POINTS TO REMEMBER

1. The first step in preventing infection is recognition of a break in technique and immediate correction of that break.
2. Hold contaminated glove away from the field. Do not use contaminated hand to pass instruments while waiting for soiled glove to be removed.
3. The open-glove method is the *only* acceptable method used for changing gloves during a procedure.

1.

2.

Fig. A. Removing soiled gown

1.

2.

Fig. B. Removing soiled gloves

Self-assessment Exercise 2

Directions: *Complete the following exercises. Answers are found at the end of the module.*

1. Cuffs of a sterile gown, the neckline, shoulders, underarms, and back are not considered sterile.

    True   False

2. Sitting during a surgical procedure in sterile gown and gloves is acceptable, as long as the procedure is performed while sitting.

    True   False

3. Name the two acceptable antimicrobial agents used for a surgical scrub procedure.

4. A surgical hand scrub procedure should be the same for all personnel.

    True   False

5. When removing the gown and gloves after the case is completed, the gloves are removed first, then the gown.

    True   False

6. When changing gloves during a procedure, the _____ method should be used.

UNIT 2

Preparation of Surgical Supplies
Mary Ann Brooks

The perioperative nurse is responsible and accountable for many of the activities that occur during the perioperative period, which include preserving and protecting the patient from infection and providing a safe environment for the health-care staff.

Instruments, supplies, and other equipment used during surgery must be properly prepared and processed according to acceptable practices. Three processes known as *preparation and packaging, sterilization,* and *disinfection* are of vital importance during the perioperative period. All personnel must know how to properly execute these tasks and be able to distinguish the process of sterilization from other processes that approach sterility, but do not achieve it.

METHODS OF ASSURING ADEQUATE PROCESSING

Medical and surgical equipment and supplies are categorized into three different groups based on the potential risk of infection associated with their usage. These categories dictate the type of processing required for the specific object or item.

Category I: Critical Items

Critical items are instruments or objects that are introduced directly into the bloodstream and/or into any normally sterile area or cavity of the body.

EXAMPLES: Examples include, but are not limited to, surgical instruments and devices, specialty trays and sets, irrigation solutions, catheters, tubes and drains, IV solutions, and internal defibrillator paddles.

Process

Critical items must be *sterilized* by either steam, chemical, or physical methods.

Category II: Semicritical Items

Semicritical items contact intact mucous membranes, and/or may or may not penetrate body surfaces.

EXAMPLES: Examples include, but are not limited to, cystoscopes, flexible and/or rigid endoscopes,

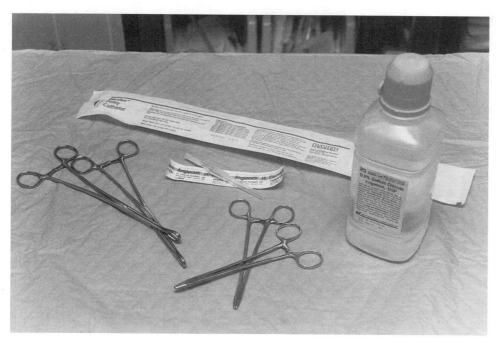

Critical items require sterilization

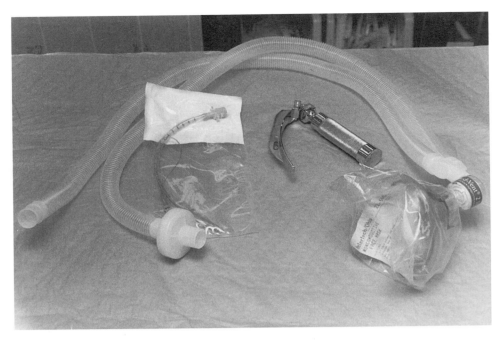

Semi-critical items: sterilization preferred but disinfection acceptable

thermometers, endotracheal tubes, anesthesia re-breathing circuits, and respiratory therapy equipment.

Process

Sterilization is preferred, but disinfection is acceptable, but only when using a high-level disinfectant solution.

Category III: Noncritical Items

Noncritical items are those which either do not ordinarily touch the patient or contact *only* intact skin.

EXAMPLES: Examples may include such items as bedpans, crutches, EKG electrodes and lead wires, blood pressure cuffs (automatic or manual), external defibrillator paddles, and grounding pads for the electrosurgical unit.

Process

These items only require a thorough cleaning and decontamination depending on their use, since with intact skin, microbial entry is rare.

PREPARATION OF SURGICAL SUPPLIES

Two common processes associated with the initial preparation of surgical supplies are (1) decontamina-

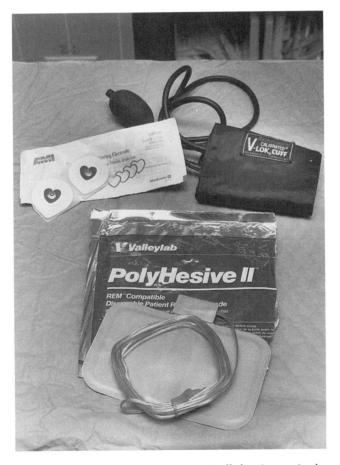

Noncritical items: decontamination is all that is required

tion and (2) packaging. All items must be thoroughly cleaned (decontaminated) before packaging and preparation for terminal processing, since effectiveness of the terminal process is directly correlated to the amount of *bioburden* on the object at the time of processing.

Decontamination Process

Decontamination is the first step toward reducing the potential hazard or direct contact with blood, fluids, or tissues left on contaminated instruments. Decontamination refers to a process by which the contaminants are removed, either by manual or mechanical methods, using specific solutions capable of rendering the blood and debris harmless and removing it from the surface of an object or instrument.

The decontamination process begins in the OR, following the completion of the surgical procedure. All instruments used during the procedure should be inspected for gross dirt and debris, and cleaned with water and/or a scrub brush soaked with an antimicrobial or bleach solution. This process must be done under the water level, preventing splash dissemination of harmful microorganisms. The instruments, along with the other nondisposable supplies exposed to the patient/procedure are then placed in a proper receptacle and covered for transference to the decontamination room. It is important to note that the contaminated instruments and nondisposable equipment should be covered when traversing hallways leading into the decontamination area.

If a *case cart* system is used, the initial cleaning should still be performed, and the instruments returned to the cart for transport to the designated decontamination area. Additionally, remember to remove all remaining sterile items from the cart before placing contaminated items back on the cart. These remaining sterile items can then be returned to their proper place to be reused in another case, as long as their protective wrappers are intact.

Once the instruments and other nondisposable items used at the field arrive in the decontamination area, the second step in the process begins, which involves the terminal cleaning of the instruments and initial sterilization before assembly of the tray. A manual cleaning procedure, for delicate and heat sensitive items, is recommended to preserve the life of the instruments and to decontaminate them before the sterilization process. If manual washing is required, all personnel must be protected from exposure to contaminants during the cleaning process.

The most common cleaning method is mechanical cleaning which can be accomplished using several different tools: *ultrasonic washer, washer–sterilizer,* or the *washer–disinfector.*

Ultrasonic Washer

All items must first be cleaned before being placed in the ultrasonic washer. The ultrasonic cleaning process removes hidden blood and debris that is left on the instrument by a process known as *cavitation,* which occurs when sound waves are passed through water, creating gas bubbles. These bubbles grow in size until they become unstable, and this generates a vacuum, which is responsible for the actual cleaning process. The smaller particles float to the top, while the larger particles settle on the bottom of the tank, and are eventually flushed away.

The particles will remain in suspension as long as the water and detergent are fresh. For this reason, it is recommended that the water be changed frequently, especially whenever soil or blood is visible.

Washer–Sterilizer

When a washer–sterilizer is used, the soiled instruments are cleaned by mechanical agitation in a bath containing a detergent, rinsed, and then sterilized for 3 minutes. Washer–sterilizers of this type are advantageous, since they reduce the bioburden, may save labor costs, and conserve time all in one process. However, soiled instruments must undergo an initial cold cycle or be washed first by hand, before the process. This prevents the "banking on" of dried blood on the instrument.

Washer–Disinfector

Another tool for decontaminating instruments is the washer–disinfector, which removes excessive amounts

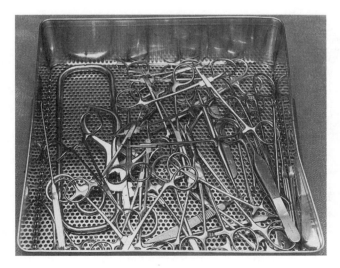

Tray wth soiled instruments awaiting cleaning and decontamination before sterilization

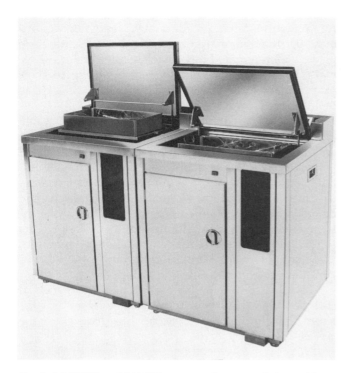

Castle 2415UW and 2415RD—sonic cleaner and rinser/dryer

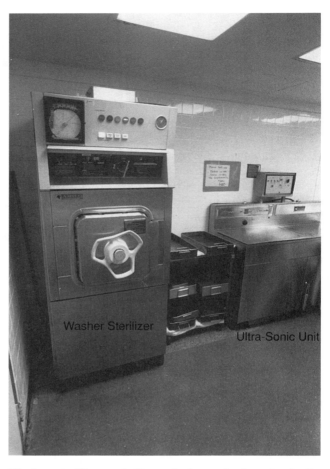

Washer–sterilizer and ultrasonic cleaner in decontamination area of surgery

of debris from the instrument, eliminating the hand-cleaning phase of the decontamination process. The numerous water jets and the increased pH of the detergent allow for thorough cleaning of even grossly soiled instruments, which is followed by a neutralizing rinse to quickly restore the pH to its neutral state. Since the agitation of the water is minimal, it cleans without tossing the instruments around in the tray, thereby reducing the risk of damage, even to delicate instruments. There is no steam injected into the chamber; however, if steam is available, it can be used to speed up the heating temperature of the water.[11]

The washer–disinfector cleans instruments so thoroughly that it may not only eliminate the need for hand cleaning, but could also replace the ultrasonic washer, which is a definite cost-effective factor in today's practice setting.

Regardless of which mechanical process is used, the decontamination phase is critical to the terminal processing, since without proper cleaning, the process cannot be effective in reducing the potential biologic hazards associated with contaminated instruments.

STERILIZATION AND DISINFECTION

Once the decontamination process is completed, the final (terminal) phase of the preparation process be-

gins. This involves one of two distinct processes: (1) sterilization or (2) disinfection.

Sterilization Principles

The modern process of sterilization has come a long way since Robert Koch first created the sterilizer in 1881, but the principles and importance of the process toward the goal of an infection-free surgical procedure has not changed in the last 100 years.

To *sterilize* means to render an item or object completely free of all living microorganisms, including spores, through one of three processes:

1. steam sterilization
2. chemical sterilization
3. physical sterilization

Each method has its own characteristics and requires specific parameters for effective completion of the process. Additionally, the process must be continu-

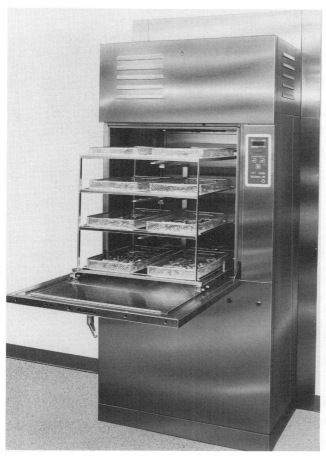

Castle 7550 washer–disinfector

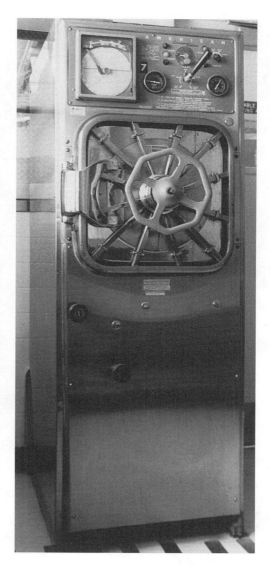

Old steam-sterilizer model

ously monitored to assure that all parameters and specifications of the process have been met, thus assuring the sterility of the item and the proper functioning of the equipment.

OVERVIEW OF STERILIZATION PROCESSES

Steam Sterilization

Steam alone is incapable of sterilizing an item. However, when steam is placed under pressure, the temperature rises, and the moist heat produces changes in the nature of the protein within the cell, rendering it harmless. It is, therefore, the relationship between temperature, pressure, and time of exposure that becomes a crucial factor in destroying microbes, and it is these principles that are used in the operation of the steam sterilizer.

Steam under pressure is the most common and economical method of sterilization for supplies used in the OR and elsewhere in the hospital. If the item is heat and moisture stable, then the item should be steam sterilized, since this is always the method of choice.

Chemical Sterilization

Not all equipment or instruments can withstand the extremes of temperature and pressure required during the steam sterilization process. Therefore, an alternative method, just as effective, must be used for these instruments or equipment.

One type of common chemical sterilization utilizes a gas known as *ethylene oxide* (EO) to accomplish this process. This gas is capable of penetrating most known substances, a criterion for effective sterilization. EO in its natural state is extremely flammable and toxic, but when mixed with carbon dioxide or fluorinated hydro-

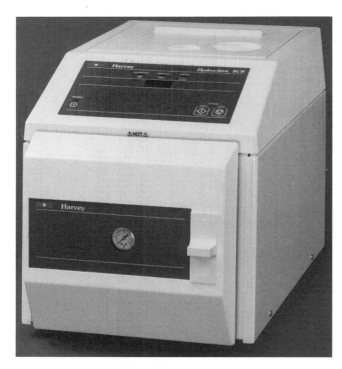

Harvey SC8 hydroclave steam sterilizer

use. These items must state the exact number of times the item can be resterilized, and these recommendations must come from the manufacturer of the product.

Physical sterilization is cost prohibitive for a hospital. Therefore this process is always associated with commercially prepared items. The sterility of the item is guaranteed until the package is opened or the integrity of the package has been compromised.

STERILIZATION EQUIPMENT

Steam Sterilizers

Sterilizers designed to use steam under pressure are referred to as autoclaves. They are generally manufactured to perform this task by one of three methods:

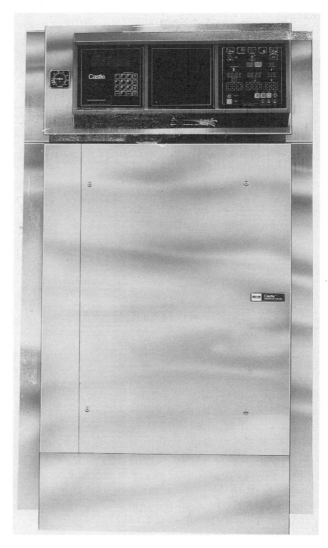

Modern Hi-vac steam sterilizer (Courtesy of MDT Corporation)

carbons, it is rendered nonflammable for hospital use. Yet it still remains toxic to body tissues, which necessitates aeration of the item. EO is expensive and requires a longer time to complete the sterilization and aeration process (up to 20 hours). Therefore, it should only be used when absolutely necessary, and with advanced planning in order to assure that the item being sterilized is available when needed. One hundred percent EO is also used by hospitals, but in smaller amounts. It is contained in a sealed canister and used indirectly for each load.

Two additional sterilants come under the heading of chemical sterilization: peracetic acid and hydrogen peroxide plasma solutions. Both will be briefly discussed later on in this chapter.

Physical Sterilization

In today's practice setting, many of the items used in the sterile field are available as prepackaged sterile items from the manufacturer. The sterilization process used for these items is *ionizing radiation (cobalt 60)*, and thereby falls into the category of physical sterilization.

Most of these items are disposable and are designed for single-use only, since resterilization may change or deteriorate the item's composition and possibly render it hazardous to the patient. If a single-use item is opened and not used, it *cannot* be resterilized. Other items have been specifically designated for multiple

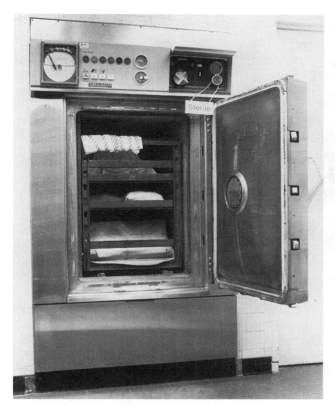

Steam sterilizer

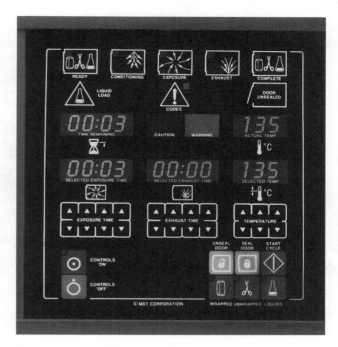

Steam autoclave control panel (Courtesy of MDT Corporation)

(1) gravity air displacement, (2) prevacuum or high-vac, and (3) special purpose high speed.

Components of the Autoclave

Regardless of the autoclave used for the process, the components of the sterilizer are basically the same. The metal casing, housing the elements, contains a *jacket* surrounding the chamber where the items are placed. A control panel (indicator panel) housing gauges that show the specific cycle is in view above or beside the door. The unit has a hinged door that is automatically locked during the cycle and, depending on the model, the unit may have a second door as a pass-through from one area to another.

A *monitoring* component, either a graph or computerized read-out, contained in the control panel, confirms that the sterilization process is proceeding according to specifications set by the manufacturer.

Most steam sterilizers can be run from 3 minutes to 99 hours, depending on the type of sterilizer and the temperature being used to sterilize the item(s).

Gravity Air Displacement Sterilizer

The gravity air displacement sterilizer utilizes the principle that air is heavier than steam. There is an inner chamber where the goods are sterilized and an outer heated jacket that ejects steam into the chamber and acts as a gravity steam separator, which removes entrapped droplets of water from the steam before admission into the actual chamber.

When the sterilizer is activated, pressurized steam enters the top of the inner chamber from the jacket, and exerts pressure on the air inside the chamber, displacing the air downward to the bottom of the chamber where it is released through a temperature-sensitive valve (Fig. 8-1).

As the pressure increases, due to steam build-up, the sterilization temperature is reached, the valve closes, and the timing of the cycle begins.

Operating Temperature and Length of Cycle   The length of cycle is dependent on the temperature reached inside the jacket. Most gravity displacement sterilizers work in a range from 250°F (121°C) to 254°F (123°C) at 15–17 pounds per square inch (psi), and takes anywhere from 15 minutes for a conventional pack to 55 minutes for sterilization of fluids.[12] Following the sterilization process, you must have a cooling period from 15 minutes to 1 hour.

NOTE: The higher the temperature, the shorter the cycle duration required.

Prevacuum (High-Vac) Sterilizer

The automatic prevacuum, high-temperature sterilizer has generally replaced the gravity air displacement

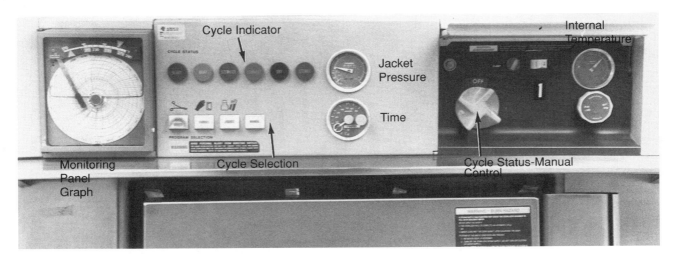

Close-up of control panel on a steam sterilizer

method, since it does not rely on gravity to remove the air from the chamber.

Instead, the air is removed by a vacuum pump that simultaneously draws the air out while steam is injected into the chamber, replacing the air. This mechanism reduces the time necessary to accomplish the sterilization cycle to as little as 20 minutes, but the time varies with the size of the sterilizer, the adequacy of the steam, and the supply of the water.

This sterilizer is efficient in preventing air pockets and has greater penetrating abilities than the gravity displacement type.

Because it relies on vacuum to begin the timing cycle, a test to ensure its proper vacuum capabilities must be performed at the beginning of each day. This test is called a *Bowie-Dick test* and is performed using a test pack of prewashed surgical towels with a commercially prepared monitoring sheet placed between the towel pack. A commercially prepared Bowie-Dick test pack that meets current recommended standards is also available.

If a hospital-prepared pack is used, it should be wrapped and labeled "test pack." Regardless of which pack is used it is placed on the rack, directly over the

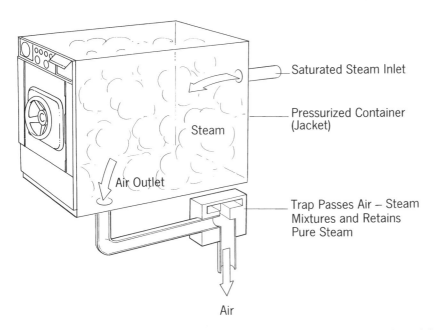

Fig. 8-1. Basic components required for pressure steam sterilizer (Adapted from Perkins, JJ. *Principles and Methods of Sterilization in Health Science* [3rd ed.]. Springfield, IL: Charles C. Thomas, 1983. P. 30.)

steam drain, in an empty sterilizer. Upon completion of the cycle, the paper is removed and observed for a uniform color change, indicating a satisfactory test result. It does not, however, measure the efficacy of the sterilization process, only the efficient workings of the vacuum established during the process.

Length of Cycle and Temperature Range The recommended exposure time for prevacuum steam sterilizers is 4 minutes, at temperatures ranging from 270°F (132°C) to 274°F (134°C), 15–20 psi.[13] This sterilizer, like the gravity air displacement sterilizer, is used primarily for wrapped goods. Faulty packaging and overloading or incorrect placement of objects may interfere with the air removal, thus negating the sterilization process. Although this is not as critical on a Hi-Vac sterilizer, it should still be a consideration. Prevacuum sterilizers permit more supplies to be sterilized within the specified period of time than do gravity air displacement sterilizers of similar size.

Special Purpose High-Speed (Flash) Sterilizer

The high-speed or *flash* sterilizer is a smaller version of the gravity air displacement sterilizer, and is used exclusively for emergency sterilization of unwrapped items that may have been contaminated during a surgical procedure.

Items are placed in a wire-mesh tray or "flash pan" after cleaning, and are sterilized for a shorter cycle at a high temperature. The flash cycle will bypass the drying phase and fast exhaust on completion of the cycle. Therefore, the length of the process is greatly reduced.

Because the items are unwrapped and do not give an indication as to their exposure to the process, as do wrapped items, a steam integrator strip is placed in the tray with the items being flashed to show that the item(s) were exposed to the sterilization process. Each integrator strip should be marked with the name of the patient or case, the date, time, and autoclave number being used (some have a place for this information, some do not). These integrator strips should be maintained with other sterilization records that demonstrate the efficiency of the equipment being used.

Length of Cycle and Temperature The flash sterilizer is adjusted to operate at 270°F (132°C) and 27 psi. The time of exposure begins when the temperature reaches 270°F, and can be set for 3 minutes, 10 minutes, or whatever is needed, depending on the number of instruments being flashed and their composition. For example, air-powered drills or a full tray of instruments would require a longer time for adequate exposure to the steam than would two or three clamps placed in a flash pan.[14]

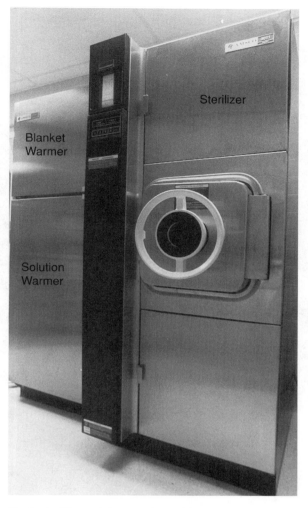

Flash sterilizer with warming cabinet

Chemical Sterilization

Chemical sterilization can be achieved through one of three processes:

1. gas (EO), for heat- and moisture-sensitive items
2. peracetic acid, for immersion of items
3. low temperature hydrogen peroxide plasma, for moisture-stable and moisture-sensitive items

Gas Ethylene Oxide Sterilization

Gas sterilization, using ethylene oxide (EO) is dependent on (1) the concentration of the gas being used, (2) the temperature inside the chamber, (3) the humidity level, and (4) the exposure time.

In general, EO gas concentrations range between 450 to 800 mg per L of chamber space, and operate at a temperature of 120°F (49°C) to 140°F (60°C), with at least 50 percent humidity, but not less than 30 percent

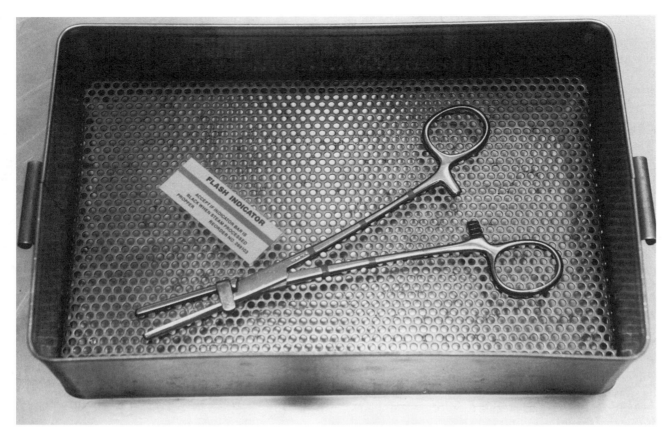

Flash pan for emergent sterilization

in order to hydrate the items during the process. (A relative humidity of 40–80 percent is recommended during the sterilization cycle.)[15]

EO sterilizers can be in the wall or on a rack in the open recess of the wall depending on the need of the area it serves. These chambers can be automatically or manually operated, and range in size from 16 × 16 × 29 inches to very large units that will accommodate several patient mattresses.

The timing of the cycle varies, but it usually takes between 3 and 6 hours for the sterilization part of the cycle to be completed. The total process does not end here, however. The items must be *aerated* before returning them for patient use, and this aeration must be part of the overall sterilization process.

Aeration of Gas Sterilized Items Ethylene glycol, a toxic carcinogen, is formed by a reaction of EO gas with water or moisture. Additionally, ethylene chlorhydrin can form when a chloride ion is present in combination with EO (i.e., PVC plastic.) If either of the substances is left on the item, it could cause immeasurable damage, including destruction of red blood cells and/or massive blistering of the skin that comes in contact with an unaerated item. Both patient and staff are therefore at risk for injury.

Because of its peculiar properties, and possible toxic effects, the sterilizer must be vented to the outside at least 20 feet from any air intake and far away from any heavy traffic areas/walkways. Therefore, for control purposes, most EO sterilizers are located in the central processing area of the hospital, unlike the steam sterilizers, which can be located both in or outside the operating room suite, and all loads *must* be aerated for a specified period of time.

Personnel working with EO must be specifically trained to effectively and safely execute this process, following acceptable standards established by the Occupational Health and Safety Administration (OSHA) and the Association for the Advancement of Medical Instrumentation (AAMI). These recommendations concern the handling, removal, and aeration process for gas sterilization:[16]

1. There must be limited exposure time for each employee working in or around the gas sterilizer.
2. EO sterilizers must be vented to outside atmosphere.
3. Gloves, resistant to EO penetration, must be worn when transferring items from the sterilizer to the aeration chamber if items are not contained in a stainless steel basket.

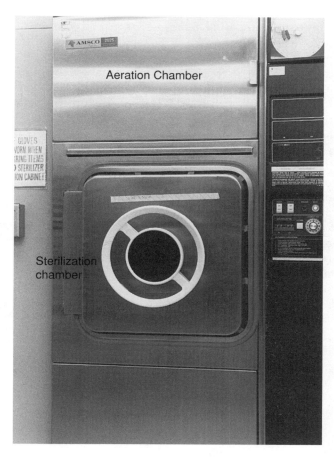

EO sterilizer for chemical sterilization process

4. All items must be placed in an aeration chamber before release for usage.
    a. ambient temperature: 7 days (in a cabinet room) Note: This method should not be used in a health-care facility.
    b. elevated temperature in aeration chamber 120°F (49°C): 12 hours
    c. elevated temperature in aeration chamber 140°F (60°C): 8 hours Note: Manufacturer's recommendations must always be followed.
5. When sterilization cycle is complete, the door should be immediately opened (3–6 inches). Either immediately remove the item, or wait 15 minutes before removing the load, depending on the manufacturer's recommendations.[17]

Preparing Items for EO Sterilization Items to be sterilized by this method require special preparation before being exposed to the sterilant. All items must be cleaned and dried, since water may unite with EO, thus forming ethylene glycol, which is not eliminated by aeration, and may result in toxic reactions in patients and personnel.

Lumens of tubings, needles, and so on, should be air dried, and open at both ends to avoid accumulation of gas inside the item. Packaging material should be specific for EO sterilization or indicated that both processes, steam and gas, are acceptable for that item.

Additional Methods— Chemical Sterilization

Sterilization by Peracetic Acid

Peracetic acid sterilization uses a sterilant solution of peracetic acid. This system is used when an item cannot be immersed in fluid, especially fiberoptic endoscopes and rigid endoscopes. Each time the process begins, a new container of single-use sterilant concentrate is used. There is no aeration time required, but the process does require that the items be rinsed with large amounts of sterile water following the sterilization process.

This system, like all sterilization systems, must be monitored for sterility with live spores. It is recommended that items sterilized by this method be used immediately.

Hydrogen Peroxide Plasma

Hydrogen peroxide is a bactericidal, viricidal, sporicidal, and fungicidal agent. This agent has been used mostly in commercial environments (i.e., laboratories, pharmaceutical agencies), but has been accepted in surgical suites. Because low concentrations of hydrogen peroxide plasma solutions have been shown to be an effective sporicidal agent, it may gradually be used as an alternative to EO sterilization for specific items.

Additionally, several other sterilants are currently under investigation for use in health-care facilities. Ozone (used in European countries), microwave, and propylene oxide are other methods of sterilization currently under study. Each has its advantages and disadvantages. After all is said and done, EO will probably remain the alternative method of sterilization for heat-sensitive and moisture-sensitive items in this century.

Perioperative Nursing Considerations—Sterilization

Bioburden relates to the number of actual or suspected microorganisms, of whatever type, found on a specific article at the same time. In order to ensure that the item has been properly sterilized, all gross dirt, blood, and tissue debris must be removed, before the item can undergo the sterilization process. This can be accomplished through proper decontamination procedures, discussed earlier in this chapter.

AORN Recommended Practices: Sterilization

I. Items to be sterilized should be decontaminated in a controlled environment, using universal precautions.

II. Items to be sterilized should be packaged according to the guidelines established in the AORN ''Recommended Practices for Selection and Use of Packaging Materials.''

III. Saturated steam under pressure should be used to sterilize heat- and moisture-stable items.

IV. Flash (steam) sterilization should be carefully selected to meet special clinical situations.

V. Ethylene oxide (EO) gas sterilization may be used for sterilization of heat- and moisture-sensitive items.

VI. Items sterilized with EO must be properly aerated in a mechanical aerator.

VII. A program for monitoring occupational exposure to EO must be established.

VIII. Low-temperature hydrogen peroxide plasma sterilization may be used for moisture-stable and moisture-sensitive items.

IX. Automated equipment using peracetic acid as a liquid sterilant may be used for items that can be immersed.

X. Every sterilized item should have a load identification.

XI. Items should be transported so as to maintain cleanliness and sterility and to prevent physical damage.

XII. Sterilized items should be stored in a well-ventilated, limited access area with controlled temperature and humidity.

XIII. Shelf life of a packaged sterile item is event related.

XIV. A quality control program should be established within the practice setting.

XV. Preventative maintenance of sterilizers should be performed on a scheduled basis by qualified personnel using manufacturer's written service instructions.

XVI. Policies and procedures for sterilization should be developed, reviewed annually, revised as necessary, and readily available within the practice setting.

Source: AORN. Standards and recommended practices, Denver, CO: The Association, 1995, Pp. 267–276.

Properly preparing instrument trays and equipment is just as important as the sterilization cycle itself, since proper preparation ensures exposure to all facets and areas of the item. Instruments which have joints (box locks) or rachets should be opened to allow the agent to penetrate all surfaces. The use of instrument racks or pegs are well suited for this purpose, and should be used whenever possible.

Instrument sets should be contained in perforated or wire mesh bottom trays, and the total weight of the tray (metal mass) should not exceed 16 to 17 pounds; otherwise, written weight recommendations from the manufacturer should be followed. If a rigid container system is used, the filter papers must be discarded after each use, and new ones inserted, to ensure proper filtration and protection of items inside the tray. When preparing basin sets, they should be *nested* with an absorbent towel, separating the metal surfaces to prevent contact and moisture buildup.

Instruments should not be strung or arranged on a *closed loop*, since the steam/gas cannot penetrate hollow items which are closed at one end. Heavier instruments should be at the bottom, with lighter or delicate instruments on top. An instruments worksheet or count sheet should be placed in the tray showing the amount of instruments, the date assembled, and the initials of the person who assembled the tray.

Packaging Materials

Materials used to wrap instruments and basins should allow for the penetration of the sterilizing agent and be compatible with the process to be utilized. Packaging materials can include reusable and single-use fabrics, peel-back pouches, and rigid container systems. The rigid container systems require no additional wrap-

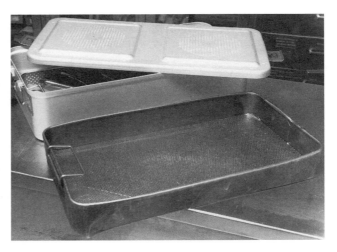

Conventional instrument tray and rigid container system used for sterilization

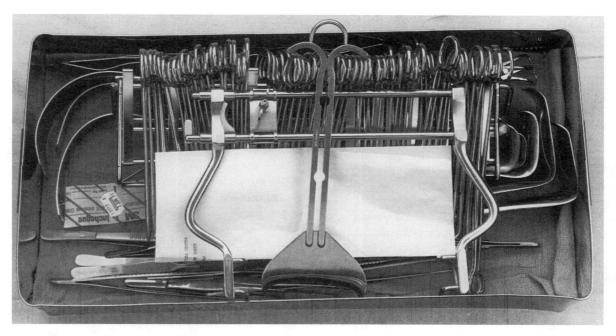

Assembled instrument tray for sterilization (note instrument count sheet in tray)

pers, but need to designate the process to be used on the outside of the container.

Since the sterility of an item is event-related, the packaging material should be strong enough to maintain its integrity following the sterilization process and protect the item from loss of sterility.

When using the disposable fabric, the wrapper must be of double-thickness, equaling a minimum of a 270 to 280 thread count per layer, and each layer must be wrapped sequentially, making the item easy to dispense to the sterile field without compromise to sterility.

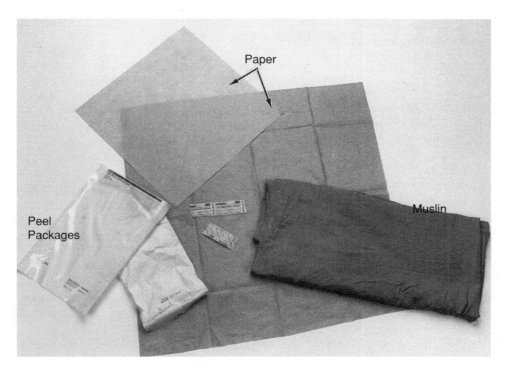

Sterilization wrapping material

Chemical Indicators and Load Identification

Before the item is wrapped for the sterilization cycle, a chemical indicator, corresponding to the sterilization process, is placed inside the tray, item, or package and stamped with a load indicator label stating the load number, sterilizer expiration/sterilization date, and the person preparing the item (Table 8-1).

The item is then wrapped using either the envelope style or square method (Figs. 8-2 and 8-3), and taped with the appropriate pressure tape for the process. The pressure tape serves as the outside indicator for the package, and signifies that the item has been exposed to one or more specific physical conditions during the cycle.

A load indicator seal is placed on the tape (as on the inside indicator), with a description of the item for easy retrieval when needed. To avoid confusion, the sterilization date should be recorded according to the Julian calendar date (day 1–365) and the expiration date according to the Gregorian calendar (month/date/year). The lot control number should be placed both inside and outside the package for visibility both in a sterile area and the storage area for sterile supplies/instruments.

When a peel-back package is used, one indicator with a load indicator seal is placed on the inside of the package, while the outer package is heat-sealed to prevent the package from opening. An external chemical indicator strip should be clearly visible on every package prepared for sterilization.

It is important to note that chemical indicators do not guarantee sterility of the item, only that the process is complete.

Biologic Monitors

It is necessary to have a reliable, inexpensive method of checking the effectiveness of the sterilization process. This is accomplished through the use of *biologic monitors*, commercially prepared according to the U.S. pharmacopeia minimum performance criteria, and used according to the manufacturer's recommendations.

As each sterilization method is different, so too are the biologic substances used to test the sterilization cycle.

Spores Used to Test the Process

A highly resistant, nonpathogenic, spore-forming bacteria, contained in a glass vial or impregnated strip, is placed in the sterilizer load. When the cycle is completed, the spore and a control ampule, not exposed to sterilization, are sent to the lab or central processing in the OR for incubation.

Bacillus stearthermophilus is used with a steam sterilizer and *Bacillus subtillis* is used with a gas sterilizer. When using a closed system (ampule), the incubation period is 24 hours for steam and 48 hours for gas.

Frequency of Spore Testing   The frequency for testing is based on the following recommendations from CDC, AAMI, and JCAHO (Table 8-2).

1. steam sterilizers: at least weekly and as necessary, should steam pressure be lost or interrupted, or following down-time due to repairs.
2. gas sterilizers: at least weekly, and as needed, as stated above.

If an implantable object is sterilized, regardless of the method, a biologic indicator should accompany each load, and these objects should not be used until the incubation period is completed, revealing destruction of the spores.

Refer to the institutional policy governing the biologic testing interval in order to ensure compliance within the institution, since sources may vary in their frequency recommendations for biologic testing.

Recommended Procedure for Positive Spore Test

In the event of a positive spore test occurring with either the gas or steam sterilizers, immediate action must be taken to prevent harm to the patient. Institutional policies and procedures dictating acceptable protocols should be well known by all personnel involved with the sterilization process. The following guidelines are recommended:

1. The suspect sterilizer should be taken out of service immediately until a qualified person can perform an operational inspection of the sterilizer.
2. The items processed by that sterilizer need not be recalled, except implantables, but the epidemiology department should be notified in order to provide closer monitoring of patients on the OR schedule for that day.
3. If sterilizer malfunction is discovered, all available items from the suspect sterilizer should be recalled, and an incident report should be filed with the risk management department, noting an unusual occurrence has taken place.
4. Once the malfunction has been corrected, another biologic indicator test *must* be performed before the sterilizer is placed back into service. If this test is negative, the suspect sterilizer may be placed back into full service.
5. Items sterilized by the suspect sterilizer must be stripped, rewrapped, and re-labeled for resterilization.

Table 8-1 Chemical Indicator Guidelines

Agency	Purpose	Require-ment	Placement External	Placement Internal	Record-keeping System
AAMI					
Good Hospital Practice: Steam Sterilization and Sterility Assurance, 1988 Good Hospital Practice: Performance Evaluation of EO Sterilizers—EO Test Packs, 1985	Adjunct to biologic indicator, never as a replacement	Should be used	On all packages (except if internal indicator is visible)	Within each package, in center or area least accessible to steam penetration	Yes
AHA					
Guidelines for the Hospital Central Service Department, 1978		Should be used	With each package; can be used inside or outside		Yes
AORN					
Recommended Practices for Sterilization and Disinfection, 1987	Show items exposed to sterilization conditions; do not replace BI or prove sterilization achieved	May be used	Visible on every package	Placed in area that is most difficult to sterilize	Yes
CDC					
Guidelines for the Prevention and Control of Nosocomial Infections, 1980	Do not indicate sterility but show item did not bypass a sterilization procedure	Should be used	Attached to each package	Inside large pack to verify steam penetration	—
JCAHO					
Standards adopted, 1990		Are used	With each package, no designation to inside or outside		Yes
Army regulations (AR-40-19), 1982	—	—	—	—	—
VA manual MP-2					
Change 107, July, 1975	Visual indicator that package exposed to physical conditions of a sterilizing cycle, not evidence of sterility	Will be used	Each package or item	—	Yes

AAMI = Association for the Advancement of Medical Instrumentation; AORN = Association of Operating Room Nurses; JCAHO = Joint Commission on Accreditation of Healthcare Organizations; AHA = American Hospital Association; CDC = Centers for Disease Control; VA = Veteran's Administration; BI = biologic indicators.
Adapted from Reichert M, Young J. Sterilization Technology for Health-Care Facility. Manual published by AMSCO Sterilizer Co., Pennsylvania.

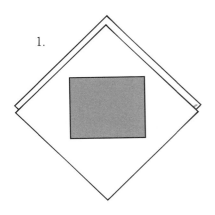
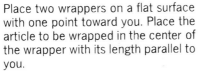

1.

Place two wrappers on a flat surface with one point toward you. Place the article to be wrapped in the center of the wrapper with its length parallel to you.

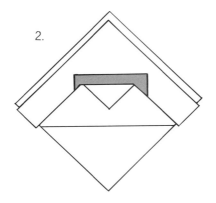

2.

Fold the corner nearest you over the article until it is completely covered. Fold the corner back toward you 2 to 3 inches.

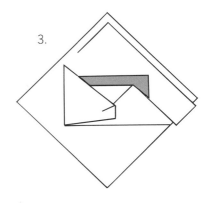

3.

Fold the left side of the wrapper over and parallel to the article. Fold the end of the corner back 2 to 3 inches.

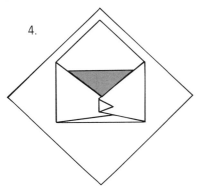

4.

Repeat with the right side. Lap center folds at least one half inch.

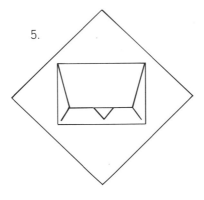

5.

Tuck in side edges of remaining corner to eliminate any direct opening to the article. Bring top corner down to bottom edges and tuck in leaving point for opening.

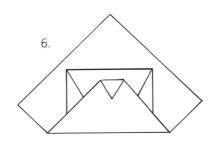

6.

Repeat step 2.

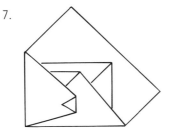

7.

Repeat step 3.

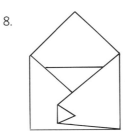

8.

Repeat step 4.

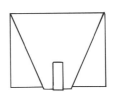

9.

Bring point of wrapper completely around. Package and seal with appropriate tape.

Fig. 8-2. Envelope wrap technique (Modified from the Association for the Advancement of Medical Instrumentation. National Standards and Recommended Practices for Sterilization [2nd ed.]. Arlington, VA, 1988.)

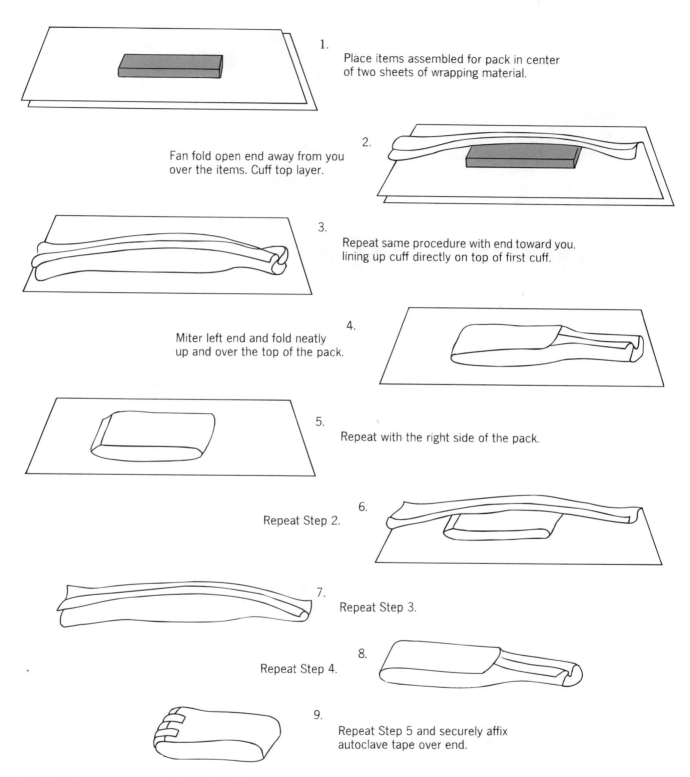

1. Place items assembled for pack in center of two sheets of wrapping material.

2.

Fan fold open end away from you over the items. Cuff top layer.

3. Repeat same procedure with end toward you, lining up cuff directly on top of first cuff.

4.

Miter left end and fold neatly up and over the top of the pack.

5. Repeat with the right side of the pack.

6. Repeat Step 2.

7. Repeat Step 3.

8. Repeat Step 4.

9. Repeat Step 5 and securely affix autoclave tape over end.

Fig. 8-3. Square wrap technique (Modified from the Association for the Advancement of Medical Instrumentation. National Standards and Recommended Practices for Sterilization [2nd ed.]. Arlington, VA, 1988.)

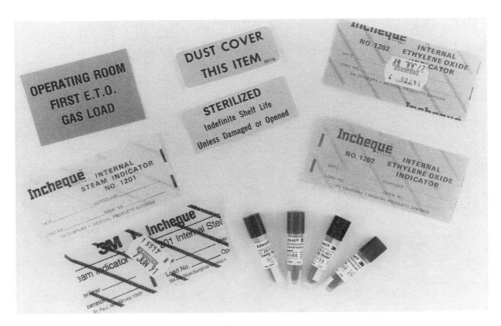

Sterilization labels and biologic monitors

Biologic monitors are the only method for assuring that all microorganisms have been destroyed during the sterilization process, and an accurate record of the test results must be maintained, using an appropriate recordkeeping system, according to institutional/manufacturer's recommendations (JCAHO/AAMI requirement).

A list of items that can be routinely steam sterilized should be available with the practice area, and new items added according to the manufacturer's recommendations for the specific procedures.

Those items requiring EO sterilization should be listed and available within the practice area, and updated as necessary. Adequate time must be provided for the sterilization/aeration cycle. Therefore, careful planning of the use of the item is essential, since once the cycle has started, it cannot for *any reason* be interrupted to retrieve an item, even from the aeration chamber.

EO sterilizers and aeration designs and venting guidelines should be available within the practice area for the specific unit being used, and OSHA and the manufacturer's recommendations for additional requirements should be obtained and kept with the official safety officer with the institution.

Loading and Handling of Steam Sterilized Items

Repeated handling of sterilized items forces air in and out of the wrapper and this could shorten the shelf life of the item.

Because sterilization depends on the direct contact of the sterilization agent with all surfaces of goods, the sterilizer must be loaded so that the sterilizing agent will penetrate through each package. This is best accomplished by placing packs, trays, and basins on their sides.

For a *gravity displacement sterilizer*, wire mesh or perforated metal shelves should be used to separate layers of packages, and for the best result, the following loading guidelines should be followed:

1. flat packages: placed on edge so that flat surfaces are vertical
2. large packages: should be placed in only one layer on the cart (nothing on top of it), and packages should not be touching each other
3. small packages: when placed on top of one another, should be in a criss-cross position
4. basins or solid containers: placed on their sides to allow air to flow out of them and prevent water accumulation; basins and packs should be placed on the bottom shelves when a mixed-size load is prepared

When using a prevacuum sterilizer, follow the recommended guidelines from the manufacturer for loading, since the principle of operation is slightly different.

Drying/Unloading the Steam Sterilizer

Once the cycle is completed, the sterilizer door should be *cracked* to allow steam to escape, then opened com-

Table 8-2 Biologic Indicator Guidelines

Agency	Requirements	Frequency Steam	Frequency EO	Placement in Sterilizer Steam	Placement in Sterilizer EO	Quarantine	Recall System	Record-keeping System	Subculture: Positive BI's
AAMI Good Hospital Practice: Steam Sterilization and Sterility Assurance, 1988 Good Hospital Practice: Performance Evaluation of EO Sterilizers—EO Test Packs, 1985	Should be used	At least weekly, and preferably daily	Recommend each load and to test new packaging	Inside the test pack that is placed in "cold point," normally the front bottom of the sterilizer	Inside the pack in the geometric center of the load	EO—yes	Yes	Yes	Should do
AHA Guidelines for the Hospital Central Service Department, 1978	Should be used	Once a day	Each load	—	—	—	Yes	Yes	—
AORN Recommended Practices for Sterilization, 1995	Should be used	Daily and with each load of implantables	Each cycle	Follow manufacturer's recommendations	Follow manufacturer's recommendations	EO—sterilized implantables or intravascular devices	Yes	Yes	Will do
CDC Guidelines for the Prevention and Control of Nosocomial Infections, 1980	Should be used	At least once a week and each load if it contains implantable objects	At least once a week and each load if it contains implantable objects	—	—	Implantable objects (EO or steam sterilized)	Yes, if implantable objects	—	—
JCAHO Standards adopted, 1990	Are tested	At least weekly, recommended daily	Used at least weekly, recommended daily; used each cycle if it contains implantable or intravascular material	—	—	Implantable or intravascular material	Yes	Yes	—
Army regulations (AR-40-19), 1982	Shall be used	Minimum of once a week	—	—	—	—	—	—	—
VA manual MP-2 Change 10, December, 1991	Will be used	Minimum of once daily	Each cycle	—	—	—	Yes	Yes	—

AAMI = Association for the Advancement of Medical Instrumentation; AORN = Association of Operating Room Nurses; JCAHO = Joint Commission on Accreditation of Healthcare Organizations; AHA = American Hospital Association; CDC = Centers for Disease Control; VA = Veteran's Administration; BI = biologic indicators.

Adapted from Reichert M, Young J. Sterilization Technology for Health-Care Facility. Manual published by AMSCO Sterilizer Co., Pennsylvania.

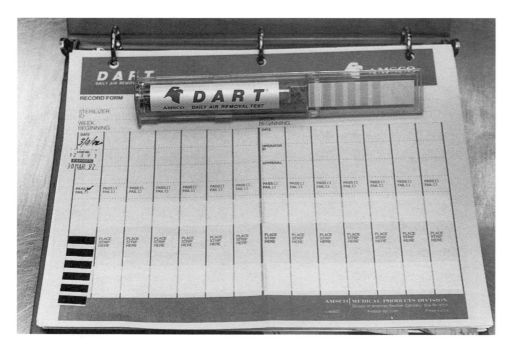

Air-removal monitor and record sheets for gravity displacement sterilizer

pletely. The wrapped packages should be removed from the sterilizer, and left untouched to dry for 15 to 60 minutes, depending on the size of the load.

Time can be saved when the wire shelves can be placed on a *transfer carriage* and then rolled into the sterilizer and removed in the same manner, avoiding the actual handling of the packages before total cooling.

Packages should be completely dry after cooling at room temperature of 68°–75°F (20°–24°C) for a minimum of 1 hour. If packages are still warm they should not be transferred to a solid metal shelf, since they may sweat, causing condensation, which in turn results in a wet pack that can no longer be considered sterile.

Storage of Sterile Items

When storing sterilized items, a method for routine rotation of stock should be employed to avoid using outdated supplies or instruments. Older supplies should be used first and new supplies placed behind them (F-I-F-O: First In–First Out). In accordance with JCAHO recommendations, cabinets used for storing sterile items should have doors, that should be closed at all times.

Additionally, the storage area should be shielded from extreme changes in temperatures and maintained as dust free as possible, and should not be used as a cross-over between two areas of the OR suite.

Shelf Life

Shelf life is described as the length of time a wrapped sterile package remains sterile while in storage. Those items continuously used are dated at the time they are prepared, indicating the time interval for safe use. For those items infrequently used, however, another system is available. By applying a sealed plastic cover over the wrapper, an indefinite shelf life can exist, as long as the integrity of the package is not compromised in any manner.

The sterility of an item is *event-related, not time-related*. Contamination of that item(s) can occur only when the contents have been exposed due to faulty preparations or compromise of the protective wrapper (container). This is the same principle behind commercially prepared items, and why an out-date or expiration dates do not usually appear on the packages, only the indication of *"guaranteed sterility until package is opened or compromised."*

Monitoring the Sterilization Process

Most sterilizers are equipped with an automatic or microcomputer time-temperature control for recording operational data and/or a graphic recorder. For both, the time-temperature is recorded for a 24-hour period, noting each time the sterilizer was used, for what duration (timing of cycle), and what temperature was reached and maintained during the cycle.

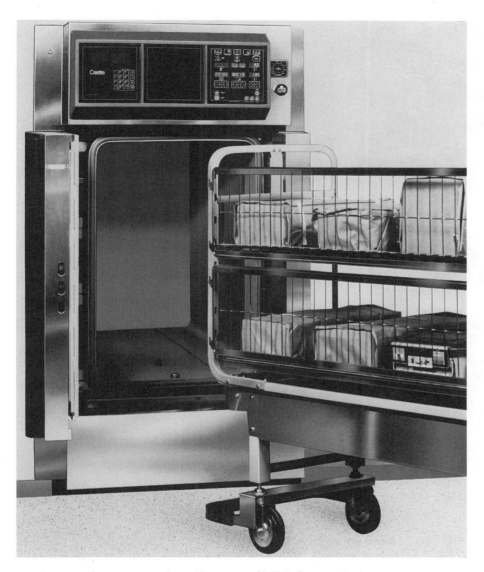

Loading cart for steam sterilizer (Courtesy of MDT Corporation)

These records should be collected at a prescribed, routine time each day (before the first run of the sterilizer), and a new record started for the next 24 hours. The information should be maintained in individual envelopes within the OR, and should be used as a reference base, should the sterilization process be questioned.

Institutional policies, describing the collection and storage of these records, should be explicit and standardized throughout the institution wherever a sterilizer is located. The performance record book should include the following data: (1) sterilizer number, (2) cycle number, (3) contents of each load, (4) temperature/time graphs per sterilizer, (5) results of biologic tests performed on each sterilizer, and (6) any additional testing performed on the sterilizer, and the results (e.g., Bowie-Dick test, etc.).

Flash Sterilization

Since speed works against the sterilization process because it reduces the margin of safety, flash sterilization should be the exception, not the routine method, for steam sterilization. Flash sterilization should be employed only for clean, unwrapped instruments and porous items. The unwrapped method should be used in emergency situations for individual items, such as a dropped instrument, during the procedure. Complete sets of trays of instruments should not be

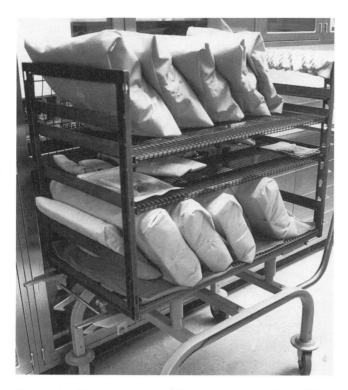

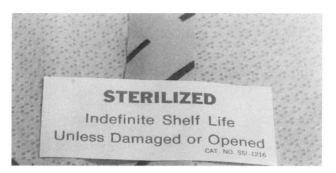

Sterility is event-related, not time-related

Proper loading ensures complete penetration of sterilizing agent

sterilized in this manner unless all of the following conditions are present:

1. There is urgent need.
2. the physical layout ensures direct delivery of a tray to the OR
3. transfer procedures ensure the sterility of the item
4. items have been properly decontaminated before the sterilization cycle is initiated

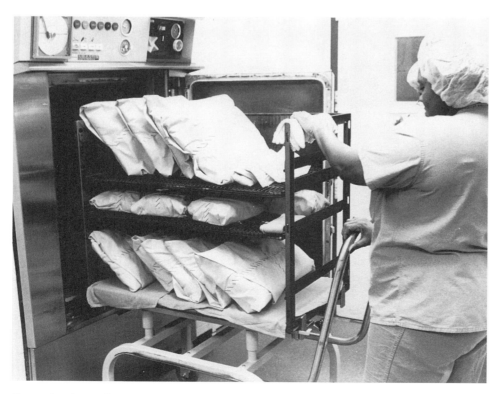

Removing items from steam sterilizer on transfer carriage

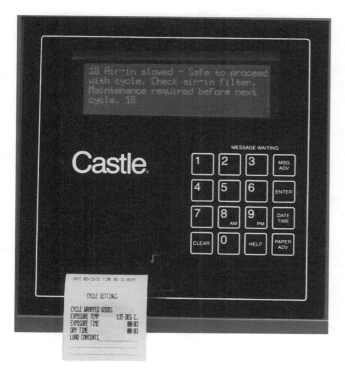

Computerized control panel for flash steam sterilizer (Courtesy of Castle)

Cycle Parameters for Flash Sterilizers (Unwrapped)

GRAVITY DISPLACEMENT

Metal only (a few instruments)	3 minutes at 270–275°F
Mixed load or full tray	10 minutes at 270–275°F

PREVACUUM

Metal only	3 minutes at 270–275°F
Mixed load	4 minutes at 270–275°F

Specialty Instruments and Devices

Sterilization of specialty instruments, such as drills, perforators, power batteries, and so forth, may require different exposure times via the flash method. In most instances, follow the written manufacturer's recommendations for time-temperature using the unwrapped method (Table 8-3).

Under no circumstances can implantable devices be flash sterilized.

(See Critical Element Task 8-6, p. 188 for handling items for flash sterilization.)

Preventive Maintenance Program

Like any piece of equipment, the steam and gas sterilizers need preventative maintenance and cleaning on a routine basis. A thorough cleaning removes concealed organisms that may be present, affecting the sterilization process.

Routine maintenance is an effective method for preserving the life of the sterilizer, and should include daily cleaning of the gasket door and the strainers located in the opening of the discharge line. The inside chamber should be cleaned weekly.

Time-temperature graphs or charting devices should be recalibrated after each maintenance check or any repairs performed on the sterilizer and/or at least every 6 months, which ever comes first.

Table 8-3   **Guide to Common Sterilization Parameters**

	Temperature		
Item	(°F)	(°C)	Time[a] (min)
Gravity displacement sterilizer			
Wrapped or containerized	270	132	15
	250	121	30
Powered instruments	270	132	Per manufacturer's instructions
	250	121	
"Flash" sterilization[b]			
Unwrapped, nonporous	270	132	3
Unwrapped, porous	270	132	10
Prevacuum (High-Vac) Sterilizer			
Wrapped	270	132	4
Powered instruments	270	132	Per manufacturer's instructions
"Flash" sterilization			
Unwrapped, nonporous	270	132	3
Unwrapped, porous	270	132	4

[a] Or per manufacturer's instructions. When following manufacturer's instructions, documentation providing evidence of efficacy within stated parameters should be available.
[b] Sterilization using the unwrapped method.

Procedure for Loading and Unloading
a Flash Autoclave

RATIONALE

To prepare and retrieve items sterilized for emergency use maintaining the sterility of the item during transfer.

PREREQUISITES

- **A.** Clean items
- **B.** Items with multiple parts disassembled
- **C.** Flash integrator strip or rapid attest
- **D.** Appropriate instrument tray/Flash pan

PROFICIENCY

One hundred percent accuracy at the time of performance

PROCEDURAL STEPS

- **I.** LOADING FLASH AUTOCLAVE
  - **1.** Clean and arrange all items in proper receptacle for steam sterilization
    - **a.** Instrument tray
    - **b.** Flash pan
  - **2.** Place Flash integrator or rapid attest inside tray/pan and place on shelf inside chamber. Close and seal door.
  - **3.** Set cycle time for appropriate duration:
    - **a.** Full metal tray and/or mixed load: 10 minutes (longer if needed depending on the load)
    - **b.** Flash pan (individual instruments): 3 minutes

NOTE: The greater the metal mass, the longer the duration required.

- **II.** UNLOADING THE FLASH AUTOCLAVE
  - **1.** On completion of the cycle, a buzzer will sound. Turn the handle of the chamber door, and "crack" the door to allow steam to escape.

NOTE: Avoid contact with steam by standing on the hinge side of the door. Remember, steam temperature is at 270°–275°F.

  - **2.** Open the chamber door completely for the retrieval process.

- **A.** Retrieval of an instrument tray (performed by scrub person)
  - **1.** Scrub person enters substerile area with two sterile towels.
  - **2.** Door is opened by circulator.
  - **3.** Scrub person reaches into chamber, avoiding contact with the chamber, and using a sterile towel grabs the tray handle and pulls tray toward self.
  - **4.** Using other towel, scrub person spreads towel over top of tray and other handle, and pulls remainder of tray out of autoclave.
  - **5.** Circulator opens OR door.
  - **6.** Tray is placed on double-draped ring stand, and towels are discarded.
  - **7.** Scrub nurse changes gloves.

NOTE: During the process, should the scrub nurse's gown touch any unsterile surface, it must be changed also.

  - **8.** Circulator removes and checks the Flash integrator, and places it in designated location for record keeping.

B.   Using a Flash pan (performed by unsterile person only)
    1.   With door completely open, and using the handle, pick up Flash pan by inserting handle into the designated slot on the side of the Flash pan.

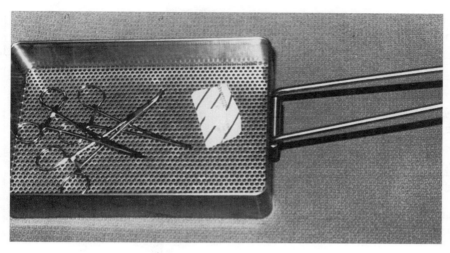

Fig. A.   Flash pan with handle

NOTE: Do not let edge of pan come in contact with hands.

    2.   Backing into the room, present the item to the scrub, keeping a safe distance to avoid contact.
    3.   Remove Flash integrator, inspect it to verify a "safe" change, and place it in the designated location for record keeping.

PERFORMANCE CHECK SHEET

NAME:	TASK # ____8-6____
	RATING: A Acceptable
	N/I Needs Improvement

PROCEDURE: Loading and Unloading a Flash Autoclave

PROCEDURAL STEPS	A	N/I
I. LOADING PROCEDURE		
1. Assures instruments/items are clean prior to process		
2. Places appropriate integrator in tray/Flash pan		
3. Avoids overloading tray/Flash pan		
4. Sets controls for appropriate time cycle, depending on size/components of load		
II. UNLOADING PROCEDURE		
A. RETRIEVAL OF AN INSTRUMENT TRAY		
1. Scrub person maintains aseptic technique during retrieval		
2. Verifies Flash integrator has changed, indicating cycle complete		
3. Grasps handle of tray with sterile towel(s) to remove tray		
4. Covers tray with sterile towel during transfer to procedure room		
5. Places tray on a prepared sterile surface other than instrument table		
6. Discards towel and changes gloves, using proper technique		

TASK # ____8-6____

PROCEDURAL STEPS	A	N/I
B. RETRIEVAL OF FLASH PAN 1. Nonsterile person maintains principles of asepsis during retrieval 2. Attaches handle to Flash pan for aseptic removal 3. Verifies Flash integrator has changed, indicating sterilization process complete 4. Enters procedure room and presents item for removal by scrub person, maintaining a safe distance 5. Collects Flash indicator and records appropriate information 6. Disposes of Flash indicator in prescribed manner, according to institutional policy/protocol		

COMMENTS: _____

_____

In accordance with JCAHO recommendations, a maintenance log should be kept within the suite, and accurate entries of all service visits and the results of the visit should be made. Included in this log book should be the:

1. date of service and description
2. model number of the sterilizer
3. serial number of the sterilizer
4. location of the equipment (OR, L&D, CS, etc.)
5. technician performing the service (name and signature)

Creating a Reference Library

A thorough knowledge of the concepts of the sterilization process helps protect the patient from infection. Maintaining current reference books and manuals concerning the sterilization process should be part of every surgical suite, and maintaining current knowledge is every person's responsibility in order to maintain an infection-free surgical environment.

Self-assessment Exercise 3

Directions: Complete the following exercises. The answers are given at the end of this module.

1. Name the two types of steam sterilizers and briefly describe how they differ from each other.

2. All instruments to be sterilized should be hand washed first.

True   False

3. Instruments that have been disassembled for cleaning should be reassembled before sterilizing them so that parts will not be lost.

True   False

4. Describe why we need biologic monitors/testing, and name the two sources and their respective usages.

5. Instrument sets should weigh no more than _____ pounds.

6. Chemical indicators are used to show that sterilization has been achieved.

True   False

7. List three items that are appropriate for gas sterilization.

8. Name two other sterilants that can be used in a hospital setting. State advantages and disadvantages of each.

9. When a 270°F, 3-minute exposure cycle is used, it is referred to as a _____ cycle.

10. Sterile is defined as _____.

11. During the decontamination phase, if the ultrasonic cleaner is used, sterilization is not required.

True   False

DISINFECTION PROCESS

There are two major purposes for disinfection used in the OR:

1. to kill pathogenic microorganisms on inanimate surfaces and objects that cannot be sterilized
2. to prevent or arrest growth of microorganisms on body surfaces through the application of an *antiseptic* solution (discussed in Chap. 11)

The disinfection process requires the use of an agent that can destroy infection-producing organisms. Disinfectants are liquid chemical compounds that destroy the microbes by either physical or chemical means. These agents are utilized on inanimate objects such as furniture, floors, walls, equipment, and some heat-sensitive items.

Disinfectants are identified as *bacteriostatic,* which act by inhibiting growth, or as *bactericidal,* which will kill bacteria (sporicides, viricides, fungicides). For a disinfectant to affect microorganisms, it must act on some vital part of the cell. Some alter the cytoplasmic membrane, some react directly with certain enzymes, nucleus, or the cell wall, while others are effective against specific types of microbes and not others.

Of some 8000 disinfectants available in the United States, most have both advantages and disadvantages. A good disinfectant is one that is noncorrosive, read-ily available, relatively pleasant-smelling, nonirritating to breathe, effective on most microorganisms, and economical. In other words there is no *one* good disinfectant available today. Solutions used to disinfect walls and furniture are not interchangeable with solutions used to disinfect instruments. Therefore the perioperative nurse must be able to distinguish between the two in order to provide maximum protection for the patient.

Types (Levels) of Disinfectants

Disinfectants are usually available in three levels or strengths, depending on their ability to affect specific types of microbes (Table 8-4).

Like sterilization, the larger the number of organisms contaminating the object, the longer it takes for the disinfectant solution to destroy them or render them harmless to the body.

High-Level Disinfectant

Description: High-level disinfectants can kill spores, bacteria, and viruses if contact time is sufficient.

The terms *germicide* and *bactericide* may be used synonymously, but the tubercle bacillus has a waxy envelope that makes it, along with some other forms of vegetative bacteria, comparatively resistant to disinfectants. The solution should be labeled as such if it has

Table 8-4   Disinfectant Solutions

Agent	Classification	Mechanism of Actions	Comments
High Level			
2% activated alkaline glutaraldehyde	Vegetative microorganisms Tubercle bacilli Spores—10 hr	Denaturation of proteins	Disinfection of instruments in 10 min; used for lensed instruments; effective chemosterilizer in 10 hr; unpleasant odor, tissue reaction may occur; rinse instruments well before use; wear nitril gloves when working with agent; cover soaking pan at all times
Intermediate Level			
Alcohol/formalin 8% Formalin with 70% isopropyl alcohol	Tuberculocidal Viricidal Sporicidal—12 hr	Coagulation of proteins	Instruments: dissolves cement mounting on lensed instruments; toxic to tissue; irritating fumes; not commonly used in today's practice settings
Alcohol, isopropyl (70%)	Bactericidal Pseudomonicidal Fungicidal Tuberculocidal	Denaturation of proteins	Spot cleaning; damp dusting of equipment; inactivated by organic debris; ineffective when it evaporates; dissolves cement mounting on lensed instruments and fogs lenses
Iodine compounds (iodine + detergent iodophores)	Bactericidal Pseudomonicidal Fungicidal Tuberculocidal in high iodine concentration	Oxidation of essential enzymes	Not used as disinfectant; may corrode instruments; inactivated by organic debris; aluminum excellent as antiseptic
Quaternary ammonium compounds	Bactericidal Pseudomonicidal Fungicidal	Surface active. Disrupts cell membrane with deactivation of enzymes and denaturation of proteins	Neutralization by soap; limited hospital use since these agents do not destroy gram-negative pathogens/tubercle bacilli
Low Level			
Mercurials	Bacteriostatic	Oxidation combines with proteins	No practical usage
Phenolic compounds	Bactericidal Pseudomonicidal Fungicidal Tuberculocidal	Same as quaternary ammonium compounds	Walls, furniture, floors, equipment; should not be used on instruments; unpleasant odor; tissue reaction on skin and mucous membranes; gloves must be worn when working with agent; should not be used on stretchers
Chlorine compounds	Viricidal Most gram-negative bacteria and *Pseudomonas*	Oxidation of enzymes	Spot cleaning for walls, floors, and furniture; in 1:10 bleach/water, can deactivate hepatitis and AIDS viruses; corrosive to metals; unpleasant odor; not for instruments

this capability. For spores, however, only an extended exposure time can render an object sterile (10 hours or more, depending on the agent) and then only when using a high-level disinfectant.

EXAMPLE: 2% activated alkaline gluteraldehyde aqueous solution

Intermediate-Level Disinfectant

Description: Intermediate-level agents kill the more resistant bacteria and viruses.

Some intermediate-level disinfectants may be capable of exhibiting sporicidal action, but these must be labeled as such by the manufacturer.

EXAMPLES: Alcohol (70% or isopropyl)

Quarternary ammonium compounds

Alcohol/formalin (8% formalin with 70% isopropyl alcohol)

Low-Level Disinfectant

Description: Low-level disinfectants kill only less resistant bacteria and viruses.

Low-level disinfectants are usually used for housekeeping purposes, and should not be used to disinfect direct patient care objects. Neither intermediate nor low-level disinfectants kill spores.

EXAMPLES: Mercurial compounds

Phenolic compounds

Chlorine compounds

Recommended Practices—Chemical Disinfection

I.   The selection and use of a chemical germicide should be scientifically based.
II. Items should be thoroughly cleaned before disinfection.
III. Chemical germicides should be used according to the manufacturer's written instructions.
IV. Practice settings should provide safe environments for personnel when using chemical germicides.

Source: AORN. Standards and recommended practices, Denver, CO: The Association, 1995. Pp. 147–149.

Implications for Perioperative Nursing Practice

1. All items to be chemically disinfected should be thoroughly cleaned, rinsed, and dried before beginning the process.
2. Chemical disinfectants must contact all surfaces of the item (including lumens and channels) in order for the process to be effective.
3. The disinfection process should be performed:
    a. before storage
    b. immediately before use
4. Following the recommended immersion time, the item should be aseptically removed, rinsed with generous amounts of sterile water, and dried in such a manner as to reduce the risk of contamination.
5. Immersion time for the item should follow the manufacturer's recommendations and should be reinforced by policy or protocol for all items, regardless of the area, if the same disinfectant solution is used.
6. Gloves and protective eyeware should be worn by persons working directly with the solution, avoiding contact with skin or mucous membranes, since contact irritation can occur.
7. An expiration date, as recommended by the manufacturer, should be highly visible on all containers of the solution currently in use.
8. The agent should be registered with the EPA and should be compatible with the type of device to be disinfected.
9. Parameters for chemical disinfection include:
    a. time of exposure
    b. concentration of the solution
    c. the amount and type of organic debris
    d. the temperature (an increase in temperature will accelerate the rate of the chemical reaction)
10. Disinfectant solutions should be covered following reconstitution to avoid noxious odors/fumes and remain covered when not in use.
11. Disinfectants should be monitored daily for effective strength.
12. If highly contaminated or large amounts of gross soil are present in the solution, it must be changed following the procedure.

It is important to remember that chemical disinfection is just that—disinfection. It is *not* sterilization. Therefore, this process should be reserved for semicritical, noncritical, and carefully selected critical items used during the surgical procedure.

Self-assessment Exercise 4

Directions: Complete the following exercises. Answers are given at the end of this module.

1. List three semicritical items that would be appropriate to disinfect.

2. All disinfectants can be used for sterilization purposes provided immersion time is sufficient.

                                    True   False

3. Only items that have been thoroughly cleaned, rinsed, and dried should be placed in a disinfectant.

                                    True   False

4. Immersing an item in a 2% solution of glutaraldehyde for 45 minutes is sufficient for sterilization to be achieved.

                                    True   False

5. Semicritical items do not require sterilization. They do require disinfection. Define a semicritical item.

References

1. Adams Francis. The genuine works of Hippocrates (translated from the Greek). New York: W. Wood & Co., 1929. P. 4.
2. Zimmerman LM, Veith I. Great ideas in the history of surgery. New York: Dover, 1967. Pp. 21–22.
3. Miller BF, Keane CB. Encyclopedia and dictionary of medicine, nursing and allied health, 2nd ed. Philadelphia: W.B. Saunders, 1978. P. 61.
4. Ibid, p. 92.
5. Cartwright F. The development of modern surgery. New York: T. Crowell Co., 1968. P. 5.
6. Francis ME. Asepsis for the nurse. London, 1889.
7. Steward I. Education for nurses. New York: Macmillan, 1944. P. 87.
8. AORN. Standards and recommended practices for perioperative nursing. Denver: The Association of Operating Room Nurses, 1995. Pp. 135–139.
9. Ibid., p. 274.
10. Ibid., p. 138.
11. AMSCO. Decontamination, sterilization, disinfection and sanitation: The concept—the fact. Erie, PA: American Sterilizer Co., 1988.
12. AMSCO. Sterilization aids. Erie, PA: American Sterilizer Co., Education Division, 1982.
13. Ibid.
14. AAMI Recommended Practice. The unwrapped method: Flash sterilization. 1986. Pp. 170–171.
15. Perkins JJ. Principles and methods of sterilization in health sciences, 2nd ed. Springfield, IL: Charles C. Thomas, 1988. P. 30.
16. Occupational Safety and Health Administration. Occupational exposure to ethylene oxide. Federal Register 57: 1989.
17. AORN. Standards and recommended practices. Denver: The Association of Operating Room Nurses, 1995. Pp. 267–276.

Foundations of Surgery

9

UNIT 1

Sutures, Needles, and Instruments

HEMOSTASIS AND WOUND CLOSURE MATERIALS

Effective *wound healing* is a major goal of all surgical procedures. The judicious choice of wound-closure materials and the application of good surgical tech-

nique can make the difference between a smooth and complicated recovery. The primary purpose of all wound-closure material is to hold tissues together until healing is completed; this purpose is applicable to both internal and external structures.

Hemostasis, on the other hand, is the arrest, control,

197

or reduction of bleeding, which can assist in the wound-healing process. Hemostasis can be accomplished by the natural clotting of blood; by the use of artificial means, such as cautery, sutures, clamps, staples, and so on; by chemical methods, using specially treated materials impregnated with a hemostatic substance; or by a combination of all three techniques. Hemostasis during a surgical procedure is essential to prevent hemorrhage, allow for visualization of the surgical field, and promote wound healing.

Historical Overview

From ancient times, warfare made necessary some means of controlling hemorrhage. It was well known even then that the loss of blood could mean a loss of life; thus, using crude methods, bleeding was stopped before the life processes faded.

From Egyptian and Assyrian writings dating back to 2000 B.C. and archeologic discoveries, mummies have been found that reveal traumatic and incisional wounds sewed together with what appears to be suture material of some type, and other ancient writings have documented the use of tourniquets and compression to control hemorrhage and assist in the wound-closure process.

Hemostasis, as practiced by early surgeons in their attempts to save the patient from hemorrhaging, combined styptics (an astringent solution) with fire, cold, pressure bandages, and the elevation of the affected part; some had great success, while others had little.

To control bleeding and achieve wound closure, Celus, early in the first century B.C., used cotton lint wet with vinegar over the wound, while Arabian surgeons used harp strings made from sheep or camel intestines that were twisted and sun dried.

Searing the wound using oil and hot irons to stop bleeding and close the wound goes back as far as the ancient Hebrews, and was again practiced by Hippocrates (460–370 B.C.). This technique is practiced today, only in a refined method, and is referred to as *electrosurgical cautery.* Although the knowledge of suturing was known to Hippocrates, through the writings on ancient Egyptian papyrus, he still preferred the searing method for hemostasis and wound closure.

Other surgeons attempted to control bleeding using various types of materials, including Galean (A.D. 200), a surgeon to the Roman Gladiators, and physicians and healers to the Pharaohs of ancient Egypt, but none had any great success.

As patients died more frequently owing to the inability to control bleeding, surgical procedures declined at a rapid rate, until a sixteenth-century barber-surgeon, Ambroise Pare, pioneered a number of advances in surgery. As field doctor to the French army, in 1545 he developed safe methods for treating wounds by controlling bleeding vessels using the *ligature,* a technique still practiced today. In addition, he championed a more humane treatment in medicine, speaking against the barbarity of searing with hot oils to close a wound, a practice that was used during that time.

Because of his continued persistence, many scientists in the middle 1800s began using animal tissue to conduct research relating to suture materials and techniques. Since the body absorbed these tissues, the door was opened to the usage of suture materials internally, with little adverse reaction to the patient.

Dr. William Halstead, well known for his surgical technique, first advocated the use of silk sutures in 1883. Using an *interrupted* method, in which each stitch was taken and tied separately, giving the wound greater strength, the healing process improved; his technique is still used today.

By 1901, processed catgut (sheep intestine) was available to the surgeon in sterile glass tubes, and in the early part of the twentieth century, surgical gut, silk, and cotton emerged as the most commonly used suture materials.

Since the early 1950s, sutures have become available in individualized, presterilized packages, with or without needles attached to the suture strand (*atraumatic*), and today there are a variety of materials for a variety of applications, depending on the needs of the patient, the surgeon's preference, and the type and location of the wound.

METHODS OF HEMOSTASIS

Blood clotting is a normal defense mechanism whereby the soluble blood protein (fibrinogen) is changed into a soluble protein (fibrin). When the natural mechanism is interrupted, and clotting does not occur, some artificial method of hemostasis must be employed. This can be accomplished by either (1) mechanical methods or (2) chemical methods.

Mechanical Methods

Instruments

Clamping the end of a bleeding vessel with a hemostat is the most common method of achieving hemostasis. The bleeder can then be ligated or sutured to accomplish the stoppage of blood flow.

Heat

Heat, in the form of electrocautery, sears the blood, allowing dilation of the vessel, which stimulates the platelets and tissues to liberate more natural hemostatic agents (thromboplastin).

Bone Wax

Bone wax is a refined beeswax that is used to control bleeding in bone marrow. Pieces of bone wax are rolled into small balls and handed to the surgeon for direct application on the bone.

Ligating Clips

Small clips made of tantalum or stainless steel are used to ligate arteries, veins, or nerves. The clip comes in various sizes with a corresponding applicator, which, when applied, stays permanently on the vessel, stopping the flow of blood from the area.

Ligature

A ligature, commonly called a *tie*, is a strand of material that is tied around a blood vessel to occlude the lumen and prevent bleeding. Large, pulsating vessels may require a *transfixion* suture.

Chemical Methods

Absorbable Gelatin Sponges

Available in either powder or compressed pad foam, gelatin sponges (Gelfoam) are absorbable hemostatic agents. When placed on the area, fibrin is deposited on the pad, and the pad swells, forming a substantial clot.

The sponge may be used either dry or soaked in a hemostatic agent (thrombin or epinephrine) for a greater hemostatic effect.

Collagen Sponge

Hemostatic sponges of collagen origin (Colostat, Superstat, Helostat) are applied dry to oozing or bleeding sites. Sponges dissolve as hemostasis occurs, and residual sponges, left in the wound, will eventually be absorbed.

Microfibrillar Collagen

Microfibrillar collagen hemostat (Avitine) is an off-white "fluffy" material prepared from purified bovine collagen used as a topical hemostatic agent. It achieves hemostasis by adhering to platelets and forming thrombi with the interstices of the collagen. It functions

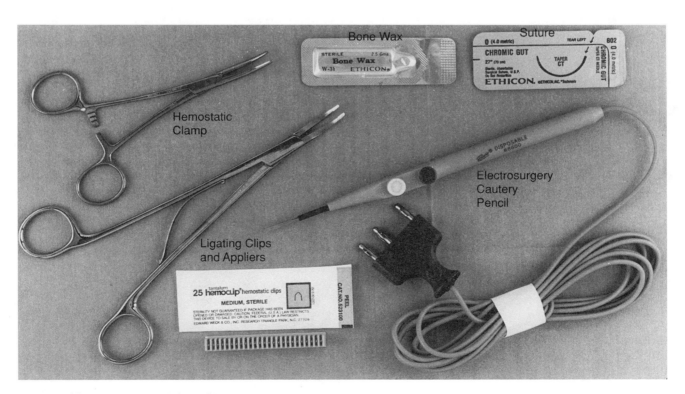

Variety of hemostatic materials and instruments

as a hemostatic when applied directly to the source of bleeding, including bone and friable tissue or from around a vascular anastomosis. Since it adheres to wet gloves and instruments, it should be presented on a dry, smooth forcep, followed by applying pressure over the site with a dry sponge.

Oxidized Cellulose

Oxidized cellulose (Oxycel, Surgicel) is a specially treated gauze that is placed directly over the bleeding area. As it absorbs the blood, it swells to seven or eight times its normal size and forms coagulum.

The hemostatic effect of oxidized cellulose is created when it is dry; therefore, it should not be moistened with water or saline before use.

Oxidized cellulose may be left in the wound, as it is absorbed in 7 to 14 days with minimal tissue reaction, except when applied to areas such as the spinal cord, optic nerve and its chiasm, or bone.

Thrombin, USP (Thrombostat)

Thrombin is an enzyme extracted from dried beef blood, and is used as a topical hemostatic agent. Thrombin accelerates coagulation of blood and controls capillary bleeding. Thrombin is available as a powder, which is reconstituted with its own diluent, or it can be sprayed on the surface, or used in conjunction with an absorbable gelatin sponge. The sponge is immersed in the thrombin and presented to the surgeon with a clean forcep after excess solution has been squeezed from the sponge. Depending on the manufacturer, thrombin may or may not need refrigeration.

Thrombin must never be injected or allowed to enter large vessels, as extensive intravascular clotting may occur.

Styptic

One category of styptics includes chemicals that cause a blood vessel to constrict. Examples of this include epinephrine, tannic acid, and silver nitrate.

Epinephrine (1:1000) may be added to local anesthetic agents to decrease the amount of bleeding or may be used to soak gelatin sponges before application.

Tannic acid is a powder used on the mucous membranes of the nose and throat to control capillary bleeding, as is silver nitrate, which when mixed with silver chloride solution and molded into pencils (sticks), creates a topical hemostatic agent.

Additional Methods of Hemostasis

In addition to the mechanical and chemical methods used to control bleeding, several other means of hemostasis are available during the intraoperative period, including the use of tourniquets, digital compression, cryosurgery (extreme cold), hypothermia technique, photocoagulation (used in ophthalmology), the heated scalpel (hot knife), which is used to cut and coagulate small vessels, and the laser, which has coagulation capabilities.

Hypotension, induced and controlled by anesthesia, is another method that can reduce the amount of blood loss and provide a dry field. It is frequently used in orthopedic, vascular surgery, and neurosurgery. When compatible blood is not available or blood transfusions are against the patient's religious beliefs and the autologous method, using the cell saver, is not available for direct transfusion of the patient's own blood, induced hypertension may be used.

Self-assessment Exercise 5

Directions: Complete the following exercises. The answers are given at the end of this module.

1. List the natural methods of hemostasis.

2. Gelfoam is a fluffy white material made from purified bovine dermis.

    True   False

3. Thrombin is an enzyme made from dried beef blood used to control capillary bleeding.

    True   False

4. Mechanical or chemical methods used to control bleeding are _____ .

WOUND CLOSURE MATERIALS: SUTURES AND NEEDLES

What Is a Suture?

According to the dictionary,[1] a suture is a thread, wire, or other material used in the operation of stitching parts of the body together; to suture is to unite by stitching (sewing).

Suture materials can be used in many different ways, such as *ligating* a bleeding vessel, *suturing* internal structures, or *closing* the skin of a wound. The "ideal" material used for these purposes would have certain characteristics, including:

- Versatility that would permit its use in any operation, the only variable being its size as determined by its strength
- Ease of handling, both comfortable and natural to the surgeon
- Minimal tissue reaction and inability to create favorable conditions for either infection, rejection, or both
- A high tensile (breakage) strength, even in small-caliber suture; the knot should not fray or break off while in place
- A material that is easy to thread, easily sterilized, and will not shrink in the tissue
- A material that is nonelectrolyte, noncapillary, nonallergenic, and noncarcinogenic in its make-up
- A material that absorbs with minimal tissue reaction once it has served its purpose

Technically, the ideal suture has not yet been manufactured, and so today there are over 10 different suture materials to choose from, and over 25 different types of sutures for a variety of surgical needs, with more being developed and manufactured each year.

Tensile Strength and Diameter

The term *tensile strength* was first described by the United States Pharmacopeia (USP), and refers to the knot-pull strength of the suture rather than the straight-pull strength. Minimum knot-pull strengths are specified for each size, and as the suture diameter decreases, so too does the tensile strength.

Suture diameter or size identifies the size of the strand, which ranges from a heavy size 7 to a very fine size 11-0. The diameter of the suture strand usually determines its effective usage in addition to its size.

A basic rule for remembering suture sizes is based on the premise that *Size 0* is smaller than *Size 1*, and the more 0's added the smaller and more fragile the suture (Fig. 9-1).

Suture Lengths

The length of the suture is standardized to two sizes: Standard length—54 or 60 inches, and Precut length—17, 18, or 24 inches. Both of these lengths are available for sutures with or without needles, and the choice of length is usually determined by the suturing technique being used by the surgeon—for example, ligating or tying, interrupted or continuous stitching, and by the depth of the wound.

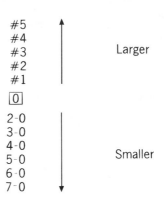

Fig. 9-1.   Size progression chart

Suture Packaging and Identification

Suture packaging has made identification of the contents easy to distinguish.

Sutures are supplied sterile from the manufacturer in a double envelope package. The inner package contains the sterile suture, and its sterility is ensured as long as the package has not been opened. The outer package is a see-through peel package designed to permit delivery of the suture to the sterile field.

Aseptic Transfer of Sutures

To transfer the suture package to the sterile field, the suture must be opened and dispensed using aseptic technique. Two techniques are considered appropriate.

Method I: Retrieval by Scrub Person

Holding the packet flaps between extended thumbs, the circulating nurse rolls his or her hands outward to peel the outer packet apart. The end of the sterile inner packet is then exposed and is offered to the scrub person, who grasps the inner packet with either gloved fingers or a sterile instrument (Fig. 9-2).

Method II: "Flipping" Suture Packet

The "flipping" procedure should be used only during the initial set-up of the sterile field, when the scrub person has not yet donned sterile gown and gloves.

Standing a safe distance from the sterile instrument table or designated receptacle, the circulator rolls the flaps of the outer package backwards, and projects (flips) the inner package onto the sterile surface, being careful not to reach over the sterile field (Fig. 9-3).

Color Coding and Package Information

To reduce the confusion associated with the various suture materials, each major category of suture material is color coded, and this coding is standard through the industry, regardless of the manufacturer. This is the first step in suture package recognition; the colors are as follows:

SUTURE TYPE	COLOR
Chromic Gut	Brown
Plain Gut	Yellow
Silk	Light blue
Nylon	Green
Prolene	Royal blue

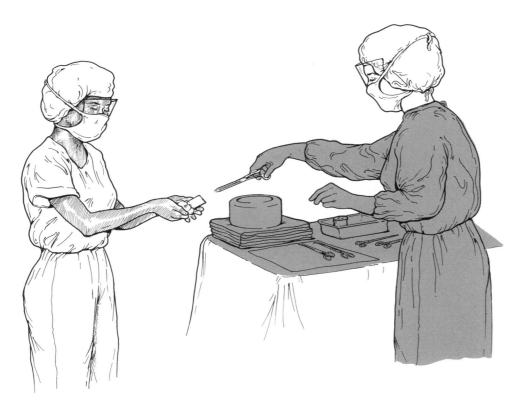

Fig. 9-2.   Method I: Retrieval by scrub person (Adapted from Wound Closure Manual. Sommerville, NJ: Ethicon, Inc., 1994)

Vicryl	Purple
Cotton	Pink
Ethibond	Orange
Mersilene	Turquoise

In addition to identifying the type of material, the suture package and its shipping box are marked with the trade name, generic name, catalog number, size, length, color of the strands, number of sutures per package, description of the needle, whether the suture is braided or monofilament, coating material (if used), classification, date manufactured, expiration date, and compliance with the USP standards.

Sutures are supplied in boxes containing 1 to 3 dozen packages of suture, and additional information about the suture is printed on each box.

Classification of Suture Materials

Surgical sutures as defined by the USP[2] are divided into two major classifications based on their reactions with body tissue: (1) absorbable and (2) nonabsorbable. Further subdivisions may also be used to describe suture materials: (1) natural or synthetic, and (2) monofilament or multifilament. Regardless of what type of suture is used, the body reacts as if it were invaded by a foreign substance. Attempts are made, therefore, by body tissue enzymes to rid the body of this substance.

Specific Suture Types and Characteristics

Absorbable Sutures

Description
Suture strands become dissolved or digested by body enzymes or hydrolyzed by tissue fluids (Table 9-1). There are basically three types of absorbable sutures:

1. plain or chromatized surgical gut
2. collagen (plain or chromic)
3. glycolic acid polymers (Vicryl; Dexon; PDS)

The first two, surgical gut and collagen, are natural materials. Glycolic acid polymers are synthetic.

Tissue Interaction
Absorbable sutures are digested by enzymes by first losing their strength, then gradually disappearing from the tissue.

Nonabsorbable Sutures

Some suture materials cannot be dissolved by tissue enzymes. These are called nonabsorbable sutures (Table 9-2). This group should be called "slowly absorbable." Only two materials, polyester and polypropylene, are truly nonabsorbable and considered permanent.

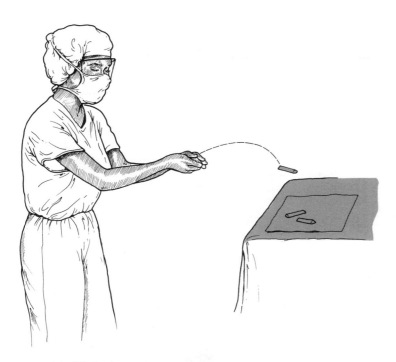

Fig. 9-3. Method II: "Flipping" suture packet (Adapted from Wound Closure Manual. Sommerville, NJ: Ethicon, Inc., 1994)

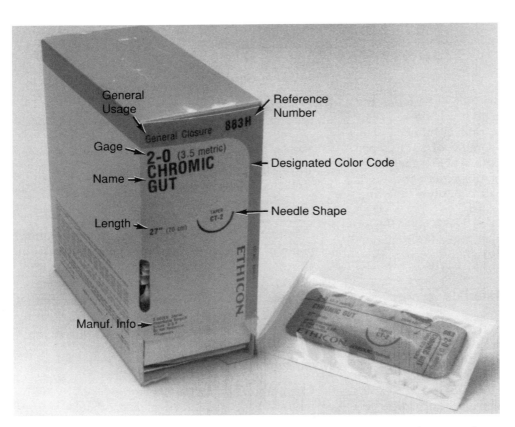

Identifying suturing material—package and box contain same information for easy reference

Table 9-1 Comparison of Absorbable Sutures

	Trade Name	Company	Material	Tensile Strength	Tissue Reactivity	Handling	Absorption
Natural	Collagen (plain)	Davis and Geck	Beef flexor tendon	Poor (0% at 2–3 weeks)	Moderate	Fair	Unpredictable (12 weeks)
	Collagen (chromic)	Davis and Geck	Beef flexor tendon	Poor (0% at 2–3 weeks)	Moderate	Fair	Unpredictable (12 weeks)
	Surgical gut (plain)	Ethicon; Davis and Geck	Animal collagen	Poor (0% at 2–3 weeks)	High	Fair	Unpredictable (12 weeks)
	Surgical gut (chromic)	Ethicon; Davis and Geck	Animal collagen	Poor (0% at 2–3 weeks)	Moderately high	Fair	Unpredictable (14–80 d)
Synthetic	Coated Vicryl	Ethicon	Polyglactin 910 (coated with calcium stearate and polyglactin 370)	Good (50% at 2–3 weeks)	Low	Good	Predictable (80 d)
	Dexon "S"	Davis and Geck	Polyglycolic acid	Good (50% at 2–3 weeks)	Low	Fair	Predictable (90 d)
	Dexon Plus	Davis and Geck	Polyglycolic acid (coated with poloxamer 188)	Good (50% at 2–3 weeks)	Low	Good	Predictable (90 d)
	PDS	Ethicon	Polydioxanone	Good (50% at 2–3 weeks)	Low	Poor	Predictable (180 d)

Modified from Bennett R. G. *Fundamentals of Cutaneous Surgery.* St. Louis: Mosby, 1988.

Table 9-2 Comparison of Nonabsorbable Sutures

	Generic or Trade Name	Company	Material	Tensile Strength	Tissue Reactivity	Handling
Natural	Cotton	—	Cotton	Good	High	Good
	Silk	Ethicon; Davis and Geck	Silk	Good	High	Good
Nylon	Ethilon	Ethicon	Polyamide (nylon)	High	Low	Poor
	Dermalon	Davis and Geck	Polyamide (nylon)	High	Low	Poor
	Surgamid	Look	Polyamide (nylon)	High	Low	Poor
	Nurolon	Ethicon	Polyamide (nylon)	High	Moderate	Good
	Surgilon	Davis and Geck	Polyamide (nylon) (coated with silicone)	High	Moderate	Fair
Polypropylene	Prolene	Ethicon	Polyolefin (polypropylene)	Fair	Low	Poor
	Surgilene	Davis and Geck	Polyolefin (polypropylene)	Fair	Low	Poor
	Dermalene	Davis and Geck	Polyolefin (polypropylene)	Good	Low	Poor
	Novafil	Davis and Geck	Polybutester	High	Low	Fair
	Mersilene	Ethicon	Polyester	High	Moderate	Good
	Dacron	Deknatel; Davis and Geck	Polyester	High	Moderate	Good
Polyesters	Polyviolene	Look	Polyester	High	Moderate	Good
	Ethibond	Ethicon	Polyester (coated with polybutilate)	High	Moderate	Good
	Ti-Con	Davis and Geck	Polyester (coated with silicone)	High	Moderate	Poor
	Polydek	Deknatel	Polyester (coated with Teflon-light)	High	Moderate	Good
	Tevdek	Deknatel	Polyester (coated with Teflon-heavy)	High	Moderate	Poor
Wire	Stainless steel	Ethicon	Stainless steel	High	Low	Poor

Modified from Bennett R. G. *Fundamentals of Cutaneous Surgery*. St. Louis: Mosby, 1988.

Description

Suture strands that become encapsulated or walled-off within the tissue during the healing process. They remain buried in the tissue unless removed surgically. When used externally, such as skin closure, they must be removed postoperatively.

Nonabsorbable suture materials can also be subdivided into several categories: (1) natural or synthetic, and (2) monofilament or multifilament.

- Class I—silk or synthetic fibers of monofilament, twisted, or braided construction
- Class II—cotton or linen fibers or coated natural or synthetic fibers. The coating forms a thickness, yet does not contribute to its strength

Tissue Interactions

Nonabsorbable sutures could also be called "slowly absorbable" since two materials, polyesters and polypropylene, are the only materials that cannot be absorbed.

Monofilament versus Multifilament

A monofilament suture is a single strand that is non-capillary (resistant to fluids soaking into the suture); it is designated by the USP as Type B.

Multifilament, on the other hand, is multiple strands of suture held together by a process of twisting, braiding, or spinning the materials. All multifilament sutures have a certain capacity to absorb body fluids (capillarity), which elicits a higher degree of tissue reaction, and are classified by the USP as Type A.

Choosing Appropriate Suture Material

Absorbable Suture Materials

Absorbable suture materials are primarily used on fast-healing tissue. Natural sources of absorbable sutures include surgical gut (chromic and plain) and collagen (Table 9-3).

1. *Surgical gut* formerly called *catgut*, which comes from the submucosa of sheep intestine or the serosa of beef intestine; it is about 98% collagen.

Table 9-3   Commonly Used Suture Material

Suture	Type	Color	Raw Material	Interaction	Frequent Uses
Surgical gut	Plain	Yellowish-tan	Collagen derived from healthy mammals	Absorbed relatively quickly by body tissues	Ligate superficial vessels; suture subcutaneous and other tissues that heal rapidly, may be used in presence of infection
		Blue (dyed)			Ophthalmology
	Chromic	Brown	Collagen derived from healthy mammals; treated to resist digestion by body tissues	Absorbed more slowly by body tissues due to chemical treatment	Fascia and peritoneum for support; most versatile of all materials for use in practically all tissues; may be used in presence of infection
		Blue (dyed)			Ophthalmology
Coated Vicryl (Polyglactin 910)	Braided	Violet (undyed)	Copolymer of lactide and glycolide coated with polyglactin 370 and calcium stearate	Absorbed by slow hydrolysis in tissues	Ligate or suture tissues where an absorbable suture is desirable except where approximation under stress is required
Surgical silk	Braided	Black	Natural protein fiber spun by silkworm	Very slowly absorbed; remains encapsulated in body tissues	Most body tissues for ligating and suturing
		White			Ophthalmology and plastic surgery
Surgical cotton	Twisted	White, blue, pink	Natural cotton fibers	Nonabsorbable; remains encapsulated in body tissues	Most body tissues for ligating and suturing
Surgical steel	Monofilament or multifilament	Silver	An alloy of iron	Nonabsorbable; remains encapsulated in body tissues	General and skin closure; retention; tendon repair; orthopedic and neurosurgery
Ethilon nylon	Monofilament	Green	Polyamide polymer	Nonabsorbable; remains encapsulated in body tissues	Skin closure; retention, plastic surgery; ophthalmology, microsurgery
Nurolon nylon	Braided	Black	Polyamide polymer	Nonabsorbable; remains encapsulated in body tissues	Most body tissues for ligating and suturing; general closure; neurosurgery
Mersilene polyester fiber	Braided	Green, white	Synthetic material made from chemicals	Nonabsorbable; remains encapsulated in body tissues	Cardiovascular and plastic surgery
Ethibond polyester fiber	Braided	Green, white	Polyester fiber material treated with polybutilate	Nonabsorbable; remains encapsulated in body tissues	Abdominal closure; cardiovascular and plastic surgery
Prolene polypropylene	Monofilament	Clear, blue	Polymer of propylene	Nonabsorbable; remains encapsulated in body tissues	General, plastic, and cardiovascular surgery

Source: Modified from Wound Closure Manual, Sommerville, NJ: Ethicon, Inc., 1985.

Characteristics
Tissue reactivity
   Plain   High
   Chromic   Moderately high
Tensile strength
   Plain   Poor (0% at 2–3 weeks)
   Chromic   Poor (0% at 2–3 weeks)
Handling
   Plain   Fair
   Chromic   Fair

Absorption rate
   Plain   Unpredictable (12 weeks)
   Chromic   Unpredictable (12 weeks)

2. *Collagen*   purest form of "gut"; infrequently used; comes in both plain and chromicized preparation

Characteristics
   Tissue reactivity   Moderate
   Tensile strength   Poor (0% at 2–3 weeks)

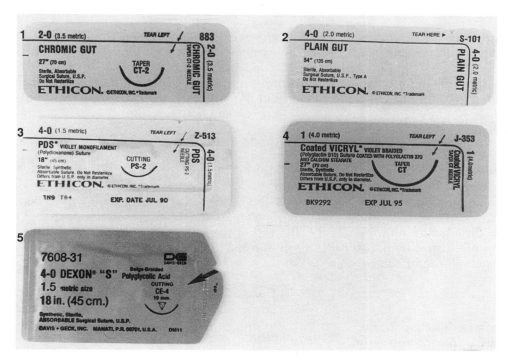

Suture packets: 1. Chromic; 2. Plain; 3. PDS; 4. Vicryl; 5. Dexon

Handling   Fair
Absorption rate   Unpredictable (12 weeks)

General Usage
Plain gut   subcutaneous (Sub-Q) layer for subcuticular closure or as ligatures—oral mucosa; eyes; small vessels
Chromic gut   mucosal layer in anastomosis; large vessel ties/ligatures, muscle, fascia; general purpose
Collagen   ophthalmology; uterine cervical banding

Contraindications
When extended or prolonged approximation is required

Nursing Implications
1. Use immediately after opening the package
2. Unwind carefully and handle as little as possible
3. Rinsing is necessary only for surgical gut or collagen being used in the eye, but others may be "dipped" in saline to facilitate handling

Synthetic sources include polymers, either dyed or undyed, and are absorbed by a slow hydrolysis process in the presence of tissue fluids. The tensile strength of synthetic absorbable sutures exceeds that of surgical gut, and it can be used in the presence of infection since absorption time and loss of tensile strength are not affected by the proteolytic enzymes in the gastrointestinal tract. Examples include

Polyglycolic acid (Dexon)
Polydioxanome (PDS)
Polyglactin 910 (Vicryl)

Characteristics (Vicryl; Dexon; PDS)
Coated Vicryl

Tissue reactivity	Low
Tensile strength	Good (50% at 2–3 weeks)
Handling	Good
Absorption rate	Predictable (80 days)

Dexon

Tissue reactivity	Low
Tensile strength	Good (50% at 2–3 weeks)
Handling	Fair
Absorption rate	Predictable (80 days)

PDS

Tissue reactivity	Low
Tensile strength	Good (50% at 2–3 weeks)
Handling	Poor
Absorption rate	Predictable (180 days)

General Usage
Can be used for the same purpose as chromic gut; general purpose; any type of tissue

Advantage
Longer period of strength (4–6 weeks) before absorption. Can be coated or noncoated depending on area and usage

Handling Characteristics
1. Synthetic absorbable suture has an expiration date; therefore, stock must be rotated to avoid outdated suture
2. Sutures are packaged to use dry. Do not dip into solution or they will loose tensile strength

Nonabsorbable Suture Materials

Nonabsorbable suture materials are primarily used with tissues that heal slower owing to their location, tissue type, or general healing factors. Like absorbable sutures, the suture materials come from both natural and synthetic sources. Natural sources include silk and cotton. Silk is made from the threads spun by silk worm larvae. Cotton sutures are formed by twisting long cotton fibers into smooth multifilament strands.

General Usage
Cotton: infrequently used today; most reactive in situ; tends to split. Used for muscle/fascia; appendix stump. Umbilical tape also classified as cotton; used to retract delicate structures or as marker

Silk: most commonly used; may be twisted, braided, or single filament; ties most easily; available in black, virgin silk, white, or dyed. Usually well tolerated. Used in ophthalmology, the gastrointestinal tract, the brain, cardiovascular system, and as skin closure. Dermal silk has added protein; therefore, it is extremely reactive.

Characteristics
Cotton
Tissue reactivity	High
Tensile strength	Good
Handling	Good

Silk
Tissue reactivity	High
Tensile strength	Good
Handling	Good

Contraindications
The presence of infection or contamination; in biliary and urinary tract (can precipitate stone formation). Should not be used if long-term support is vital since it loses substantial strength 90 to 120 days after implantation.

Advances in suture manufacturing have resulted in decreased usage of natural substances and an increase in synthetic substances adaptable for suturing material. Examples of these substances include nylon, polyester, polyethylene, polypropylene, and surgical steel/wire.

General Description and Usage
Nylon (Polyamide Derivative)
Available as monofilament or multifilament. Monofilament is available in clear, blue, black, or green; texture is very smooth and inert; used on skin; plastic surgery in fine gauges; in ophthalmic, microvascular, and peripheral nerve repairs.

EXAMPLES (trade names)
   Ethilon; Surgilon; Dermalon; Neurolon

Polyester
Very inert; may be coated or impregnated with Teflon, silicone, polybutilate; has the highest tensile strength of all synthetic absorbable materials, even after prolonged implantation with minimal tissue reaction

EXAMPLES (trade names)
   Ti-Con; Dacron; Tevdeck; Ethiflex; Polydek; Ethibond; Mersilene

Polypropylene
Extremely inert and newest of synthetics. Handles like silk with good properties of silk; smooth passage through tissue and vascular prostheses with minimal tissue reaction; high tensile strength over extended time. Can be used when delayed or retarded healing is anticipated, in the presence of infection, or when extended support is required (cardiovascular surgery). May be difficult to handle, since it has memory, and may kink. Used in plastic surgery, tendon repairs, microsurgery, and cardiovascular (CV) surgery.

EXAMPLE (trade names)
   Prolene; Surgilene; Dermalene

Characteristics
Tissue reactivity
Nylon	Low to moderate
Polypropylene	Low
Polyester	Low to moderate

Tensile strength
Nylon	High
Polypropylene	Fair (Prolene; Surgilene)
	Good (Dermalene)
Polyesters	High

Handling
Nylon	Poor to fair
Polypropylene	Poor
Polyesters	Good

Surgical Steel/Wire
Very inert and permanently strong; made from an alloy of iron (stainless steel or silver wire); available

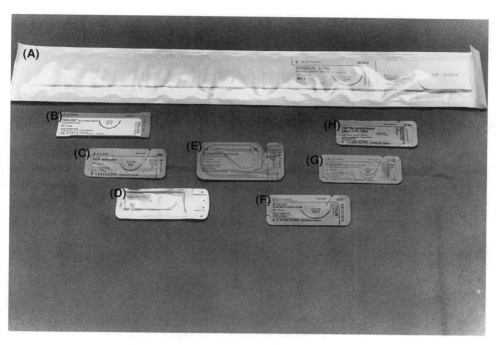

Nonabsorbable suture material: (A) Surgical steel; (B) Prolene; (C) Silk; (D) Tevdeck; (E) Mersilene; (F) Nylon; (G) Ethibond; (H) Cotton

in monofilament and multifilament. May be twisted or tied depending on gauge. Extremely difficult to handle (kinks easily) and has a "sawing" effect on tissue, causing possible tissue reaction. Can be used in the presence of infection, to hold bone together, in the abdominal region when extreme strength is required (repairs of wound disruption or evisceration), or as retention sutures.

NOTE: When used with implantable metal prostheses, knowing the composition of metal is important in order to prevent unfavorable electrolytic reactions between the two metals; therefore, stainless steel sutures should not be placed close to the metal prosthesis or the wound.

Characteristics

Tissue reactivity	Low
Tensile strength	High
Handling	Poor to fair

Silver wire is soft and pliable, and easy to handle with antibacterial characteristics and high tensile strength. Used for closure following dehiscence or for added strength for recurrent inguinal hernias with or without mesh application, such as surgical steel, polyester fiber, polypropylene, or synthetic absorbable.

Availability

Spools; packages of precut surgical lengths, with or without needles; usually multistrand when in precut packages

Handling Characteristics

1. To avoid a "kink," leave wire sutures in package until ready to use
2. To prevent "spring-back" effect, clamp open end with Kelly clamp and pass both needle holder and clamp to surgeon
3. Requires the use of a *heavy* needle holder and a *wire scissors*

Self-assessment Exercise 6

Directions: Complete the following exercises. The answers are given at the end of this module.

1. A suture that is dissolved by body enzymes is classified as _____.

2. Standards and classifications of sutures are set by the USP.

    True   False

3. _____ and _____ are two examples of synthetic absorbable sutures.

4. A 4-0 suture has less tensile strength and is finer than a 5-0 suture.

    True   False

5. Identify the following type of suture stating its:

    a. classification _____

    b. trade name _____

    c. size _____

    d. general use _____

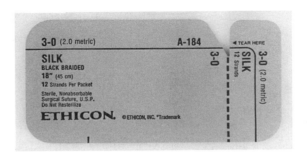

SURGICAL NEEDLES

Surgical needles are made of a steel alloy with a high carbon content. Surgical needles are precision-made instruments, and must be handled gently in order to achieve maximum effectiveness.

At one time, in surgical history, reusable eyed needles were used exclusively. These needles were available in many shapes and sizes and required sterilization before each use. In specific instances, these needles are still being used.

Today, many of these needles have been replaced by either a needle-suture combination prepared by the manufacturer (*atraumatic*) or are available as a disposable, presterilized *free needle*, requiring the user to thread the suture strand to the needle, and both are available in a variety of shapes, sizes, and points.

Components of a Surgical Needle

All surgical needles have three basic sections: the *point*, the *body* or *shaft*, and the *eye*.

The body or shaft determines the shape of the needle; either straight or curved. Needle points range from a *taper* (noncutting) to a *cutting* (one side or both have a cutting edge) to a *blunt* tip (neither cuts nor pierces). The eye of the needle is where the suture strand is attached or threaded, and may be round, oblong, or square (Fig. 9-4).

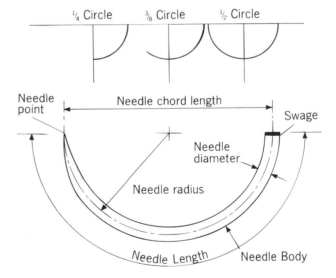

Fig. 9-4. Components of a surgical needle (Adapted from *Davis and Geck: Perspectives on sutures.* O. Stroumtos, ed. Pearl River, NY: American Cyanamid Co., 1978.)

CLASSIFICATION OF SURGICAL NEEDLES

Needles are classified according to their *shape*, the *type of point*, the *shaft*, and the *eye* (Table 9-4).

Shape

Needles come straight or curved. The amount of curvature of the needle or lack of it determines its type and

Table 9-4   Surgical Needles

Types and Appearance		General Uses	Examples
Needle Points			
Blunt		Spongy tissues that are easily penetrated and/or torn	Liver; kidney
Taper		Delicate to substantial tissues that are easily penetrated and torn	Intestines; subcutaneous; muscle/fascia; veins; nonarteriosclerotic arteries
Cutting-spear		Tissues that are tough to penetrate	Skin; sclera; tendons; arteriosclerotic arteries
Cutting-trocar		Extremely tough tissues to penetrate and pass through	Cartilage; cervix (uteri)
Needle Shafts			
Straight		Where suturing can be done in a flat or shallow depth	Skin; any anastomosis in which the tissues may be elevated to the top level of the wound
Circle, 3/8		Shallow depths	Essentially the same as straight and skin
Circle, 1/2		General purpose, usually in wounds of some depth	The interior of any wound
Circle, 5/8		Deepest, smallest maneuvering-room wounds	Any interior of any seep, small wound, where exposure is difficult—vaginal hysterectomy; hemorrhoidectomy
Circle, 1/4		Same as half circle	
Needle eyes			
Round (threaded)		Gross general purpose, where tissue trauma is not a factor	Muscle/fascia approximation; subcutaneous; suture-ligatures
French (threaded)		Delicate tissues; precursor to swaged; infrequent today	Similar to swaged, half circle taper point
Atraumatic (swaged)		Where least tissue trauma is desired	Fine/delicate anastomoses anywhere in the body; GI, ducts, cavity linings, etcetera; plastic repairs

From Fairchild S. Surgical Technician Student Workbook. Unpublished manuscript, 1982, p. 64.

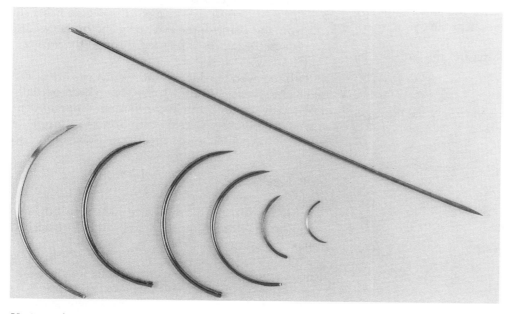

Variety of surgical needles

can dictate its primary use. There are five common shapes associated with surgical needles, regardless whether they are attached to a strand of suture or free: straight and ¼, ⅜, ½, and ⅝ circle. The deeper the tissue, the greater the need for a sharper curve (Fig. 9-5).

Full curved needles are used with a needle holder, while the straight needle is held in the hand. Straight needles are generally reserved for superficial surfaces, including skin.

Points and Shafts

The delicacy of the tissue determines which point is most suitable to use. There are three basic needle points, with variations of each (Fig. 9-6).

Taper Point

Taper points are used on delicate tissues that are easily penetrated. These areas include the peritoneum, the heart, or the intestines. A taper-point needle is designed so that the shaft gradually tapers to a sharp point, which results in a very small hole in the tissue.

Cutting Point

A cutting-point needle is designed with a razor-sharp tip and is used for tissue such as skin or tendons. There are three types of cutting needles:

1. *Taper cut* used for tough, fibrous tissue
2. *Conventional cutting* two opposing cutting edges with a third edge on the *inside* curve of the needle
3. *Reverse cutting* two opposing cutting edges with a third edge on the *outside* curve of the needle. The triangular shape extends from the point to the eye of the needle; only the edges near the tip are sharp

Generally, the tougher the tissue, the greater the need for a cutting-type shaft.

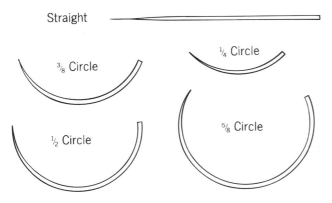

Fig. 9-5. Shapes of surgical needles (Adapted from Wound Closure Manual. Sommerville, NJ: Ethicon, Inc., 1994)

Blunt Point

Blunt-tip needles have a rounded end and are used in friable tissue, such as liver or kidney, when neither piercing nor cutting is appropriate.

Additional points include the *precision point, micropoint reverse cutting,* and *micropoint spatula,* to name just a few.

The Eye of the Needle

The eye, or head, of the needle is designed to cause minimal trauma to the tissue.

There are three types of eyed needles, each a variation of the other:

1. *Atraumatic or swaged* one or two needles attached to the suture strand at the factory, eliminating the need for threading. This causes the least amount of tissue trauma, since the suture and needle are a continuous unit in which the needle size and suture diameter are matched as closely as possible.

    A modification of the permanently swaged suture is the *control-release* suture, sometimes referred to as "pop-off." The needle and suture begin as one unit; however, they may be separated by means of a light pull on the needle, allowing the surgeon to tie without a needle remaining on the end of the suture (Fig. 9-7). Control-release sutures allow for faster interrupted suturing.
2. *Eyed needles* the needle must be threaded with the suture strand, thus making it necessary to pull two strands of suture through the tissue, creating a larger hole and possibly more tissue trauma
3. *Spring or French eyed needles* the needle has a slit from the inside of the eye to the end of the needle, where the suture is secured through the spring

Both the eyed needle and the French eye are classified as *free needles*. Although they have been partially replaced by the control-released suture, some surgeons may still prefer them for specific uses or as a type of suture not available in the preattached format.

Free Needles

Free needles come in the same size and shape, but have been named to differentiate them from those attached at the factory, and include:

Keith needle	Straight, medium weight, with cutting point
Milner needle	Straight; delicate; taper shaft and point

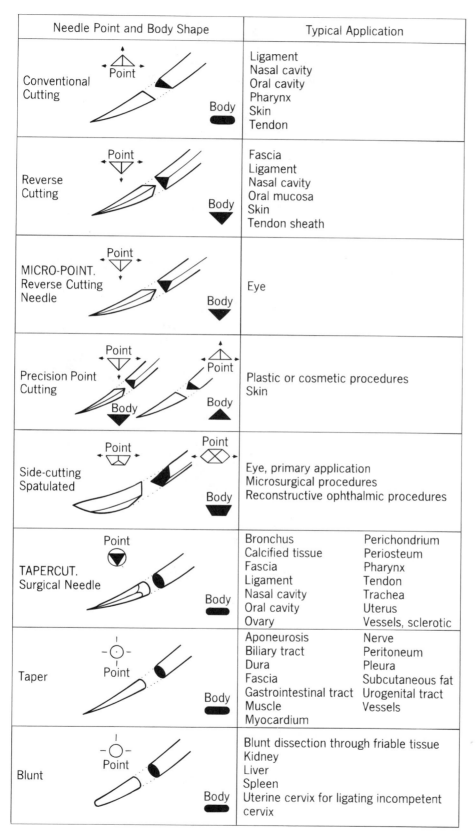

Needle Point and Body Shape	Typical Application
Conventional Cutting	Ligament Nasal cavity Oral cavity Pharynx Skin Tendon
Reverse Cutting	Fascia Ligament Nasal cavity Oral mucosa Skin Tendon sheath
MICRO-POINT. Reverse Cutting Needle	Eye
Precision Point Cutting	Plastic or cosmetic procedures Skin
Side-cutting Spatulated	Eye, primary application Microsurgical procedures Reconstructive ophthalmic procedures
TAPERCUT. Surgical Needle	Bronchus Perichondrium Calcified tissue Periosteum Fascia Pharynx Ligament Tendon Nasal cavity Trachea Oral cavity Uterus Ovary Vessels, sclerotic
Taper	Aponeurosis Nerve Biliary tract Peritoneum Dura Pleura Fascia Subcutaneous fat Gastrointestinal tract Urogenital tract Muscle Vessels Myocardium
Blunt	Blunt dissection through friable tissue Kidney Liver Spleen Uterine cervix for ligating incompetent cervix

Fig. 9-6. Glossary of needle points (Adapted from Wound Closure Manual. Sommerville, NJ: Ethicon, Inc., 1994)

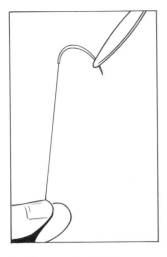 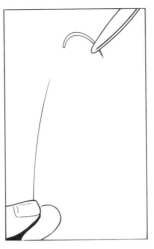

1. The needle is held securely in holder. Suture is grasped securely just below needle, pulling strand taut.

2. The needle is released with a straight tug of the needleholder.

Fig. 9-7. Control-release suture and needle (Adapted from Wound Closure Manual. Sommerville, NJ: Ethicon, Inc., 1994)

Ferguson needle	Half circle; delicate; taper shaft and point
Mayo needle	Half circle; heavy; taper shaft and point
Surgeon's regular	Half circle; medium weight; cutting point with taper shaft
Trocar	Half circle; heavy; spear-shaped point; taper shaft
French eye	Half circle; delicate; taper point shaft

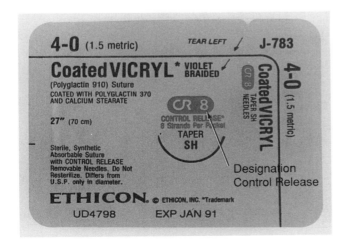

Control-release suture pack

WORKING WITH SUTURES AND NEEDLES

Advanced preparation is the key to a smooth surgical procedure, and preparation of sutures used during the case is an important component of this phase.

Sutures should be prepared in their order of use, but certain preliminary preparations are necessary to ensure sterility and prevent prolonged exposure, unnecessary handling, and excess waste (Fig. 9-8).

Sutures will first be used to ligate or tie off bleeding vessels; therefore, sutures without needles (*ligatures*) should be prepared first.

The use of suture materials in dry packages requires no special preparation, but those contained in solution must be opened carefully to avoid contamination of the field from the liquid contents. Sutures that need to be straightened for easy handling should be prepared first, and placed in a "suture book," created from a sterile towel, and leaving the ends extended to reduce time and wasted motion. Remember, chromic, plain, nylon, and prolene sutures require only slight straightening, which is accomplished by grasping the two ends, using the thumb and forefinger, and pulling gently.

When using a multiple-suture packet, such as *Labyrinth Design,* the packet should be torn open along the dotted line and the sutures nudged forward from the package so that individual strands can be obtained as needed. The design of the labyrinth package allows for single-strand selection without disturbing the other strands in the package.

Suture ligatures may be handed as a free tie, placed in the open hand of the surgeon, or placed on the end of an instrument for a deep tie. When a dispensing reel is used, both the free end and the spool are passed to the surgeon simultaneously.

If the ligatures are pre-cut strands, no further preparation is required. However, if ligatures are available only in the standard length, the scrub person may have to cut the strands for ease of handling. To prepare the individual ligatures, the strand is folded in equal parts and held between the fingers, and the strand is divided into desired lengths—approximately 12 to 15 inches for superficial ties and 24 to 30 inches for deep ties.

Handling Eyed Needles and Sutures

To prepare a suture–needle combination, the scrub person grasps the exposed needle with fingertips or a needle holder and gently pulls the strand to remove it from the package, or if not immediately used, can leave the needle holder on the needle with the suture in the package for easy identification when the suture is requested.

1. Continuous ties
   on plastic disk-type reel

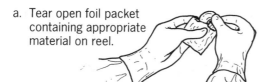

a. Tear open foil packet
   containing appropriate
   material on reel.

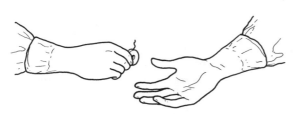

b. Hand to surgeon as needed, being certain end
   of ligating material is free for grasping.

2a. Single-strand ties–Labyrinth pack

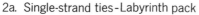

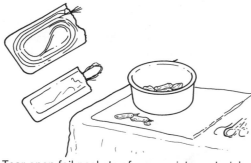

a. Tear open foil packets of appropriate material.

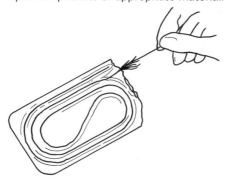

b. Remove nonabsorbable pre-cut length one
   strand at a time from the Labyrinth packet when
   the surgeon is ready to use it.

2b. Single strand–pre-cut

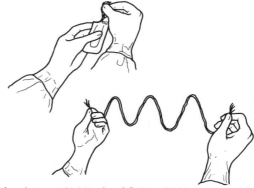

a. Extract pre-cut strands of Sutupak sterile
   sutures, either absorbable or nonabsorbable.
   Straighten surgical gut with gentle pull.

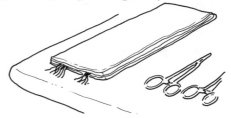

b. Place packets or strands in "suture book" with
   ends extended far enough for rapid extraction.

Presentation technique

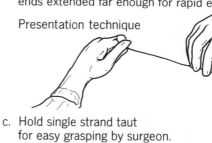

c. Hold single strand taut
   for easy grasping by surgeon.

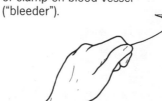

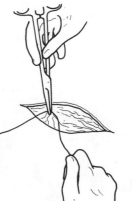

d. Surgeon places single-
   strand tie around tip
   of clamp on blood vessel
   ("bleeder").

Fig. 9-8. Preparing and handling ligatures (Adapted from Wound Closure Manual. Sommerville, NJ: Ethicon, Inc., 1994)

Mounting the Needle

The curved needle is mounted on a needle holder. In mounting the needle, it should be placed nearest the eye, about one third of the total length of the shaft away from the eye end. When swaged needles are mounted, it is important that the needle holder is not clamped directly over the swage itself, since this weakens the area and can cause the suture to detach unexpectedly from the needle.

Threading the Needle

The suture may be threaded through the eye from either side of the curve. The suture strand is drawn through the eye about one third of its length. Both ends of the suture may be drawn between the jaws of the needle holder (or only one end depending on surgeon preference), and the instrument is passed to the surgeon.

Passing the Needle Holder

When mounting the needle on a needle holder, it should be positioned so that the surgeon does not have to reposition it for suturing. The outside curve of the needle should be aimed downward, with the point aimed for the ceiling, in the direction of the surgeon's chin or thumb.

The instrument is passed handle first, tip pointed toward the surgeon's opposite thumb, while the scrub person gently holds onto the loose end to avoid contact with the surgeon's palm as the instrument is transferred. Suture needles must be passed on a one-to-one basis, and the previous needle retrieved before passing another. To avoid delay, two needles should be mounted so that as one is returned, another is ready to use.

When passing a straight needle, the tip is covered by the scrub person's hand, and the swaged portion of the needle is handed to the surgeon.

Using Multiple-Needle Packs

If more than one needle is contained in the package, all needles should be seen and counted by the scrub and circulator before use.

Multiple-strand needles can be placed in a towel fold, similar to multistrand ligatures, with needles exposed on top for ease of handling.

Maintaining a Suture Inventory

After the suture has been used, the needle, on the needle holder, is returned to the scrub person, who places it into the needle counter for future confirmation of the needle count. To avoid loss, needles must never be allowed to lay loose on the field.

Maintaining a running, silent count of all needles used is the responsibility of the scrub person. Therefore, empty suture packets must stay on the sterile field until the final needle count is confirmed in case there is a misplaced needle.

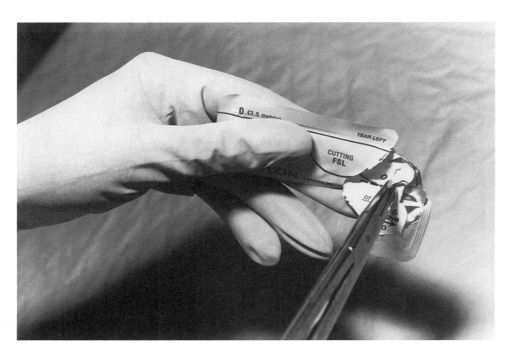

Removing suture

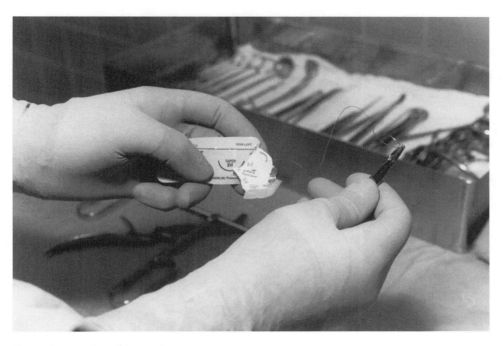

Preparing a suture for passing

METHODS OF SUTURING

There are two basic methods of suturing, and various ways to use the two techniques. The suture is either *running*, using a single continuous suture, or it is *interrupted*, placed separately and tied separately. The running suture saves time, but if the suture breaks during the healing process, the wound could open along the entire length of the incision.

The following paragraphs describe some stitches commonly used in surgery (Fig. 9-9).

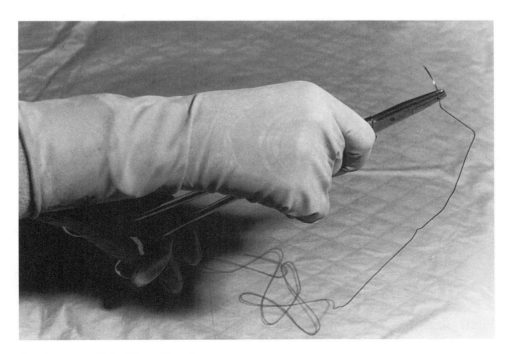

Passing a needle holder with suture

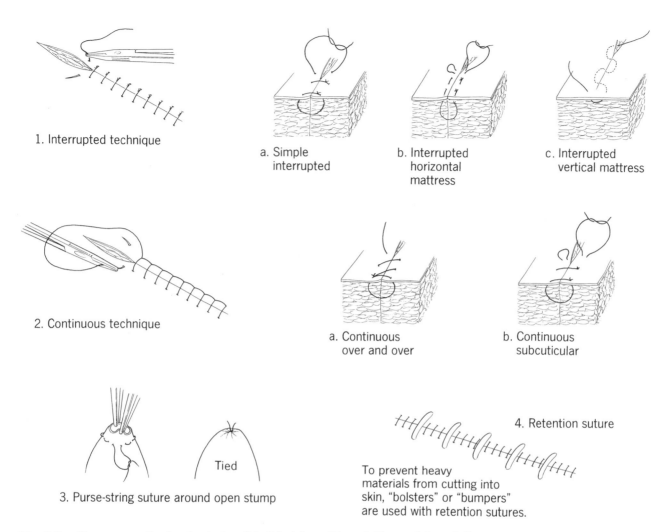

1. Interrupted technique

a. Simple interrupted

b. Interrupted horizontal mattress

c. Interrupted vertical mattress

2. Continuous technique

a. Continuous over and over

b. Continuous subcuticular

3. Purse-string suture around open stump

Tied

4. Retention suture

To prevent heavy materials from cutting into skin, "bolsters" or "bumpers" are used with retention sutures.

Fig. 9-9. Common methods of suturing (Modified from Wound Closure Manual. Sommerville, NJ: Ethicon, Inc., 1994)

Interrupted Suture

Interrupted stitches are formed by placing the suture in such a manner that each stitch is placed separately and tied independently of the other stitches. This method is widely used and is generally considered to be the most efficient.

A variation of this technique is called the *mattress stitch,* which is created by taking a second "bite" with the needle through the tissue vertically, horizontally, or crossed in a figure-of-eight stitch.

Continuous Suture

A continuous stitch is made with a single strand of suture material. Each stitch follows one after the other without interruption, and only the first and last are

tied. This stitch is not widely used, since a break at any point may mean wound disruption of the entire suture line.

A variation of this suture is the *over/under* stitch. It is used primarily to close tissue layers such as peritoneum, which do not have great strength but require a close closure to lessen the chance of an intestinal loop penetrating through the suture line.

Purse-String Suture

When a continuous stitch is placed around an aperture to create a closure, such as before the removal of an organ (e.g., the appendix, cecum, gallbladder, or urinary bladder), it is referred to as a *purse-string* technique. Once the suture is in place, the end is drawn closed, causing the opening to close tightly.

Retention or Stay Sutures

Retention or stay sutures provide a secondary suture line. These sutures, placed at a distance from the primary suture line, relieve undue pressure and help to remove dead space. They are placed in the wound in such a way that they include most if not all of the layers of the wound.

This technique is used to close long vertical abdominal wounds and lacerated or infected wounds. Suture material is usually heavy, nonabsorbable material such as silk, nylon, polyester fibers, or wire. To prevent the suture from cutting into the skin, a rubber tubing or "bumper" is passed over or through the exposed portion of the suture.

Self-assessment Exercise 7

Directions: Complete the following exercises. The answers are given at the end of this module.

1. A taper point needle is mostly used on internal structures.

                                  True   False

2. List two factors that may influence the selection of a surgical needle. _____

3. Describe the advantage of using an atraumatic suture. _____

4. A continuous stitch is preferred over the interrupted technique since it provides more strength.

                                  True   False

5. Retention sutures may be used along with other methods of routine skin closure.

                                  True   False

6. Vicryl is classified as a nonabsorbable suture.

                                  True   False

ALTERNATIVE METHODS TO SUTURING

Skin clips, surgical strips (tape), ligation clips, and internal and external staples are alternatives to conventional suturing materials, and have several applications in today's surgical practice setting. The advantage of these methods include time saved under anesthesia and close approximation of wound edges, promoting greater and faster healing with less tissue loss or reaction. The use of these methods, however, requires additional education of both the surgeon and the surgical team to achieve maximum efficiency when using these alternative methods.

External Devices

Surgical Strips (Tapes and Steri-Strips)

Surgical strips are made of a reinforced, micropore surgical tape that is adhesive on one side. They are used to approximate skin edges following a subcuticular closure or superficial lacerations in conjunction with skin sutures, permitting the skin sutures to be removed 36 to 48 hours postoperatively. They can be used for any type of surgery, but are most often associated with plastic and pediatric surgery, since they leave no mark on the skin. Tapes are available in various sizes ranging from $\frac{1}{8}$ inches to 2 inches wide and are $1\frac{1}{2}$ to 4 inches long, which can be cut to meet the needs of the wound or patient (synonym = steri-strips).

Skin Clips

Skin clips are made of noncorroding metal, and may be used for skin closure, with or without sutures. Skin clips can be steam sterilized, or be disposable, and can be applied in the presence of infection or drainage and applied quickly using a specific application instrument.

Because they are bulky and uncomfortable postoperatively, they have been replaced by the disposable skin staples.

Skin Staples

Skin staples are the fastest method of skin closure and have a low level of tissue reactivity.

The edges of both cuticular and subcuticular layers must be everted (aligned with the edges slightly raised), and the stapler is positioned over the line of the incision so that a staple will be placed evenly on each side.

Skin staples come preloaded and disposable with different quantities of staples and different widths (35 regular/wide — 35 staples, regular or wide width). More may be needed to close an abdomen than to close a herniorrhaphy in the inguinal region.

Skin staples must be removed, usually 5 to 7 days postoperatively, and a staple extractor is used for this purpose. Because the skin flattens as it heals, staples provide an excellent cosmetic result if they have been properly placed lightly over the incision.

Internal Devices

Ligation Clips

Ligation clips were first devised in 1911 by Dr. Harvey Cushing for use in brain surgery. The metal Cushing clips or Frazier clips are made of silver or stainless steel; those made of PDS (a synthetic material) and titanium are more commonly used today.

As mentioned earlier, ligation clips are used for hemostasis or to ligate nerves and ducts. The clips come preloaded or are placed on a special applicator, placed

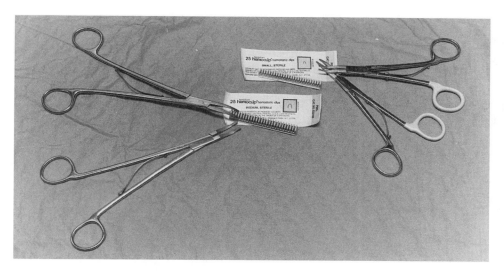

Internal ligation clips and instruments

around the vessel or structure, and the handle is squeezed so the jaws of the applicator are closed with the clip secured around the structure.

Ligating clips (trade names: Hemoclip, Ligaclip, Surgiclip) are available in several sizes, and when using the nonautomatic instrument, a corresponding applicator is needed for each size clip.

Surgical Staples

Included in most surgical suite inventory lists are a group of mechanical stapling devices for internal ligation and division, resection, and anastomosis, skin, and fascia closure.

The first surgical staple was introduced in Hungary in 1908 for closing the stomach. This was followed in 1924, also in Hungary, by a mechanical device for gastrointestinal anastomosis developed by Aladar von Petz.[3] Although cumbersome and heavy, the von Petz clamp was widely acclaimed as more general surgeons began using the instrument. But a large drawback was the fact that before each use, the instrument had to be hand loaded with each staple, a time-consuming ordeal, resulting in a subsequent refinement of the instrument by the Russians during the 1950s.

In the United States, a reusable stapler became available in the 1960s through patents licensed from the Soviet Union, and in 1978, a disposable stapling instrument was developed and is currently in use today. It is preassembled, thus reducing the workload of the surgeon and surgical team.

Advantages of Internal Stapling The mechanical application of the stapling instrument significantly reduces tissue manipulation and handling, thus reducing surgical and anesthesia time and permitting a more natural wound healing process to occur in a shorter period of time. The staple produces an airtight, leakproof closure and can be safely used in many types of tissues.

Stapling Instruments Each stapler is designed for stapling specific tissues, and is named after its application techniques. For example:

1. thoracic/abdominal stapler
2. gastrointestinal anastomosis stapler
3. intraluminal stapler
4. *LDS Instruments* ligation stapler
5. *Skin stapler*

Several companies that manufacture internal staplers have different names for these instruments, but their usage is generally the same.

Staplers fire either a single staple or simultaneously fire one or two straight or circular rows of staples, in addition to cutting or separating edges and stapling the edges closed.

When fired, the staples are shaped like a capital "B," and are noncrushing; thus, nutrition is permitted to pass through the staple line to the cut edge of the tissue. This promotes healing and reduces the possibility of necrosis.

The staples are essentially nonreactive; therefore, the occurrence of tissue reaction or infection is reduced, permitting an anastomosis created with staples to function sooner than one created with manual technique.

The surgeon selects the correct instrument for the desired application, and may use two or three stapling devices during one surgical procedure, as necessary.

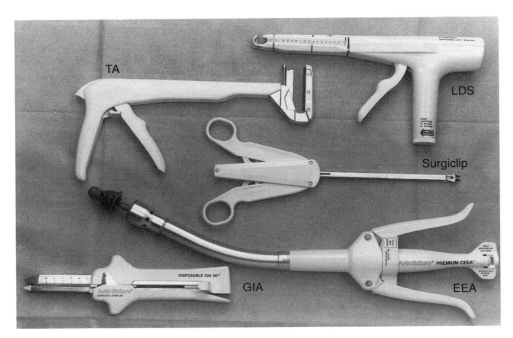

Examples of internal stapling devices—alternative to suturing (Courtesy of Autosuture, Inc.)

Disadvantages of Surgical Stapling

Although the positives outweigh the negatives, the reusable and disposable instruments are expensive and are not always reliable, due mainly to the user's unfamiliarity with the operation of the instrument.

The surgeon and the assistants (scrub persons) should receive instructions outside the operating room regarding the proper use and function of the instrument, since inappropriately placed staples are much more difficult to correct than manually placed sutures.

The nursing personnel must know how to assemble, disassemble, and sterilize the reusable instruments, since improper cleaning and assembly could cause misfiring, rendering the instrument useless. Second and third generation, totally disposable and preassembled instruments have greatly reduced this problem, and will open new avenues for a variety of surgical procedures. However, the need for education of surgeons and staff remains the key element for effective application of surgical staples.

Self-assessment Exercise 8

Directions: Complete the following exercises. The answers are given at the end of this module.

1. A continuous suture, placed beneath the epithelial layer of the skin in short lateral stitches, is known as a subcuticular stitch.

    True   False

2. Bumpers or guards are used with retention sutures to _____.

3. List five pieces of information found on a suture package.
    a. _____
    b. _____
    c. _____
    d. _____
    e. _____

4. A surgical mesh is used when additional strength is needed for repairs.

    True   False

5. A *blunt* needle would be appropriate for suturing liver tissue.

    True   False

6. Identify the following internal staplers, and briefly state their clinical application.

1.

2.

SURGICAL INSTRUMENTATION: TOOLS OF THE TRADE

Introduction and Historical Overview

The key to any successful surgical procedure is the efficiency of the material you are using. Surgical instruments are the most important tools the surgeon uses, and therefore they must be handled carefully and with respect.

OR personnel are responsible for the use, handling, and care of hundreds of surgical instruments each day. This activity requires a basic knowledge of how these instruments are manufactured, maintained, and properly used in order to prolong their usefulness. Surgical instruments are expensive and represent a major investment for every institution, regardless of its size, type, or the number of procedures performed each day.

The history of surgical instruments dates back to around 350,000 B.C. Archeologists found a skull from that time revealing evidence of a surgical procedure known as *trephining* (opening of the skull), probably performed to release the demons believed to be trapped inside the patient. A sharp flint and hammer were needed to create a hole in the skull, and fine animal teeth were used as probes; later, they were used for bloodletting and drainage of abscesses.

The ancient Greek, Egyptian, and Hindu instruments, when compared with some used today, show a remarkable resemblance in design, but even with these societies' advanced knowledge of the arts, the instruments were very crude, cumbersome, and nonversatile (Fig. 9-10).

In the late 1700s surgical instruments used in the

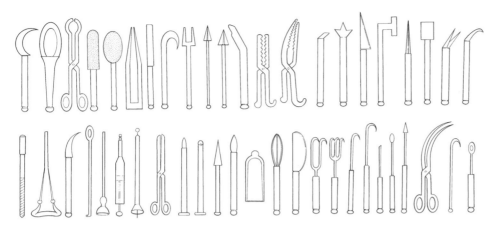

Fig. 9-10. Variety of ancient surgical instruments

United States were either imported from Europe or made by skilled American artisans, such as silversmiths, workers in wood or bone, coppersmiths, and glass blowers, under the supervision of the surgeon requesting the instrument.

The surgeon would explain how the instrument was to be used, and each instrument was specifically created for a particular surgeon, some with intricately carved ivory handles or initials carved into the blade or jaws of the instrument. Custom-designed instruments became a status symbol in the surgical community, and surgeons traveled and performed their profession with their own instruments.

In the mid 1800s, surgeons were scarce and medical instruments were almost nonexistent, so kitchen knives, carpenter's saws, and table forks were used until the late 1800s and early 1900s, when surgical specialties were beginning to emerge and the demand increased for smaller and more delicate instruments.

World War I to the Present

In Germany, during World War I, the development of stainless steel provided a superior material for the manufacturing of surgical instruments, since it did not rust easily or chip or dent with normal handling, as did instruments made with other materials. In 1924, instrument craftsmen were brought to the United States from Germany, Sweden, and England, and the manufacturing of precision instrumentation was under way.

Today, surgeons and OR nurses have assisted in the design of new and better surgical instruments, in addition to recommending methods in which the instruments' longevity can be increased, even after repeated sterilization, decontamination, and usage in all types of surgery.

As the art of surgery grows, so too does the need for improved instrument design, and since an instrument set represents a major investment (somewhere in the range of $1500 to $5000, depending on the set), proper care and handling should be a primary concern for all persons working with surgical instruments.

USAGE OF SURGICAL INSTRUMENTS

A surgical instrument—any surgical instrument—is designed to do one of the following tasks.

To Cut, Incise, Dissect
Cutting instruments, frequently called "sharps," include knives, scalpels, blades, and scissors of all types.

To Retract
Such instruments include handheld and self-retaining retractors, skin hooks, and tenacula, all designed to hold tissues or organs away from the incision to provide better visualization.

To Grasp or Hold
This category includes clamps and forceps used to hold or grasp tissue and/or structures, and are designed with either serrations or projecting teeth, depending on the specific need and type of tissue being held.

To Suture
Besides needle holders designed to accommodate very heavy to very light suture material, this category includes instruments used to apply wound clips, he-

mostatic/aneurysm clips, and stainless steel wire suture.

To Dilate, Probe, Cannulate, or Drain

These instruments occupy a miscellaneous category, since they perform multiple tasks; they include suction tips, syringes, gall duct probes, trocars, cannulas for drainage of blood or fluids from an area, catheters, tubes, and drains, even to shunt blood flow around an operative site.

IDENTIFYING SURGICAL INSTRUMENTS

Unfortunately there is no standard nomenclature for the instruments used in surgery. The names change not only from region to region, but also from hospital to hospital and manufacturer to manufacturer. What any particular surgical team may call their instruments depends greatly on the surgeon and where he or she was educated.

Design and Structure

Each instrument, by its design and structure, is made to do a particular job and to function in a particular fashion; thus, it should be used only for that function, to preserve its longevity.

Of the literally thousands of instruments available to surgeons today, each falls into one of the five categories mentioned earlier, regardless of their differences (characteristics) in pattern and/or size.

Differences in lengths, weights, and shapes of surgical instruments and differences in size, curves, or angulations of jaws, blades, or handles are specific to each instrument to perform its specific function, and to improve, shorten, or simplify an operative procedure for the ultimate benefit of the patient.

Anatomy of an Instrument

The clamp or forcep is the most common type of instrument found in any set, since it not only provides hemostasis, but also serves as the basic generic instrument for any procedure (Fig. 9-11).

Each of these instruments has specific identifiable parts. The *point* of the instrument is its tip. When closed, it should fit tightly, unless its function requires that the tissue be compressed only partially (e.g., intestinal or vascular clamps). The *jaws* of the instrument hold tissue securely. Jaws are either smooth or serrated. The serrations allow greater gripping strength

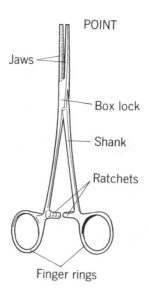

Fig. 9-11. Parts of a clamp

and prevent slippage. The *box lock* is the hinge point of the instrument, and the pin within the box lock should be flush against the instrument. The *shank* is the area between the box lock and the *finger rings*. The *ratchets* interlock to keep the instrument locked shut when the instrument is closed, and they should mesh together smoothly. Forceps, which resemble a tweezer, are held between the thumb and index finger; the tissue is held between the jaws.

THE BASIC INSTRUMENT SET

Persons who use surgical instruments must know and recognize the names, uses, and care of the instruments used for a variety of surgical procedures. A basic or foundation tray is the starting point for becoming familiar with these instruments, since all instrument trays are similar except for size, shape, or numbers of specific instruments in the tray.

Using the five basic categories of instruments, we can create or modify any instrument tray.

MAJOR/LAPAROTOMY TRAY

Since general surgery is considered a "foundation" specialty, the *major tray* or *laparotomy tray* has been designated as the foundation instrument tray for any operating room.

The following list of instruments and their usage (depending on the surgeon's preference) will help create a useful classification system.

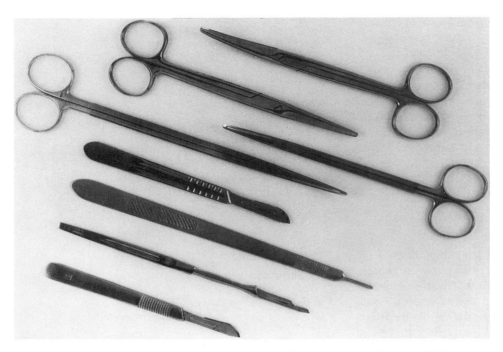

Category I: Cutting and dissecting instruments such as scissors, scalpels, and blades

CLASSIFICATION OF SURGICAL INSTRUMENTS

Category I: Cutting/Dissecting Instruments

Sharps, as they are called, are exactly what their name implies, and the usable part of the instrument has a sharp or cutting edge.

> *SCISSORS: designed in short, long, medium, and heavy; may be blunt or sharp with straight or curved tips (cutting edge)*

INSTRUMENT	COMMON USAGE
Straight Mayo	Suture scissors
Curved Mayo	Heavy/tough tissue
Metzenbaum	
Short	Superficial; delicate tissue
Long	Deep; delicate tissue

> *SCALPELS/BLADES: the oldest of all the instruments; handles are suited to attachment of corresponding disposable blades*

INSTRUMENT	COMMON USAGE
No. 4 Handle/20 Blade	Skin knife; deep puncture wounds
No. 3 Handle/10, 11, 15 Blade	Second knife; minor; delicate structures
No. 7 Handle/11, 15 Blade	Deep; small areas
No. 3L Handle/10, 11, 15 Blade	Deep; abdomen
No. 3LA Handle/10, 11, 15 Blade	Angled; deep; abdomen

Category II: Holding/Grasping Instruments

Clamps and forceps are part of this category, and are designed for specific uses, including hemostasis and assisting with suturing or holding tissue. Forceps are mostly used in pairs.

> *Holding Clamp/Forcep: serrated jaw*
> *Grasping Clamp/Forcep: projected tooth/teeth*

INSTRUMENT	COMMON USAGE
Mosquito Hemostat Curved/Straight	Smallest; superficial Minor/plastic, pediatric surgery Holding clamp
Crile Hemostat Curved/Straight	Medium; first two layers of abdomen Holding clamp
Kelly Hemostat Curved/Straight	Larger Crile; heavier abdominal tissue; long or standard length Holding clamp

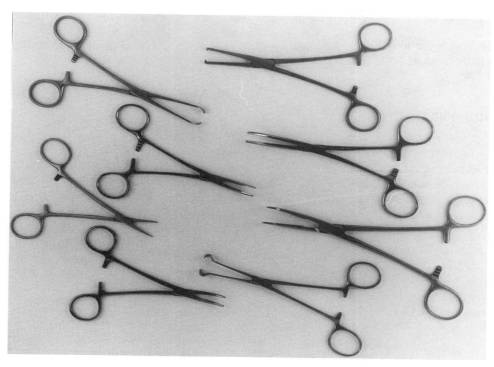

Category II: Holding and grasping clamps

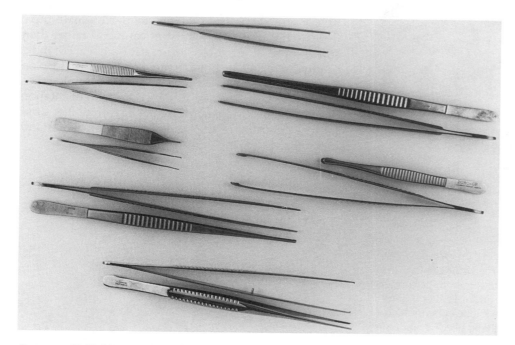

Category II: Holding and grasping forceps

INSTRUMENT	COMMON USAGE	INSTRUMENT	COMMON USAGE
Pean Clamp Curved/Straight	Heavy, large Kelly; same usage as Kelly holding clamp	Allis Clamp (Medium/Long)	Intestinal; delicate structures Grasping clamp
Babcock Clamp (Medium/Long)	Intestinal; delicate structures; noncrushing Holding clamp	Kocher Clamp (Medium/ Long) Curved/Straight	Internal/external structures; tough fibrous tissue Grasping clamp

INSTRUMENT	COMMON USAGE
Tissue Forceps Smooth or with teeth	Short, regular, or long length; grasp or hold tissue

Category III: Retracting Instruments

Retractors are used to hold tissue away from the operative site. Retractors are either self-retaining via a bridge or metal bar keeping the edges apart, or handheld, requiring a team member to retract using the instrument. Handheld retractors are primarily used in pairs.

INSTRUMENT	COMMON USAGE
Handheld Retractors	
Army-Navy; Parker; Eastman	Superficial; used to open/close first two layers of abdomen

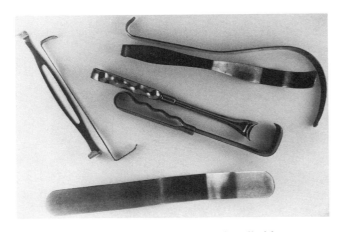

Category III: Retracting instruments—handheld

Richardsons Small, medium, large blade	Used inside abdomen to retract organs
Deavers Narrow/medium/wide blades	Curved blades; used inside abdomen to get under and/or retract organs
Malleable (Ribbons) Narrow/medium/wide blades	Flexible; can be molded to shape needed; abdomen
Skin Hooks (single-double) Senn Retractors	Superficial; skin; minor/plastic surgery; sharp/dull prongs

Self-retaining Retractors

Balfour Abdominal Retractor Regular/Deep Blades	Abdominal surgery

O'Sullivan-O'Connor Retractor	Dominant in GYN or pelvic surgery
Weitlander; Gelpi; Mastoid	Small-to-medium structures; dull or sharp

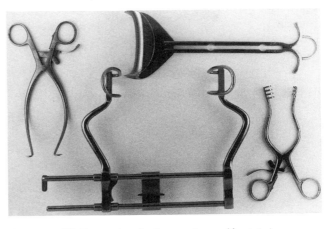

Category III: Retracting instruments—self-retaining

Category IV: Suturing Instruments

Suturing instruments consist of *needle holders,* ranging in size and shape from a long standard to extremely delicate tips. Since they must grasp metal rather than soft tissue, they are subject to greater damage. For maximum usage, needle holders must retain a firm grip on the needle. The so-called *diamond jaw* needle holder has a tungsten carbide insert designed to prevent rotation of the needle. Needle holders may have a ratchet similar to a hemostat or they may be a spring action and lock type.

INSTRUMENT	COMMON USAGE
Mayo-Hegar Short/medium/long	Standard; used in general surgery

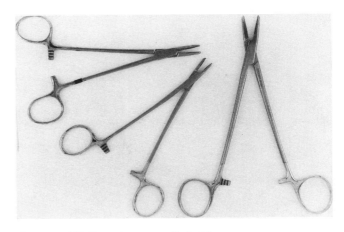

Category IV: Suturing—needle holders

INSTRUMENT	COMMON USAGE
Webster	Smaller than Mayo-Hegar; plastic surgery; pediatric surgery
Castroviejo	Spring with lock; vascular; eyes; plastic; extremely delicate
Heany; Rogers	GYN surgery; used for hysterectomy (closure of surgical os)
Needle-Nose	Heavy, blunt tip; used for surgical steel, wire sutures

Category V: Miscellaneous Instruments

The miscellaneous category contains instruments that do not fit into any other category by virtue of their function. These include towel clips, rings forceps, suction tips, probes, grooves, trocars, and so on.

INSTRUMENT	COMMON USAGE
Suction tips (steel or disposable)	
Yankauer (tonsil)	Standard; narrow or medium areas
Pool (abdominal)	Abdominal; thick or heavy fluids
Frazier/Anthony	Diameter of tip determines size; used in small delicate areas
Probe and groove	Dilate and probe lumens of vessels or ducts
Towel clamps Small/medium/large	Used with towels to wall off an incisional site or to hold tubing or drapes
Ring forcep (sponge stick) Short/medium/long	Available curved or straight for prepping, when used with a sponge for blunt dissection of delicate tissue, or mopping up of fluids/blood

Care and Handling of Surgical Instruments

Few things cause greater frustration in the OR than instruments that do not function as they should during a procedure. As a member of the OR team, entrusted with the provision of surgical sets ready for use, you can do much to avoid many such problems.

Instruments must be handled gently. Bouncing, dropping, and setting heavy equipment on top of the delicate instruments should be avoided. At the end of a procedure, they must be handled individually and not thrown together in a tangled heap. Sharps and deli-

cate instruments should be set aside and individually cleaned, then the tips protected with either an individual tip protector or a holding pouch.

Each instrument should be inspected before and after cleaning to spot chips, breaks, cracks, or imperfections. Forceps, clamps, and other hinged instruments should be inspected for alignment of jaws and teeth and for stiffness. Edges of scissors should be tested for sharpness. To cut effectively, they must be filed smoothly, and maintained sharp by careful observation and usage. It is further recommended that all instruments be periodically lubricated in special instrument "milk," which contains silicone, following the cleaning process to preserve their ease of use and prevent sticking of boxlocks and/or ratchets.

In addition, some basic guidelines for proper use and handling include:

1. Know the names and proper use of each instrument
2. Constantly observe the sterile field for loose in-

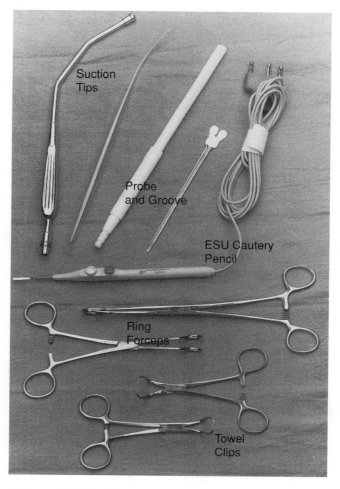

Category V: Miscellaneous

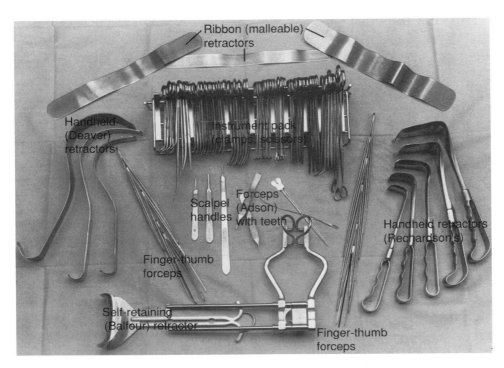

Major laparotomy tray—complete

struments. Remove used instruments promptly to original location for easy retrieval

3. Keep instruments clean during procedure by periodically cleaning instruments using a damp cloth (towel or lap sponge)
4. Protect the edges of sharp instruments during and after a procedure. Remove all blades and needles to a designated sharps container, and close the lid for further protection
5. A no-touch or "hands-free" technique should be used to prevent accidental sharp/needle sticks during the procedure. Sharps should be placed in a designated "neutral zone" by the surgeon(s) and scrub personnel when delivering or exchanging instruments.

STANDARDIZED INSTRUMENT SETS

Standard basic instrument sets, containing the minimum number and types of instruments, will facilitate an instrument count. A basic instrument set should include instruments needed to open and close the incision along with instruments needed to complete the surgical procedure.

A kardex or pictorial reference book for each tray, with the vendor's name, numbers of specific instruments and the cost, and any cross referencing information will assist personnel in preparing the instrument trays.

The kardex book should be routinely updated as instruments are added or deleted from the tray. A count sheet specific to the tray should also be part of this reference book.

By grouping the instruments within the reference book according to service and/or by the specialty tray or set, a complex process can become an ongoing learning experience for those responsible for using and assembling the instrument trays.

Proper selection of additional instruments is based on information obtained during the preoperative assessment and includes the age and size of the patient, the selected surgical approach, the anatomy, the possible pathologic condition, and the surgeon's preference.

Self-assessment Exercise 9

Directions: *Complete the following exercises. The answers are given at the end of this module.*

INSTRUMENT IDENTIFICATION*
Identify the following instruments by:

A. Category

B. Name

C. General Usage

* Composites created courtesy of Muller V. *The surgical armamentarium.* Chicago: Rand-McNally, 1989.

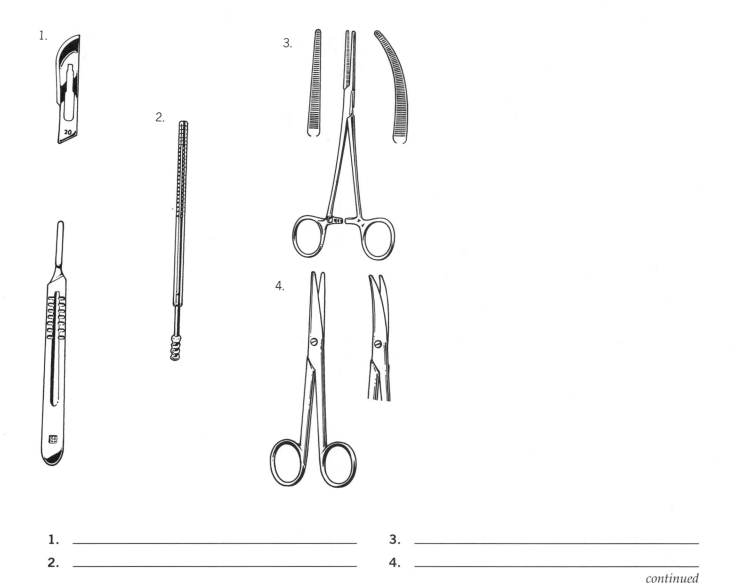

1. _____   3. _____

2. _____   4. _____

continued

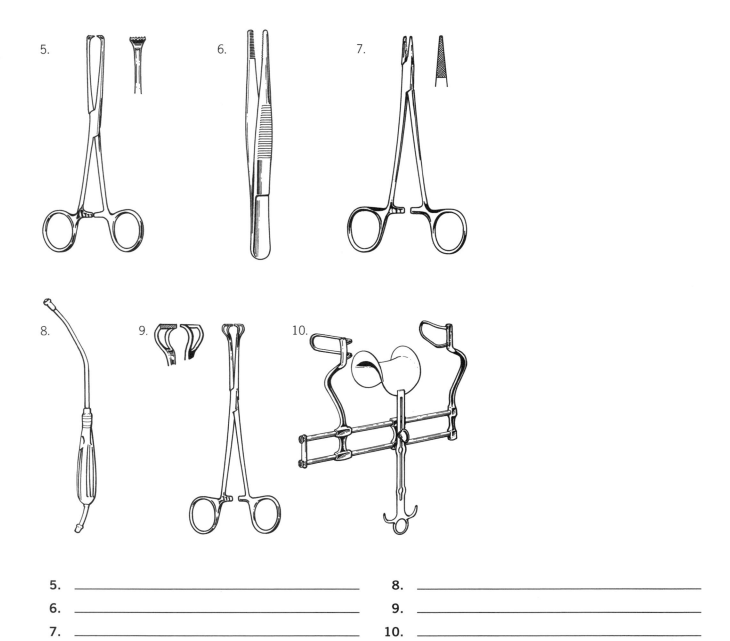

5. _____

6. _____

7. _____

8. _____

9. _____

10. _____

UNIT 2

Procedural Supplies and Equipment

PREPARING FOR A SURGICAL PROCEDURE

The scrub and circulator receive their daily case assignments from the surgical schedule board and begin to prepare the procedure room for the upcoming procedures. Part of this preparation includes the selection and assembly of supplies and equipment needed for each case, both sterile and nonsterile, by using a preference card or computer print-out.

But before starting any case, you must "assemble yourself mentally." This process begins long before you enter the procedure room, regardless of the role you are performing. Some of the questions you should ask yourself during this preparation time include your knowledge of:

- the anatomy involved
- the proposed incision site and surgical approach
- the physiologic status of the patient
- the preferred supplies and equipment requested and how to use them safely and effectively

Knowledge of these and other aspects of the procedure will help to prepare you for any type of surgery and assist you in performing professionally and efficiently.

There are four factors that will help you become a secure member of the surgical team. These factors must be considered as listed, in correct sequential order, to avoid omission in the preparation for a surgical procedure.

1. Surgical Approach
    a. How will the anatomic area involved be exposed?
    b. How will the patient be positioned to provide maximum exposure?
    c. Where is the incision site; what area needs to be prepped; are there any allergies that would prevent the use of the routine prep solution?
2. Surgical Procedure
    a. What is the sequential order of the procedure?
    b. When are the counts to be performed?
    c. What additional supplies might be requested?
    d. How should the specimens, if any, be prepared?
3. Surgical Complications
    a. What unforeseen difficulty might arise during surgery that may require additional supplies

or equipment?
    b. What is your role during an emergency situation, and how can you best meet the needs of the patient and team during this time?
4. Surgical Closure
    a. What types of dressings will be used for the procedure?
    b. What are the special needs of the patient during the immediate postoperative period?

It is practically impossible to anticipate every single aspect of every procedure and possible deviations from the routine, but what you must do is be alert and totally aware of what is happening from the moment you begin planning for the procedure until the patient has been safely transported to the designated postoperative area. At that time, and not before, your responsibility for that patient ends, as other professionals assume the care of the patient.

PLANNING INTRAOPERATIVE PATIENT CARE

Perioperative nursing practice is based on the Nursing Process format, and the third phase of that process is identified as the *planning phase.*

Quality assurance requires evidence that a specific care plan for each patient has been proposed and implemented during the intraoperative phase, and in order to be in compliance, the following prerequisites of knowledge and skill are needed.

1. Knowledge and assessment of the patient's individual needs related to pathophysiology, the surgical procedure, and the surgeon's preferences
2. Knowledge of surgical supplies and instrumentation and of cost-effective methods for selection and assembly of these items
3. Knowledge of those items considered "standard" for all surgical procedures, including sterile and nonsterile supplies
4. Knowledge of appropriate procedure room preparation, including acquisition, usage, and placement of furniture and special equipment needed for the procedure
5. Knowledge and management of available resources, both material and personnel

By planning perioperative patient care using these broad concepts, you can establish and maintain a therapeutic environment; one that is safe for both the patient and the staff.

THE STERILE FIELD

Use of the sterile field is composed of three distinct phases: (1) creation of the sterile field, (2) maintenance of the sterile field, and (3) termination of the sterile field.

The implementation of intraoperative nursing activities is directly related to the organization and coordination of sterile supplies, instruments, equipment, and health-care team members, and is based on priority setting and an ongoing assessment of the surgical environment.

Preliminary Preparation

The first step in creating a suitable environment is related to the preparation of the procedure room, including the physical layout of furniture and equipment and the placement of supplies in a convenient location, since wasted motion is not only time-consuming but also can add to physical and mental fatigue.

Preliminary preparation of the room is done before each patient enters the room, and is a team effort by both the circulating nurse and the scrub person. To be effective, it must be a cooperative effort that can also include assistance from aids, orderlies, and environmental services personnel.

The following is a checklist for preparing the procedure room:

Step 1.   Damp dusting/arranging furniture
   a.   Damp dust all flat surfaces and all portable or mounted equipment (PRN).
   b.   Position the operating room table under the overhead light fixture.
   c.   Arrange the furniture needed for the specific procedure (e.g., instrument table, Mayo stand, and ring stands).

Furniture and Equipment

Some of the more common pieces of furniture and equipment found in a procedure room include:

1. *The OR table*   The operating table is an expensive, sometimes complex, and essential piece of furniture that is used for all surgical procedures. There are several types of operating tables, some for general usage, others specifically designed for surgical specialties, such as urology, orthopedics, or cataract surgery.

   The table is fully adjustable in all directions to create the positions needed for various surgical procedures, and all personnel should be totally familiar with its operation and its corresponding accessories. The table should be positioned directly under the overhead light fixture, and once in position, should be locked for patient and staff safety.

2. *Instrument (back) table*   Once it is draped with a bacterial barrier, the instrument table provides a set-up area for sterile supplies to be used during the procedure. The table is made of a noncorrosive metal, and has a top and bottom shelf. The bottom shelf can be used for storage of extra supplies not immediately needed. The table is on wheels, and can be positioned wherever necessary to provide maximum efficiency during the procedure.

   The instrument table should be at least 18 inches away from walls and cabinets, away from linen hampers, doors, garbage receptacles, anesthesia equipment, and paths of traffic.

3. *Ring stand*   The ring stand is round or square, and is used to hold basin sets and/or instrument trays. The ring stand, once draped, should be placed close to the instrument table, since it will become part of the sterile field during surgery.

4. *Mayo stand*   The Mayo stand is used to hold instruments that will be used frequently during the procedure. It is draped with a bacterial barrier, and then placed directly over, but not in contact with, the patient once the patient drapes have been applied. It is adjustable in height, and is totally portable, since it moves on wheels. During the set-up period, the stand should remain close to the other furniture to avoid possible contamination or accidental bumping of the stand.

Step 2.   Placement of packs and supplies
   a.   Put sterile drape pack on the instrument table.
   b.   Place wrapped sterile basic set into one of the ring stands.
   c.   Put the wrapped sterile instrument tray on top of the other ring stand.
   d.   Place the scrub's gown and gloves on the Mayo stand.

Additional Furniture and Equipment

The use of *kick buckets* (a bucket on wheels) is restricted to soiled sponges during surgery. It is lined with a

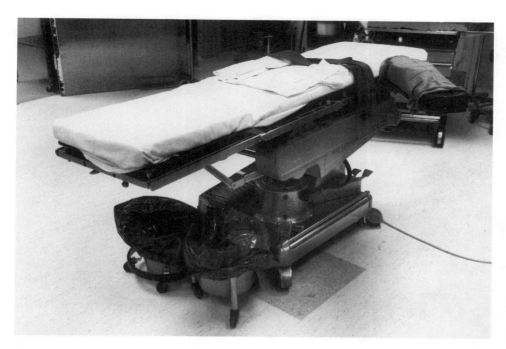

Standard operating room table

disposable liner which can be removed and exchanged as required during the procedure without jeopardizing the sterility of the surgical field.

All other trash should be placed in a larger trash receptacle. However, once the procedure has started, no trash may leave the room.

In addition, anesthesia machines, electrosurgical units (ESU), suction cannisters/tubing, IV poles, linen receptacles for nondisposable linen, and adjustable stools (rolling or permanent) are usually found in a procedure room.

All furniture and equipment should be in their proper position before opening and creating the sterile field to avoid possible contamination of the field during moving activities.

Step 3. Collection of remaining items
   a. Collect additional instruments and supplies according to procedural need, including drugs and special items (specialty cart).
   b. Collect positioning devices, positional aids, and special equipment, such as the ESU, laser, microscope, and so on.
   c. Choose the proper suture and amounts for the procedure according to the surgeon's preference.
   d. Collect the irrigation fluids and prep solutions needed.

STANDARD AND ACCESSORY SUPPLIES

Surgical supplies can be divided into two major categories: sterile supplies and nonsterile supplies. Each category can then be subdivided into those items that are considered essential, or standard supplies, and those that are not required for every case (accessory supplies).

To select the proper packs, drapes, and supplies for a surgical procedure, it is necessary to follow some general guidelines:

1. Determine the required supplies based on the anatomy and proposed procedure.
2. Use the Physician's Preference Card to select the specialty/accessory items needed for the procedure.
3. Carefully select the proper amount of supplies, to be cost-effective, following a logical sequential order of selection.

Standard Sterile Supplies

Imagine this scenario: *You have been asked to select the supplies and equipment required for an emergency procedure, but the surgeon does not have a preference card on file for that procedure. How would you choose the proper supplies and what would be your rationale?*

By having a working knowledge of standard sup-

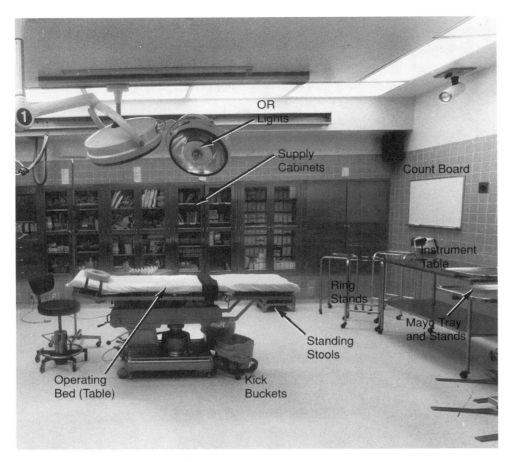

Operating (procedure) room with standard equipment

plies and equipment that could be used for each broad category of surgical specialties, and then adding the specific instrumentation based on the nature of the procedure, you can effectively assemble the supplies needed, even without the use of a preference card.

Sterile Packs and Drapes

Many different types of packs and drapes are available today designed for specific surgical procedures. Packs are the primary supply needed to create a sterile field. In some institutions, the use of a *customized pack*, one that contains specific items needed according to institutional preference, has been created, thus eliminating the need for obtaining additional items. The packs and drape sheets are made of disposable, fluid-resistant material, which acts as a bacterial barrier against microbial infiltration. At the end of the procedure, all disposable items are discarded, reducing the possibility of cross-contamination with another patient and the surgical environment.

Sterile Packs

Three primary packs are commonly associated with surgical procedures. The surgical team member, choosing the appropriate pack, should be familiar with its contents in order to avoid "pulling" extra supplies, which could be wasted. Each pack has a list of the contents conveniently printed on the reverse side of the pack.

The following is a list of common packs used in surgery, and their contents. (Contents may vary depending on the manufacturer.)

Laparotomy Pack (Major Pack)

General usage: flat body surfaces with a vertical fenestration (hole) in the patient drape sheet. Appropriate for general abdominal, pelvic, and spinal surgery, or any instance when a vertical incision line is used.

Contents (depending on manufacturer):

1. Overwrap/table cover
2. Absorbent towels

3. Utility towels (small)
4. Plastic Mayo stand cover
5. Laparotomy sheet with fenestration
6. Disposable gowns and absorbent hand towels
7. Ray-Tec X-ray–detectable sponges

Basic Pack (Minor Pack)

General usage: to create a "customized" pack for special procedures that require a specific fenestrated sheet or drape an additional instrument table, or use when a fenestrated sheet is not required.

Contents:

Same as a laparotomy pack, minus the fenestrated sheet and sponges. Usually only contains one surgical gown.

Additional Surgical Packs

Each specialty pack usually contains a fenestrated sheet and additional items needed for the procedure:

GYN pack
   Usage: vaginal procedures (lithotomy position)
Laparoscopy pack
   Usage: laparoscopy procedure
Cysto pack
   Usage: closed urologic procedures (lithotomy position)
Extremity pack
   Usage: upper/lower extremity surgery
Head and neck pack
   Usage: ophthalmologic, facial, and throat procedures
Cardiovascular pack
   Usage: vascular surgery, open heart surgery
Hip pack
   Usage: hip repair/replacement procedures
Arthroscopy pack
   Usage: arthroscopic procedures
Cesarean section pack
   Usage: abdominal obstetric procedures
Universal pack
   Usage: emergency/trauma cases (generic contents)

Sterile Drape Sheets

Sterile drape sheets come in various sizes and forms, with or without fenestrations, and are usually used in conjunction with either a basic pack or as an added bacterial barrier for specific draping needs.

Some examples include *transverse lap sheet, split sheet, pediatric lap sheet, thyroid sheet, craniotomy incise sheet, eye/ear sheet, plastic adherent incise sheets (Vi-Drape)* (plain or impregnated with iodine), and *stockinette cuffs* to cover extremities such as toes, fingers, or hands, in addition to three quarters and one half table drape sheets for patient drape or table cover, to name just a few.

Basin Sets

Basin sets are available in either a reusable or a disposable format, and contain the "pots and pans" needed for surgery. Three types of basin sets are usually found in the surgical suite; they may be used interchangeably or for a specific purpose. The contents will vary depending on the needs of the institution, and can be "customized" like the custom packs mentioned earlier.

A. **Major Basin Set**
   General usage: for procedures requiring large supplies of instruments, sponges, and so on (general, vascular, ortho).
   Contents: (per institutional preference)

   1. Large round basins (1 or 2)
   2. Round basins (T & A basin) (2 or 3)
   3. Kidney basin (emesis basin) (1)
   4. Prep cups/medicine glasses (2)
   5. Graduated pitcher (optional)

B. **Minor Basin Set**
   General usage: procedures not requiring extra basins or graduated pitcher, such as hernia repairs, peripheral vascular procedures, and plastic surgery.
   Contents: (per institutional preference)

   1. Large basin (1)
   2. Round basin (1–2)
   3. Medicine glasses (2)

C. **Single or Hand Basin**
   General usage: to clean instruments.

NOTE: A single basin should not be used as a "splash" basin, since contamination from this basin, when used to clean gloves during surgery, can cause contamination of the sterile field.

Surgical Sponges

Surgical sponges are manufactured in a variety of shapes and sizes and serve three general purposes:

1. to absorb fluid and blood
2. for blunt dissection of delicate tissue
3. to protect tissue from injury

Only those sponges with an X-ray–detectable feature should be used at the sterile field once an incision has been made, and all sponges must be counted at

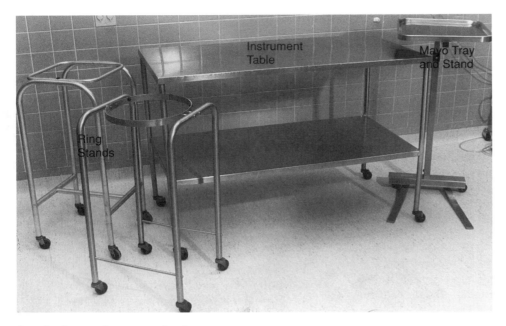

Standard procedure room furniture

proper intervals during the surgical procedure, according to acceptable protocol by both the scrub and circulating nurse.

Surgical sponges are available in specific numerical increments, depending on the type of sponge being used, and all increments are standardized, regardless of the manufacturer.

Common Surgical Sponges

Ray-Tec (4 × 4)
Prepackaged in increments of 10 per box. Used in all procedures. Ray-Tec should be removed from the surgical field once any deep cavity has been entered, unless it is folded and used on a "sponge stick" for blunt dissection purposes.

Laparotomy Sponge (18 × 18 "Lap Sponge")
Prepackaged in increments of five per package. Used during major surgery or for absorbing fluid in large areas.

Small Laps (Tapes) (4 × 18)
Packaged in increments of five per package. Used in smaller areas when large sponges may not be applicable or advisable due to the nature of the incision, or in place of the Ray-Tec sponge.

Cottonoids (Neuro Patties)
Prepackaged in increments of 10 per package, and are available in a variety of sizes ranging from ¼ × ¼ to 3 × 3 inches. Each patty has a string attached that is left outside the wound during its use. They are made of a soft, lint-free material so they will not injure or scratch delicate tissue/structures.
Used predominantly in craniotomies and spinal procedures.

Dissecting Sponges
Available in many different sizes and shapes, dissecting sponges are used to absorb blood in very small areas or "push" away delicate tissue. They have a variety of names that may change from hospital to surgeon to manufacturer. Examples include *Cherry, Peanut, Pushers, Kittners.*
Prepackaged in increments of five, dissecting sponges should always be mounted on a clamp, and may be used wet or dry.

Tonsil/Dental Sponges
Tonsil sponges are round, gauze sponges with a thread attached that is kept outside the mouth during surgery. Prepackaged in increments of five, they are used for tonsillectomies.
Dental sponges (rolls) are tubular in shape, and are non–X-ray detectable. They are used for packing the mouth during teeth extractions. Although they are not X-ray detectable, they must be counted as any other sponge. Packaged either in-hospital or prepackaged, and usually in increments of 5 or 10.
Depending on physician preference, surgical sponges may be wet (soaked in saline) or dry.

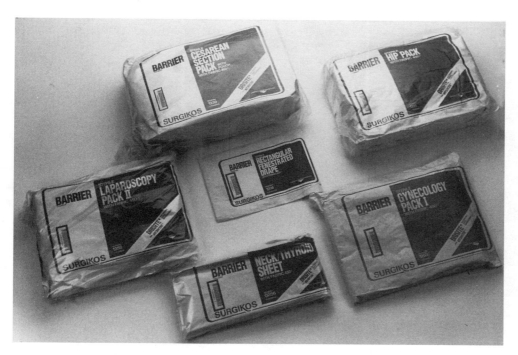

Examples of disposable linen packs and drape sheets

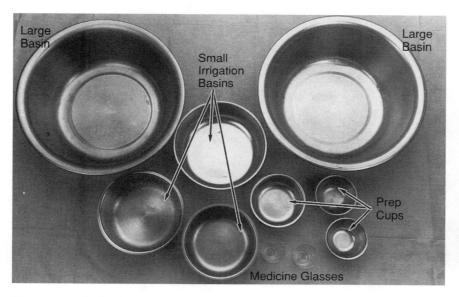

Contents: major basin set

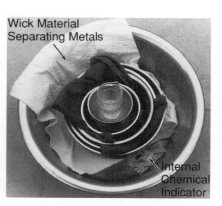

Preparation of multiple basins (basin set) for sterilization

Additional Standard Sterile Supplies

1. *Irrigation solutions* sterile water and saline are available in 500 or 1000 mL "pour" bottles. Saline is always used on back table for irrigation. Sterile water is poured into the large round basin for instrument cleaning, since salt water will corrode the instruments, resulting in rust stains.

2. *Gowns, gloves* (surgeon and assistants).
3. *Prep tray* preassembled wet (with solution) or dry.
4. *Sterile towels* packaged four to five per package; can be linen or a disposable linen fabric, prepackaged and sterilized by the manufacturer or hospital created.
5. *Suction tips/tubings* metal or disposable tips.

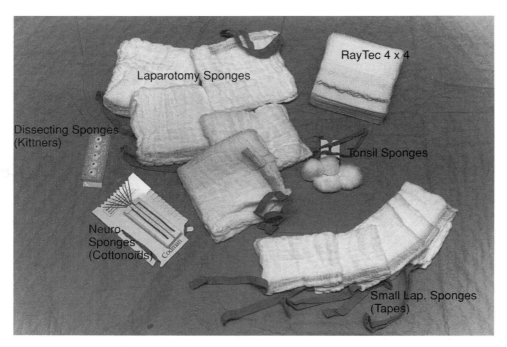

Variety of surgical sponges

Sterile Accessory Supplies

Accessory supplies are those items not required for every procedure, or specifically requested by the surgeon. These include such items as:

1. Cautery devices
   a. Monopolar pencils/tips
   b. Bipolar forceps
2. Syringes: irrigation/hypodermic
3. Needle counter (sharps container)
4. Sutures/needles (specific to surgeon request)
5. Catheters/tubes/drains
6. Dressing supplies: non–Ray-Tec 4 × 4's; ABD's; Telfa

Nonsterile Supplies and Equipment

In addition to the furniture and equipment mentioned earlier in this unit, other nonsterile supplies must

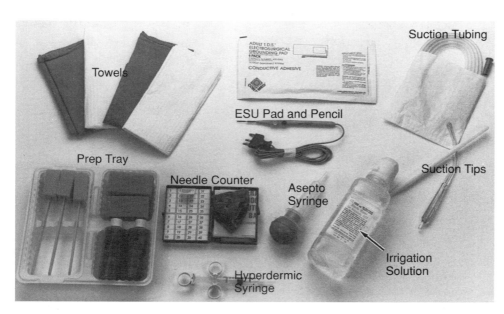

Sterile accessory items

be selected for each case, and these supplies either complement or assist in the usage of the sterile supplies.

For example, you cannot use an electrocautery unit without a grounding pad, nor apply a dressing without tape.

Positioning devices, special table pads, suction cannisters, connecting tubings, and medications to be administered at the sterile field; all these items are needed during the procedure and must be a part of the initial preparation phase, in order to avoid leaving the room to collect them during the procedure.

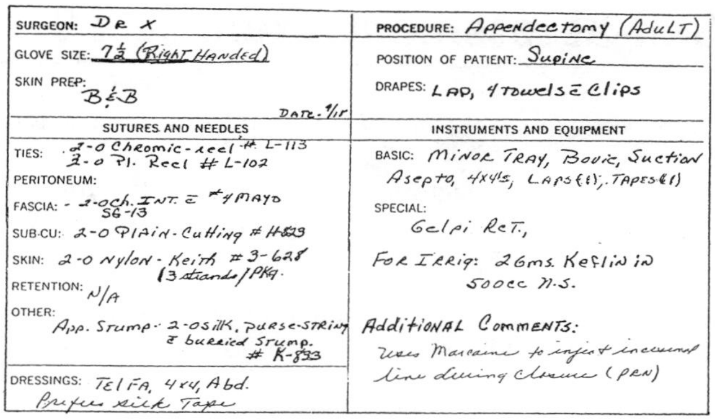
SURGEON: Dr X
GLOVE SIZE: 7½ (Right Handed)
SKIN PREP: B & B
DATE: 9/15
SUTURES AND NEEDLES
TIES: 2-0 Chromic-reel # L-113; 2-0 Pl. Reel # L-102
PERITONEUM:
FASCIA: 2-0 ch. INT. c̄ #4 MAYO SG-13
SUB-CU: 2-0 Plain-Cutting # H-829
SKIN: 2-0 Nylon-Keith # 3-628 (3 strands/PKG.
RETENTION: N/A
OTHER: App. Stump: 2-0 silk, purse-string c̄ burried Stump. # K-833
DRESSINGS: Telfa, 4x4, Abd. Prefers silk Tape
PROCEDURE: Appendectomy (Adult)
POSITION OF PATIENT: Supine
DRAPES: LAP, 4 Towels c̄ Clips
INSTRUMENTS AND EQUIPMENT
BASIC: Minor Tray, Bovie, Suction Asepto, 4x4's, LAPS (1), TAPES (1)
SPECIAL: Gelpi Ret.,
For Irrig: 2 Gms. Keflin in 500cc N.S.
Additional Comments: Uses Marcaine to inject incisional line during closure (PRN)

Fig. 9-12. Sample physician's preference card

THE PHYSICIAN'S PREFERENCE CARD

For every surgical procedure performed in the OR by a specific surgeon, a corresponding reference list of all supplies and equipment used for the procedure in addition to the supplies and equipment requested by the surgeon, should be created, and should be readily available wherever the cases are assembled, be it the OR or in the instance of case cart assembly, in the central processing area. This card or computerized listing is referred to as a *physician's preference card/list* (Fig. 9-12), and can serve multiple purposes, including maintaining an inventory/charging list for a specific procedure by a specific surgeon for a specific patient.

It is vitally important that all information remains current and that any changes that occur during the procedure are noted and communicated to the staff and personnel responsible for assembling and using the supplies, thereby avoiding delays in the procedure owing to improper selection.

Not all supplies and equipment are specified on this preference list, but by knowing and understanding the standard and accessory supplies needed for the procedure, the surgical team can effectively prepare the procedure room for the planned surgical procedure.

Self-assessment Exercise 10

Directions: Complete the following exercises. The answers are given at the end of this module.

1. List the four factors associated with the mental preparation for a surgical procedure, and briefly describe each.

2. Prior to the first case of the day, the perioperative nurse should prepare the procedure room by _____ .

3. List the furniture and items that should be present before beginning any surgical procedure.

4. Differentiate between sterile *standard* and *accessory* supplies, and give an example of each.

5. An excellent source to assist the surgical team in selecting the appropriate supplies and equipment for a procedure is the _____ .

6. There are three phases inherent to all surgical procedures related to the sterile field. Name them:

   1.

   2.

   3.

PHASE I: CREATING A STERILE FIELD

Once the equipment and supplies have been gathered and placed on their respective surfaces, and the procedure room has been properly prepared, the surgical team can begin the task of creating the sterile field through a process of organized steps and procedures.

Opening Sterile Supplies

Before any sterile supplies are opened, the integrity of each package must be checked. Packages not meeting acceptable criteria should be placed aside, since they cannot be considered sterile, and new ones chosen.

Each package must be opened under strict aseptic technique, thereby guaranteeing the sterility of the sterile field.

The following steps can serve as a guideline for opening sterile supplies in preparation for a surgical procedure:

1. Remove the tape from a CSR wrapped package and check the indicator tape to be certain the item has been properly exposed to the sterilization process.
2. Open the linen pack on the instrument table so that the inside of the wrapper becomes the sterile table cover. (See Critical Element Task 9-1.)
3. Open sponges, gowns, gloves, drape sheets, and towels on the back table. Open blades on the right corner of the table.
4. Open basin sets and the instrument tray on ring stands. If sequentially wrapped, both layers are opened.
5. Place small items and extra instruments in the basin or in the instrument tray. Maintain object in inner wrapper.
6. Open scrub gown and gloves on the Mayo stand.

Delineation of the Scrub and Circulator Roles

Although all surgical procedures require a cooperative effort, from the time the surgical scrub begins until the operation is finished and the dressings are applied, there is a definite line of demarcation between the duties and responsibilities of the scrub person and the circulating nurse that neither may cross. The *circulating nurse* performs those functions associated with the management of the room before, during, and after the procedure, while the *scrub person* (nurse or technician) performs all tasks related to the creation and maintenance of the sterile field before and during surgery, in addition to the care of the instruments when surgery is completed (Table 9-5).

Standardized Basic Set-Up

Each institution may have its own "standard set-up" for the instrument table and Mayo stand. The need for a standard set-up is evident for two basic reasons:

1. Decreasing the actual set-up time.
2. Ease of transition during relief of scrub personnel.

Table 9-5   Comparative Division of Duties

Scrub Nurse/Technician	Circulating Nurse

A. PREOPERATIVE
  1. Checks the card file for surgeon's special needs/requests
  2. Opens sterile supplies
  3. Scrubs, gowns, and gloves and sets up sterile field.
    Obtains instruments from flash autoclave if necessary. Checks for proper functioning of instruments/equipment
  4. Performs counts with circulator
	1. Assists in assembling needed supplies
	2. Opens sterile supplies
	3. Assists scrub in gowning
	4. Performs and records counts
	5. Admits patient to surgical suite

B. PREINCISIONAL
  1. Completes the final preparation of sterile field
  2. Assists surgeon with gowning/gloving
  3. Assists surgeon with draping and passes off suction/cautery lines
	1. Transports patient to procedure room
	2. Assists with the positioning of the patient
	3. Assists anesthesia during induction
	4. Performs skin prep
	5. Assists with drapes; connects suction and cautery

C. DURING THE PROCEDURE
  1. Maintains orderly sterile field
  2. Anticipates the surgeon's needs (supplies/equipment)
  3. Maintains internal count of sponges, needles, and instruments
  4. Verifies tissue specimen with surgeon, and passes off to circulator
	1. Maintains orderly procedure room
	2. Anticipates needs of surgical team
	3. Maintains record of supplies added
	4. Receives specimen and labels it correctly
	5. Maintains charges and OR records
	6. Continually monitors aseptic technique and patient needs

D. CLOSING PHASE
  1. Counts with circulator at proper intervals
  2. Organizes closing suture and dressings
  3. Begins clean-up of used instruments
  4. Applies sterile dressings
  5. Prepares for terminal cleaning of instruments and nondisposable supplies
  6. Reports to charge nurse for next assignment
	1. Counts with scrub at proper intervals
	2. Finalizes records and charges
	3. Begins clean-up of procedure room
	4. Applies tape
	5. Assists anesthesia in preparing patient for transfer to PACU
	6. Takes patient to PACU with anesthesia and reports significant information to PACU nurse
	7. Disposes of specimen and records
	8. Reports to charge nurse for next assignment

As a member of the surgical team, it is your responsibility to know and use the proper set-up as directed by the *Surgical Policy and Procedure Manual*.

The following procedure and illustrations can serve as a guide for a basic set-up if one does not already exist. Both the instrument table and Mayo tray set-ups are adaptable to any surgical procedure with slight modification.

Draping the Surgical Patient

To isolate the surgical wound from bacterial contamination, the patient must be covered with sterile drapes so that only the incisional site is exposed.

The actual draping procedure is usually performed by the surgeon, with assistance from either the scrub person or the assistant. (See Critical Element Tasks 9-2 through 9-9.)

PHASE II: MAINTAINING THE STERILE FIELD

According to the principles of basic aseptic technique mentioned earlier, a sterile field, once established, must be constantly monitored and maintained. This monitoring process is the responsibility of every member of the surgical team, and each must watch for events that may compromise the sterility of the field, and take appropriate corrective action.

Once the patient is placed on the operating table, prepped and draped, he or she becomes the center of

**CRITICAL ELEMENT
TASK 9-1**

Procedure for Opening and Dispensing
Sterile Supplies

PURPOSE

To assure proper technique when preparing a room for surgery by opening and dispensing sterile supplies.

PREREQUISITE

Application of mask; arrangement of equipment and supplies in the procedure room.

PROFICIENCY

One hundred percent accuracy at the time of performance.

PROCEDURAL STEPS

A. PREPARATION
    1. Place sterile supplies on respective holders.
    2. Check integrity of packages; dates on tape.
B. OPENING LINEN PACK (See Fig. A)
    1. Place Laparotomy pack in center of instrument table and remove outside (paper) wrapper (part 1 below).

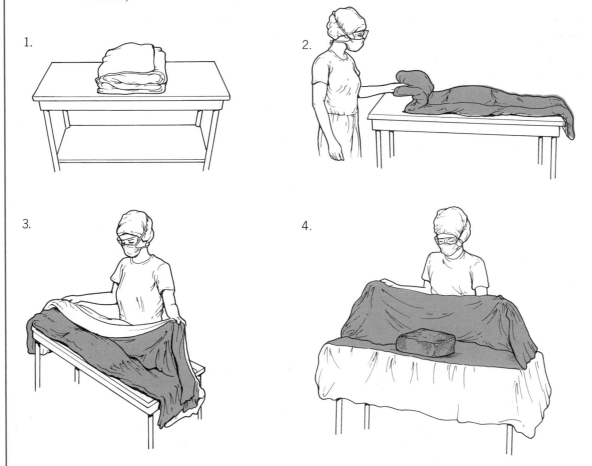

Fig. A. Opening linen packs

2. Break seal holding sides together and open the pack following the directions on the folds as indicated (part 2).

3. Standing behind the table, place hands under the protective cuff of the wrapper, sliding them away from the center of the pack, and lift up and out so that half of the pack covers the length of the table, letting the sides fall below table level. Repeat the same process from the other side of the table (parts 3 and 4).

C. OPENING INDIVIDUAL ITEMS (See Fig. B)

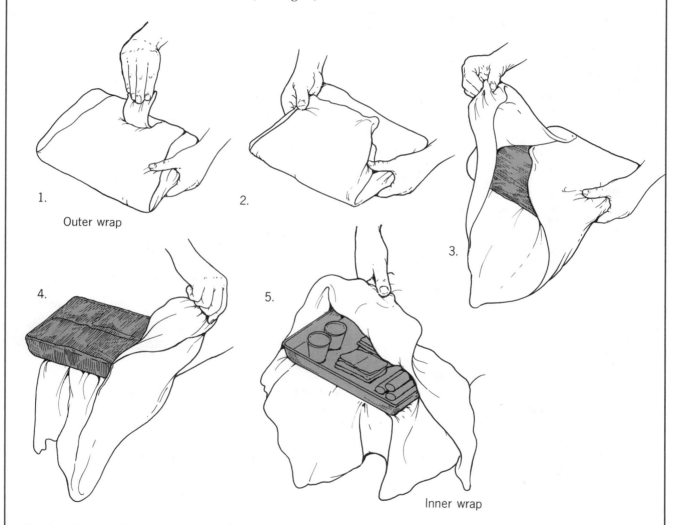

Fig. B. Opening and dispensing individual items (**Note:** Small objects must be protected from unsterile hands while being dispensed)

**CRITICAL ELEMENT
TASK 9-1** *cont.*

Presenting a sterile item

6.

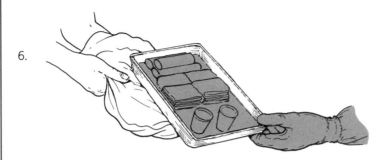

Fig. B. *(continued)*

1.   Open individual instruments or small supplies in an envelope wrap by holding the item in one hand, then breaking the seal (1) and grasping the corner of the wrapper. Unwrap away from you (2), letting the wrapper edge fall (3 and 4). Do the same with each corner, and for each layer (5). Covering your hand with the tails of the wrapper (6), present the sterile item to the scrub person, being careful not to contact sterile to nonsterile surfaces during the process.
2.   Open sterile basin set on ring stand by peeling back both layers of the wrapper, allowing the sides to fall below the edge of the ring stand.
3.   Open the instrument tray on the ring stand by peeling back both layers of the wrapper in the same manner as for the basin set.

D.   DISPENSING STERILE SUPPLIES DURING A CASE
1.   Using proper technique and maintaining a safe distance from the field, present the sterile unwrapped item to the scrub person, covering your hands with the wrappers.
2.   If scrub cannot take the item, place the unwrapped item on the proximal side of the table to you, or "flip" the item into the Mayo stand or back table, maintaining a safe distance.
3.   When pouring sterile solutions into a basin or cup, keep the label facing up while holding the bottle a safe distance from the edge of the receptacle. Hands should not be over the sterile surface.

POINTS TO REMEMBER

1.   A sterile package should be opened by a nonsterile person from the far side first and near side last.
2.   Never reach over a sterile field when you are unsterile.
3.   Do not overload the instrument table with supplies. Only gowns, gloves, drape sheets, towels, sponges, and blades should be opened on the table.
4.   Scalpel blades should be opened onto the right corner of the instrument table, and scrub person informed of location.
5.   Whenever possible, both layers of the wrapper should be opened, when it does not risk the possibility of contamination of the item.
6.   When opening a peel-package, grasp the two sides of the wrapper, and peel back to expose the item.

PERFORMANCE CHECK SHEET

NAME: _____	TASK # _____9-1_____
	RATING: A Acceptable
	N/I Needs Improvement
PROCEDURE: Opening and Dispensing Sterile Supplies	

PROCEDURAL STEPS	A	N/I
A. PREPARATION		
1. Compares physician's preference to items picked for accuracy		
2. Checks integrity of all sterile item wrappers, and replaces those in question		
3. Distributes items to proper place for opening sequence		
4. Applies mask and closes procedure room door		
B. OPENING SEQUENCE: Packs and Packages		
1. Opens linen pack on instrument table maintaining aseptic technique		
2. Opens basin set on ring stand; both layers		
3. Opens instrument tray(s) on ring stand(s); both layers		
4. Opens individual items in proper place, avoiding overload of any surface/instrument table		
5. Opens and arranges prep tray		
6. Maintains aseptic technique during opening sequence		

TASK # ___9-1___		Page 2 of 2
PROCEDURAL STEPS	A	N/I
C. DISPENSING STERILE SUPPLIES DURING A PROCEDURE		
1. Pours sterile solutions without contamination (strike-through)		
2. Presents sterile item(s) to scrub person maintaining safety distance		
3. Presents sterile item(s), unwrapping both layers, and covering hands with wrapper tails		
4. Dispenses items from flash sterilizer in aseptic manner		
5. Dispenses sponges as requested and waits for confirmation count		
6. Dispenses sutures and needles as requested, and waits for confirmation count		
7. Maintains neat, orderly work environment		
8. Anticipates needs of sterile team by careful observation of procedure		
9. Maintains accurate, visible count of sponges and needles dispensed during procedure		
10. Dispenses medication/solutions in aseptic manner to sterile field		

COMMENTS: _____

Procedure for Basic Set-up

PURPOSE

To assist in standardizing instrument table and Mayo stand set-ups in order to increase proficiency.

PREREQUISITE

Sterile scrub; gown and gloves.

PROFICIENCY

One hundred percent accuracy at the time of performance.

PROCEDURAL STEPS

I.   LINEN PACK ASSEMBLY (see Fig. A)
1.   Remove linen pack for center of table, and discard any supplies not needed. Maintain three disposable towels.
2.   Remove Mayo stand cover from pack and drape Mayo stand.
3.   Arrange the linen pack in the order of usage starting from the last item to be used on the bottom of the pack.
     Proper Order of Linen Pack:
       Bottom: • Fenestrated or specialty drape sheet
                      • Folded green towels for incision
                      • Gown and gloves for surgeon/assistant
       Top: • Cloth towels for hand drying (surgeon)
4.   Remove instrument tray from ring stand, and place on left corner of instrument table.
5.   Place assembled linen pack on ring stand. (It is recommended that these items be kept on ring stand so that entire contents can be brought up to the operating table during the draping procedure.)

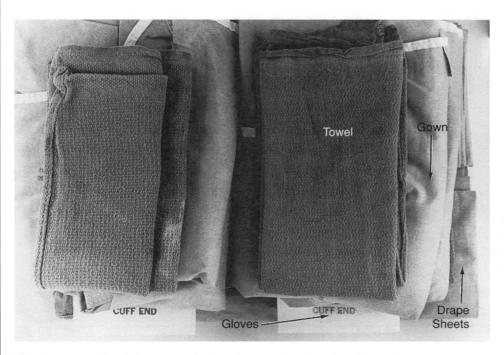

Fig. A.   Assembly of linen pack (bottom layer to top in order of usage)

II.   INSTRUMENT TABLE SET-UP (Fig. B)
1.   Place green towel on right side of instrument table and place contents of basin set on the towel.
2.   Arrange towels and sponges next to instrument tray.
3.   Remove instrument rack/string and place it in front of instrument tray, then arrange retractors and forceps for easy retrieval as needed.
4.   Arrange sutures according to usage, and if free ties are needed, construct a "suture book" from a green towel.
5.   Pass off the Instrument Count sheet from the tray and perform preincisional counts (sponges, sutures, and instruments).
6.   Unstring instruments, and place needle holders and skin forceps by suture packet.
7.   Open suture packets (nonabsorbable), and place packages in garbage bag provided in pack.

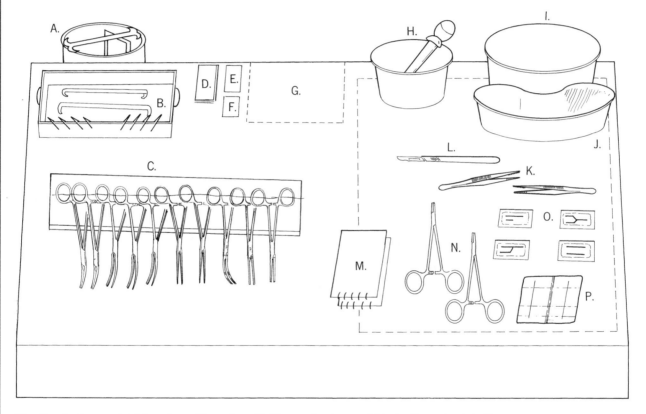

Fig. B.   Instrument table set-up. Key: A = Balfour retractor and blade (large basin); B = instrument tray (retractors and forceps); C = instrument string (rolled towel or rack); D = extra towels; E = lap sponges or tapes; F = Ray-Tec sponges (4 × 4's); G = specialty instrument tray (prn); H = small basin with Asepto syringe (for irrigation); I = medium basin (for saline); J = kidney basin (with medicine glasses); K = Adson forceps with teeth (for skin); L = knife handles with blades: No. 7–15 or No. 3L–11; M = suture book (for free-tie strands, optional); N = needle holders; O = suture packets (in order of usage); P = needle counter (Note: green towel under basin area of table)

III. MAYO TRAY SET-UP (see Fig. C)

    1. Drape the Mayo stand. Using the cover like a pillow case, which is fan folded with a wide cuff to protect gloved hands, slide the cover over the tray, guiding it with gloved hands toward the base end of the stand. Do not allow your hands to go beyond the top of the tray. Place green towel over draped Mayo stand cover and secure towel and cover under the tray to prevent slippage.

    2. Place knife handles with blades (No. 4 w/20 and No. 3 w/10) on right side of Mayo tray.

    3. Roll a green towel, and place it three quarters of the way toward end of Mayo tray for instruments. Place handheld or small self-retaining retractors behind towel.

    4. If Labyrinth suture packets are used, place between towel and Mayo stand cover, leaving end protruding. Place dispensing reel near retractors.

Draped adjustment bar

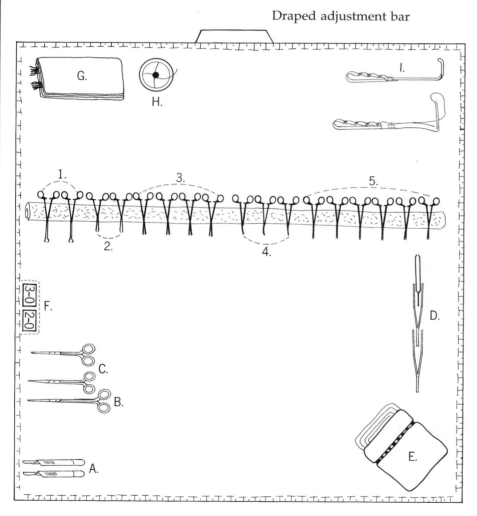

Fig. C. Mayo stand set-up. Key: A = knife handles with blades (No. 4 and 3); B = scissors (dissecting)—Cr. Metzenbaum; C = scissors—Cr. and St. Mayo; D = forceps (smooth and with teeth) in pairs; E = Ray-Tec 4 × 4 sponges (one pack); F = suture ligatures (Labyrinth package); G = suture book (optional for ligatures and multineedle packages); H = suture dispensing reel; I = retractors (handheld, in pairs). Instrument string (amounts will depend on procedure being performed); 1 = (2) short Babcocks; 2 = (2) short Allis clamps; 3 = (4) short Cr. Kellys; 4 = (2) short Kochers and (1) short Rt. angle; 5 = (6) hemostats (cr. and straight)

5. Place straight Mayo scissors near rolled towel, to separate from the other scissors.
6. Place dissecting scissors (Mayo and Metzenbaum) near knife handles.
7. Arrange forceps (in pairs) at the back of the tray (far side from scrub); smooth and with teeth together.
8. Place minimum number of instruments on rolled towel with tips facing the end (sharps end) of tray.
9. Place green towel over assembled Mayo tray, and place suction tubing/tip, cautery pencil, and light handles on top of green towel. (Green towel will be used at the end of fenestration of drape sheet.)

General Recommendations*

6	Cr. Hemostats
4	Cr. Kellys (short)
2	Long Kellys
2	St. Kochers (short)
2	Babcocks (short)
4	Allis Clamps (short)
2	Rt. Angle clamps (short)

* Numbers will vary according to procedure and usage of electrocautery for hemostasis.

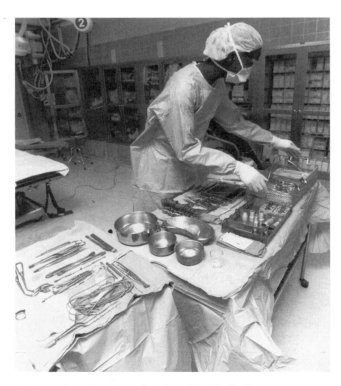

Putting it all together: Creating the sterile field

PERFORMANCE CHECK SHEET

NAME: _____	TASK # ___9-2___
	RATING: A Acceptable
	N/I Needs Improvement

PROCEDURE: BASIC SET-UP: Instrument Table and Mayo Tray

PROCEDURAL STEPS	A	N/I
I. INSTRUMENT TABLE		
1. Maintains aseptic principles during set-up procedure		
2. Works in a logical, orderly progression		
3. Correctly assembles linen pack		
4. Drapes Mayo stand correctly		
5. Arranges suture in order of usage; maintains outer foil packages		
6. Prepares suture ligature in efficient manner		
7. Prepares instruments in a logical, orderly progression		
8. Performs counts correctly		
9. Completes set-up within a reasonable time frame		
II. MAYO TRAY		
1. Maintains aseptic principles during set-up procedure		
2. Assembles knife handle/blade with an instrument; maintains point downward		
3. Selects/arranges instruments according to procedural need in logical, orderly progression		
4. Completes set-up within a reasonable length of time		

COMMENTS: _____

_____

Draping the Surgical Patient

PURPOSE

To provide a sterile bacterial barrier against microbial invasion into the surgical wound.

PREREQUISITE

Sterile gown and gloves; linen pack prepared. Surgical skin prep performed.

PROFICIENCY

One hundred percent accuracy at the time of performance.

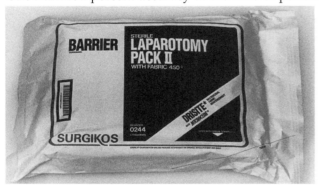

Laparotomy drape pack

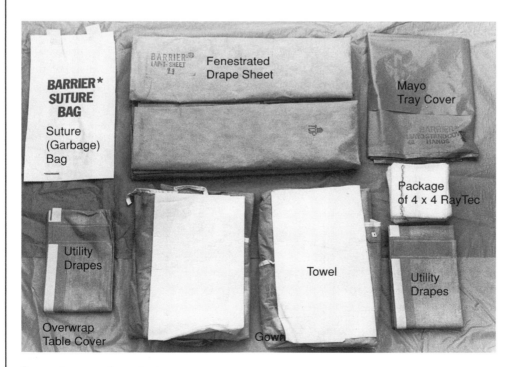

Laparotomy pack contents

**CRITICAL ELEMENT
TASK 9-3** *cont.*

PROCEDURAL STEPS

A. LAPAROTOMY DRAPE (see Fig. A)
  1. Towels are placed to "square-off" incision site.
  2. Half sheet (if used) is placed over foot of patient.
  3. Fenestrated sheet is brought to table, folded, and opening is placed over towels with TOP portion toward the head. Sides are allowed to fall below table level.
  4. Sheet is opened over lower portion of the table, then the upper portion is extended over the head of the patient, being secured to IV poles (by anesthesia personnel).

NOTE: Steps may be added or deleted depending on surgeon's preference.

B. GYN/GU DRAPE IN LITHOTOMY POSITION (see Fig. B)
  1. Position under buttocks drape, protecting gloved hands.
  2. Place leggings over the stirrup holders and cover legs to inguinal area.
  3. Place abdominal drape sheet across top.

NOTE: Cysto drape may come with or without separate leggings. Check contents before draping to avoid contamination.

POINTS TO REMEMBER

  1. Gloved hands must be protected during the draping procedure by use of cuff created by drape.
  2. Never flourish drapes. Dust and lint are then released into the air, creating a vehicle for airborne bacteria.
  3. Be aware of defined areas of sterility.
  4. Allow time for draping procedure.
  5. Keep drapes folded until time of use, and do not allow drapes to touch the floor or become tangled in floor equipment or lines extending from the table.
  6. Once a drape has been placed, *it cannot be repositioned.* Either reinforce the drape or discard it and begin with a new drape sheet.
  7. If incise drape is used, the area must be blotted dry before the drape is applied. Towels are applied, then the incise drape, and last the fenestrated drape.
  8. All cables, tubings, and so on for equipment should be secured on the sterile field with a nonperforating clamp. If towel clips are used, the tips are considered contaminated once they have perforated the drape, and cannot be removed or touched until the end of the procedure when the drape sheets are removed.

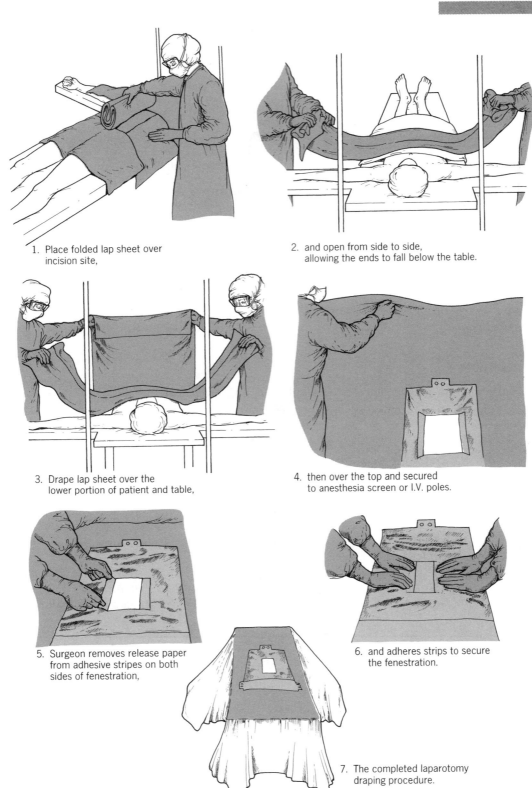

1. Place folded lap sheet over incision site,

2. and open from side to side, allowing the ends to fall below the table.

3. Drape lap sheet over the lower portion of patient and table,

4. then over the top and secured to anesthesia screen or I.V. poles.

5. Surgeon removes release paper from adhesive stripes on both sides of fenestration,

6. and adheres strips to secure the fenestration.

7. The completed laparotomy draping procedure.

Fig. A. Creating and maintaining the sterile field (courtesy of Devon Industries, 1995)

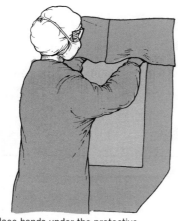

1. Place hands under the protective cuff of the under buttocks drape,

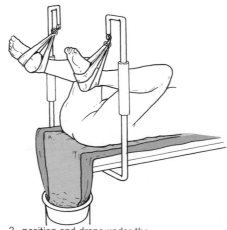

2. position and drape under the patient so that tail falls into kick bucket.

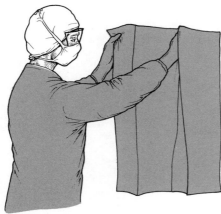

3. Holding the leggings so that one hand is grasping the toe, open leggings to full length and place over stirrup holders.

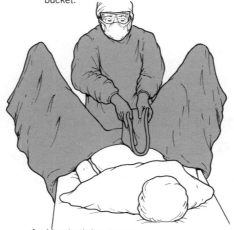

4. After both leggings are in place, place abdominal drape on abdomen,

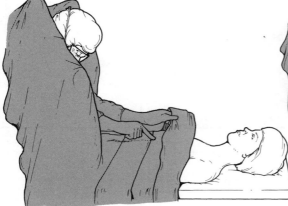

5. and open first from side to side, then toward the patient's head.

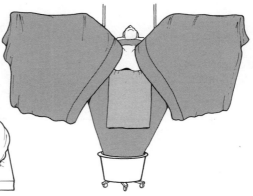

6. The completed lithotomy draping procedure.

Fig. B.   Draping for lithotomy position

PERFORMANCE CHECK SHEET

NAME: _____	TASK # _____9-3_____
	RATING: A Acceptable
	N/I Needs Improvement

PROCEDURE: Draping the Surgical Patient

PROCEDURAL STEPS	A	N/I
1. Prepares linen pack in proper sequential order		
2. Presents drape sheets folded to surgeon/assistant		
3. Protects gloved hands during draping procedure		
4. Avoids "flourishing" of drapes		
5. Follows correct sequence for application of plastic incise drape		
6. Unfolds fenestrated sheet (patient drape) over feet first, then head, protecting hands with cuff of drape sheet		
7. Secures tubings with nonperforating clamps in proper fashion		
8. Does not readjust drape sheet once in place		
9. Avoids contact with nondraped areas		
10. Reinforces drapes as necessary to maintain sterility of field		

COMMENTS: _____

_____

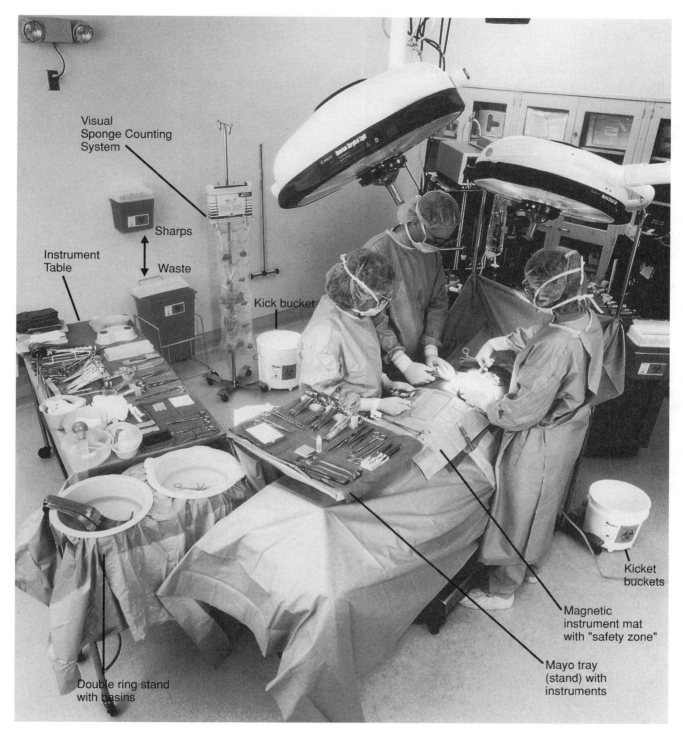

Creating and maintaining the sterile field (Copyright © 1996. Devon Industries, Inc. Used by permission. May not be reproduced without written consent.)

the sterile field, and all movement and activities in and around that field must be performed without compromise to that field.

All sterile supplies and equipment should be grouped around the patient, and must be kept in view at all times by both the sterile and nonsterile members of the team.

Sterile items should be presented to the scrub person or placed securely on the sterile field without reaching over the field, which would cause immediate contamination. Sharp or heavy objects should be opened on a separate surface to avoid injury or possible contamination of the object during transfer.

Some materials appear resistant to moisture, but should liquid be spilled, creating *strike-through*, the area must be reinforced with a sterile towel or drape, since strike-through of fluids constitutes contamination of that sterile surface.

As always, if the sterility of an item, be it a towel, instrument, or needle, is in doubt it must be considered contaminated, removed from the field, and replaced by another sterile item.

Unsterile equipment, furniture, and personnel should remain a safe distance from the sterile field (at least 12 inches) to avoid accidental contact with the field. Unsterile personnel should approach the field facing it and never walk between two sterile fields.

Sterile supplies should never be opened and then covered or left unguarded during the preliminary phase of the sterile field's creation. Chances for contamination of an unguarded sterile field are numerous, and without direct observation, there is no way to ensure sterility.

For additional guidelines, review Chapter 8 in this module. These principles and practices should become part of your everyday activities, since the safety of the patient rests solely on the ability to maintain the sterile field during the surgical procedure, in addition to maintaining an aseptic environment.

PHASE III: TERMINATION OF THE STERILE FIELD

It is important to terminate the sterile field in a safe and logical manner, and at the proper time.

Until the patient has been prepared for transfer to the postoperative area, the environment must be maintained in an aseptic manner, in case an unforeseen emergency occurs that necessitates immediate action. Therefore, all members of the surgical team should keep their masks in place during this transition period.

After the last stitch is in place, and the area cleaned, the sterile dressing is applied by the scrub nurse and held in place while the drape sheets are removed with assistance from the circulator, rolling the drape sheet inside out toward the foot of the table. The scrub nurse, with the equipment, should then step back to a position away from the operating table, where the actual termination procedure will take place.

The criteria for disassembling the sterile set-up calls for the *patient to have left the room,* but this is not realistic, since room turnover time is usually limited to 15 minutes maximum after a procedure is over (and may be longer for complicated procedures with excessive equipment).

The next best approach is to begin the clean-up process during the closing phase of the procedure, leaving the Mayo stand intact until the very end. This would still allow for the use of sterile equipment should an emergency situation arise necessitating reentry into the wound.

All instruments, whether used or not, are considered contaminated and must be decontaminated according to acceptable protocol. However, instruments that have been used during the procedure should be hand cleaned using a basin of sterile water and a lap sponge or brush before terminal decontamination. This action provides safety for those persons handling the instruments during the cleaning phase. Before disposing of drape material, it should be checked for instruments, since they may be still attached to the drapes during the dismantling phase. Disposable linen and cloth items are then placed in their respective bags for disposal. Gloves must be worn during this process, even by the circulating nurse, since blood and fluids may still be present on the drape sheet. All sharps, including cautery tips, blades, and hypodermic needles should be placed in a container (a needle-counter box can serve this purpose) and disposed of according to acceptable protocol.

To avoid any unsightly transfer of instruments to the decontamination area, the tray(s) should be covered. The last step is the removal of the scrub's gown, gloves, and mask.

Environmental services begin the interim cleaning process by removing the trash and linen from the room, followed by cleaning the floor and all surfaces according to institutional procedure.

By following the process of creating, maintaining, and terminating the sterile field, the patient and personnel working in and around the sterile field can be assured of a safe and therapeutic environment, before, during, and after the surgical experience.

Protecting the patient and personnel from harm is the responsibility of everyone, and by practicing the principles of basic aseptic technique, effectively monitoring the environment, and selecting, organizing, and safely utilizing the supplies and equipment during surgery the surgical experience can become a rewarding experience for both the patient and the surgical team.

References

1. Miller BF, Keane CB. Encyclopedia and dictionary of medicine, nursing and allied health. 3rd ed. Philadelphia: Saunders, 1983. P. 970.
2. The United States Pharmacopeia, 22nd revision. Rockville, MD: USP Convention, 1990.
3. U.S. Surgical Corp. Stapling techniques: general surgery with autosuture instruments. 3rd ed. Norwalk, CT: 1988. P. 6.

Questions for Review for Module III

1. The instrument (back table) becomes contaminated with solution as the surgeon is closing the peritoneum. The *first* course of action as a scrub person would be to:
   a. use the Mayo stand only
   b. cover the contaminated area with a sterile towel and proceed with the procedure
   c. redrape the instrument table before proceeding with the procedure
   d. avoid that part of the table which is contaminated

2. Halfway through the surgical procedure, the surgeon, who has been standing, requests a sitting stool. The perioperative nurse should:
   a. give the surgeon the stool since he or she requested it
   b. give the surgeon the stool and document the incident on the operative record
   c. remind the surgeon that a change of position alters the sterile field boundaries, and then give the surgeon the stool
   d. remind the surgeon about the correlation between changing positions and the maintenance of the sterile field and refuse to give him or her the stool

3. According to the AORN's Recommended Practices, the area of a surgical gown considered sterile includes _____.

4. It is proper aseptic technique for two gowned persons to pass each other back to back.

   True   False

5. According to current concepts regarding the *shelf-life* of a package, sterilization is:
   a. time-related and contamination can occur in 60 days using nonwoven wrappers
   b. time-related and contamination can occur in 120 days when using peel packages
   c. event-related, not time-related
   d. time-related, not event-related

6. The penetration of moisture through a bacterial barrier or vice versa is known as:
   a. transmission
   b. fallout
   c. strike-through
   d. denaturation

7. When performing an *anatomic timed hand scrub*, the required time following a contaminated procedure is:
   a. 3 minutes per extremity
   b. 7 minutes total time
   c. 10 minutes total time
   d. no different than any other scrub

8. Which statement regarding sterile technique is *FALSE?*
   a. Tables are sterile at table level only.
   b. Wrapper edges of a sterile item are considered unsterile once the package is opened.
   c. Fluid contents remaining in a bottle, once opened and poured, cannot be used later, and must be discarded.
   d. A sterile package is opened from the near side first, and then the far side.

9. Which methods are used to check the sterilization process but do not guarantee sterility of an item?
   1. chemical indicators
   2. biologic indicators
   3. indicator strips
   4. recording graphs/temperature charts
      a. 1, 2
      b. 1, 2, 4
      c. 1, 3, 4
      d. all of the above

10. The two types of scissors most often used in general surgery are the _____ and the

    _____ .

11. Match the following instruments with their correct description:
    a. Kocher   1. _____ right-angled clamp
    b. Army-Navy   2. _____ heavy hemostat
    c. Mixtner   3. _____ single-tooth clamp
    d. Kelly   4. _____ handheld retractor

12. Only the instruments actually used during a procedure must be washed.

    True   False

13. Cutting needles are appropriate for suturing a liver bed.

    True   False

14. List the five categories of surgical instruments and give an example in each category.

1. _____

2. _____

3. _____

4. _____

5. _____

15. Sutures that are assimilated by body enzymes during the healing process are classified as _____ and would be used on tissue that _____ .

Glossary

Absorbable Suture a material that is attacked, broken down, and eventually absorbed by body tissue

Ambient Air surrounding room air

Antisepsis prevention of infection through a reduction of microbial contamination on animate surfaces/areas

Antiseptic any substance that inhibits growth of bacteria

Approximation bringing together two sides or edges of an open wound or incision

Asepsis absence of septic matter; freedom from infection or infectious materials

Aseptic Technique a series of procedures that reduce the possibility of microbial contamination

Atraumatic Suture a strand of suture material with an eyeless needle that is attached by the manufacturer (syn: swaged)

Autoclave sterilizer designed to use steam-under-pressure as sterilizing agent

Bacterial Barrier any material that prevents microorganisms from coming in contact with a sterile surface or aseptically prepared areas; used to create and maintain a sterile field (e.g., gowns, gloves, drapes, etc.)

Bactericidal agent that destroys bacteria

Bioburden microbial population of a specified item or device at a specific time

Biologic Indicator commercially prepared device with a known population of highly resistant microorganisms (spores) used to test the sterilizing efficacy of the sterilizer being monitored; *Bacillus stearothemophilus, B. subtilis*

Bowie-Dick Test method for monitoring adequacy of air removal from a high vacuum sterilizer chamber during prevacuum stage of cycle; not considered a test for sterility

Buried Suture Technique any stitch made and tied so that it remains completely under the skin

Capillary characteristic of suture materials that allow the passage of tissue fluid along the strand

Cauterizing the act of searing a bleeder using heat

Cautery electrosurgical means of searing bleeders to control hemostasis; monopolar or bipolar methods (syn: Bovie)

Chemical Indicator commercially prepared device used to monitor all parts of the physical condition of the sterilization process; used internally and externally

Contaminated soiled with microorganisms; unsterile

Continuous Suturing Technique one strand passed back and forth between two edges of the wound to close tissue layers, tied only at each end of suture line

Control-Release Suture–Needle suture–needle combination that permits fast and controlled separation of needle from suture material (syn: pull-off; pop-off)

Cross-Contamination transmission of microorganisms from patient to patient; from inanimate objects to patient or vice versa

Decontamination a process whereby the number of microorganisms on an item is reduced or eliminated, using a specified agent

Disinfection chemical or physical process of destroying all pathogenic microorganisms, except spores, on inanimate objects/surfaces

Flash Sterilizer smaller version of gravity displacement sterilizer used to sterilize unwrapped items for emergency use during surgery; preset at 270°F

Flora bacteria/fungi normally inhabiting the body; often delineated as *transient* or *resident*

Interrupted Suturing Technique single stitches, separately placed, tied, and cut

Ligate to tie off

Ligature strand of material, usually without a needle, used to tie off structure/blood vessels (syn: ties)

Medical Asepsis destruction of organisms *after* they leave the body, to avoid spread of infection from one person to another (e.g., isolation technique)

Monofilament suture strand consisting of single thread

Multifilament strand made of more than one thread, held together by "twisting" or "braiding"

Natural Fiber Source suture material made from natural fibers

Nonabsorbable Suture suture material that cannot be dissolved by tissue enzymes but remains encapsulated when buried in tissue, or one that is removed after wound strength has been returned (e.g., skin suture)

Noncapillary characteristic of nonabsorbable suture in which specific processing meets tests establishing them as resistant to "wicking" transfer of body fluids

Permeation to pass through the openings in a bacterial barrier or interstices, causing a hole or breakage in a protective layer

Primary Suture Line sutures or staples used to approximate wound edges; mostly referenced to skin

Secondary Suture Line retention sutures, placed about 2 inches away from wound edges, to reinforce primary suture line and protect suture line from undue stress

Sepsis severe toxic febrile state, resulting from infection with pyrogenic microorganisms, with or without associated septicemia

Sterile free of all living microorganisms, including spores

Sterile Field area surrounding the site of incision into tissue or introduction of any instrument/device into a body cavity, prepared and protected by use of sterile supplies and/or equipment. Includes furniture covered with sterile drapes and personnel in proper sterile attire

Sterile Technique methods by which contamination of sterile items is prevented during invasive procedures requiring the maintenance of sterility

Sterilization process by which all microorganisms, including spores, are killed using steam, chemical, or physical methods

Strike-Through soaking and/or penetration of moisture through a bacterial barrier to unsterile layers or vice versa

Subcuticular Closure suture placed under the skin for a cosmetic closure effect; skin suture or stapling may not be necessary with this closure method

Surgical Asepsis destruction of organisms *before* they enter the body through sterilization procedures

Surgical Conscience a self-discipline which dictates that appropriate action has been taken to correct deviation from acceptable practice, whether observed or unobserved; foundation for the practice of *aseptic technique*

Surgical Needle an instrument used to carry strands of suture material through tissue; atraumatic or free

Surgically Clean mechanically cleaned, but unsterile, reducing the number of microorganisms by chemical and/or mechanical means

Synthetic Fiber Source suture material made with fibers created from artificial (man-made) sources

Tensile Strength amount of tension or "pull strength" against a knot, measured in pounds, which determines breaking point

Terminal Sterilization procedure carried out at the end of a procedure, reducing the number of pathogens on inanimate objects

Unsterile inanimate object or device that has not been subjected to a sterilization process

USP United States Pharmacopeia. Official agency that sets standards for purity, strength, and/or dosages of drugs and suture material. Official reference of *Food and Drug Administration* when this agency tests drugs

Bibliography for Module III

Aldrete JA, Kroulik D. A postanesthetic recovery score. *Anesth Analg* 49:924, 1970.

Assoc. for the Advancement of Medical Instrumentation (AAMI) National Standards and Recommended Practices for Sterilization. 2nd ed. Arlington, VA: 1988:157–171, 173–200. The Assoc. (pub.)

American Society for Hospital Central Service Personnel. Training Manual for Central Service Technicians. Chicago: American Hospital Association, 1986.

American Sterilizer Company. Decontamination, Sterilization, Disinfection and Sanitation: The Concept—the Facts. Erie, PA: The Company, 1988.

Association of Operating Room Nurses. Standards and Recommended Practices for Perioperative Nursing Practice. Denver: The Association, 1991.

Atkinson LJ. Berry & Kohn's Introduction to Operating Room Nursing. 7th ed. New York: McGraw-Hill, 1992.

Brooks SM. Fundamentals of Operating Room Nursing. 2nd ed. St. Louis: Mosby, 1979.

Brooks SM. Instrumentation for the Operating Room: A Photographic Manual. 3rd ed. St. Louis: Mosby, 1988.

Codman & Shurleff, Inc. The Care and Handling of Surgical Instruments. Randolf, MA: Codman & Shurleff, Inc., 1975.

Ethicon, Inc. Wound Closure Manual. Sommerville, NJ: Ethicon, Inc., 1994.

Fuller JR. Surgical Technology: Principles and Practices. 2nd ed. Philadelphia: Saunders, 1994.

Gruendemann B, et al. Alexander's Care of the Patient in Surgery. 8th ed. St. Louis: Mosby, 1987.

Kneedler J, Dodge G. Perioperative Patient Care: The Nursing Perspective. 3rd ed. Boston: Blackwell Scientific, 1994.

Lach J. Operating Room Nursing: Perioperative Care and Draping Techniques. Chicago: Kendall Co., 1974.

Meeker M, Rothrock J. Alexander's Care of the Patient in Surgery. 10th ed. St. Louis: Mosby, 1995.

Miller BF, Keane CB. Encyclopedia and Dictionary of Medicine and Nursing. 3rd ed. Philadelphia: Saunders, 1983.

Perkins J. Principles and Methods of Sterilization in Health Sciences. 2nd ed. Springfield, IL: Charles C Thomas, 1983.

Roth RA (ed). Perioperative Nursing Care Curriculum. Denver, CO: AORN, Inc., 1995.

Stroumtos O. Perspectives on Suture. New York: The American Cyanamid Co., 1974.

Surgikos, Inc. Asepsis: A Programmed Instruction in Asepsis. Arlington, TX: Surgikos, Inc., 1980.

U.S. Surgical Corp. Stapling Techniques in General Surgery with Autosuture Instruments. 3rd ed. Norwalk, CT: The Corporation, 1988.

United States Pharmacopeia, 22nd revision. Rockville, MD: U.S.P. Convention, 1990.

V. Muller, Inc. The Surgical Armamentarium. Chicago: Rand McNally, 1988.

Answers for Module III

Self-assessment Exercise 1

1. A series of procedures by which contamination of a sterile field/area is prevented.
2. Sterile technique prevents contamination of a sterile item by maintaining its sterility throughout a series of aseptic procedures.
3. Surgical conscience
4. 1. Scrubbed persons should wear sterile gown and gloves.
    2. Sterile drapes should be used to establish a sterile field.
    3. All items used within a sterile field must be sterile.
    4. All items introduced to the sterile field should be dispensed by methods that maintain sterility and integrity of the item/field.
    5. A sterile field should be constantly monitored and maintained.
5. Monitoring the environment; maintaining a safe distance from the sterile field; checking the packaging of sterile items before using the item; recognizing contamination when it occurs and implementing corrective action; properly dispensing sterile supplies by maintaining the principles of aseptic technique
6. FALSE: it is necessary to maintain aseptic technique whenever and wherever a patient's natural defenses are compromised and/or an invasive procedure is performed.

Self-assessment Exercise 2

1. TRUE
2. TRUE
3. iodophor; chlorohexidine gluconate
4. TRUE
5. FALSE: this would cause contamination of hands with the blood and debris from the gown
6. open glove

Self-assessment Exercise 3

1. *Gravity displacement* air is displaced by gravity; therefore, the time necessary for steam to contact all surfaces is longer.
   Prevacuum air is removed and a vacuum is created before steam fills the chamber. Steam entering the vacuum almost instantly contacts every surface.
2. TRUE
3. FALSE: instruments must be open and parts separated so that the steam can be displaced evenly, covering all parts of the instrument/device.
4. Only through biologic testing, by resistant spores, can there be assurance that all conditions necessary for sterilization have been achieved.

Bacillus stearothemophilus	Steam
Bacillus subtilis	EO Gas

5. 15 to 17 pounds
6. FALSE: chemical indicators reflect that the physical conditions of the process have been achieved, but do not guarantee sterility of the item.
7. Telescopic instruments; plastic goods with low melting points; rubber items; delicate instruments (to preserve their precision)
8. Flash sterilization
9. The absence of all microorganisms, including spores achieved through steam, chemical, or physical methods.
10. FALSE: terminal sterilization should be performed on all instruments as part of the decontamination process.

Self-assessment Exercise 4

1. Bronchoscope; cystoscope; thermometer; endotracheal tube
2. FALSE: high-level disinfectants are only appropriate for disinfecting patient-care items.
3. TRUE
4. FALSE: cold sterilization can only be achieved by soaking an item for 10 hours; anything less is *disinfection*.
5. A semicritical item is one that makes direct contact with intact mucous membranes, but is not introduced beneath the skin or mucous membranes.

Self-assessment Exercise 5

1. Platelet plug formation; vasoconstriction; formation of fibrin clot
2. FALSE: this substance is a microfibullar collagen (Avitine).
3. TRUE
4. Instruments; suture; bone wax; specially treated gauzes, sponges, and foams; electrocautery; thrombin

Self-assessment Exercise 6

1. Absorbable suture
2. TRUE
3. Dexon; Vicryl; PDS
4. FALSE: a 5-0 suture has a smaller diameter and less tensile strength than a 4-0.
5. a. Nonabsorbable (natural)
   b. Silk (black braided)
   c. 3-0 (18 inches)
   d. ligature (ties) in Labyrinth packaging used to tie off bleeding vessels

Self-assessment Exercise 7

1. TRUE
2. Size and properties of suture materials; nature of surgery; surgeons' preference

3. Less tissue trauma; smaller hole to heal; convenient
4. FALSE: a break at any point may lead to wound disruption since one strand is used during the suturing process.
5. TRUE
6. FALSE: Vicryl is used internally as an absorbable suture.

Self-assessment Exercise 8

1. TRUE
2. Reduce the possibility of heavy suture cutting into the skin.
3. Trade name; generic name; catalog number; size; length classification (type); color; number of sutures/needles per package; braided or monofilament; coating material; date of manufacture; expiration date (if applicable); compliance with USP standards
4. TRUE
5. TRUE
6. 1. TA internal stapling instrument
   2. Ligating clip appliers

Self-assessment Exercise 9

1.
   A. Cutting/dissecting
   B. No. 4 Knife handle (scalpel) with No. 20 blade
   C. Skin knife; deep puncture wounds
2.
   A. Miscellaneous
   B. Poole abdominal suction tip
   C. Abdominal cavity; heavy bleeding
3.
   A. Holding clamp
   B. Hemostat (Crile)
   C. Superficial tissue; first two layers of abdomen
4.
   A. Cutting/dissecting
   B. Mayo scissors (curved/straight)
   C. Curved: tough, fibrous tissue
      Straight: suture scissors
5.
   A. Grasping clamp
   B. Allis clamp
   C. Grasps nondelicate tissue in tight areas
6.
   A. Holding clamp
   B. Smooth tissue forceps (thumb forceps)
   C. Holds delicate tissue
7.
   A. Suturing instrument
   B. Needle holder (diamond jaw)
   C. Used with eyed/eyeless suture; medium needle
8.
   A. Miscellaneous
   B. Yankauer (tonsil) suction tip
   C. Normal suctioning; superficial
9.
   A. Holding clamp

B. Babcock
C. Noncrushing; delicate/tubular structures
10.
   A. Retracting instrument
   B. Balfour retractor with bladder blade
   C. Self-retaining; abdominal structures

Self-assessment Exercise 10

1. Surgical approach
   Surgical procedure (sequence)
   Surgical complications
   Surgical closure
2. Damp dusting all flat surfaces; collecting and placing necessary furniture/supplies; assembling positioning devices/aids
3. Operating table; instrument table; Mayo stand; ring stand; prep table; etc.
4. Standard: needed for every surgical procedure linen pack; sponges; gowns/gloves; basin sets; prep tray
   Accessory: items needed only when requested by surgeon or by virtue of the procedural needs: suture; ESU with hand component; syringes; catheters/tubes/drains
5. Physician's preference card/computer listing
6. 1. Creating
   2. Maintaining
   3. Terminating

Questions for Review

1. B
2. C
3. In front, shoulders to table level and sleeves to 2 inches above elbow
4. TRUE
5. C
6. C
7. D
8. D
9. C
10. Mayo; Metzenbaum
11. 1. C
    2. D
    3. A
    4. B
12. FALSE: all instruments must be washed and decontaminated after each procedure.
13. FALSE: a blunt needle is used to suture the liver bed.
14. 1. Cutting/dissecting (scissors; scalpel)
    2. Grasping/holding (clamps and forceps)
    3. Retracting (Deaver; Richardsons)
    4. Suturing (needle holder)
    5. Miscellaneous (suction tip, probe, groove)
15. Absorbable; tissue that heals slowly or requires extra support during healing process

MODULE IV Perioperative Nursing Practice

Chapter Outline

Content Overview

The role of the perioperative nurse as practiced today has changed from the old concept of the "technically oriented nursing practice" to a *patient-centered*, individualized practice, the basis of which stems not only from the psychomotor skills required, but also from a scientific foundation using the Nursing Process as its format.

This module correlates the scope of perioperative nursing practice with the Nursing Process during the three phases of surgical intervention: preoperative, intraoperative, and postoperative, and discusses the legal aspects related to this specialty nursing practice.

Module Objectives

Upon completion of this module, you will be able to:

1. Discuss the Nursing Process as it relates to perioperative nursing practice.
2. Discuss the preoperative preparation of a surgical patient, including the psychological and physiologic aspects and admission criteria to surgery.
3. Identify and discuss the perioperative nurses' role as it relates to the five aspects of professional nursing practice and the phases of surgery, including the usage of specialized equipment and supplies during the intraoperative phase.
4. Discuss the procedures and protocols associated with the immediate postoperative phase of surgical intervention.
5. Describe the professional and legal obligations and accountabilities related to patient management and the maintenance of a safe, therapeutic environment during the perioperative period.

Perioperative Nursing Process

Kathleen Blais

Nursing is the diagnosis and treatment of human responses to actual or potential health problems.

—ANA, 1980

The *nursing process* offers the nurse a system for planning and providing patient care. The goal of the nursing process is to identify the patient's actual or potential problems, to develop a plan to mediate the identified problems, to provide specific nursing actions or interventions, to resolve problems, and to evaluate continually the patient's response to care so that appropriate changes can be made in the plan to ensure an effective outcome. Hence, the nursing process is a dynamic and cyclical activity (Fig. 10-1), continually changing in response to the patient's status.

The perioperative nurse uses the nursing process to plan and provide care during the three stages of surgical intervention: preoperative, intraoperative, and postoperative.

The scope of perioperative nursing practice encom-passes all three phases of surgical intervention. These activities begin when the client (patient) makes a conscious decision to have surgery (or an invasive procedure) and discusses those prospects with the surgical team members (preoperative), proceeds through the actual performance of the surgical (invasive) procedure (intraoperative), to the resolution of the presenting problem (postoperative).

"Perioperative nurses interact with both the patient and/or the patient's significant others throughout the continuum of patient care."[1]

While the three stages of the perioperative experience are easily defined, the nursing process provides a care plan that includes the patient's needs in each stage and crosses all three stages. Once the patient has made the decision to have surgery, it is essential for the nurse to determine the current or actual and potential problems in all three stages of the perioperative period. After identifying patient problems, the perioperative nurse implements appropriate interventions to prevent untoward outcomes. The nursing process is an interactive process which, to be effective, requires the active participation of the patient.

STANDARDS OF PRACTICE AND THE NURSING PROCESS

Surgical patients may interact with many nurses during the perioperative experience. To provide continuity of care during the three phases of surgical intervention, the *standards of nursing practice,* as they relate to the management of the surgical patient, are used as a reference for all nurses during the perioperative period.

AORN developed (1975) and reaffirmed (1995) the *standards of nursing practice* to ensure that guidelines are available for delivering quality patient care during the perioperative period. According to AORN (1995), "...standards of perioperative clinical practice describe a competent level of perioperative nursing..."[2] through the use of the nursing process. According to standards:[3]

The Perioperative Nurse:
  I.   Collects patient health data.
  II. Analyzes the assessment data in determining diagnoses.
  III. Identifies expected outcomes unique to the patient.
  IV. Develops a plan of care that prescribes interventions to attain expected outcomes.
  V.   Implements the interventions identified in the plan of care.
  VI. Evaluates the patient's progress toward attainment of outcomes.

Source: AORN. Standards and recommended practices. Denver, CO: The Association, 1995. Pp. 107–109.

In assisting the patient as he or she prepares for surgery, the surgical unit nurse may develop an initial care plan, often in consultation with the perioperative nurse or the nurses who will care for the patient following surgery. The perioperative nurse relies on information provided by the floor nurse to continue the plan of care during surgery. The recovery nurse relies on

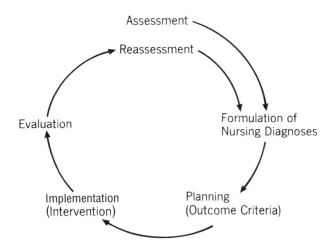

Fig. 10-1. Cyclical nature of the nursing process

information provided by the floor nurse and the perioperative nurse to provide care during the immediate postoperative period.

As the patient returns to the surgical unit to recover, the floor nurse will review the notes of the perioperative nurse and recovery room nurse to plan for the postsurgical care of the patient so that continuity of care continues (Fig. 10-2).

All the nurses providing care use the nursing process to plan the patient's care. Each phase of the nursing process—*assessment, diagnosis, planning, implementation (intervention)* and *evaluation*—will be discussed in detail as it relates to the perioperative event.

ASSESSMENT

Assessment is the first phase of the nursing process. It involves collection and validation of information about the patient. While assessment is identified as the first stage, the nurse continues to assess the patient in all stages of the nursing process as he or she determines the appropriateness of decisions about the nursing diagnoses, plan, and interventions. Evaluation, in fact, becomes a reassessment of patient responses to the nursing care plan and the basis for future patient care planning.

Collection of Data

The information gathered about the patient is called *data.* It is further broken down into *subjective* data and *objective* data.

Subjective data is that which only the patient can experience—that is, it is not readily observable to the nurse or other caregivers. Examples of subjective data are pain, nausea, and itching. Another term for subjective data is *symptoms*. The perioperative nurse may collect subjective data from the patient when taking the admission health history (e.g., in the outpatient setting).

Objective data is data that is observable or measurable by the caregiver. Examples of objective data include vital signs, observations made during the physical examination, and the results of laboratory or diagnostic studies. Another term used for objective data is *signs*.

AORN Standard I for clinical practice states that "assessment is the systematic and ongoing collection of data, guided by the application of knowledge of physiologic and psychological principles and experience, and is used to make judgments and predictions about a patient's response to illness or changes in life processes."[4] Criteria used for meeting this standard should include such data as current medical history, physiologic and psychological status, understanding and perception of the planned surgical event, and previous medical and surgical history.

For the surgical patient, assessment may begin before admission. Information about the past health history of the patient may be obtained in the physician's office and forwarded to the hospital, or in the case of outpatient surgery be sent to the ambulatory surgery unit.

In many hospitals, perioperative nurses visit the prospective surgical patient to conduct a preoperative assessment and interview. No matter how minor the surgical procedure, a thorough health history is essential and should be available to the operating room staff at all times during the patient's surgical experience. Information about allergies, preexisting medical problems (e.g., heart condition, hypertension, diabetes, blood dyscrasias and coagulation problems, chronic respiratory or renal problems), medications that the patient is currently taking, previous surgical experiences, and previous responses to anesthesia may have great significance for the present perioperative plan.

In addition to previous health information, patient feelings and concerns about the proposed surgery may have an impact on the outcome. Fear, anxiety, and depression can affect the patient's ability to cooperate with the proposed care plan.

Preoperative Patient Assessment

> The first consideration in prevention is the careful and complete evaluation of the patient.
> —*Rogers and Sturgeon, 1985*

Before surgery the patient must be assessed both physiologically and psychologically. Carpenito[5] states that preoperative focus assessments should be done to determine factors that can influence the patient's risk for intraoperative or postoperative complications.

Such focus assessments should include: the patient's understanding of events, any acute or chronic conditions experienced by the patient, the patient's previous surgical experiences, and the patient's nutritional, fluid and electrolyte, and emotional status. Parameters of physiologic assessment should include the physical examination and review of the current diagnostic studies and laboratory values that will be used as baseline data.

Physical Examination

The physical examination is a valuable part of the patient assessment. Baseline data regarding vital signs, cardiopulmonary function, bowel function, urinary function, nutritional status, and physical limitations are all important in developing the care plan for the perioperative experience.

Laboratory and diagnostic studies help to validate the information obtained through the nursing history and physical examination. Most hospitals require specific diagnostic studies to determine the patient's ability to tolerate the surgical procedure. Additionally, the studies serve as a baseline for comparing laboratory and diagnostic findings obtained during and after surgery. Some of these studies, discussed in detail on the following pages, include hemoglobin and hematocrit levels, blood typing, complete blood counts, urinalysis, chest x-ray, and electrocardiogram.

It is important for the perioperative nurse to know that one can never have too much information about the patient who is about to undergo surgery. What may initially appear to be trivial information may subsequently have great significance for the patient's optimal outcome.

Baseline Assessment Components

Vital Signs Baseline vital signs including temperature, pulse, respirations, and blood pressure should be obtained. In addition to the pulse rate, the quality of the pulse and any irregularity in the pulse should be noted. In addition to the respiratory rate, the lungs should be assessed to determine the extent of preoperative lung expansion, breath sounds, and any difficulty the patient has with ventilation, deep breathing, or coughing. The blood pressure should be taken on several occasions before surgery to establish an accurate baseline for the intraoperative and postoperative phases. Obtaining one blood pressure reading on a patient who is anxious may provide an inaccurate determination of hypertension.

Hemoglobin and Hematocrit The hemoglobin (Hgb) and hematocrit (Hct) are obtained before surgery to determine the blood's ability to carry oxygen. A low hemoglobin or hematocrit may be reason to delay an elective procedure.

White Blood Cell Count   The white blood cell (WBC) count is obtained to identify any preexisting infectious process. An elevated WBC count may also be reason to delay or cancel elective surgery.

Blood Typing and Cross-Matching (Screening)   The patient's blood is typed and cross-matched in the event that replacement blood is required. If indicated, the patient's own blood can be filtered and returned to him or her in surgery via the *cell saver*. Patients may elect to bank their own blood for *autotransfusion* when there is sufficient time before an elective procedure. In recent years many patients preferred to bank their own blood to minimize the risk of exposure to HIV and other blood-borne pathogens, but newer blood testing and screening techniques have decreased the risk of transfusion-borne infections.

Serum Electrolytes   Electrolyte studies (Na, K, Cl, Ca, Mg) are done preoperatively to determine any actual or potential imbalances. The three studies most often reviewed during the preoperative assessment are potassium, sodium, and calcium. These electrolytes may be affected if the patient becomes dehydrated during the procedure or loses excessive amounts of blood or plasma through suctioning or intraoperative blood loss. A deficit state of electrolytes could produce potential intraoperative and postoperative complications.

Urinalysis   A routine urinalysis is done to identify a urinary tract infection, and to determine whether glucose is present in the urine.

Chest X-Ray   The chest x-ray identifies lung pathology and the patient's postoperative ability to perform deep breathing exercises. The physician and nurse may plan the postoperative respiratory support equipment and treatment according to the chest x-ray findings. Additionally, the chest x-ray shows heart size and location, an important factor in assessing cardiac function.

Pulmonary function studies (arterial blood gases [ABGs]) may be ordered for a patient who has significant lung disease. This study is an important factor in the intraoperative management of anesthesia and the postoperative management of the patient.

Electrocardiogram   The ECG is routinely done preoperatively to detect any cardiac disease that may affect the patient either intraoperatively or postoperatively. Patients with cardiac disease are at greater risk for problems during surgery than are noncardiac patients. Cardiac conditions that may be contraindications to elective surgery include recent angina pectoris, unstable angina, severe aortic stenosis, uncontrolled hypertension, and a myocardial infarction within the past 6 months.

Additional studies may be done preoperatively according to the specific procedure planned (e.g., CT scan, cardiac catheterizations, arteriogram, and diagnostic x-rays). The results of all studies should be available on the patient's record when he or she goes to the operating suite. Often the surgeon will request the diagnostic x-rays be sent to the operating suite to be used as a reference during the procedure.

Psychological Assessment   The patient's understanding of and response to the proposed surgical procedure needs to be assessed. Most patients will experience some degree of anxiety when undergoing surgery, therefore, the nurse must not only identify the reasons for the anxiety or fear, but also determine the support systems and coping mechanisms the patient has for dealing with these feelings. In some cases, anxiety may be incapacitating to the point of placing the patient at risk. In such situations, surgery may be postponed until the patient is better able to cope.

As all information obtained during the preoperative assessment will be used in planning for care during the preoperative, intraoperative, and postoperative phases of patient care, it is essential that it be transmitted completely and accurately to all potential caregivers. To facilitate communication of the preoperative assessment findings, many hospitals use a separate preoperative assessment form (Fig. 10-3) or combine it with a perioperative assessment form, reflecting all three phases of surgical intervention.

Intraoperative Assessment

The assessment of the patient continues into the intraoperative phase, and is usually associated with admission to the operating suite.

Initial assessment in the operating suite will determine the patient's preparedness for surgery, and primarily consists of the following observations:

- Identification/verification of the patient
- Confirmation of consents and permits for surgery and anesthesia
- History and physical report by the physician(s)
- Laboratory and diagnostic testing results
- Status of parenteral fluid administration
- Urinary output
- Responses to preoperative medications
- Emotional status of the patient

In the procedure room, assessment continues in order to compare the patient's status with preoperative parameters and expected postoperative outcomes. Ongoing assessment during the surgical procedure will routinely include vital signs, blood loss, skin color, and

Name Patient Responds to: _____

PRE-OP ASSESSMENT	INTRA-OP ASSESSMENT	POST-OP ASSESSMENT

A MENTAL/EMOTIONAL STATUS
☐ Alert ☐ Sedated
☐ Apprehensive ☐ Comatose
☐ Confused
☐ Oriented _ _ _ _ _ _ X _____
☐ Other Comments _____
_____
 	
B COMMUNICATION LIMITATIONS
☐ N/A
☐ Retardation
☐ Language Barrier
 	
C MOBILITY
☐ Moves Well ☐ W/Assist
☐ Mobilizer Used ☐ Traction
☐ Painful Joints _____
☐ Joint Prothesis _____
 	
D SKIN
(1) COLOR
☐ Normal ☐ Cyanotic
☐ Flushed ☐ Pale
☐ Jaundiced ☐ Other _____
(2) INTEGRITY
☐ Intact ☐ Bruises ☐ Other
☐ Mottled ☐ Rash
☐ Reddened Areas
Describe _____
(3) TEMP/CONDITION
☐ Cool ☐ Warm ☐ Hot
☐ Diaphoretic ☐ Dry
 	
E RESPIRATORY STATUS
☐ Unlabored
☐ Minimum Distress
☐ Oxygen @ _____ L/min
☐ Ambu Bag
☐ Ventilator
☐ Endotracheal Tube
☐ Tracheostomy
 	
F CATHETER PRESENT
☐ No
☐ Yes Emptied _____ cc
 	
G COMMENTS
 	
H RN Sig. _____
	A POSITIONS
	☐ Supine ☐ Prone
	☐ Lithotomy ☐ Jackknife
	☐ Lateral ☐ Sitting
	  ☐ L Side Up ☐ Other
	  ☐ R Side Up _____
	
	B POSITIONED BY _____
	
	C ARM POSITION
	LEFT RIGHT
	☐ By Side ☐
	☐ Armboard ☐
	☐ Across Chest ☐
	☐ Other ☐
	
	D POSITIONAL AIDS
	☐ Axillary Roll ☐ Donut/Foam H'Rest
	☐ Bean Bag ☐ Eggcrate Mattress
	☐ Chest Rolls ☐ Montreal Positioner
	☐ Kidney Rests ☐ Shoulder Roll
	☐ Pillows ☐ Wilson Frame
	☐ Head Holder ☐ Other _____
	
	E PREP ☐ Shave in O.R.
	☐ Betadine Scrub ☐ Gel
	☐ Betadine Paint ☐ Alcohol per MD Order
	☐ Other _____
	
	F EQUIPMENT USED
	(1) Anesthesia Machine # _____
	(2) Cautery Unit # _____
	   Ground Pad _____
	(3) Hypet/Hypothermia Unit
	   Unit # _____ Temp. Set _____
	   Time PT. ON _____ OFF _____
	
	G TOURNIQUET UNIT # _____
	(1) Location _____
	(2) Positioned By _____
	(3) Padded ☐ YES ☐ NO. Per MD Order
	(4) Monitored By _____
	(5) Extremity Condition
	   (A) Pre-Op _____
	   (B) Post-Op _____
	
	H URINE OUTPUT _____ cc at _____
	
	I MEDS. ON FIELD OR GIVEN BY
	CIRCULATOR ☐ NONE
	
	J STANDARD CARE PLAN FOLLOWED?
	☐ Yes ☐ No. List Exceptions
	
	K RN Sig. _____
		A TRANSFERRED TO:
		VIA ☐ Mobilizer
		☐ PACU ☐ Guerney
		☐ _____ ICU ☐ Bed
		☐ Other _____ ☐ Other _____
		
		B LINES/DRAINS
		☐ Same as Pre-Op
		☐ Peripheral IV
		☐ Arterial
		☐ CVP/Swan
		☐ NG Tube
		☐ Foley Catheter
		☐ Others _____
		
		C SKIN INTEGRITY
		☐ Same as Pre-Op
		☐ Other _____
		☐ Ground Site Clear ☐ N/A
		
		D DRESSINGS
		☐ Dry, Intact
		☐ None
		☐ Other _____
		
		E RESPIRATORY STATUS
		☐ Endotracheal Tube
		☐ Oral Airway
		☐ Resp. Assisted
		☐ Tracheostomy
		☐ Spontaneous
		☐ Ambu Bag
		☐ Oxygen @ _____ L/Min
		
		F EBL _____ cc
		
		G TOTAL INTAKE
		(1) Crystalloids _____ cc
		(2) Colloids _____ cc
		(3) Bld Products _____ cc
		(4) Other _____ cc
		   Total _____ cc
		
		H TOTAL URINARY
		OUTPUT _____ cc
		
		I COMMENTS
		
		J RN Sig. _____

Fig. 10-2. Perioperative assessment form (From Fairchild S. Perioperative nursing update-90 [unpublished manuscript]. 1990 Educational Design Systems, Inc.)

drainage. Additionally, before final suturing, all sponges, instruments, and sharps will be counted as the perioperative nurse assesses the final outcome of the surgical procedure.

Before discharge from the procedure, the perioperative nurse, along with the anesthesia practitioner/nurse anesthetist, will assess the patient's wound dressings, respiratory status, drainage tubes for patency, collection chambers for amounts, status of parenteral infusion lines, and general readiness to be transferred to the postanesthesia area.

Postoperative Patient Assessment

In the immediate postoperative area; either the postanesthesia care unit (PACU) or in some instances the ambulatory care unit or the patient care unit, the initial assessment should include vital signs, color, activity level, and neurologic status using the Aldrette Recovery Scoring System (see Chap. 11). Subsequently, additional parameters of patient function will be assessed throughout the immediate postoperative period, including level of consciousness, dressings and drainage, pain level, parenteral infusion, patient safety, and any specific assessments directly related to the type of procedure that was performed.

Before discharge from the PACU, the patient is again assessed using the Aldrette Scoring System, and using a preestablished criteria for discharge. Discharge from PACU requires a physician's order, which is usually given after he or she has reviewed the Aldrette score and assessed the patient.

Assessments conducted and care provided in the postanesthesia care unit are documented to ensure adequate communication to the floor nurse.

The PACU nurse will usually accompany the pa-

PROPOSED SURGICAL PROCEDURE: _____

PROPOSED DATE OF SURGERY: _____ SURGEON: _____

PROPOSED ANESTHESIA: ☐ General   ☐ Regional   ☐ Local MAC   ☐ Local

* *

I.   PHYSIOLOGICAL ASSESSMENT DATA

Lab Values (enter values if abnormal)

☐ Hct. _____   ☐ Hgb. _____   ☐ K+ _____

☐ Coag. Studies _____   ☐ Type & Screen _____ (# of units)

Other: _____

Diagnostic Studies (on the chart)

☐ EKG (↑ 40)   ☐ CXR (↑ 60)   Waived by: _____

II. PSYCHOLOGICAL ASSESSMENT (✓ those applicable)

☐ Calm   ☐ Anxious   ☐ Confused   ☐ Fear   ☐ Withdrawn

☐ Cooperative   ☐ Unresponsive

Orientation: ☐ Person   ☐ Place   ☐ Time

III. PRE-OP TEACHING PROGRAM (to include but not be limited to:)

☐ Sequence of Events   ☐ Pre-Anesthesia Visit

☐ Catheters, Tubes, Drains   ☐ IV Therapy

☐ Post-Op Regime/Excercises   ☐ Post-Op Pain Management

☐ Family/Significant Other   ☐ Discharge Instructions (ACU)

IV. PRE-OP CHECKLIST (check those applicable)

☐ Proper ID   ☐ Allergies Listed _____

Consent Forms: ☐ Operative   ☐ Anesthesia   ☐ _____

History & Physical: ☐ Report on Chart   ☐ Dictated Date _____

Surgical Procedure confirmed with Schedule ☐ Yes   ☐ No

V.   SPECIAL CONSIDERATIONS (Intraoperative)

Communication Ability: ☐ Deaf   ☐ Blind   ☐ Response Appropriate

                       ☐ Language Barrier   ☐ _____

Mobility Limitations: ☐ None   ☐ Specific: _____

Additional Comments: _____

DATE: _____ TIME: _____ NURSE's SIGNATURE: _____

Fig. 10-3. Preoperative assessment form (From Fairchild, S. Perioperative nursing update-90 [unpublished manuscript]. 1990 Educational Design Systems, Inc.)

tient to the floor to give a verbal report, and the assessment continues as the floor nurse, using the same parameters as the PACU nurse, continues to monitor the patient's progress through the next phase of the surgical experience (see Fig. 10-3).

NURSING DIAGNOSES

Standard II for clinical practice relates to the determination of *nursing diagnoses*, which are derived from information accumulated during the assessment activities.

These statements reflect current problems that may or may not be specifically identified; they are communicated to other members of the health-care team to maintain continuity of care.

The nursing diagnosis is the judgment or conclusion of the patient's health problem(s) made after reviewing all assessment data.

Nursing diagnoses may represent *actual* or *potential* problems. An actual problem is one the patient currently exhibits during assessment. Potential problems are those that the patient is not presently experiencing, but is at risk for developing if appropriate interventions are not implemented. Examples of potential problems for the surgical patient in the intraoperative phase are the risk for skin breakdown during prolonged procedures, or the risk of trauma from a fall if transport cart siderails and safety belts are not used for a patient who is confused, unconscious, or sedated.

Nursing diagnoses are different from medical diagnoses in that medical diagnoses identify specific disease processes, while nursing diagnoses identify the patient's responses to a disease, injury, or situation (Fig. 10-4).

Other differences are that nursing diagnoses focus on the *patient*, not the disease, and that they change as the patient's condition changes, while medical diagnoses usually remain the same during the course of treatment.

A patient may have many nursing diagnoses at any one time. Nursing diagnoses are prioritized by their relative importance for being resolved. For example, a nursing diagnosis of alteration in gas exchange would normally take priority over a nursing diagnosis of knowledge deficit, since gas exchange problems can be life-threatening. New nursing diagnoses are added and prioritized as the patient's health status changes. As new ones are identified, old ones that have been resolved are deleted, thus providing accurate and current data regarding potential or actual problems during the continuing process.

Nursing diagnoses guide and direct independent nursing activities. They may be an expression of a patient's physiologic, psychological, social, developmental, or cultural needs. Table 10-1 lists the current nursing diagnoses approved by the North American Nursing Diagnosis Association (NANDA) as of October 1994.

A nursing diagnosis not only is a statement of the problem, but includes the causative factor. Manifesting data that support the diagnostic statement may also be included. An example of an appropriately worded nursing diagnosis for the perioperative patient is *Pain related to surgical incision*. Manifestations of the nursing diagnosis may include verbal expression, increased pulse, and increased respirations.

Preoperative Nursing Diagnoses

Figure 10-5 includes several nursing diagnoses that may be identified during the preoperative phase. They may also occur during the other phases of the perioperative period.

Additional preoperative nursing diagnoses are related to the specific physical disease or injury process requiring surgical intervention. An example of such a nursing diagnosis might be *Gas exchange, impaired, related to cancer of the lung*. Coexisting medical problems may necessitate additional nursing diagnoses.

Intraoperative Nursing Diagnoses

General factors that may guide the nurse's thinking about the intraoperative patient's nursing diagnoses include the specific procedure being performed, the type of anesthesia being used (i.e., local, general, regional), and the patient's general preoperative health status. Figure 10-6 lists some common nursing diagnoses appropriate for the intraoperative patient.

Additionally, more specific nursing diagnoses may

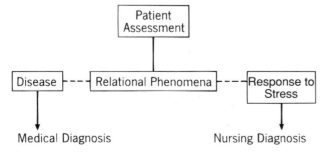

Fig. 10-4. Medical model versus nursing model

Table 10-1   Nursing Diagnoses: North American Nursing Diagnoses Association (NANDA)*

Activity intolerance
  high risk for
Adjustment, impaired
Airway clearance, ineffective
Anxiety
Aspiration, high risk for
Body image disturbance
Body temperature, high risk for alerted
Breastfeeding
  effective
  ineffective
  interrupted
Breathing pattern, ineffective
Cardiac output, decreased
Caregiver role strain
  high risk for
Communication, impaired verbal
Constipation
  clonic
  perceived
Coping
  defensive
  ineffective individual
Decisional conflict (specify)
Denial, ineffective
Diarrhea
Disuse syndrome, high risk for
Diversional activity deficit
Dysreflexia
Family coping
  compromised, ineffective
  disabling, ineffective
  potential for growth
Family processes, altered
Fatigue
Fear
Fluid volume deficit
  high risk for
Fluid volume excess
Gas exchange, impaired
Grieving
  anticipatory
  dysfunctional
Growth and development, altered
Health maintenance, altered
Health-seeking behaviors (specify)
Home maintenance management, impaired
Hopelessness
Hyperthermia
Hypothermia
Incontinence
  bowel
  functional
  reflex
  stress
  total
  urge
Infant feeding pattern, ineffective
Infection, high risk for
Injury, high risk for
Knowledge deficit (specify)

Noncompliance (specify)
Nutrition, altered
  less than body requirements
  more than body requirements
  potential for more than body requirements
Oral mucous membrane, altered
Pain
  chronic
Parental role conflict
Parenting
  altered
  high risk for altered
Peripheral neurovascular dysfunction, high risk for
Personal identity disturbance
Physical mobility, impaired
Poisoning, high risk for
Posttrauma response
Powerlessness
Protection, altered
Rape trauma syndrome
  compound reaction
  silent reaction
Relocation stress syndrome
Role performance, altered
Self-care deficit
  bathing/hygiene
  feeding
  dressing/grooming
  toileting
Self-esteem
  chronic low
  situational low
Self-esteem disturbance
Self-mutilation, high risk for
Sensory-perceptual alterations (specify, visual, auditory,
  kinesthetic, gustatory, tactile, olfactory)
Sexual dysfunction
Sexuality patterns, altered
Skin integrity
  high risk for impaired
  impaired
Sleep pattern disturbance
Social interaction, impaired
Social isolation
Spiritual distress
Suffocation, high risk for
Swallowing, impaired
Therapeutic regimen, ineffective management of
Thermoregulation, ineffective
Thought processes, altered
Tissue integrity, impaired
Tissue perfusion, altered (specify type, renal, cerebral,
  cardiopulmonary, gastrointestinal, peripheral)
Trauma, high risk for
Unilateral neglect
Urinary elimination, altered
Urinary retention
Ventilation, inability to sustain spontaneous
Ventilatory weaning response, dysfunctional
Violence, high risk for
  self-directed or directed at others

* Current as of October 1994.
Adapted from the North American Nursing Diagnosis Association.

be required, depending on the patient's status or the specific surgical procedure.

Fig. 10-5. Possible nursing diagnoses—preoperative phase

Anxiety
- Related to unfamiliar environment
- Related to impending surgery and/or diagnosis

Body image disturbance related to surgical procedure (e.g., mastectomy, amputation, etc.)

Activity intolerance

Decisional conflict related to surgical choices

Anticipatory grieving related to possible changes in body image

Sleep pattern disturbance related to anxiety

High risk for injury-trauma
- Related to sedation
- Skin integrity related to positioning

Knowledge deficit related to
- Sequence of events; perioperative period
- Surgical procedure
- Effective techniques for deep breathing, coughing, turning, and ambulation

Fig. 10-6. Possible nursing diagnoses—intraoperative phase

Hypothermia

High risk for injury-trauma
- Neuromuscular damage related to improper positioning
- Burns related to chemical or electrical hazards
- Nosocomial infection
- Infection related to retention of foreign objects
- Physical hazards

Impaired skin integrity related to
- Surgical incision
- Immobility
- Improper positioning

Fluid volume; deficit or excess, high risk for

Impaired gas exchange related to general anesthesia

High risk for altered tissue perfusion
- Decreased peripheral circulation
- Related to interrupion of flow by outside constricting factors

Decreased cardiac output related to improper positioning and/or anesthesia

Fig. 10-7. Possible nursing diagnoses—immediate postoperative phase

High risk for ineffective airway clearance related to decreased level of consciousness

High risk for infection
- Related to poor incision healing
- Related to inadequate lung expansion
- Related to impaired mobility

Alteration in comfort related to surgical incision

Body image disturbance related to surgery

High risk for injury related to sedation

High risk impaired gas exchange related to incisional pain

Postoperative Nursing Diagnoses

Most potential postoperative patient problems can be identified preoperatively and appropriate interventions planned. Other postoperative patient problems may evolve related to complications of surgery. Some of the common postoperative nursing diagnoses associated with the immediate postoperative phase are listed in Figure 10-7.

The importance of anticipating patient problems and formulating high risk nursing diagnoses during the entire postoperative period cannot be overemphasized. Early recognition of potential problems and early intervention can provide the patient with a smooth postoperative course and swift recovery. Nursing diagnoses therefore are the judgment statements that reflect the patient problems as identified by the assessment data. They then become the foundation upon which to develop a plan for patient care and specific nursing interventions.

Regardless of their format, nursing diagnoses must be documented to enhance communication between health-care providers.

PLANNING

Planning is the third phase of the nursing process, and involves cooperation between the nurse, the patient, the patient's support systems, and other health-care providers involved in the patient's care. Planning involves the establishment of specific goals and/or outcome criteria for the individual patient.

Some important points to remember about patient outcome criteria are:

1. Patient outcome goals are patient-focused; that is, they state clearly what the patient will be able to do.
2. Patient outcomes are the observable and measurable physiologic and psychological responses to planned nursing interventions.
3. Outcome criteria include an expected time of accomplishment or completion.

General patient care standards, developed by specialty organizations, provide guidelines for judgments concerning patient responses.

The AORN identifies six patient outcome standards for perioperative nursing (1995), which have been derived from Standard III of the Standards of Clinical Practice, and state: Patient outcomes are derived from nursing diagnoses and direct the interventions to correct, alter, or maintain the nursing diagnoses.[6] These outcome standards focus on potential high-incidence problem areas of the surgical patient, including absence of infection, maintenance of skin integrity, absence of adverse effects, maintenance of fluid and electrolyte balance, knowledge by the patient and significant others of the physiologic and psychological responses to surgical intervention, and participation by the patient and significant others in the rehabilitation process.

Each of these outcome standards have specific criteria to assist the perioperative nurse in determining whether the standards have been met, but it is the individual nurse's responsibility to adapt, modify, and add outcome criteria that are appropriate to the individual patient's situation.

Documenting the Care Plan

Most institutions still require a patient care plan to be completed for each patient. These care plans serve as a guide for managing and directing patient care. The Joint Commission for Health Care Organizations (JCAHO) currently requires written, outcome-directed care plans to indicate that quality patient care, according to acceptable standards, has been administered to all patients.

Patient care plans should contain the following elements (Fig. 10-8):

1. What nursing actions are to be performed.
2. How the nursing actions are to be performed.
3. When the nursing actions are to be performed.
4. Where the nursing actions are to be performed.
5. Who is to perform these actions.

IMPLEMENTATION (INTERVENTION)

Implementation, the fourth phase of the nursing process, takes place only after thoughtful planning has taken place.

According to the AORN Standards of Clinical Practice, **Standard V** states: The perioperative nurse implements the interventions identified in the plan of care.[7] As with all aspects of the nursing process, interventions are documented and communicated to appropriate personnel.

During implementation, the nurse continues to assess the patient's responses to surgical/medical treatment and nursing care.

Included among nursing interventions for the perioperative patient are promotion of physical and psy-chological comfort, support of cardiopulmonary function, promotion of safety, promotion of skin integrity, support of elimination functions, maintenance of fluid and electrolyte balance, promotion of nutrition, personal hygiene care, functional rehabilitation, and education of the patient, family, and significant others who are part of the patient's support system. Implementation includes all the nursing interventions directed toward resolving the patient's nursing diagnoses.

Nursing interventions are those activities carried out by the nurse to assist the patient to achieve the outcome criteria. Nursing interventions may be *independent, interdependent* (collaborative), or *dependent,* and may be written in the form of *protocols* (Fig. 10-9).

Independent nursing interventions are activities the perioperative nurse institutes based on her or his own judgment; that is, a physician's order is not required (e.g., conducting a sponge count at specified intervals during the procedure).

Interdependent or collaborative interventions are activities performed jointly with another health-care provider (e.g., physician, perfusionist, etc.) or instituted after a decision made by the nurse with another health-care provider (e.g., positioning the patient with the physician's assistant [PA] and/or RN first assistant [RNFA]).

Dependent interventions are those that require physician direction either in the form of a written order, direct supervision, or standard protocols. Implementation includes all the nursing interventions that are directed toward resolving the patient's nursing diagnoses (e.g., specific instruments requested by the surgeon for a selected case or blood administration directed by the anesthesia practitioner).

Characteristics of Nursing Interventions

Examples of interventions that can be related to each phase of the perioperative period include, preoperative, intraoperative, and postoperative intervention.

Preoperative

Preoperative interventions are primarily directed toward preparing the patient for the proposed surgical intervention, including

- Patient and family education
- Patient preparation, including care of preexisting health problems
- Obtaining required baseline assessment data, laboratory and diagnostic work, and consent for surgical procedures

STANDARD OF CARE STATEMENTS ON
PATIENTS WITH: ___Cesarean Section___

OUTCOME STANDARDS	Date Met & R.N. Int.
1. The patient will recover without infection.	
2. The patient will verbalize/demonstrate desire for independence through post-op activities.	

SUBJECT HEADINGS / POTENTIAL CARE PROBLEMS	Initiated		NURSING INTERVENTIONS	Discontinued	
	Date	R.N.		Date	R.N.
1. Anxiety related to unfamiliar environment, loss of the birthing experience and/or impending surgery.			1. A. Assess patient and family knowledge base of procedure upon admission. B. Explain procedures in understandable terms prior to performing. C. Allow time for questions and clarifying information.		
2. High risk for injury, related to improper positioning on operating table.			2. A. Place safety strap above knees over blanket. B. Align extremities in anatomical position. C. Assess for pressure points by checking circulation after positioning. D. Provide anesthesia with free access to airway and IV lines.		
3. High risk for impaired skin integrity, related to improper placement of electrosurgical ground pack.			3. A. Position ground pack away from bony prominences. B. Check all connections prior to activities. C. Assess site after pack is removed and document.		
4. High risk for infection, related to surgical incision and procedure.			4. A. Insert and maintain foley catheter per policy at all times. B. Perform sponge, needle and instrument counts prior to, during and after procedure per policy. C. Perform abdominal prep per policy prior to surgery. D. Maintain aseptic technique throughout the operation. E. Apply sterile dressing to incision before sterile field is broken. F. Document		
5. High risk for fluid imbalance related to NPO status and loss of body fluids.			5. A. Assess IV fluid, rate and site prior to and following procedure. B. Request estimated blood loss from surgeon, after procedure. C. Assess urine output prior to and following procedure D. Assess uterine clots and tone following procedure. E. Document		
6. Alteration in body temperature, decreased related to surgical exposure.			6. A. Assess temperature upon admission and following surgery. B. Expose only surgical area during procedure. C. Place warm blankets on patient at end of procedure D. Record and report deviations from normal.		
7. Knowledge deficit, related to surgical procedure and separation from family.			7. A. Instruct patient in turn, cough and deep breathing techniques prior to surgery. B. Inform patient's family when surgery has begun. C. Allow family to view infant prior to transport to nursery D. Inform family when patient may be seen in Recovery Room.		

Fig. 10-8.   Example of standards of care—intraoperative phase "C" section (Courtesy of the Broward General Medical Center, Ft. Lauderdale, FL, 1992)

TITLE: Electrosurgical Safety Management .... Protocol for

PURPOSE: To provide information relating to the safe and effective use of the electrosurgical unit (ESU) and its components during a surgical procedure.

Supplemental Data: 1) <u>Dispersive Electrode:</u> The accessory item that directs current flow from the patient back to the generator (ground pad).

2) <u>Active Electrode:</u> The accessory which directs current flow to operative site (pencils, with various types of tips, bi-polar forceps, rectoscopes, fulgeration tips, etc.).

LEVEL: Independant.

CONTENT AREA

Key Words

Initial Inspection

1) Prior to initial use, the ESU should be inspected and tested by the BioMedical Department.
2) Each ESU is assigned an ID number and current inspection sticker.
3) Each component of the ESU is inspected (foot pedal, connectors, alarm connectors, etc.).
4) Each ESU is mounted on a stand that will not "tip" and can be easily cleaned and is moveable.

Per Case Inspection

5) Prior to each use of the ESU, the Circulating Nurse inspects and tests the unit.
   a) electrical plug/outlets
   b) connectors
   c) foot switch control
   d) alarms (sound activated)
   e) lights
6) If the ESU is not working to 100% efficiency, it is removed from the procedure room and returned to the BioMedical Department for further testing/inspection.

Dispersive Electrode

7) The dispersive electrode (ground pad) cord should be of adequate length and flexibility to reach the positioned patient without stress on any connection.
8) The dispersive electrode pad is placed on the patient following positioning procedure.
   a) clean, dry skin
   b) over a large muscle mass
   c) close to operative site as possible without interference
   d) avoid bony prominences, metal implants, monitoring leads
9) The dispersive electrode must maintain uniform body contact and must be rechecked should repositioning be required.
10) The dispersive electrode site is documented on the intraoperative record.
11) At the conclusion of the surgical procedure, the site is inspected and condition of patient's skin is documented on the intraoperative record.

Active Electrode

12) The active electrode (hand piece) should be inspected at the sterile field by the scrub person for damage before use.
13) The reusable active electrode should be inspected for damage before each processing, and be periodically inspected by the BioMedical Department for conductive electrical damage.
14) The active electrode cord should be adequate in length and flexible to reach operative site and generator without stress.
15) During the procedure, the active electrode should be placed in a clean, dry, non-conductive and highly visable area to prevent accidental activation.
16) The active electrode cord should be impervious to fluids and the tips placed securely in the electrode handle.
17) Periodic cleaning of the tips should be employed to remove charred tissue.

Fig. 10-9. Example of nursing protocol—intraoperative phase, electrosurgical safety (Courtesy of the Broward General Medical Center, Ft. Lauderdale, FL, 1992)

Intraoperative

Interventions during the intraoperative phase are generally directed to providing a safe environment and protecting the patient from injury. As all members of the surgical team are present, the patient care provided is generally of a collaborative nature, with each member assuming responsibility for predetermined activities, including

- Performance in the scrub person's role
- Performance in the circulating nurse's role
- Management of personnel, materials, and environment
- Maintenance of a safe, aseptic environment

Although the responsibilities of the scrub and circulating nurses may seem to be a series of tasks, it is

```
┌─────────────────────────────────────────────────────────────────────────────┐
│    Electrosurgical Safety Management              PAGE _2_ OF _2_             │
├─────────────────────────────────────────────────────────────────────────────┤
│                                                                               │
│                      18)  If the active electrode does not function properly, │
│                           it should be removed and                            │
│                           a) sent to BioMedical Department (reusable)          │
│                           b) saved for product inspection by manufacturer      │
│  Termination of Use  19)  At the conclusion of the procedure, the ESU should  │
│                           be cleaned, cords properly stored, and unit moved    │
│                           to an area out of traffic within the procedure room. │
│                                                                               │
│                                                                               │
│                                                                               │
│  APPROVAL:                                                                    │
│          Standards / Protocol Council: _____        │
│          Nurse Practice Council: _____          │
│          Council of Directors: _____          │
│  REVIEW / REVISION: _____                                │
│  REFERENCE:  A.O.R.N. Standards & Recommended Practices - Perioperative        │
│              Nursing (1990) pp. III: 5 1-5                                     │
│  DISTRIBUTION:   Standards / Protocol Manual ....                              │
│                  - Department of Surgery                                       │
│                  - Labor & Delivery                                           │
│                                                                               │
└─────────────────────────────────────────────────────────────────────────────┘
```

Fig. 10-9. *(continued)*

important to remember that they are interventions based on professional judgment aimed at maintaining the goals of patient safety, keeping the patient free from harm and infection, and assuring optimal recovery.

Postoperative

Postoperative interventions are directed toward preventing infection, promoting optimal healing, and preventing complications, both during the *immediate* and *intermediate* phases of recovery. Some of the activities related to this phase include

- Monitoring and evaluating the patient's status
- Managing patient care, including pain, fluid status, cardiopulmonary status, and positioning
- Assessing nutritional status and needs
- Providing rehabilitation, counseling, and emotional support

The specific interventions for every surgical patient are too numerous to list here, and so the reader is referred to the subsequent chapters in this text in addition to medical–surgical or standard care plan books to obtain more information about nursing interventions for specific surgical procedures.

The nurse is responsible for implementing sufficient and appropriate interventions to achieve the identified patient outcomes related to the established nursing diagnoses, with the ultimate goal: providing quality patient care.

EVALUATION

Standard VI of the AORN Standards of Clinical Practice states that: *The perioperative nurse evaluates the patient's progress toward attainment of outcomes.*[8] Evaluation, the last phase of the nursing process, is the basis for modifications to the overall plan of care. During evaluation, the nurse compares the patient's postintervention status with the expected outcomes or outcome criteria. This phase includes communication with the patient, other health-care providers, and the patient's family and significant others to determine the patient's postintervention health status and to identify resolved, ongoing, or new problems. Evaluation findings are also communicated through written documentation on the patient's record.

The nurse documents patient progress toward the attainment of expected outcomes in the patient's record, on the patient's care plan, and on other appropriate forms consistent with the policies of the institution. Communication of evaluation findings with the patient, the patient's family, and significant others may be done verbally or in writing depending on the policies of the institution and the judgment of the patient's physician and nurse.

Evaluation is a systematic and continuous process, and evaluation is therefore the last step, as well as the first step, in ongoing care planning. The criteria used to achieve this standard are based on observation of patient responses. The patients, their family and significant others, and other health-care providers are involved in the evaluation process when appropriate.

Evaluation must be conducted in an organized way, looking first at each nursing diagnosis, the prescribed patient outcomes, and the patient's level of accomplishment for each expected outcome.

If the patient outcome is that he or she will be free of infection, the nurse would look at whether or not he or she has any infectious problems or complications associated with an infection. If the wound is clean, but the patient has developed a postoperative pneumonia, the nurse would maintain the existing care plan relative to the incision, and develop a more aggressive plan of care with specific interventions related to the nursing diagnosis altered gas exchange to resolve the postoperative pneumonia.

Generalized outcome criteria, developed by the AORN, have been mentioned earlier in the planning section of this chapter.

Assessment and evaluation are interlocking steps of the nursing process, leading the nurse through the cycle in a repeated fashion until the patient has returned to optimal health.

Assessment, diagnosis, planning, implementation (intervention), and *evaluation,* the heart of nursing practice, have become an important aspect in the management of patient care during the perioperative period. By integrating the steps of the nursing process with nursing activities performed in the perioperative role, the nurse ensures the continuous provision of quality patient care.

PATIENT CARE PLANS FOR THE PERIOPERATIVE PERIOD

A plan of care could be described as a portrait of a patient's surgical experience, and describes the nursing interventions the patient needs to attain the expected outcome.

There are a number of proposed formats for care plans, ranging from individual documents in kardex form to those incorporated into the operative record, but they have one common factor; they must be flexible and be individualized to meet the specific needs of the patient.

Joint Commission: Statement of Quality

Before 1987, nursing service activities and interventions directed toward assuring quality of care relating to perioperative nursing practice were part of the Nursing Service chapter of the Joint Commission Accreditation Manual.

In 1988, through joint efforts of the AORN and the commission, a separate chapter was introduced entitled *Surgical and Anesthesia Services,* which became the evaluation tool that would help to establish the minimal acceptable criteria for this specialized area of practice. In 1994, JCAHO revised its accreditation procedure and created standards that focus on process. The standards appropriate to perioperative nursing and patient care are contained in Section 1: Care of Patients, subsection Operative and Other Invasive Procedures.[9] The standards in this section focus on providing operative and other invasive procedures necessary for: (1) diagnosis; (2) cure or palliation of disease, impairment, or disability; (3) restoration or improvement of function; and (4) relief of symptoms. The processes described in the standards which relate to nursing are: (1) preparing the patient for the procedure, (2) performing the procedure and monitoring the patient, and (3) providing postprocedure care.

The Operative and Other Invasive Procedures subsection makes the following recommendations:

> Standard TX.5.3. The plans of care for the patient are formulated and documented in the patient's medical record before the procedure(s) is performed and include at least:
> TX.5.3.1. a plan for nursing care
> TX.5.3.2. a plan for the operative or invasive procedure
> TX.5.3.3. a plan for the level of postprocedure care
> TX.5.3.4. an assessment of the need for additional diagnostic data
> TX.5.3.5. an initial assessment of the patient relative to the acuity of needs to determine the appropriate level of postprocedure care
> TX.5.3.6. an initial assessment of the patient's physical, mental, and neurologic status and needs.

Additionally, TX.5.4 identifies standards related to the patient's postprocedure period requiring monitoring of: (1) the patient's physiologic and mental status, (2) pathologic findings, (3) IV fluids and drugs administered, including blood and blood components, (4) any unusual events or postoperative complications and the management of those events or complications, and (5) the patient's impairments and functional status.

The process of developing a care plan that meets the needs of the individual and institutional criteria has become an on going process; one that is still evolving, and although the format or type is not specified in the Joint Commission Manual, the care plan should be integrated with the AORN patient outcome standards, and contain certain key elements:

1. The plan should reflect coordination with the overall plan of medical care.
2. The plan should include actions that will ensure maximum physical and emotional safety and security for the patient during the intraoperative period.
3. The plan should be based on both scientific knowledge and patient information derived during the preoperative assessment, and be therapeutically effective.
4. The plan should reflect the immediate health and emotional needs of the patient having surgery and should include long-term planning in order to help the patient achieve or maintain optimum health status.
5. The plan should include patient–family preparation in the rehabilitation process, including self-care and discharge planning.
6. The plan should reflect and/or include outcome goals revised to meet the individual patient needs.

CREATING STANDARDIZED CARE PLANS

Planning for perioperative nursing care is an ongoing process, and documentation for planning individualized patient care is mandated by the Joint Commission.

Although an individualized care plan must be developed, the format, or *style*, of the care plan has never been specified, only that the components reflect the nursing process: assessment, planning, implementation, and evaluation.

Standards of Care

Throughout this chapter we have referred to the *AORN Standards of Practice* as the basis for implementing perioperative nursing care. Now, let's discuss the concept of how these practices can be reflected in the planning of patient care.

First, what is the difference between *standards of practice* and *standards of care?* The major difference lies in the terms *practice* and *care*.

A standard refers to a criterion used by general agreement to decide exactly what something should be or how it should be expressed (performed). It is considered to be a recognized level of safe and effective performance. Therefore, a standard of practice defines how the nurse should practice (perform) his or her designated role and is usually predetermined by a national, state, or specialty organization involved with the practice of nursing, such as the ANA, AORN, or the Nurse Practice Act for a particular state.

For perioperative nursing, the standards of practice form the basis for acceptable or recommended nursing practice during the three phases of surgical intervention.

Standards of *care*, however, are different. According to Marker,[10] Standards of Care define the level of practice that directly relates to the quality of care a patient receives. They are developed through a *systematic* approach, which uses a hierarchical structure to define and delineate nursing practice, referred to as the *Marker Model for Standard Development* (1988).

In this model, Marker refers to three types of standards: *structure, process,* and *outcome*,[11] and in order to use the model effectively, the nurse must be aware of how these standards impact the practice of nursing. Therefore, a brief description of each standard will be presented.

Structure Standards

Structure standards form the basis for all activity within a given institution. They describe how the system operates and the mechanisms needed to operate that system; for example, standards applicable to the department of nursing within the hospital, or how a specific nursing unit operates within the department.

Process Standards

In contrast, *process standards* define the actions or behaviors used to provide care to the patient, and the criteria for performing that care effectively, safely, and proficiently. Examples include the *position description of the RN, procedures used for nursing care,* and *standard care plans* that reflect the planning and management of the nursing care provided.

Outcome Standards

Outcome standards are the end result of nursing intervention, and are expressed either as what the nurse should accomplish (nursing goals) or what the patient should be able to do (patient outcomes). Examples include patient outcomes and nursing goals related to patient teaching or the planning of patient care.

Standards of care, then, according to the Marker model, are the highest level of process standards,[12] since they represent a written plan of care developed to assist the nurse in providing effective nursing care.

Standards of care can be created in two different

styles, depending on the type of patient and/or the area involved with the care of the patient.

For patients requiring hospitalization for 48 hours or longer, the Marker model recommends the use of a *standard care plan (SCP)*, which provides for periodic evaluation of the patient's progress and the care given to accomplish the patient outcome goals listed. However, since some areas are a transitional area, where patients are only in the area for a short period of time (less than 48 hours), the Marker model recommends the use of the *standard care statement (SCS)* as a means for describing the nursing care provided.[13] As always, it is up to the individual facility to create its own model for patient care.

DOCUMENTING THE CARE PLAN

Regardless of the format, a standard care statement uses a two-column approach to documentation; a *subject heading/patient problem* column and a *nursing interventions* column. The patient outcome statements are not written for each problem, as when using the standard care plan, but represent the three domains of individuality: cognitive (self-care), psychological (coping mechanisms), and physiologic (body).

AORN's Patient Outcome Standards[14] can serve as an excellent source for creating standardized care plans for the surgical patient. For example:

Standard I   The patient demonstrates knowledge of the physiologic and psychological responses to surgical intervention.
Related Nursing Diagnoses/Patient Problem:
- Anxiety related to lack of knowledge of surgical procedure
- Fear related to risk of death, alteration of body image, or change in lifestyle

Standard II   The patient is free from infection.
Related Nursing Diagnoses/Patient Problem:
- High risk for infection related to:
    type of operative procedure
    wound classification
    length of procedure

Standard III   The patient's skin integrity is maintained.
Related Nursing Diagnoses/Patient Problem:
- High risk for skin impairment related to:
    diabetes
    obesity
    immobility

Standard IV   The patient is free from injury related to positioning; extraneous objects; or chemical, physical, and electrical hazards.
Related Nursing Diagnoses/Patient Problem:
- High risk for injury related to:
    electrical hazards
    positioning
    nosocomial infection
- Impaired gas exchange related to:
    positioning
    inadequate airway

Standard V   The patient's fluid and electrolyte balance is maintained.
Related Nursing Diagnoses/Patient Problem:
- Fluid volume deficit related to hemorrhage, diuresis, medications
- Alteration in tissue perfusion

Standard VI   The patient participates in the rehabilitation process.
Related Nursing Diagnoses/Patient Problem:
- Activity intolerance related to results of surgery
- Alteration in comfort related to incision pain

It is highly recommended that care plans should be preprinted, individualized, and used for the duration of the patient's stay, although the standard care plan will be reviewed and revised as needed.

It is obvious, then, that the utilization of a specific format or model offers an innovative method for organizing and defining the standards of care. By standardizing and differentiating the variety of activities performed by the perioperative nurse for the benefit of quality patient care, this systematic approach can individualize a plan of care, using the standards of practice. In addition to the accurate documentation on the intraoperative record, the care plan creates a comprehensive picture of how the patient's care was planned and executed during the perioperative period, and the patient's response to that intervention (see Fig. 10-9).

Other types of care plans can be used, besides the Marker model, that will accomplish the same goal, though not in the same way.

For example, a care plan could be designed around a specific procedure, position, patient outcome, or a specific nursing diagnosis, using a generic concept for design, and modifying the plan as needed to fit the individual patient.

The specific type of care plan designed should enable the perioperative nurse to plan the patient's care effectively, using the nursing process format for generic terminology and the perioperative standards of practice, patient outcome standards, and competency statements as a basis for the implementation and evaluation of the plan.

By combining the appropriate model for patient care planning with precise documentation, routine nursing care activities are identified and a foundation for nursing action can be evaluated.

The patient care plan should be referred to on the intraoperative nurse's notes, since most "care plans"

Table 10-2 Standard Perioperative Nursing Care Plan: Intraoperative Phase

Nursing Diagnoses	Expected Outcome	Nursing Interventions	Evaluation
1. Anxiety related to: impending surgical procedure knowledge deficit: sequence of events	1a. Patient verbalizes anxiety to perioperative nurse before surgery 1b. Patient verbalizes and/or demonstrates decreased anxiety	1. Assess current knowledge of sequence of events 2. Instruct patient as to sequence of events: pre-, intra-, postoperative 3. Allow patient/family to verbalize fears, anxieties, concerns 4. Remain with patient as much as possible 5. Communicate to appropriate personnel patient's concerns, anxieties, unresolved questions 6. Offer emotional support as needed 7. Document teaching, patient's responses on appropriate forms	
2. High risk for injury to musculoskeletal and/or neurologic systems related to transfer, moving, lifting, positioning, and/or length of procedure	2. Patient will not experience injuries, falls, redness, bruises, or evidence of skin abrasions before, during, after surgery	1. Assess skin preoperatively and document condition 2. Keep side rails up on bed/stretcher during transport 3. Lift or roll patient with adequate help when transferring or moving 4. Pad pressure points and bony prominences. Check for adequate protection 5. Place patient in proper body alignment and position 6. Assess skin condition after surgery 7. Document findings and procedures used to ensure safety measures have been met	
3. Potential for loss of privacy/dignity related to physical exposure and/or disclosure of confidential information	3. Patient will not experience loss of dignity. Confidentiality will be maintained	1. Prep patient in private area avoiding any undue exposure 2. Expose only area needed for adequate skin prep 3. Limit traffic of personnel 4. Make chart available to only authorized personnel 5. Limit discussion of patient to information pertinent to surgical procedure and current patient status	
4. Potential impairment of skin integrity related to: pooling of prep solutions, improper placement of electrosurgical ground pad, unprotected pressure points	4. Patient will not experience unusual impairment of skin integrity. Absence of redness, bruises, abrasions; blisters and/or burns	1. Assess for allergies before skin prep 2. Place towels along skin edges of prep site to absorb excess solution and remove when prep is completed 3. Use minimum amount of solution on prep sponges to avoid excess solution pooling under patient 4. Correctly position ground pad avoiding bony areas and tenting 5. Pad all unprotected/bony areas 6. Assess skin after procedure and document findings on operative record	
5. High risk for injury related to retained foreign objects associated with surgical procedure	5. Patient will be absent of all foreign objects: sponges needles instruments	1. Count and document all sponges, needles, and instruments according to established protocols 2. Count and document additional items used during surgery 3. Take and record counts during relieves and at change of shift 4. Verbally confirm counts with physician 5. Report immediately any incidents or incorrect counts. Take appropriate actions	

(continued)

Table 10-2 *(continued)*

Nursing Diagnoses	Expected Outcome	Nursing Interventions	Evaluation
6. Potential alteration in body temperature related to: fluids, anesthesia, surgical exposure	6. Patient's body temperature will remain within normal parameters	1. Place hyperthermic blanket on OR table prn. Record temperature at regular intervals 2. Limit patient's physical exposure before and during procedure 3. Use warm blankets postoperatively 4. Provide anesthesia with blood warmers prn 5. Provide warmed irrigation solutions	
7. High risk for fluid and electrolyte imbalance related to blood loss or shift of body fluids and electrolytes	7. Patient's body fluid and electrolyte balance will be maintained	1. Monitor and record intake and output 2. Estimate blood loss on sponges in suction containers. Report estimated losses to appropriate personnel 3. Assess availability of blood and blood products. Record type of blood and blood products used 4. Record type and amount of irrigation used during surgery	
8. High risk for infection related to: wound contamination; break in aseptic technique; catheters, tubes, and drains	8. No evidence of contamination of sterile field, wound, invasive lines, tubes, or drains	1. Ensure aseptic environment through procedure. Correct any breaks in technique 2. Record breaks in technique and corrective actions taken 3. Follow prescribed sterile procedures for insertion of catheters, tubes, and drains 4. Determine and record CDC Wound Classification	
9. High risk for injury related to: positioning immobility	9. Patient will not experience injury related to positioning and/ or immobility	1. Assess patient before surgery 2. Position patient using proper alignment and adequate padding 3. Assess areas at risk during and after surgery. Record findings 4. Document positioning devices used and patient's physical response 5. Use floatation devices (egg crates, gel pads, etc.) prn	
10. Potential alteration in tissue perfusion and/or peripheral circulation related to: external constricting factors, prolonged immobility, hypothermia	10. Patient will not experience cardiovascular compromise or decreased tissue perfusion	1. Place body in proper alignment 2. Apply restraints without compromise to circulation 3. Apply antiembolitic hose prn 4. Utilize hyperthermic blankets 5. Apply tourniquet cuff on limb with adequate padding. Monitor limb and tourniquet pressure according to protocols 6. Use warmed solutions (blood and irrigation and IVs) as needed	

Source: Adapted from NANDA: Nursing diagnoses: Definitions and classification, 1995–1996. Philadelphia: NANDA. 1994.

are not part of the patient's permanent record. For example:

```
Standard Care Plan Followed?
Yes ☐   No ☐   If no, list exceptions:
```

Table 10-2 represents an example of a standardized care plan that could be used during the intraoperative period.

CRITICAL PATHWAYS

More recently, critical pathways have been developed as guidelines for multidisciplinary coordinating, plan-

Table 10-3 **Critical Pathway for Client Following Laparoscopic Cholecystectomy***

	DATE _____ Preoperative	DATE _____ First 24 h following surgery
Daily outcomes	Client verbalizes understanding of preoperative teaching including: turning, coughing, deep breathing, incentive spirometer, mobilization, and pain management Client verbalizes ability to cope	Client is afebrile Client has a dry, clean wound with edges well-approximated, healing by first intention Client manages pain with non-pharmacologic measures or oral medications Client is independent in self-care Client is fully ambulatory Client has resumed preadmission urine and bowel elimination pattern Client verbalizes home care instructions Client tolerates usual diet Client verbalizes ability to cope with ongoing stressors
Tests and treatments	CBC Urinalysis Baseline physical assessment: with a focus on respiratory status and gastrointestinal function Anesthesia consult	Vital signs and O_2 saturation, neurovascular assessment, dressing and wound drainage assessment q15 min × 4; q30 min × 4; q1h × 4 and then q4h if stable. Assess lung sounds and gastrointestinal function q4h and pm. Intake and output every shift Assess voiding—if unable to void, try suggestive voiding techniques or catheterize q8h or pm if unable to void
Knowledge deficit	Orient to room and surroundings Provide simple, brief instructions Review preoperative preparation including hospital and surgical routines Reinforce preoperative teaching regarding specific postoperative care: turning, coughing, deep breathing, incentive spirometer, mobilization, and pain management	Reorient to room and postoperative routine Review plan of care and importance of early mobilization Begin discharge teaching regarding wound care/dressing change
Psychosocial	Assess anxiety related to pending surgery Assess fears of the unknown and surgery Encourage verbalization of concerns Provide information regarding surgical experience Minimize external stimuli (e.g., noise, movement)	Assess level of anxiety Encourage verbalization of concerns Provide information and ongoing support and encouragement
Diet	NPO Baseline nutritional assessment	Advance to clear liquids, if tolerated advance to full liquids/soft diet morning following surgery
Activity	OOB ad lib until premedicated for surgery	Provide safety precautions Bathroom privileges with assistance evening after surgery and begin progressive ambulation to tolerance the morning following surgery until fully ambulatory
Medications	NPO except ordered medications	IM or PO analgesics Antibiotics if ordered IV fluids until adequate PO intake then intermittent IV device Discontinue before discharge
Transfer/ discharge plans	Assess discharge plans and support system	Probable discharge within 24 h of surgery Complete discharge home care teaching when fully awake and oriented and before discharge Provide a written copy of discharge instructions

* Expected length of stay: less than 24 hours.
Adapted from Kozier, B, Erb G, and Wilkinson, J. *Fundamentals of Nursing: Concepts, Process, and Practice*. Redwood City, CA: Addison-Wesley, 1995.

ning, and documenting of patient care. Critical pathways are also called critical paths, multidisciplinary action plans, and action plans. Members of the institution's health-care team collaborate to develop critical pathways for specific medical/surgical diagnoses that occur with frequency. The goals of critical pathways are: (1) to achieve realistic, expected patient and family outcomes, (2) to promote professional and collaborative practice and care, (3) to ensure continuity of care, (4) to guarantee appropriate use of resources, (5) to reduce costs and length of stay, and (6) to provide a framework for continuous quality improvement.[15] According to Kozier et al., the overall goal of critical pathways is "to improve the quality and proficiency of patient care by designing pathways that facilitate a reproducible standard of care for specific patient populations."[16] Many agencies are replacing nursing care plans with critical pathways as they provide for collaborative care, are outcome-driven, and provide a time line, consistent with DRG standards, to achieve the predetermined goals. An example of a critical pathway for a same day surgery patient is provided in Table 10-3.

Self-assessment Exercise 1

Directions: Complete the following exercises. The answers are given at the end of this module.

1. List three assessment methods used for collection of data.

   1. _____

   2. _____

   3. _____

2. Write a Patient Outcome Goal for the following Nursing Diagnosis: Impaired skin integrity.

   _____

3. Match the Nursing Diagnosis with the corresponding patient condition.

   1. __ restriction interfering with movement   A. sensory perception alterations

   2. __ disorientation to time/place   B. alteration in comfort

   3. __ increased respiratory pulse rate, and verbalization   C. impaired skin integrity

   4. __ complains of pain/ discomfort   D. impaired mobility

   E. moderate anxiety

4. Medical and nursing diagnoses identify potential as well as actual health problems.

   True   False

5. *Limit exposure to only that which is necessary* would be a nursing intervention for which Nursing Diagnosis?

References

1. AORN. Standards and recommended practices. Denver: The Association, 1995. P. 70.
2. AORN. Standards and recommended practices. Denver: The Association, 1995. P. 97.
3. Ibid, pp. 107–109.
4. Ibid, p. 107.
5. Carpenito LJ. Nursing care plans and documentation: Nursing diagnoses and collaborative problems. (2nd ed.). Philadelphia: J.B. Lippincott, 1995. P. 43.
6. AORN. 1995. P. 108.
7. Ibid, p. 109.
8. Ibid, p. 109.
9. AHA. Accreditation manual for hospitals. Chicago: Joint Commission of Accreditation of Health Care Organizations, 1994. Pp. 160–166.
10. Marker CGS. Setting standards for professional nursing: The Marker model. St. Louis: Mosby, 1988. P. 4.
11. Ibid.
12. Ibid. Using the Marker model: Developing guidelines and standards of care in the OR. *O.R. Manager*, 4: 1988.
13. Rothrock JC. Perioperative nursing care planning. St. Louis: Mosby, 1990. Pp. 29, 30.
14. AORN. 1995. Pp. 125–126.
15. Kozier B, Erb G, Blais K, and Wilkinson J. Fundamentals of nursing: Concepts, process, and practice. Redwood City, CA: Addison-Wesley 1995. Pp. 75–77.
16. Ibid op. cit., p. 14.

11 Patient Care Management

THE PERIOPERATIVE NURSE'S ROLE: MANAGING PATIENT CARE

The traditional nursing roles of patient advocate and health-care teacher have assumed new importance in today's health-care climate, and this change has affected all areas of nursing practice.

During the early days of surgery, the nurse's role was primarily that of an assistant to the surgeon. It included such activities as maintaining an aseptic environment, passing instruments, and other general nonnursing tasks, with little direct contact or involvement with the patient either before, during, or after surgery.

Today, the perioperative nurse practices his or her specialty during all three phases of surgical intervention in an expanded role: that of (1) caregiver, (2) patient advocate, (3) leader, (4) research consumer, and (5) teacher. The combination of these roles results in effective management of patient care during the perioperative period.

As the primary *caregiver* during the intraoperative phase, the perioperative nurse uses acquired knowledge and skills related to the surgical experience, which encompass the management of supplies, equipment, and personnel, in addition to providing psychological support to the patient, family, and significant others.

As a *patient advocate,* the perioperative nurse assures a safe, therapeutic environment by maintaining the standards of practice associated with nursing care during the perioperative period. As the primary manager of patient care, the nurse's role encompasses patient safety, comfort, and an acute awareness of the surroundings. In no other setting is this role of a patient advocate more challenging, since the patient relies on the surgical team to meet physiologic as well as psychosocial needs.

The professional nurse in the operating room is responsible and accountable for actions relating to patient care. The perioperative nurse must ensure that the informed consent, given by the patient, has not been violated, since the surgical patient may be unable to take action on his or her own behalf, and relies on others for protection from harm.

As a *leader,* the perioperative nurse projects a positive role model to other members of the health-care team by remaining current in all areas of clinical practice. By focusing on the professional role of the perioperative nurse, and motivating others, the perioperative nurse can assist others to grow and develop their professional skills.

As a *research consumer,* the perioperative nurse is seeking to expand his or her knowledge relating to practice and materials (products). This knowledge is based on scientific investigation and research, in order to eliminate outdated methods, equipment, and traditions while maintaining a cost-effective work setting.

And finally, as a *teacher,* the perioperative nurse is involved with the education of not only the patient and family, but also colleagues, students, and society in general, in the hope of elevating the conceptual role of a "technical nurse" to a "patient-oriented" nurse involved with all aspects of care during the perioperative period (see Fig. 1-2).

A Practice Model for Perioperative Nursing Practice

Over the past decade there has been an explosion of interest and activity in the nursing profession toward the establishment of a theoretical basis for nursing practice. The incorporation of a theoretical-based practice model for perioperative nursing can assist in representing the unique practice of the perioperative nurse in today's complex health-care setting.

Several nursing theories can be used to further describe the practice of perioperative nursing. Dorothea Orem's Theory of Nursing Systems,[1] the third theory in her self-care deficit theory, most clearly adapts to the basic assumptions and concepts related to the definition and practice of perioperative nursing. The perioperative nursing practice model depicts the integration of perioperative nursing practice concepts and Orem's Nursing Systems Theory.

Conceptual Framework: PNPM

Orem's Self-Care Deficit Theory of Nursing utilizes several concepts as a means to plan and manage nursing activities. This general theory of nursing consists of three interrelated theories. These theories are: (1) Theory of Self-Care, (2) Theory of Self-Care Deficits, and (3) Nursing Systems Theory.[2] The first two theories describe the object of nursing and provide the basis for developing nursing outcomes.[3] The Nursing Systems Theory describes the nursing actions that will help promote the other two systems. The Perioperative Nursing Practice Model (PNPM) focuses on the Nursing Systems Theory, since this theory represents the focal point of nursing practice during the perioperative period.

According to Orem,[4] nursing systems are dynamic actions created by the nurse that occur as a result of deliberate nursing interaction between the nurse and the person (patient, family, community). The goal of this system is to help the person meet his or her own therapeutic self-care demands (i.e., independence, responsibility for self-care).

The Nursing Systems Theory utilizes the nursing process, although labeled differently, as a means to assess, plan, and manage nursing care activities. The first phase, labeled *diagnosis and prescription,* enables the nurse to acquire information and make professional judgments about the existing situation and status of the client. Prescription is the decision or conclusion about the planned nursing actions needed to be taken in order to compensate for the existing self-care deficits. This phase is similar to the *assessment and diagnosis* phases of the nursing process.

The second phase, *design and planning,* begins with the establishment of appropriate nursing actions (nursing systems) that will be needed to accomplish the care for the patient. Orem describes three types of nursing systems: (1) wholly compensatory, which requires the nurse to compensate for the client's inability to perform self-care activities, (2) partly compensatory, in which the nurse performs some of the self-care activities, but the client is able (capable) of performing most self-care activities, and (3) supportive-educative, where the nurse's role centers around assisting the client in making decisions and acquiring new skills and knowledge. This phase can be likened to the planning phase of the nursing process.

The third phase is labeled *production and control,* which refers to the actual giving of care, the management of that care, and the evaluation of that care. This phase can be compared to the implementation and evaluation phases of the nursing process.

Perioperative Nursing Practice and Orem's Nursing System Theory

Orem's Nursing System Theory can be easily assimilated with perioperative nursing practice. Nursing care during the preoperative phase is mostly supportive-educative, since the client is capable of making decisions and performing self-care. The nursing system becomes *partly compensatory* as the client receives the preoperative medications, which may diminish protective reflexes.

The nursing system becomes *wholly compensatory* during the intraoperative phase due to either unconsciousness, sedation, or immobilization, which renders the client incapable of rendering self-care. The perioperative nurse must do everything for the client in addition to serving as the client's advocate during this phase. The nursing system continues to be wholly compensatory immediately after surgery (postoperative phase) until the client's protective reflexes have returned, and gradually changes to partly compensatory as the client recovers from anesthesia and/or sedation and is capable of resuming some self-care activities.

The nursing system returns to supportive-educative before discharge. The perioperative nurse will teach the client specific tasks that need to be performed at home, while providing emotional support to both the client and family. The perioperative nurse will also evaluate the client's responses to the surgical experience through interviews and follow-up procedures with both the client and family in order to assess the outcomes of the perioperative experience.

Perioperative Nursing Practice Model

The PNPM is a visual means of providing a better understanding of how separate concepts and theories are interrelated with the whole (see Fig. 11-1). The PNPM depicts a continuous interaction between the phases of the perioperative period (pre-, intra-, and postoperative), nursing process activities during the three phases, and the areas where these nursing activities are performed. Interacting with these concepts are the nursing systems described in Orem's Theory of Nursing Systems. These systems are cyclic and dynamic, responding to the individual needs of the client throughout the perioperative period.

The roles of the perioperative nurse and client differ with each type of surgical experience and nursing system in order to meet self-care demands. It is therefore not unusual for the client to experience all or portions of the nursing systems, depending on the specific circumstances, settings, and/or individualized needs. Table 11-1 provides a comparison of nursing actions

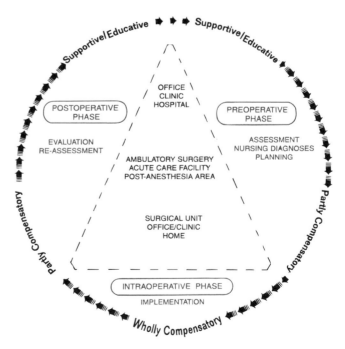

Fig. 11-1. Perioperative nursing practice model (From Fairchild, S. "Developing a Perioperative Nursing Practice Model," unpublished Master's thesis)

Table 11-1 Comparison of Nursing Activities

Orem's Nursing Systems Theory	Perioperative Nursing Practice
Nursing Systems/Nursing Actions	**Perioperative Phases/Nursing Actions**
Supportive—Educative Patient is capable of performing self-care activities Nurse provides the knowledge and therapeutic environment for the patient in order to accomplish these activities Regulates the exercise and development of self-care agency	**Preoperative Phase** Begins when decision for surgical intervention is made and ends with transference of patient to the OR table Nurse's role is to reassure the patient by explaining routines and sequence of events and providing preoperative teaching, answering questions, and clarifying concerns Nurse will perform some of the preoperative treatments that the patient cannot do Preoperative shave prep, preoperative medications, and IV, etc.
Partly Compensatory Patient is able to perform some self-care activities Nurse provides partial care and helps the patient accomplish other self-care activities Compensates for self-care limitations of the patient; regulates self-care agency	**Intraoperative Phase** Begins when the patient is transferred to the OR table and ends when patient is admitted to the postanesthesia area Nurse performs all care since patient is either unconscious, heavily sedated, or immobilized; protective reflexes absent, therefore nurse serves as client advocate
Wholly Compensatory Patient is unable to perform self-care activities Nurse will perform all nursing care activities for the patient Nurse compensates for patient's inability to perform self-care, supports and protects patient During emergence from anesthesia and the immediate postoperative phase in PACU, patient remains *wholly compensatory*; totally reliant on the nurses' actions	**Postoperative Phase** Begins with admission to postanesthesia area and ends with a resolution of surgical sequelae Following transference to second stage postanesthesia area (surgical unit; OPS) nurse encourages patient to participate in self-care activities; feeding, bathing, deep-breathing exercises, etc. Nurse performs tasks patient cannot do for self, at this time Nurse will assist the client in postoperative teaching; provide a resource once the discharge has occurred and answer questions of patient/family concerning postoperative recovery phase Postoperative evaluation of care in clinic or home by interview will be conducted by perioperative nurses (OR and OPS)
Partly Compensatory Patient is gradually able to resume self-care activities Nurse still performs selected tasks that patient is unable to do Nurse compensates for self-care limitations of patient; assists as required	
Supportive—Educative Patient is now able to resume all self-care activities Nurse will begin discharge teaching and assessment as to when the patient is ready to leave Regulates the exercise and development of self-care agency	

related to both Orem's Nursing Systems Theory and the practice of perioperative nursing.

The utilization of the PNPM provides an important focus for perioperative nurses in today's changing health-care environment. By utilizing a clinical practice model derived from a theory of nursing, the practice of perioperative nursing can be better organized and structured, which will ultimately result in the improvement of perioperative patient care. Additionally, the utilization of a clinical practice model such as the PNPM could eventually replace the traditional medical model currently used in today's perioperative setting. The integration of perioperative nursing practice concepts and a nursing theory can provide a theoretical

nursing basis for this specialized area of nursing practice.

Nursing, regardless of the area, is an *art* and a *science* and must be cultivated and learned as any other specialized practice that involves people. Each nurse has a responsibility to seek out new information and perfect his or her practice in order to manage patient care safely and effectively during the perioperative period.

NURSING ACTIVITIES IN THE PERIOPERATIVE ROLE

The nursing activities in the perioperative role are illustrated in Figure 11-2.

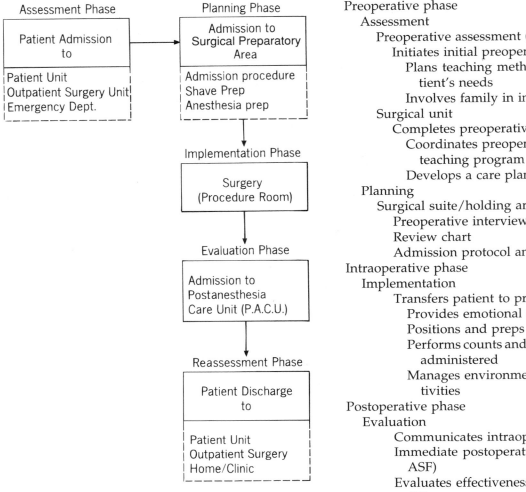

Fig. 11-2. Perioperative nursing activities

Preoperative phase
  Assessment
    Preoperative assessment (Home/ASF/ED)
      Initiates initial preoperative assessment
        Plans teaching methods appropriate to patient's needs
        Involves family in interview
    Surgical unit
      Completes preoperative assessment
        Coordinates preoperative activities and teaching program
        Develops a care plan
  Planning
    Surgical suite/holding area
      Preoperative interview
      Review chart
      Admission protocol and procedures
Intraoperative phase
  Implementation
    Transfers patient to procedure room
      Provides emotional support
      Positions and preps patient
      Performs counts and documents patient care administered
      Manages environment and patient-care activities
Postoperative phase
  Evaluation
    Communicates intraoperative information
    Immediate postoperative assessment (PACU; ASF)
    Evaluates effectiveness of nursing care in the OR
    Assists with discharge planning
  Reassessment
    Discharge planning and interview
      Patient unit/postoperative visit
      ASF/home (follow-up)

UNIT 1

Preoperative Phase
Daniel James Little

Learning makes a difference in the behavior, attitudes, and perhaps even the personality of the learner, . . . where it illuminates the dark area of ignorance he is experiencing.

—Carl Rogers (1969)

The *preoperative phase* of surgical intervention begins with the patient's decision to have surgery, and ends with the transfer of the patient to the operating table.

Perhaps in no other field is the concept of psychosomatics—the interrelationship of body and mind—so evident as in surgery. Before and after surgery, the patient's will to survive, to cooperate, and to recover can turn a major complicated surgical procedure into a smooth postoperative recovery and convalescence.

The physiologic preparation of the patient should be continuously intermeshed with the psychological preparation. Preoperative preparation often consists of explanations and teaching about the sequence of events that are about to take place. The patient, family, and significant others should be assisted in gaining accurate information that will lead to a successful conclusion of a possibly traumatic experience. The perioperative nurse must take an active part in this process in order to assure quality and continuity of patient care throughout the patient's surgical experience.

THE MEANING OF SURGERY: A CONCEPT

> Surgery . . . a planned alteration of the human organism designed to arrest, alleviate or eradicate some pathological process.
> —*LaMatrie and Finnegan (1975)*

Although no one disputes this general description, it is missing one crucial element: the patient and his or her view of this treatment modality. We each perceive events as related to our past experiences, information that has been passed down, or knowledge acquired through investigation. Therefore, patients have preconceived ideas and emotions about undergoing surgical intervention. The perioperative nurse must reflect whether these feelings are known, or lie silent within the patient, causing fear and anxiety.

Perioperative nursing practice is patient-oriented—not environment-oriented or physician-oriented. Perioperative nursing practice believes in the patient as a *whole person* with a broad spectrum of needs, and so the nursing activities must be geared to meet the patient's psychosocial needs as well as immediate physical needs.

The term *psychosocial* involves the social and psychological aspects of the patient's behavior, such as coping mechanisms, anxiety levels, self-image, personality, cultural influences, and support systems that can affect the patient during this period. By being observant, an active listener and empathic with his or her responses, the perioperative nurse can have a vital role in the activities designed to help the patient adjust to the proposed surgical therapy.

Most patients view surgery in several ways: as (1) an aggressive act directed against them, since it involves cutting into and possible removal of a body part; (2) a radical invasion of privacy; (3) a reduction or total loss of control; and (4) the subduing of their individuality. All of these can combine to produce fear, resentment, hostility, or apathy, depending on the patient's ability to adapt to stress.

On the positive side, however, patients may view surgery as an act of faith, projected as a feeling of trust in the surgeon and the perioperative nurse, and in their judgment.

As part of the total care of the patient, the perioperative nurse must understand these feelings and attempt to reduce the anxiety level through teaching, communication, and the establishment of a therapeutic nurse–patient relationship. Patients usually wish to cooperate, but stress will alter behavior patterns in most instances. Nursing care based on the individualized needs of the patient is critical to a patient's acceptance or rejection of the planned surgical procedure.

THE THEORY OF HUMAN NEEDS

A. H. Maslow, when describing a *hierarchy of human needs*,[5] emphasized that the accomplishment of self-actualization is a motivating factor in the healthy individual, but it cannot be attained until the basic needs of survival and security have been met.

From the moment a patient steps into a hospital, for whatever reason, we begin a systematic process of breaking down the individuality of the person and subsequently reducing his or her ability to think or act alone.

Maslow's theory is based on the concept of wants (needs) developing on five levels, the lowest being physiologic or biologic requirements and the highest being self-fulfillment and creativity (Fig. 11-3).

As the lower needs are gradually being satisfied, the higher needs gradually emerge. To satisfy these needs, humans expend energy (motivation). Once a need has been fairly well satisfied, it no longer acts as a motivator and efforts are then directed toward satisfying the need of the next level. Maslow focused his attention on the positive aspects of human behavior, such as happiness, contentment, and satisfaction as individuals strive toward their accomplishments.

What then is the effect of illness, and specifically the surgical experience on the attainment of these different levels?

Physical Needs

Biologic needs focus on life-sustaining necessities, such as food, water, oxygen, sleep, and warmth. In illness, the patient and family become acutely aware of these needs, and respond accordingly when any is threat-

ened. These needs must be met to achieve the next level of completeness, but should not become the total focus of patient care.

Surgical intervention, at some stage of the perioperative period, adversely affects all or some of these needs, creating an anxious state that requires supportive measures from all who are in contact with the patient and family during this period.

Psychosocial Needs

Safety and Security

Safety and *security* focus on the feelings of being safe in a nonthreatening environment, one which is familiar and comfortable, and void of harmful substances or actions.

In illness, this safety and security is replaced by the fear of the unknown, since the patient is surrounded by unfamiliarity in both the environment and the persons designated to care for him or her during the illness. Additionally, the patient may fear a loss of a body part or even death related to their illness. Therefore the nursing care should establish a protective, caring environment, and provide reassurance, comfort, and spiritual well-being during the hospitalization, especially during the perioperative period.

Social Acceptance

Social acceptance, or belonging, having an association with others, feeling affection or receiving love, friendship, and the creation of trust, are all an important aspect of this stage.

It is paramount, then, that patients and their families receive an empathic and understanding response to their feelings and attitudes, whether negative or positive. If a patient cannot trust those who are providing the care, it may result in cancellation of surgery, or high anxiety levels that require more medication to calm the patient, which can adversely affect the physiologic status of the individual both intraoperatively and postoperatively.

Self-Esteem

To feel good about one's self and to have confidence in one's own abilities leads to productivity, rational decision-making processes, and knowledgeable choices.

Confidentiality needs to be respected, since behavior patterns may change and could become an embarrassment if known. The radical invasion of privacy leads to feelings of low self-esteem, loss of control, and decreased decision-making capabilities. To many

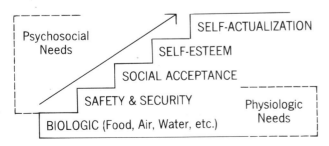

Fig. 11-3.   Maslow's hierarchy of needs

patients, this alone is reason for panic, since adults, young and old, pride themselves on their ability to function as independent individuals. Patients may be concerned with a potential change in body image related to the surgery, and how this image could ultimately affect their lifestyle. Patients may fear rejection by loved ones should the change be perceived as cosmetically unpleasant, such as a colostomy or removal of a breast.

Support systems must be activated as soon as possible to help the patient and family adjust to these feelings and/or impending changes in their lifestyle. The perioperative nurse is important in activating support systems during the preoperative assessment and interview of the patient, family, and significant others.

Self-Actualization

The final step on Maslow's hierarchical ladder focuses on being creative, self-motivated, and capable of reaching one's fullest potential, and is the ultimate motivator for the healthy individual. By allowing the patient to participate actively in health-care decisions, and providing patient education and rehabilitation programs, the goal of striving toward optimal existence can be reached. Effective and therapeutic nurse–patient relationships, created from the beginning, help the patient and family adjust and eventually achieve an optimum state of health.

By respecting the patient's individual rights and being a patient advocate, the perioperative nurse can assist the patient in feeling a sense of worth and importance, which can ultimately move the patient toward self-actualization and eventual accomplishment of his or her desired goals.

PREOPERATIVE TEACHING CONCEPTS

Education is the key to a successful conclusion.

A perioperative teaching program can provide the necessary means to assure quality and continuity of care during the perioperative period. Although the main area of the perioperative nurse's role is in the operating room during the intraoperative phase, the term *perioperative* encompasses all three phases of surgical intervention. Who is better prepared to conduct a preoperative teaching program than a professional nurse familiar with all three phases of the perioperative period?

One of the Outcome Standards for Perioperative Nursing, mentioned in Chapter 10, states:

The patient will demonstrate knowledge of the physiologic and psychological responses to surgical intervention.[6]

If the surgeon and anesthesiologist have supplied adequate information during their portion of the preoperative interview, the patient is now ready to become involved in an individualized preoperative teaching program. To make the program meaningful, the nurse must continue to assess the patient's current level of knowledge and readiness to learn. Assisting the patient in gaining additional knowledge assures the patient's awareness about the treatment he or she is about to receive.

Sharing information and answering the patient's and family's questions concerning the scheduled surgical procedure should be incorporated with the explanations from both the surgeon and the anesthesia practitioner. By doing so, the anxiety associated with the surgical procedure can be greatly reduced.

An effective preoperative teaching program includes input from all members of the surgical team, including the perioperative nurse.

A preoperative teaching program should include a general orientation to the surgical experience and instructions in anticipated postoperative activities. Research has revealed that surgical patients who receive preoperative and postoperative teaching are less anxious, more willing to participate in their own care, comply with prescribed medical regimens, and have fewer complications, thus shortening the hospitalization period.

Each program, though individualized, has certain key elements regardless of the type of surgery or patient status (inpatient or ambulatory patient). The perioperative nurse should be aware of these elements in order to create a comprehensive preoperative teaching program. These elements should include, but not be limited to, the following items:

1. Information regarding the sequence of events
2. Dietary restrictions
3. Preoperative shave (if applicable)
4. Preoperative medications
5. Postoperative activities
   a. Limitations
   b. Pain management
6. Family orientation
   a. Location of surgical waiting room
7. Self-care goals and discharge planning
   a. Follow-up visits

b. Resumption of preoperative activities, medications, lifestyle, and so on

In addition to these elements, the program should contain a teaching/learning component. To facilitate recovery, the patient should be taught techniques for specific postoperative exercises, assisted ambulation, and any other postoperative activities recommended by the surgeon. The patient should be shown the proper technique, and asked to return the demonstration with the nurse supervising the activity in order to offer any suggestions or answer any questions during the program. In this way the patient, without stress and/or pain, becomes an active participant, not just a passive observer.

Preoperative teaching is a vital component of the surgical experience. It should not be overlooked because of time limitations or lack of staff, since the ultimate outcome will be of significant benefit to the patient and family as well as the health-care team caring for patient.

Preoperative teaching, including the activities conducted and performed by the patient, should be documented on the patient's record as a means of communication to other nurses and health-care members who may care for the patient during the perioperative period. Documentation of preoperative teaching is especially important if the circulating nurse assigned to the case was not available to provide the preoperative preparation and teaching (Fig. 11-4).

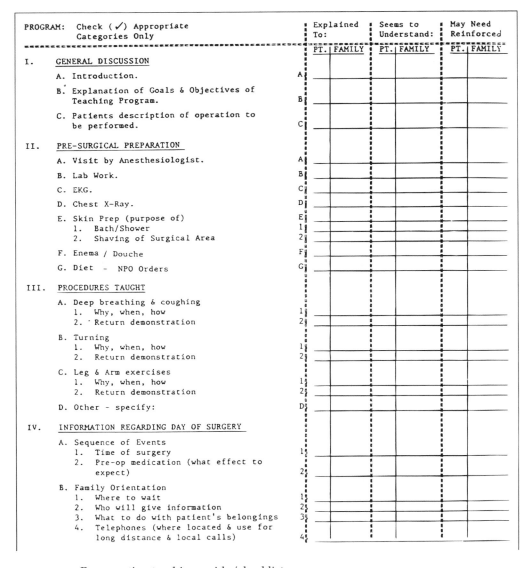

Fig. 11-4. Preoperative teaching guide/checklist

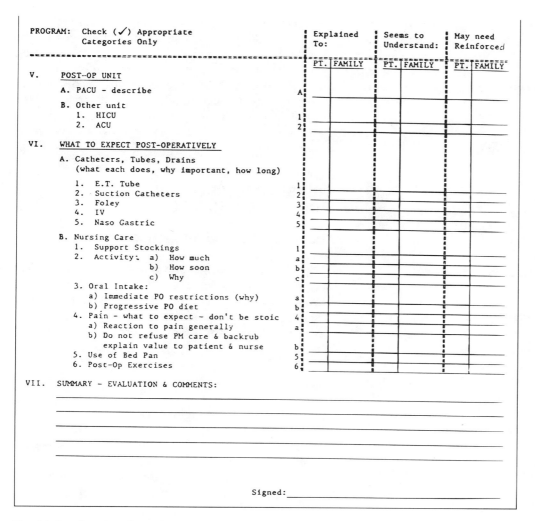

PROGRAM: Check (✓) Appropriate Categories Only		Explained To:		Seems to Understand:		May need Reinforced	
		PT.	FAMILY	PT.	FAMILY	PT.	FAMILY
V. POST-OP UNIT							
A. PACU - describe	A						
B. Other unit							
1. HICU	1						
2. ACU	2						
VI. WHAT TO EXPECT POST-OPERATIVELY							
A. Catheters, Tubes, Drains (what each does, why important, how long)							
1. E.T. Tube	1						
2. Suction Catheters	2						
3. Foley	3						
4. IV	4						
5. Naso Gastric	5						
B. Nursing Care							
1. Support Stockings	1						
2. Activity: a) How much	a						
b) How soon	b						
c) Why	c						
3. Oral Intake:							
a) Immediate PO restrictions (why)	a						
b) Progressive PO diet	b						
4. Pain - what to expect - don't be stoic	4						
a) Reaction to pain generally	a						
b) Do not refuse PM care & backrub explain value to patient & nurse	b						
5. Use of Bed Pan	5						
6. Post-Op Exercises	6						

VII.   SUMMARY - EVALUATION & COMMENTS:

_____

_____

_____

_____

_____

Signed: _____

Fig. 11-4. *(continued)*

Planning Perioperative Patient Care

Based on the assessment you have made, the planning and goal-setting phase of patient care begins. The planning stage consists of three components:

1. Individual needs of the patient
   a. Transportation needs
   b. Emotional support
   c. Moving and lifting concerns
   d. Special procedure required before incision, for example, insertion of Foley catheter; positional aides; alternate prepping solutions; area and/or shave prep
2. Possible complications
   a. Based on medical condition and diagnosis
   b. Laboratory data; nurse's notes; anesthesia evaluation
   c. Equipment and supplies anticipated
3. Actions/activities to be performed
   a. Based on assessment needs
   b. Goal-directed; patient-oriented
   c. Specialty equipment, for example, OR table; ESU; laser; microscope; monitoring devices, and so on.
   d. Surgical team needs

Perioperative nurses, as the professional nursing member of the surgical team, have a responsibility to *plan* as well as *give* care. If the planned and performed nursing activities are not documented, it could be assumed legally that the care did not take place. The nurse who creates this plan carries it out by communicating it to other members of the health-care team, thus ensuring the continuity of patient care after the perioperative period.

Although the creation of this care plan does not ensure that quality of care will be provided, it does reflect a reliable source of information for all health-care team members, and can serve as a tool for monitoring and evaluating the quality of care that the patient has received.

ADMITTING THE PATIENT TO SURGERY

The information obtained by the perioperative nurse during the preoperative assessment, such as appropriate transport methods or unusual patient problems (e.g., impaired mobility, alterations in sensory motor perception or emotional status, and any individual patient requests), should be conveyed to the individuals responsible for preparing and transporting the patient to the surgical suite.

Depending on institutional policies, a nurse may or may not accompany the patient to the presurgical waiting area or surgical preparatory unit or area, where a report should be given to the appropriate nursing personnel as the transfer of care is accomplished.

The admission procedure begins with an introduction by the surgical preparatory unit nurse and a series of questions to verify data on the chart, and ends when the patient has been cleared by area personnel and the patient is transferred to the surgical suite.

The institutional/OR policy and procedure manual should contain the protocol for admitting a patient to the surgical suite. This process should include the following elements:

1. *Verification of patient's identification*
   Verbally (if feasible); chart review and ID bracelet
2. *Verification of completion of appropriate forms*
   History and physical; results from diagnostic studies; consent forms; preoperative assessment/teaching
3. *Review of related nursing procedures performed*
   Nursing notes; physical and emotional status; vital signs; allergies
4. *Verification of physician's orders*
   Elimination; medication; nutrition; IV therapy; special procedures; NPO status
5. *Safety and comfort measures needed during the perioperative period* (removal of prosthesis, dentures, and so on)
6. *Patient's response to preoperative medication*
   Physiologic monitoring; emotional status; pain control; observation of the patient

A preoperative check sheet can assist in the documentation of this information, since it identifies, according to hospital policy, the information required on all presurgical patients. This form is completed by the surgical unit nurse, and should be started the evening before (or within a specific time for ambulatory patients). Additionally, the preoperative checklist should be completed and signed off prior to the arrival of the patient in the holding area, and is reverified by the holding area nurse and circulating nurse for completeness prior to entry into the procedure room (Fig. 11-5).

NURSING ACTIVITIES: ADMISSION PROCESS

Identification and Verification

Proper patient identification is one of the most important safety measures that can be taken by the professional nurse receiving the patient in the holding area. This identification should include verification of the patient, surgeon, surgical procedure, and type of anesthesia.

Review of Record

The patient's record usually gives a total picture of the patient and completes the identification process. Key elements include review of the patient's admission record (fact sheet); allergies; results of laboratory tests; history and physical examination; preoperative medications given; and specific preoperative orders, either by the surgeon or the anesthesia practitioner.

Pertinent Laboratory Data

Certain laboratory values are critical to the success of the proposed surgical procedure. The nurse caring for the patient should be aware of the results of these tests and their normal values according to institutional criteria.

Any deviations should be reported to the anesthesia practitioner and/or surgeon, since abnormal or unsafe levels could necessitate postponement of the procedure until the patient is in better physical condition.

Table 11-2 provides a list of normal hematologic values, including blood, plasma, and serum values most often checked before surgery.

In addition to the laboratory values and diagnostic tests used to determine the physiologic status of the patient, preoperative vital signs can be used as an excellent indicator of potential problems that could occur during the intraoperative period (Table 11-3).

The nurse should review these findings and report any concerns to the appropriate persons for immediate intervention.

Date

SECTION I. TO BE COMPLETED THE DAY BEFORE SURGERY	Checked By:	Name / Status / Time
Operative Consent — Signed & Witnessed	☐	
Anesthesia Consent- Signed & Witnessed	☐	
History & Physical — (written report on chart)	☐	
CBC (valid for two (2) weeks)	☐	
EKG (valid for 72 hours)	☐	
Chest X-Ray (Written Report on Chart; valid for one (1) month)	☐	
Physician's Order Sheet (Checked and All Orders Completed)	☐	
I.D. Bracelet ☐ Wrist ☐ Ankle	☐	
Skin Prep (May include Antimicrobial Bath) or shower, if ordered)	☐	
Blood: Type & Screen ☐ None Ordered ☐ Consent ☐	☐	
Allergies: ☐ NKA Specify: _____	☐	
Pre-Op Teaching done according to protocol;(review of Post-Op Exercises; coughing, Deep Breathing, etc.)	☐	

SECTION II. TO BE COMPLETED IN A.M. BEFORE SURGERY	Checked By:	Name / Status / Time
Dentures ☐ Upper ☐ Capped Teeth ☐ None ☐ Lower ☐ Partial Plate ☐ Removed	Location: _____	
Contact Lens/Prosthesis: ☐Yes ☐ No ☐ Removed	Location: _____	
Jewelry/Valuables: ☐ Removed	Location: _____	
Catheters & Drains ☐ Yes ☐ No Type:_____		
Pre-Op V.S.: TPR B/P		
Voided: ☐ Yes ☐ No		
Pre-Op Medications: (Type, Dose, Route, Time) 1. _____ 2. _____ 3. _____		
Pre-Op I.V. started ☐ Yes ☐ None Ordered Gauge & Location _____		
Bed lowered & side rails up	☐	
Chart Checked & Complete With Patient's Plate ☐	☐	
Special Considerations: ie: physical impairment and/or limitations; Foreign language) _____		

Fig. 11-5. Preoperative check sheet (Adapted from Broward General Medical Center, Department of Surgical Services, Ft. Lauderdale, FL)

Preoperative Interview

After the nurse reviews the patient's record, he or she is ready to begin the interview process.

The nurse should address the patient by proper name and title (where applicable), introduce herself or himself to the patient, and give a brief explanation of what will transpire during the preoperative, intraoperative, and postoperative phases of this surgical intervention. The nurse should provide individual attention to the patient, and if the family is present, include them in the interviewing process.

Special circumstances that the nurse must be aware

of during the interview process should be reviewed prior to beginning the interview. For example, elderly patients having difficulty with memory or cognitive acuity, extremely anxious patients, depressed patients, those with hearing or vision impairments, patients with a language barrier, or children with or without their parents may have difficulties with communication.

After establishing a rapport with the patient and/ or family members present, the nurse should assess the patient's understanding of the surgical procedure, using the *preoperative teaching/assessment* tool as a guide to meet the needs and concerns of the patient.

Table 11-2 **Normal Hematologic Values**

	Percentage	Absolute
Erythrocytes		
Men		4.6–6.2 million/μL
Women		4.2–5.4 million/μL
Children (varies with age)		4.5–5.1 million/μL
Leukocytes		
Total		4500–11,000/μL
Differential		
Myelocytes	0	0/μL
Band neutrophils	3–5	150–400/μL
Segmented neutrophils	54–62	3000–5800/μL
Lymphocytes	25–33	1500–3000/μL
Monocytes	3–7	300–500/μL
Eosinophils	1–3	50–250/μL
Basophils	0–0.75	15–50/μL
Platelets		150,000–350,000/μL
Hemoglobin		
Men		14–18 gm/100 mL
Women		12–16 gm/100 mL
Newborns		16.5–19.5 gm/100 mL
Children (varies with age)		11.2–16.5 gm/100 mL
Hematocrit		
Men		40–54 mL/100 mL
Women		37–47 mL/100 mL
Newborns		49–54 mL/100 mL
Children (varies with age)		35–49 mL/100 mL
Prothrombin time (PT)		12–14 sec
Activated partial thromboplastin time (APTT)		24–38 sec
Arterial Blood Gas Values		
P$_{AO_2}$		90–100 mm Hg
P$_{ACO_2}$		35–45 mm Hg
pH		7.35–7.45
Saturation		96–100%
Base excess		0
HCO$_3$		23–28 mEq/L
Electrolyte Values		
Magnesium, serum		1.5–2.5 mEq/L
Potassium, serum		3.5–5 mEq/L
Sodium		135–145 mEq/L

If problems or concerns have not been adequately addressed, the surgeon and/or anesthesia practitioner should be notified immediately for further explanation and/or clarification of concepts for the patient.

Consent Forms

All nurses involved with patient care should be aware of the state laws that govern the consent forms regarding the legal age requirement, mental competency of a patient, special surgical requirements, and appropriate signatures.

Nurses must also be aware of the institution's policies pertaining to consents. Attaining an informed con-

sent is the responsibility of the operating surgeon. An explanation should contain information regarding the proposed surgical procedure, the possible risks involved, expected benefits, available alternatives, and so on. (See Chap. 12.)

Related Nursing Procedures

During the admission process, the patient may have an IV inserted, a surgical shave prep performed, or a cast bivalved or removed. The perioperative nurse should provide support for the patient by explaining all the procedures and why they are necessary. The noise in the area should be kept to a minimum,

Table 11-3   Physiologic Status Review and Implications

Vital Sign	Abnormal Finding	Possible Indication	Possible Postoperative Complication
Temperature	Fever (above 101°F [38.3°C] in an adult)	Infection; dehydration (when accompanied by decreased skin turgor)	Systemic infection; wound infection; dehiscence/evisceration; fluid imbalance; shock
Pulse	Tachycardia (above 100 bpm)	Pain; fever; dehydration; anemia; hypoxia; shock	Poor tissue perfusion; vascular collapse; cardiac arrhythmias; renal failure; anesthetic complications
	Bradycardia (below 60 bpm)	Drug effects (e.g., digitalis); spinal injury; head injury	Spinal shock; increased intracranial pressure (also for tachycardia)
Respiration	Tachypnea (above 24 breaths/min)	Atelectasis; pneumonia; pain or anxiety; pleurisy; infection; renal failure	Tissue hypoxia; anesthetic complications; pneumonia; atelectasis
	Bradypnea (below 10 breaths/min)	Brain lesion; respiratory center depression	See tachypnea
Blood pressure	Hypotension (below 90 mm Hg systolic)	Shock; myocardial infarction; hemorrhage; spinal injury	Poor tissue perfusion; renal failure; vasodilation; shock
	Hypertension (above 140 mm Hg systolic and/or 90 mm Hg diastolic)	Anxiety or pain; renal disease; coronary artery disease	Stroke; hemorrhage; myocardial infarction

privacy maintained, and the patient never left unattended.

Preoperative Preparation of the Skin

The skin (*integument*) serves as a protective barrier and is composed of two layers: the *epidermis* (the thin surface layer) and the *dermis* (the deeper layer of skin that lies below it).

The dermis is attached through subcutaneous tissue or superficial fascia to underlying structures and is composed of blood vessels, lymphatics, nerves, the secreting portions of sebaceous glands and the sweat glands and hair follicles (Fig. 11-6).

The skin is continuously replenished by millions of new cells each day. As resilient as the skin is, though, it can fail as a protective barrier if it fails to remain intact.

Bacteria found on the skin are numerous, and generally are divided into *transient* and *resident flora*. Transient microbes are easy to remove with soap and water, while the resident flora adhere to epithelial cells and extend downward toward the glands and hair follicles.

Because the skin cannot be sterilized, it must be properly prepared in order to reduce the microbial count to as low as possible, thereby reducing the risk of infection.

Two methods used to prepare this surface are the (1) preoperative skin prep, and (2) the surgical skin prep during the intraoperative phase.

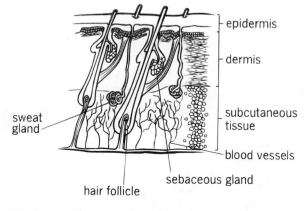

Fig. 11-6. Cross-section of the skin

Preoperative skin preparation done on the unit and/or in the holding area consists of two steps:

1. A shower/bath the night before with an antimicrobial agent, and
2. The possible removal of hair directly involved with the proposed incision site.

Removal of hair from the operative site is not necessary for all surgical procedures or for all patients. Physician's preoperative orders should indicate appropriate skin preparation.

AORN Recommended Practices for Surgical Skin Prep

I.   The operative site and surrounding areas should be clean

II. The operative site should be assessed before skin preparation

III. The operative site and the surrounding area should be prepared with an antimicrobial agent

IV. Patient skin preparation should be documented in the patients' record.

Source: AORN. Standards and recommended practices, Denver, CO: The Association, 1995. Pp. 255–257.

The ideal methods to remove unwanted hair are either by depilatory or by clipping the hair using disposable clippers. Either of these methods eliminates the possibility of cutting or scratching the skin with shaving, which may create an opening for microbial contamination of the surgical wound.

Using AORN's recommendations as a guide,[7] the removal of hair should be performed as close to the time of surgery as possible, and should be performed by qualified personnel instructed in the proper procedure regardless of what method is used, and in an area that can afford privacy. Ideally, the surgical preparatory area should be equipped to perform this task.

If the shave method is the *only* choice available, the wet shave method is *mandatory*, as it facilitates hair removal, minimizes skin trauma, and prevents dry hair and debris from becoming airborne.

If a depilatory is used, a "patch-test" should be performed first to identify a possible reaction. If no adverse effects are visible, the agent is applied following the manufacturer's instructions for application and removal.

A manual containing the procedural steps and diagrams of proposed prep areas should be available within the practice setting and referred to as necessary before beginning the skin prep.

SAMPLE: SHAVE PREP MANUAL

Note: The following areas are suggested according to the proposed incision/procedure. Check with surgeon for more specific shave prep instructions.

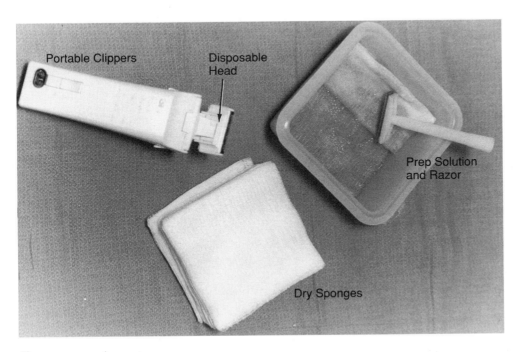

Shave prep equipment

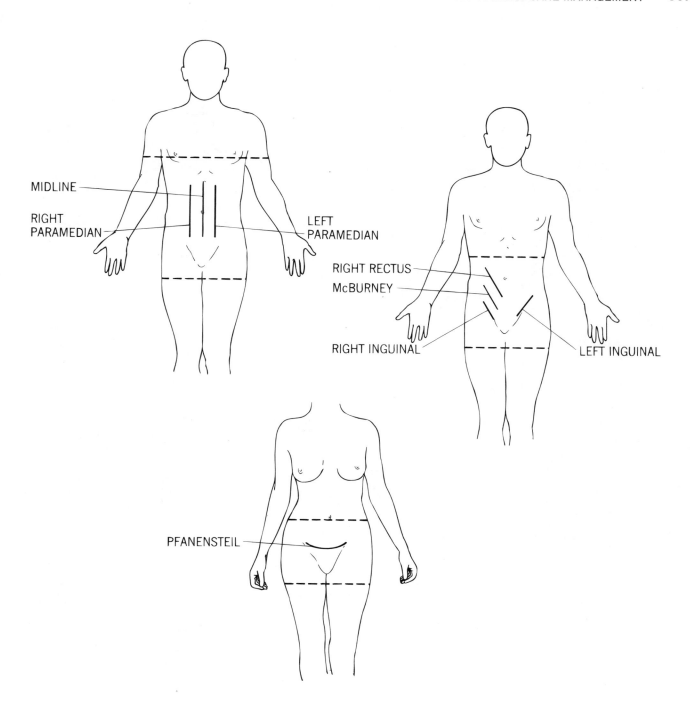

MIDLINE

RIGHT
PARAMEDIAN

LEFT
PARAMEDIAN

RIGHT RECTUS

McBURNEY

RIGHT INGUINAL

LEFT INGUINAL

PFANENSTEIL

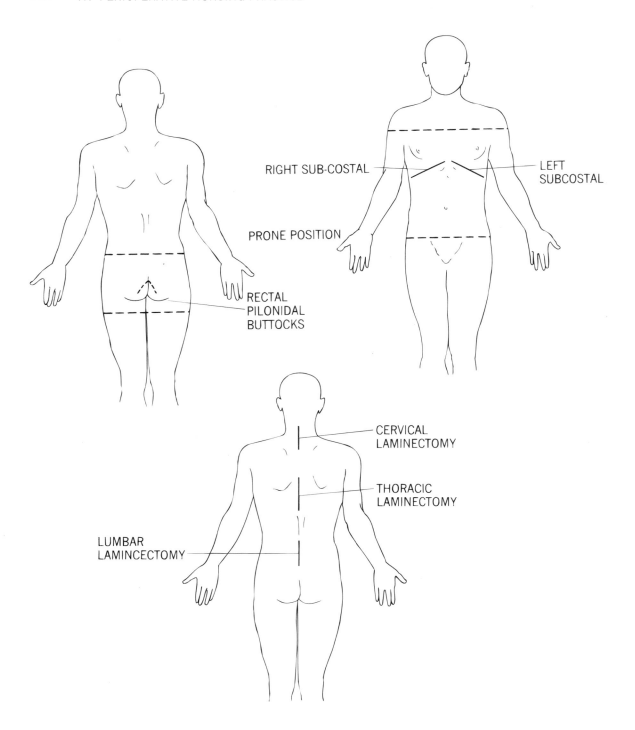

RIGHT SUB-COSTAL

LEFT SUBCOSTAL

PRONE POSITION

RECTAL PILONIDAL BUTTOCKS

CERVICAL LAMINECTOMY

THORACIC LAMINECTOMY

LUMBAR LAMINCECTOMY

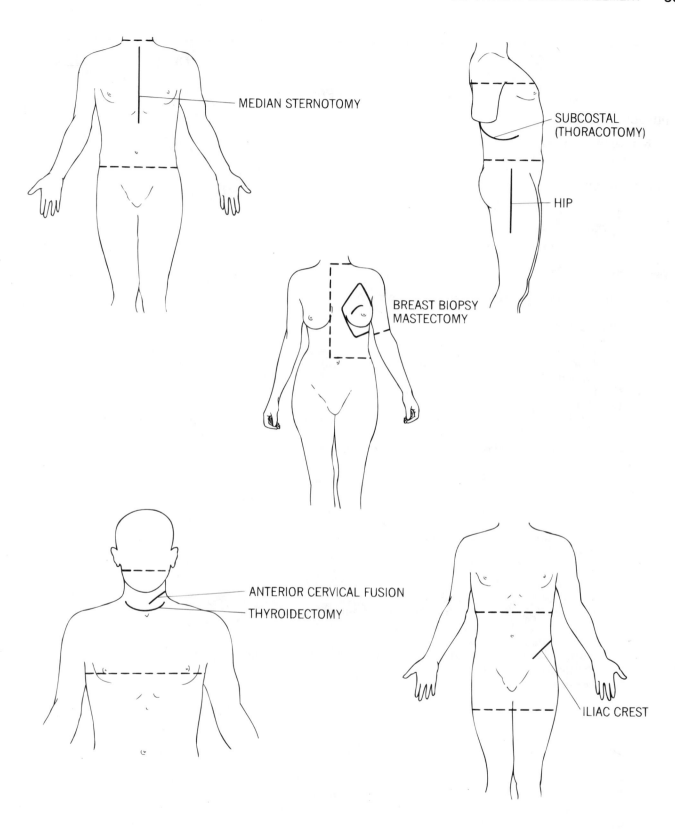

MEDIAN STERNOTOMY

SUBCOSTAL
(THORACOTOMY)

HIP

BREAST BIOPSY
MASTECTOMY

ANTERIOR CERVICAL FUSION

THYROIDECTOMY

ILIAC CREST

Preoperative Skin Preparation

PURPOSE

To reduce the number of microbes and removal of hair directly involved with the incision site, which could interfere with the surgical procedure.

PREREQUISITE

1. Appropriate equipment/supplies
2. Appropriate area; privacy provided
3. Performed no more than 2 hours before procedure

PROFICIENCY

One hundred percent accuracy at time of performance

PROCEDURAL STEPS

I. SHAVE PREP
   1. Assemble the necessary equipment and supplies.
   2. Explain the procedure to the patient, and provide privacy.
   3. Don disposable gloves and arrange supplies.
   4. Drape the patient to expose *only* the area to be prepped.
   5. Wash the skin with appropriate antimicrobial solution from incision site to periphery, creating a generous lather.
   6. Using a sharp, disposable razor, begin shaving in the direction of the hair growth by pulling the skin taut.

NOTE: Clean the razor periodically to maintain a sharp blade.

   7. Rinse off area, removing any loose hairs, and dry.
   8. Remove drape sheet, being careful not to let drape flourish or hair fly around.
   9. Document procedure on patient's record, noting condition of patient's skin pre- and postprocedure.

II. DEPILATORY CREAM
   1. Follow Steps 1–4 of shave prep.
   5. Perform "patch-test" on patient's wrist and record results.
   6. Apply cream to proposed site, according to manufacturer's instructions.
   7. Allow cream to remain on skin, untouched, for prescribed length of time.
   8. Wipe off cream with a damp cloth, and rinse area thoroughly.
   9. Remove drape sheet.
   10. Document procedure on patient's record, including condition of skin pre- and postprocedure.

III. ELECTRIC CLIPPERS (preferred method)
   1. Follow Steps 1–4 of shave prep.

Note: Clipping hair is performed dry using disposable clipper head attachment (one per patient).

   5. Clip hair in direction of hair growth, avoiding pull by holding skin taut.
   6. Wash off skin with antimicrobial solution and rinse well.
   7. Remove drape sheet, being careful not to let drape flourish or hair fly around.
   8. Document procedure on patient's record, including condition of skin pre- and postprocedure.

CRITICAL ELEMENT
TASK 11-1 cont.

POINTS TO REMEMBER

1. If using the shave method, avoid creating nicks or abrasions in the skin by allowing sufficient time for the procedure.

2. When shaving over areas such as the shin, shave across the bone, perpendicular to it.

3. Never shave the face, eyebrows, or cut eyelashes unless specifically ordered by surgeon.

4. Scalp hair is first cut, then clipped, followed by routine shaving if necessary with a safety razor. Always save hair when shaving entire scalp, since it is the patient's property, and a wig could be fashioned from the hair.

5. Rinse and dry the area thoroughly when prep is completed.

6. "Spot preps," performed in the procedure room, *must be wet* to avoid skin debris and hair from being introduced into the aseptic environment.

7. The skin harbors both transient and resident flora; *Staphylococcus epidermis* (resident flora) found on normal skin and *Staphylococcus aureus* (transient flora). Transient flora may be harmless or deadly, and if introduced into a surgical wound, could cause a serious postoperative infection. Therefore, strict aseptic technique *must* be maintained during the preoperative skin prep.

PERFORMANCE CHECK SHEET

NAME: _____	TASK # ____11-1____
	RATING: A Acceptable
	N/I Needs Improvement

PROCEDURE: Preoperative Skin Preparation

PROCEDURAL STEPS	A	N/I
GENERAL CONSIDERATIONS		
1. Explains the procedure to the patient		
2. Provides privacy and limits exposure to prep area		
3. Procedure performed prior to entry into procedure room (exceptions noted)		
4. Documents procedure on patient's record, including skin condition before and after prep		
I. SHAVE PREP		
1. Uses wet method only		
2. Avoids nicks, cuts, abrasions by pulling skin taught and shaving in direction of hair growth		
3. Maintains adequate lather during procedure for ease of technique		
4. Rinses with warm water and towel-dries area		
5. Maintains principles of asepsis		
II. DEPILATORY CREAMS		
1. Performs a "patch test" and observes skin for adverse reactions		
2. Follows manufacturer's recommendation for application and removal of cream		
3. Maintains aseptic technique		

TASK # ___11-1___   PAGE 2 of 2

PROCEDURAL STEPS	A	N/I

III. ELECTRIC CLIPPERS
 	
   1. Performs procedure dry
 	
   2. Applies new clipper head prior to each procedure
 	
   3. Applies clippers to taught skin, at proper angle, and removes hair in direction of hair growth
 	
   4. Washes off prep site with antimicrobial solution, rinses with warm water and towel dries, following procedure
 	
   5. Maintains aseptic principles
 	
Note: Skin prep procedure should be performed not more than 2 hours before the surgical procedure. Persons performing preps should be wearing gloves (sterile/nonsterile)		

COMMENTS: _____

_____

Self-assessment Exercise 2

Directions: Complete the following exercises. The answers are given at the end of this module.

1. Briefly describe the psychological benefits of adequate preoperative preparation of the patient.

2. The single most important cause of preoperative anxiety in a well-adjusted patient is the

   _____.

3. Using your answer to number 2, identify three supportive nursing interventions that may be helpful in reducing patient anxiety during the perioperative period.

4. List the three essential components of a preoperative teaching program.

5. List six information elements needed when admitting the patient to the surgical preparatory area/ surgical suite.

6. A shave prep should be done on all patients who are having surgery.

   True   False

UNIT 2

Intraoperative Phase

Where does man come closer to working hand in hand with the creator than in the operating room. . . .

—M. Gordon, *Code Care for Nurses*

The *intraoperative phase* begins with the transference of the patient to the procedure room, and ends with the admission of the patient to the designated postanesthesia area.

PERIOPERATIVE NURSING ACTIVITIES

Perioperative nursing practice has one continuous goal: *To provide a standard of excellence in the care of the patient before, during, and after surgery.*

As the only nonscrubbed member of the surgical team, besides anesthesia personnel, the circulating nurse represents the coordinating link between the scrub team and all other departments and personnel associated with the surgical patient and the procedure.

The circulating nurse, by virtue of her educational preparation and specialized skill, is responsible for managing patient care activities in the procedure room during surgery, so his or her duties begin long before the patient arrives in the procedure room and continues until the final dispensation of the patient, OR records, and specimens is completed. The following list depicts some of the activities performed by the circulating nurse before induction and on conclusion of the procedure.

1. Assisting and preparing the procedure room.
2. Supervising the transporting, moving, and lifting of the patient.
3. Assisting with anesthesia as requested during induction and reversal of anesthesia.
4. Positioning the patient for surgery.
5. Performing the surgical skin prep.
6. Conducting and maintaining accurate records of counts.
7. Maintaining accurate documentation of nursing activities during the procedure.
8. Dispensing supplies and medications to the surgical field.
9. Maintaining an aseptic and safe environment.
10. Estimating fluid and blood loss.
11. Handling special equipment, specimens, and so on.
12. Communicating special postoperative needs to appropriate persons at the conclusion of the case.

Anticipation is the key element for a successful and efficient surgical procedure.

TRANSPORTING, MOVING, AND LIFTING THE PATIENT

When the preoperative admission procedures have been completed, and the OR is prepared for the surgical procedure, the patient is transported to the designated procedure room.

The process of transporting the patient to the procedure room is often viewed by the nurse as a chore, and is usually delegated to the aide or orderly assigned to the surgical suite. It is not unusual for this transition time to be neglected by nursing personnel, yet the patient may be vulnerable, helpless, and extremely anxious during this time, and may need the support of a perioperative nurse.

Of primary importance during this time is *patient safety,* and the following guidelines can aid in maintaining a safe, nonthreatening transition for the patient:

1. Transport the patient only after the preadmission procedure has been completed.
2. Maintain the side rails in an up position during transport.
3. Assure that upper extremities are well within the framework of the stretcher.
4. Move the patient in a smooth, nonjerking motion, traveling feet first.

5. Before moving the patient to the operating table, position the stretcher by the side of the operating table, lower the side rail nearest the operating table, lock the stretcher, and lower the other side rail. If the patient is alert, caution him or her to move slowly to the table, and provide assistance as necessary. If the patient is sedated, use a *roller* to assist in the moving process.

6. When transporting a child in a crib, raise all side rails of the crib to their highest point to prevent the child from crawling over the top.

7. Never leave a patient on the operating table without immediate supervision present.

Since safety is a primary concern, assigned transporter's duties and manipulation in and out of a procedure room should be part of an orientation program designed specifically for the surgical environment. This orientation program may include principles of aseptic technique, transportation, moving and lifting awake and anesthetized patients, and assisting with patient positioning in the procedure room.

If the patient has special tubes, machines, and so on, a nurse should accompany the patient to the procedure room if the circulator is unable to assist in the transport process, and assist with moving the patient in order to manage the special equipment.

When the patient is finally on the operating table, the nurse applies the safety strap with a brief explanation of its purpose, and remains with the patient as anesthesia prepares for induction. The perioperative nurse is responsible and accountable for all nursing care, procedures, and actions performed for or with the patient. The patient and the anesthesia induction become the priorities during this phase of the surgical experience.

POSITIONING THE SURGICAL PATIENT

Patient positioning is a facet of patient-care management that is as important to the surgical outcome as adequate preoperative preparation and safe administration of anesthesia. It requires knowledge of *anatomy* and *physiology*, and requires *skill* in using the various positioning equipment and accessories.

The patient is positioned *after* induction and then only when the anesthesia practitioner believes the patient is stable and can be moved safely.

Criteria for Proper Positioning

According to the AORN's *Standards and Recommended Practices*, the following statements can be directly re-lated to the positioning of the surgical patient, and the perioperative nurse, as the patient advocate, must continuously provide a safe environment for the patient during this procedure.[8]

AORN Practice—Positioning
Policies and procedures related to positioning . . . should include but are not limited to assessment criteria, anatomic and physiologic considerations, safety and security measures, patient monitoring, and documentation of position and devices used.

A positive outcome related to positioning is based on specific criteria. The position should:

1. Not interfere with respirations
2. Not interfere with circulation
3. Not cause pressure on any nerve
4. Provide total accessibility for administration of anesthesia agents
5. Provide total accessibility to the operative site
6. Reflect proper body alignment, resulting in no unusual postoperative discomfort
7. Be based on individual anatomic considerations and/or requirements
8. Provide safety throughout the surgical procedure

The following guidelines should be used when moving and repositioning any patient who has been anesthetized or whose protective reflexes have been impaired:

1. Before moving the patient, always ask permission from the anesthesia clinician, who will ultimately be responsible for the patient's head and lines.
2. Obtain enough help to move the patient smoothly and safely.
3. Be gentle when manipulating joints into the desired position. Abducting a limb to an angle greater than 90 degrees may cause injury to the extremity.
4. Support all joints and extremities during the move, since they will be vulnerable to injury.
5. Respect the patient's dignity by avoiding any unnecessary exposure during the positioning.
6. Maintain proper body alignment, regardless of the position required for the procedure.
7. Move the patient slowly and deliberately, maintaining a total awareness of physiologic impairment that can occur related to positioning.

8. Protect from tension IV lines, catheters, and breathing circuits.
9. Provide padding for all bony prominences.
10. Protect *yourself* by using proper body mechanics during the move.
11. Have available all necessary accessories for positioning the patient in the room before the move is initiated.
12. Once in position, secure the patient with a safety strap, avoiding occlusion or pressure over an area. The safety strap should be placed on top of the blanket (sheet) covering the patient. If an electrocautery unit is to be used, place the ground pad in proper position at this time.

Positioning: A Team Concept

The responsibility for safely positioning the surgical patient involves the entire surgical team.

The surgeon determines the position for optimal exposure of the surgical site, while the anesthesia practitioner, being concerned with airway maintenance, vascular access, and cardiovascular stability, will either agree or make an alternative suggestion, trying to accommodate the surgeon while assuring physiologic stability for the patient.

The perioperative nurse, aware of this decision, coordinates the activities related to positioning, such as preparation of the positioning aids and equipment.

The related patient information, which will aid in safely positioning a patient, can be obtained from the *preoperative assessment* tool, and from there a plan of action can be formulated and executed using the principles of safe moving and lifting techniques.

Planning Considerations

Five factors should be considered when planning the position of a patient for surgery:

1. Anatomy involved with the procedure
   a. Knowledge of the area in relation to
      1. Organs, site of disease/tumor
      2. Right- or left-sided extremity
      3. Area to be grafted or repaired
2. Surgical approach and/or surgeon's preference
   a. Area must be easily accessible and provide maximum exposure to expedite surgery
3. Patient comfort
   a. Support for head and extremities
   b. Proper body alignment
   c. Avoidance of pressure points by adequate padding
   d. Avoidance of overexposure

1. Maintaining privacy
2. Avoiding hypothermic complications
   e. Proposed length of surgery
4. Patient and staff safety
   a. Proper use of safety strap
   b. Proper use and placement of positioning devices
   c. Moving and lifting using proper body mechanics and adequate personnel
   d. Protecting neuromuscular and skeletal structures
   e. Proper placement of electrosurgical ground pad
   f. Knowledge of own physical limitations
5. Respiratory and circulatory freedom
   a. Respiratory
      1. Relief of chest area from external pressure
      2. Maintenance of adequate airway
   b. Circulatory
      1. Avoidance of pressure on extremities that could decrease venous blood flow
      2. Avoidance of hyperextension of arms without proper support
      3. Avoidance of crossed ankles or legs in supine position

General Physiologic Effects of Patient Positioning

Patient positioning influences the cardiovascular, respiratory, and neurologic systems, and coupled with the effects of anesthesia, can become a potential danger for all surgical patients.

1. Respiratory system
   a. A change in position alters the pulmonary capillary blood flow volume, thereby affecting the amount of blood available for oxygenation
   b. The inspired air in the lungs may be redistributed, affecting the available air needed to oxygenate blood
   c. Lung tissue compliance is decreased, which reduces the amount of air that can be taken in for rapid exchange
   d. Expansion of the lungs is limited, either by mechanical restriction of the ribs or a reduced ability of the diaphragm to force the abdominal contents downward
2. Cardiovascular system
   a. Anesthesia (general or regional) causes the peripheral blood vessels to dilate
   b. Hypotension can occur related to positioning effects
   c. Pooling can occur in dependent areas, caused by dilated vascular beds

d. The amount of blood returned to the heart and lungs can be reduced, affecting oxygenation and redistribution of oxygenated blood

e. Usually, pressure and/or obstruction of a vessel causes the greatest amount of damage to the cardiovascular system

3. Neurologic system

a. Most of the problems related to positioning are seen during the postoperative phase

b. Peripheral and superficial nerves are vulnerable to damage from mechanical pressure

c. The majority of the problems are related to pressure, obstruction, and stretching due to faulty positioning, and are most commonly associated with nerve injury

d. Motor/sensory nerve loss can happen within minutes of improper positioning, and tissue damage can have a long-term effect

SURGICAL POSITIONS AND RELATED PHYSIOLOGIC EFFECTS

There are eight common positions that can be adapted and used for most surgical procedures, and all are variations of two basic positions, supine and prone:

1. Supine (dorsal recumbent)
2. Prone
3. Trendelenburg
4. Reverse Trendelenburg
5. Lithotomy
6. Sitting (modified Fowler)
7. Kraske (jackknife)
8. Lateral recumbent

Supine (Dorsal Recumbent)

The most common and most natural position is the supine (dorsal recumbent) position (Fig. 11-7).

Procedures
Abdominal, extremity, vascular, chest, neck, facial, ear, breast surgery

Positioning Techniques
- Patient lies flat on back with arms either extended on arm boards or placed along side of body
- Small padding placed under patient's head and neck and under knees
- Vulnerable pressure points should be padded, for example, heels, elbows, sacrum
- If procedure will be longer than 1 hour or patient is particularly vulnerable to pressure, egg crate or flotation mattress should be used
- Safety strap applied 2 inches above knees
- If head is turned to one side, doughnut or special head rest should be used to protect superficial facial nerves and blood vessels
- Eyes should be protected by using eye patch, and ointment to prevent drying

Physiologic Effects
1. Cardiovascular system
   a. Decrease of mean arterial pressure, heart rate
   b. Increase in cardiac output and stroke volume
   c. Decrease in diastolic blood pressure
   d. Potential for venous pooling in lower extremities
2. Respiratory system
   a. Compromised respiratory function
   b. Decrease in vital capacity
   c. Decrease in diaphragmatic excursion
   d. More even distribution of ventilation from apex to base of lung

Prone

See Figure 11-8 for an example of the prone position.

Procedures
Surgeries involving posterior surface of the body, for example, spine, neck, buttocks, lower extremities

Positioning Techniques
Induction of anesthesia is performed in supine position either on patient's bed or operating table. Once asleep, patient is "log rolled" onto stomach.

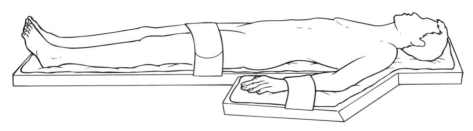

Fig. 11-7. Supine position

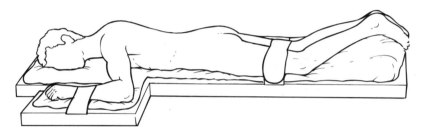

Fig. 11-8. Prone position

- Chest rolls or bolsters are placed on operating table before positioning, lengthwise on both sides
- Foam head rest or doughnut; head turned to side or facing downward
- Patient's arms are rotated to the padded armboards that face head, bringing them through their normal range of motion, elbows bent
- Padding for knees and pillow for lower extremities to prevent toes from touching mattress
- Safety strap applied 2 inches above the knees

Physiologic Effects
1. Cardiovascular system
   a. Few cardiovascular problems if positioned correctly
   b. Pressure on inferior vena cava and femoral veins, which can reduce venous return resulting in a decrease in blood pressure if improperly positioned
   c. If head turned to one side, pressure on carotid sinuses can cause hypotension and arrhythmias
2. Respiratory system
   a. Most vulnerable to respiratory problems
   b. Body weight against abdominal wall limits diaphragmatic movement, resulting in increased airway pressure with difficulty in ventilation; limits tidal volume

Trendelenburg

An example of the Trendelenburg position is shown in Figure 11-9.

Procedures
Lower abdomen, pelvic organs, when there is a need to tilt abdominal viscera away from the pelvic area

Positioning Techniques
- Patient is supine with head lower than feet
- Shoulder braces should not be used as they may cause damage to brachial plexus. If needed, they should be well padded and placed over acrominal process of the scapula
- When patient is returned to supine position, care must be taken to move leg section slowly, then the entire table to level position
- Modification of this position can be used for hypovolemic shock
- Extremity position and safety strap are the same as for supine position

Physiologic Effects
1. Cardiovascular system
   a. Blood pools in upper torso, increasing blood pressure
   b. Can produce drop in blood pressure when returned to supine position

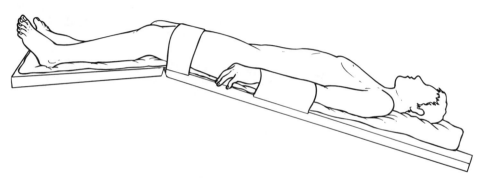

Fig. 11-9. Trendelenburg position

  c. Neck veins engorged (good for CVP/Swan line insertion)
  d. Cyanosis; increased vascular load to heart from lower extremities
2. Respiratory system
  a. Decrease in lung volume resulting in respiratory embarrassment
  b. Interference with respiratory exchanges
  c. May precipitate pulmonary congestion and edema
  d. Decrease in diaphragmatic expansion (abdominal contents pushed up)

Reverse Trendelenburg (Not Pictured)

Procedures
Upper abdominal, head and neck, facial surgery

Positioning Technique
- Patient is supine with head higher than feet
- Small pillow under neck and knees
- Well-padded footboard should be used to prevent slippage to the foot of the table
- Antiembolic hose should be used if position is to be maintained for an extended period of time
- Patient should be returned slowly to supine position

Physiologic Effects
1. Cardiovascular system
  a. Diminished cardiac return resulting in decreased cardiac output
  b. Decrease in brainstem perfusion due to gravity
  c. Pooling of blood in lower extremities
  d. Possibility of circulatory overload if returned to supine position quickly
2. Respiratory system
  a. Unimpaired respiratory movement with minimal restrictions of ventral expansion of anterior chest wall
  b. Potential reduction in the diffusing capacity of oxygen owing to perfusion of upper regions of lungs
  c. Potential for respiratory insufficiency and respiratory acidosis

Lithotomy

The lithotomy position is shown in Figure 11-10.

Procedures
Perineal, vaginal, rectal surgeries; combined abdominal-vaginal procedures

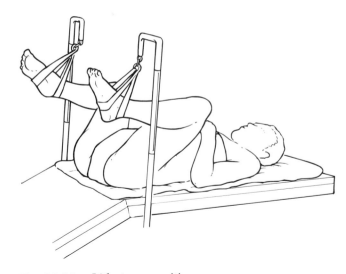

Fig. 11-10.   Lithotomy position

Positioning Techniques
- Exaggerated variation of supine position; can be dangerous and uncomfortable to patient
- Patient is placed in supine position with buttocks near lower break in the table (sacrum area should be well padded)
- Feet are placed in stirrups or knee rests attached to operating table on both sides
- Stirrup height should not be excessively high or low, but even on both sides
- Padded stirrups (knee brace) must not compress vascular structures or nerves in the popliteal space
- Pressure from metal stirrups against upper inner aspect of thigh/calf should be avoided
- Legs should be raised and lowered slowly and simultaneously (may require two people)

Physiologic Effects
1. Cardiovascular system
  a. Circulatory pooling in the lumbar region
  b. Rapid lowering of legs could cause sudden drop in blood pressure (500–800 mL of blood may shift from lumbar area to legs)
  c. Compromise to circulatory system due to compression of abdominal contents on inferior vena cava and abdominal aorta
2. Respiratory system
  a. Reduction in respiratory efficiency due to pressure from thighs on abdomen and pressure from the diaphragm on abdominal viscera, restricting respirations
  b. Lung tissue becomes engorged with blood; vital capacity and tidal volume decreased

In addition to circulatory and respiratory problems associated with this position, a major concern is nerve damage to femoral, obturator, and perineal nerves; dislocation of hip; crushing of fingers if they are left too close to the lower table break when raising table to supine position.

Modified Fowler (Sitting)

For an example of the modified Fowler (sitting) position, see Figure 11-11.

Procedures
Otorhinology (ear and nose), neurosurgery (posterior or occipital approach)

Positioning Techniques
- Variation of reverse Trendelenburg position
- Patient is supine, positioned over the upper break in the table (footboard optional)
- Backrest is elevated, knees flexed
- Arms rest on pillow placed in lap; safety strap 2 inches above the knees
- Pressure areas include the scapula, olecranon, sacrum, ischial tuberosities, and calcaneus
- Slow movement in and out of position must be used to prevent drastic changes in blood volume movement
- Antiembolic hose should be used to assist venous return
- When using special neurologic headrest, eyes must be protected

Physiologic Effects
1. Cardiovascular system
   a. Venous pooling in lower extremities
   b. Potential presence of air emboli due to negative pressure on the head and neck
   c. Hypotension related to position and effect of anesthesia
      NOTE: Doppler and/or CVP line may be used for detection and treatment should venous sinus be opened
2. Respiratory system
   a. Same as for reverse Trendelenburg

Kraske (Jackknife)

The Kraske (jackknife) position is illustrated in Figure 11-12.

Procedures
Rectal procedures, sigmoidoscopy, colonoscopy

Positioning Techniques
- Variation of prone position
- Table is flexed at center break (90-degree angle)
- All precautions taken with prone position are taken with Kraske position
- Table (safety) strap applied over thighs

Physiologic Effects
Because of its adverse effects on both cardiovascular and respiratory systems, the Kraske is considered

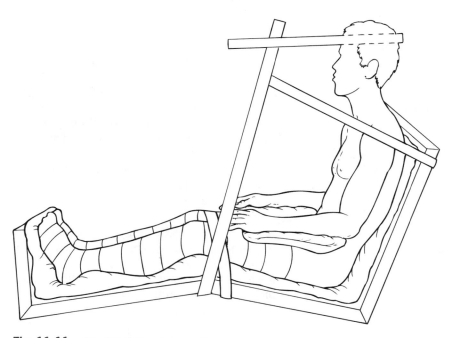

Fig. 11-11. Modified Fowler position

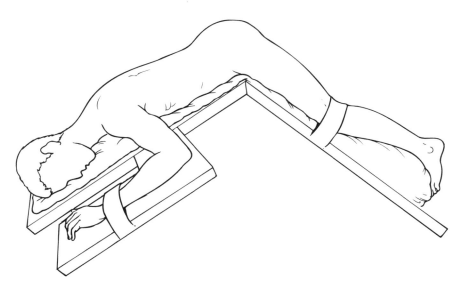

Fig. 11-12. Kraske position

the most dangerous of all surgical positions. Physiologic responses are the same as with prone, only more exaggerated.

Lateral Recumbent

See Figure 11-13 for an example of the lateral recumbent position.

Procedures
Chest and kidney surgeries

Positioning Techniques
- Special pad, "bean bag or Vac-Pac" is placed on operating table
- Initially, patient is positioned supine for induction
- Patient is then lifted and turned onto the nonoperative side (usually requires four people during the move)
- Head is supported and aligned with spinal column

Chest Surgery
- Upper arm is flexed slightly at elbow and raised above head; padded overhead armboard may be used or padded Mayo stand
- Lower arm is brought forward slightly, flexed, and placed on padded armboard
- The lower leg is flexed with a pillow placed between legs; feet are placed on pillow to maintain proper alignment
- Safety strap is applied at hip level

Kidney Surgery
- Patient is positioned over kidney elevator of operative table (beneath bony iliac crest)

- This position elevates operative area between the twelfth rib and iliac crest
- Upper extremities may be perpendicular to shoulder level; naturally flexed and supported with padded armboards (two lying side-by-side), or upper arm on overhead armboard
- Lower leg is flexed, and pillow placed between legs, with feet supported with pillow
- Safety strap across thigh (out of operative field)

Once in proper position, bean bag (Vac-Pac) is inflated; for kidney surgery, kidney elevator is raised and table is flexed.

Physiologic Effects
1. Cardiovascular system
   a. Slight change in cardiac output may be evident
   b. Circulation may be impaired by pooling of blood in dependent limb
   c. If kidney rest is elevated, additional compromise may occur owing to pressure on abdominal vessels
   d. In left lateral position, mean arterial pressure drops 24 mm Hg; and in right lateral position it drops 33 mm Hg
2. Respiratory system
   a. Respiratory efficiency may be affected owing to pressure from weight of the body on the lower chest
   b. Restricted movement of chest results in possible compromise in gas exchange
   c. When anesthetized patient is breathing spontaneously, dependent lung has better ventilation at expense of lower lung

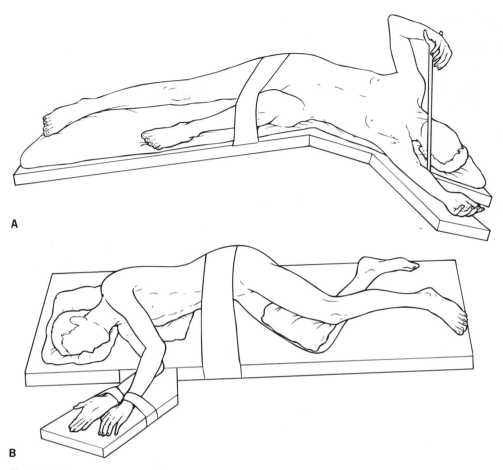

Fig. 11-13. Lateral recumbent positions. (A) chest position; (B) kidney position

d. When patient is paralyzed, upper lung assumes greater compliance and ventilations increase

e. Simple lateral position reduces vital capacity 10 percent and tidal volume 8 percent; kidney position decreases vital capacity by 14.5 percent due to impairment of chest expansion in all directions.

COMMON POSITIONING DEVICES AND CLINICAL IMPLICATIONS

Many devices are on the market today to aid in safely positioning the surgical patient. The perioperative nurse should have a working knowledge of these devices to provide optimum patient positioning, safety, and comfort.

Ideally, any materials used for positioning, especially padding, should accomplish four tasks: (1) absorb compressive force, (2) redistribute pressure, (3) prevent excessive stretching, and (4) provide support for optimum operative stability. All materials should be able to be cleaned adequately and disinfected.

Table Attachments

The following list contains some of the more common table attachments that can be used during positioning:

1. Safety table straps
2. Armboards and wrist restraints
3. Stirrup bars and popliteal knee supports
4. Head rests (specialty) and attachments
5. Kidney elevator and kidney rests
6. Shoulder braces, supports, and overhead arm rests
7. Footboards

Safety Table Straps

The safety strap is the most important positioning device, since it is used the moment a patient is placed on the operating table and remains in place during the entire procedure, as a restraining tool. It must be ap-

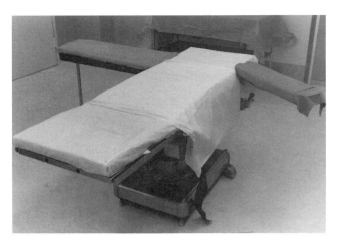

OR table with extremity table attachment

plied with specific principles in mind:

1. The strap is placed above the knees for supine position and below the knees for prone position.
2. It must be secure, yet not constricting, and must be positioned between the blanket (sheet) covering the patient and the patient to avoid any skin irritation.
3. The strap should be tightened enough to allow only a three-finger breadth beneath the strap, to avoid any possible pressure.

Some straps are attached individually on each side of the operating table, with the ends brought together and secured with a Velcro closure device. Others attach on one side of the table frame and extend and attach to the opposite side.

When the safety strap cannot be used, some measure of safety restraint must be used to protect the patient from falling, moving, or turning. Keep in mind that the operating table is very narrow, and remind the patient of this fact and the purpose of the safety restraint.

Armboards and Wrist Restraints

Armboards are used to support patients' arms and hands when they are not placed at their sides. The armboards are attached to the metal frame of the OR table approximately at the axilla level, and once in place have a self-locking mechanism to prevent movement. The angle of the board, however, can be manipulated by a rod-like projection under the board to assist in a more natural placement of the extremities.

An important concept to remember when positioning an extremity on a board is that it should not exceed a 90-degree angle to the body, regardless of the position.

Wrist restraints come in a variety of materials and closures. They should be soft and nonconstricting, yet offer security for the arm when placed around an armboard.

A modification of this armboard is the *adjustable extremity table*, which is either attached to the side of the table frame or slipped under the table mattress, extending the working surface laterally to accommodate surgeries of the upper extremities. When this extension is used, the surgical team usually sits during the procedure.

Stirrup Bars and Popliteal Knee Supports

Metal stirrup posts are placed inside holders that slide onto the table frame to support the legs and feet while in lithotomy position. The feet are placed in canvas or padded loops suspended from the stirrup, and usually cause the legs to be at a right angle to the feet.

For extensive surgery in the lithotomy position, padded knee supports can be used in which the popliteal space is supported in a padded "trough" like stirrup attached to the table. Careful positioning, and protecting the space behind the knees, can avoid pressure on the popliteal vessels and nerves.

Head Rests (Specialty) and Attachments

Commonly used for neurosurgical procedures, head rests attach to the head of the table after removing the pillow section of the table. The head rest supports and exposes areas of the head and cervical vertebrae. They can be used with the supine, prone, sitting, or lateral positions; some types use pin attachments, while others are horseshoe-shaped. The surgeon positions the head while the perioperative nurse stabilizes the head during final positioning and head rest attachment.

Kidney Elevator and Kidney Rests

The kidney elevator is part of the operating table, and can be elevated using the control panel (or crank) at the head of the table. It is used to elevate the mid-torso area of the body when a patient is lying in the lateral position.

The kidney rest is a concave padded metal attachment that is anchored to the table frame to stabilize the patient while he or she is in the lateral position. Kidney rests are placed on both the anterior and posterior sides of the patient, and should be heavily padded to avoid pressure against the body.

Shoulder Braces, Supports, and Overhead Arm Rests

The shoulder braces are attached to the head of the table and are used to prevent the patient from slipping

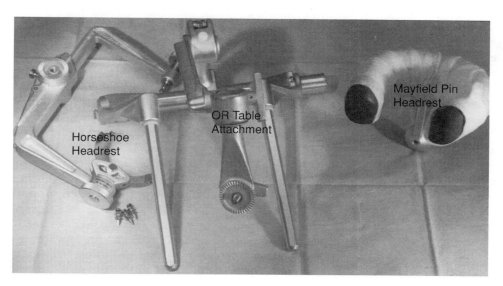

Variety of neurologic headrests and table attachments

toward the head of the table when in the Trendelenburg position. They are metal, concave, and are covered with a foam slipcover.

Shoulder braces should not be used when the arm is extended on an armboard, to avoid compression of the axillary nerve.

Similar to a double armboard, this positioning device is attached to the table in line with the upper torso, with a flat, padded surface extending over the patient's head (face). A Mayo stand, padded and covered, can be used for the same purpose. Used in the lateral position, care must be used when positioning to avoid hyperextension of the axillary region, and the surface must be well padded to prevent pressure on vessels or nerves of the upper extremity.

Footboards

The footboard can serve two purposes:

1. Left flat, as a horizontal surface extension of the table during vaginal or perineal surgeries performed in the lithotomy position, or
2. Raised perpendicular to the table and padded to support the feet, with the soles resting securely against it. This is used primarily in the Trendelenburg position.

Additional Positioning Aids

1. *Sandbags/pillows* available in a variety of shapes and sizes to accommodate anatomic structures. This category includes doughnut-shaped head rests and foam rubber/gelled support pads for stabilization and immobilization of body sections.

2. *Flotation mattresses* (*gelled/egg crate*) created in full table size or proportioned to fit specific devices. They are used to minimize pressure on bony prominences, peripheral blood vessels, and nerves during prolonged procedures (more than 2 hours), and for all cases in which the patient is awake or under conscious sedation.
3. *Chest rolls/commercial bolsters* can be manufactured or can be created by the perioperative nurse using bath blankets; primarily used when the patient is in the prone position. They are placed longitudinally between the axilla and the hip bone, bilaterally in order to maintain adequate respiratory exchange, and to prevent pressure on the chest (breasts), genitalia, and abdominal structures.
4. *Laminectomy frame* a padded metal frame used to elevate the spinal area. The frame is positioned on the table and the patient placed on the frame, being supported from the acromioclavicular joint to the iliac crest. Extensive padding must be used with this frame, and the femoral artery and nerve must be protected.
5. *Towels, tape, ace bandages, soft roll, and so on* can be used to stabilize a position, depending on the type of device being used. Additionally, the table draw sheet (lift sheet) can be used to assist in repositioning a patient or to secure the patient's arms when placed at the sides.

COMMON INJURIES RELATED TO POSITIONING

Planning and preparation can eliminate common injuries related to positioning the surgical patient. However, certain events increase the possibility of injury for all surgical patients. For example, anesthesia prevents the body's normal defense against pain from warning the patient about exaggerated stretching, twisting, and compression of body parts. Peripheral nerve damage and ischemia caused by hyperextension or preexisting disease conditions are also common positioning injuries.

Four areas are commonly susceptible to positioning complications and/or injury: (1) brachial plexus region, (2) ulnar/radial area, (3) saphenous and peroneal nerves, (4) the integumentary system, and (5) eye and facial injuries. Crushing injuries to digits (upper and lower) can also occur whenever the Mayo tray or instrument table is repositioned or resting on or exerting pressure against the patient.

Brachial Plexus Injury

Brachial plexus injury can result from improper positioning and/or hyperextension of the arm(s) or armboard(s), especially for patients in the supine position. To avoid this injury, the perioperative nurse should never allow the patient's arm to be extended to more than a 90-degree angle, and the patient's head should be turned toward the extended arm with the palm supinated or in a natural position. Brachial plexus injuries can also occur when a shoulder brace is used owing to improper positioning of the brace.

Ulnar/Radial Nerve Injury

The ulnar nerve is most commonly injured when an elbow slips off the mattress to the metal edge of the table, and the nerve is compressed between the table and the medial epicondyle.

Radial nerve injury can occur either when the arm slips off the armboard and strikes the table or when it is placed at the side and is pressed between the patient and the table surface.

To eliminate either of these possible injuries, position the hand downward along the patient's side, pad the elbow, and use the draw sheet to secure the arm and hand, and/or use wrist restraints placed loosely yet securely around the armboard and the patient's arm (especially an arm with an IV infusion catheter).

Saphenous and Peroneal Nerve Damage

Saphenous and peroneal nerve injuries are usually associated with the lithotomy position and the use of stirrups. Special care must be used when placing a patient in and out of stirrups in order to avoid these injuries.

Both legs should be raised together when placing a patient in the lithotomy position, first to the knee-chest position, then into the stirrups, to avoid strain on the hip joint and surrounding nerves. Injury to the peroneal nerve can also occur if the thigh is compressed against the stirrup bar (holder); therefore, the bar should be padded around the area of the fibula bone.

Injury to the saphenous nerve can occur if the nerve is pressed between the metal popliteal knee support stirrup and the medial tibial condyle. This pressure could result in numbness in the calf and possible paralysis. Padding of the knee support can prevent this injury, especially between the stirrup and medial aspect of the knee.

Integumentary Damage

Excessive pressure caused by any position can result in damage to the skin in the form of excoriation or actual bruises. When planning positions for any procedure, certain factors to protect the skin and soft tissue should be considered, including the patient's age, general health status, weight distribution, blood pressure, hydration status, and proposed length of immobility.

To prevent these injuries, adequate padding must be used, especially on bony prominences and those anatomic areas requiring special consideration owing to the nature of the required position.

Eye and Facial Injuries

The eyes should be closed and, if needed, an ointment used to maintain moisture and prevent scratching. Excessive pressure against the eye can cause thrombosis of the central retinal artery and can even result in blindness in some instances if the problem goes uncorrected.

Compression of facial structures can be caused by position, equipment, or the surgical team leaning or pressing against the patient's face. This can be avoided by constant monitoring of the patient's head position, and, if necessary, the use of a Mayo stand over the face to elevate the drapes, thus preventing possible injury.

Preventive measures taken before positioning surgical patients can avoid undue harm and protect patients when they cannot protect themselves: one of the primary goals of perioperative nursing practice.

Self-assessment Exercise 3

Directions: Complete the following exercises. The answers are given at the end of this module.

1. In the lateral position, one leg is flexed, while the other is extended. Which leg is flexed? Why?

2. What is the proper placement of the safety strap in the supine and prone positions? Why?

3. Nursing assessment related to positioning should include at least four aspects. List them.

4. The patient should be allowed to cross his or her ankles during surgery because it is a normal position.

    True   False

5. List six potential pressure points when lying in a supine position.

6. List three safety measures that should be used during the transfer of a patient from a stretcher to the OR table.

7. When positioned on armboards, the arm extension must be less than _____ degrees and the palm should be _____.

8. A team of four persons should be used to safely position a patient in lateral position.

    True   False

9. List the five systems that could be adversely affected by poor positioning.

10. Describe the purpose of the following positioning devices:
    a. Egg crate
    b. Bolsters
    c. Sandbags
    d. Doughnut

PREPARING THE INCISION SITE

After the patient has been checked for proper positioning, the next phase of preparing the patient for surgery begins: *first*, selection of the incision site based on the proposed surgical procedure, and *second*, preparation of the skin by removing the resident flora, dirt, and oils.

Even though nurses do not usually assist in the decision of what type of an incision to use for the surgical procedure, the knowledge of incisions in relationship to involved anatomy, positioning, instrumentation, suture choice, and skin preparation area is needed to plan for optimal patient outcomes.

Impact of Site Selection

Two of the primary factors determining where the incision will be are the patient's diagnosis and the pathology the surgeon expects to encounter.

Other factors may affect the selection of sites: these include maximum exposure, ease and speed of entry or reentry (in an emergent state), the possibility of extending the incision, maximum postoperative wound strength with minimal postoperative discomfort, and, finally, the general cosmetic effect.

For the nurse or technician assisting at the sterile field, the knowledge of anatomic layers and structures as they relate to the incision site can assist in choosing the right instruments and suture/stapling choices. Knowledge of the incision site can also be used to help

gauge the progress of the operation, thereby assisting in anticipating the needs of the surgeon/assistant during the procedure.

For the circulating nurse, knowledge of the incision site is of primary importance, since it will guide him or her in performing the surgical skin preparation. The prep should always begin at the site of the incision and work outward, toward the periphery. Additionally, gauging the progress of surgery assures the performance of counts at the proper interval and can help estimate the proper time for requesting the next patient to be premedicated.

For the anesthesia practitioner, the choice of sites can directly or indirectly affect the method and/or technique for administration of anesthesia, depending on the anatomic structure involved.

Anatomic Considerations

When discussing incisions and their locations, it is important to know anatomic directional terms, such as *median* and *horizontal* planes of the body, so that basic landmarks can be located when other directional terms are used, such as *upper quadrant*, *oblique*, or *paramedian*. For example, a *right paramedian* would be located just to the right of and perpendicular to the median (middle) line.

The illustrations (Fig. 11-14) will assist you in reviewing the common anatomic planes and areas with their corresponding structures. It is essential that the

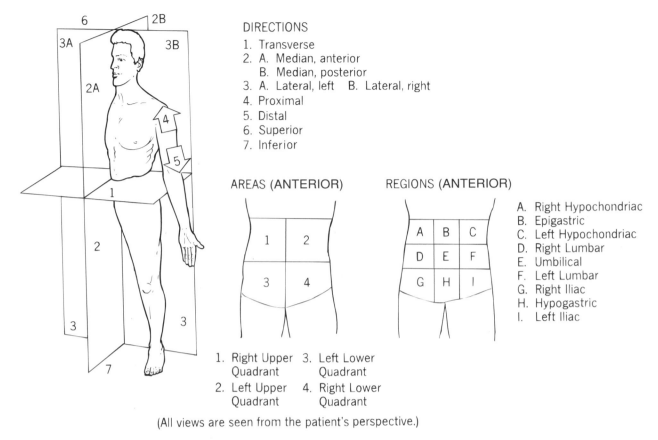

DIRECTIONS
1. Transverse
2. A. Median, anterior
   B. Median, posterior
3. A. Lateral, left   B. Lateral, right
4. Proximal
5. Distal
6. Superior
7. Inferior

AREAS (ANTERIOR)

1. Right Upper   3. Left Lower
   Quadrant   Quadrant
2. Left Upper   4. Right Lower
   Quadrant   Quadrant

REGIONS (ANTERIOR)

A. Right Hypochondriac
B. Epigastric
C. Left Hypochondriac
D. Right Lumbar
E. Umbilical
F. Left Lumbar
G. Right Iliac
H. Hypogastric
I. Left Iliac

(All views are seen from the patient's perspective.)

Fig. 11-14. Anatomic directions, areas, and regions (patient's view)

perioperative nurse become familiar with these areas/ planes to prepare the incision site effectively.

Incision Site Locations

Although it is not uncommon for surgeries to have several approaches, Table 11-4 provides the most common incision sites as they relate to anatomic structures and/or surgical procedures associated with the thoracic, abdominal, and pelvic cavities.

INCISION DESCRIPTIONS: THORACOABDOMINAL CAVITY

Midline

The midline incision is the simplest and most common abdominal incision, and is used primarily with general surgical procedures as it provides adequate exposure to nearly all the structures within the abdominal cavity. It usually extends in the upper region from the xiphoid process to the umbilicus and in the lower abdomen from the umbilicus to the symphysis pubis.

The five major layers of the midline incision from the ventral surface to the dorsal surface include (Fig. 11-15):

1. Skin
2. Subcutaneous tissue/fat
3. Fascia
4. Muscle
5. Peritoneum

If the surgeon makes the incision slightly left or right of this line, it is referred to as a *paramedian* incision, which additionally involves the *rectus abdominus* muscle.

Subcostal (Kocher's)

This incision, either right or left, follows the lower costal margin in a semicurved shape. Because the *rectus* muscles are severed, this incision can be more painful postoperatively than the midline incision. The tissues encountered include:

1. Skin
2. Subcutaneous tissue/fat

Table 11-4 Incision Reference Chart*

Incision	Reference	Use	Characteristics
Collar	A	Thyroid surgery	Provides access to thyroid; generally heals well
Sternal split	B	Cardiac surgery	Access to all thoracic structures; leaves very large scar
Lateral thoracotomy	C	Thoracic and cardiac surgery	Generally heals well; damage to an intercostal nerve can cause persistent pain in incision area
Subcostal (Kocher's) Right	D, E	Gallbladder and biliary tract surgery	Excellent exposure of the upper abdomen; difficult to extend; very painful
Left Horizontal flank	F	Surgery of the spleen Nephrectomy; lumbar sympathectomy; ureterolithotomy; inferior vena cava ligation	Allows access to retroperitoneal space; quickly executed; easy to extend and quickly closed
Upper abdominal midline (vertical)	G	Surgeries involving the stomach; exploratory laparotomy	Excellent exposure of upper abdomen; quickly opened and closed; easily extended
Lower abdominal midline (vertical)	H	Surgeries of the uterus, tubes, ovaries; cystostomy; suprapubic prostatectomy; exploratory laparotomy	Excellent exposure of pelvic organs; quickly opened and closed; easily extended; not as strong as lower paramedian or lower transverse
Paramedian Right upper	I	Surgeries of the biliary tract, stomach, pancreas, duodenum	Excellent for exposure to the specific organs; easy to open and close; easy to extend; provides firm closure
Right lower	J	Appendectomy; small bowel resection; left adnexae	
Left upper	K	Surgery of the spleen; gastrectomy; vagotomy	
Left lower	L	Sigmoid colon resection; Miles' resection; hysterectomy; left adnexae	
McBurney's	M	Appendectomy	Quick to open and close; not easy to extend; poor exposure for exploration; firm closure
Inguinal (oblique) (right/left)	N	Hernia repair; hydrocelectomy of spermatic cord	Does not enter abdomen
Infraumbilical	O	Umbilical hernia repair; laparoscopy	Curvilinear—below umbilicus
Transverse upper abdominal	P	Exploratory laparotomy; hiatal hernia repair	Difficult to extend; hard to heal and painful postoperatively
Transverse suprapubic (Pfannensteil)	Q	Surgeries on uterus, tubes, ovaries, prostate	Difficult to extend; limited exposure; good cosmetic closure

* See p. 331, Fig. 11-16.

3. Rectus muscle
4. Fascia
5. Peritoneum

Obliques

The term *oblique* refers to a slanting or inclined line, which is usually associated with the inguinal regions,

or when performing an appendectomy (McBurney's). However, it can be used to denote any incision created on this angle.

Inguinal

The right/left oblique in the inguinal region gives excellent exposure of the structures located in the groin

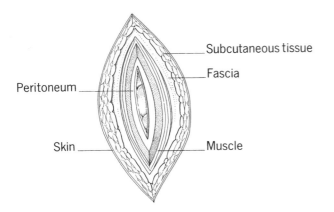

Fig. 11-15. Layers of the abdomen (From Anatomical insights: The abdomen. Sommerville, NJ, 1987. Reprinted with courtesy of Ethicon, Inc.)

area. The muscle layers associated with this incision include:

1. External oblique
2. Internal oblique
3. Transversus abdominis
4. Conjoined tendon
5. External inguinal ring

McBurney's

The McBurney incision is traditionally associated with an exploration of the appendix, but can be used for exploration of any other structure located in the right lower quadrant of the abdomen, although visibility is limited.

This incision is commonly called a "muscle splitting" incision, because the muscle fibers split naturally, without being severed as with most. Although the exposure is limited, the incision can be lengthened if necessary. The tissue layers involved with this incision include:

1. Skin
2. Subcutaneous tissue/fat
3. Fascia
4. Oblique and transversalis muscle
5. Peritoneum

Transverse

There are two commonly used transverse incisions:

1. Lower (Pfannensteil)
2. Midabdominal

Pfannensteil

This incision, nicknamed the "bikini-cut," is frequently used in gynecologic surgery. The incision is a curved line across the lower abdomen, above the symphysis pubis. The incision allows for a strong, yet cosmetic closure, owing to the contraction of the rectus muscle, which places less strain on the fascial sutures. The tissues involved include:

1. Skin
2. Subcutaneous tissue and rectus sheath
3. Rectus muscle
4. Peritoneum (midline vertical incision)

Midabdominal

This incision is used on the right or left side, or for a retroperitoneal approach.

It begins slightly above or below the umbilicus and is extended to the lumbar region at an angle, between the ribs and the crest of the ilium. Tissue layers include:

1. Skin and subcutaneous tissue
2. Anterior rectus vessels/muscle
3. Posterior rectus sheath
4. Peritoneum (near midline)—extended laterally to oblique muscles. Lateral muscles may be excised to provide a wider exposure.

Thoracoabdominal

The thoracoabdominal, as its name implies, is used when exposure to the thoracic and abdominal cavities may be required. The incision begins at a point midway between the xiphoid process and the umbilicus, extending across to the seventh or eighth intercostal space, and to the midscapular line superiorly.

In most instances the abdominal portion of the incision is made first, allowing for initial exploration, and then, if needed, it is extended across the costal margin to the chest. Tissues involved include the rectus and oblique muscles, peritoneum, costal cartilages, and diaphragm.

Upper Abdominal

Although seldom used, this incision line extends from a point below the costal margin on one side, anterior to the axillary line, to the same point on the opposite side, and resembles a U. The midpoint usually lies between the xiphoid process and the umbilicus, preserving the intercostal nerves. If used, its application might include surgeries involving the stomach, colon, biliary, and pancreatic structures.

SURGICAL SKIN PREPARATION

> Surgery cannot be carried out without the basic principles of aseptic technique and wound care.
> —*Lord Joseph Lister*

The majority of postoperative infections results from contamination acquired in the operating room. Three factors seem to have a dominant role in the development of surgical infections:

1. Microbial contamination of the wound
2. Condition of the wound at the end of surgery
3. Patient susceptibility

Since the interaction of these factors is complex, measures intended to prevent surgical wound infections are aimed at all three.

The actual surgical technique will ultimately determine the condition of the wound at the end of surgery. Measures taken by the perioperative nurse to prevent surgical wound infections can be directly related to the preparation of the incision site.

The area to be prepped is determined by the site of the incision and the nature of the planned surgical intervention. A wide area is usually preferable, because it allows the surgeon to extend the incision and/or strategically place tubes or drains as needed within an aseptically prepared area.

Since the patient's skin cannot be sterilized, measures must be taken to reduce the resident and transient flora naturally present on the skin surface. This can be accomplished by the application of an antimicrobial agent, rendering the skin "surgically clean," and is performed before the draping procedure.

The antimicrobial agent(s) chosen for the skin preparation should be capable of removing superficial oils, dirt, and debris without causing undue tissue reaction to the agent. It should be able to decrease the microbial count while leaving a protective film or residue on the skin.

The surgical skin prep is performed by the circulating nurse (or designated person, e.g., intern) using strict aseptic technique. The area of the skin prep, the solutions used, and any undesirable patient reactions (e.g., allergenic) should be documented on the intraoperative record.

Sequence of the Surgical Skin Prep

The skin preparation is performed in three segments (Fig. 11-16):

1. Assessing and documenting skin condition and removing any hair directly interfering with the incision site

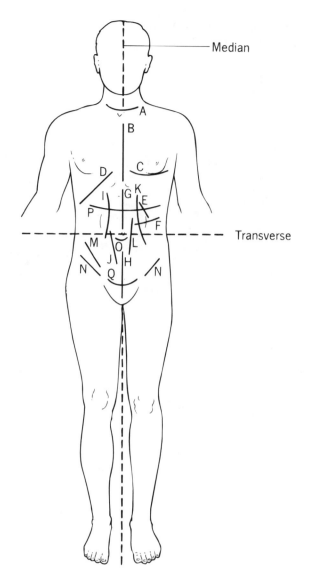

Fig. 11-16.   Incision reference chart

2. Cleansing (scrubbing) the skin with the antimicrobial scrub solution, removing the superficial dirt, oils, and debris
3. Applying the antimicrobial solution, which creates an antiseptic-like bacterial barrier

Today, there are a variety of prep solutions and prepping set-ups to choose from. Some require only one step, while others require both the scrubbing and the painting. Regardless of how the agent(s) is dispensed, the overall principles of performing an aseptic procedure remain the same: the prep begins at the site of the incision and works outward toward the periphery, never going over an area already prepared.

Association of Operating Room Nurses Recommended Practices

The following recommended practices are associated with the surgical skin prep, and should be used as a guide for effective practice:[9]

> ### Recommended Practices for Skin Preparation of Patients
>
> I. The operative site and surrounding areas should be clean.
> II. The operative site should be assessed before skin preparation
> III. The operative site and surrounding area should be prepared with an antimicrobial agent
> IV. Patient skin preparation should be documented in the patient's record.
>
> *Source:* AORN. Standards and recommended practices. Denver, CO: The Association, 1995. Pp. 255–257.

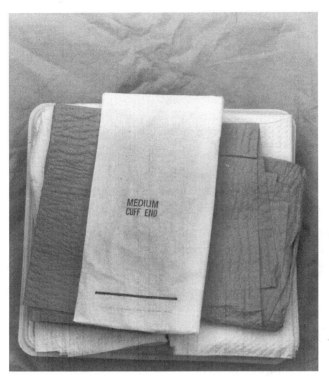

Surgical skin preparation tray

Antimicrobial Solutions

Two generic groups of antimicrobial agents are capable of reducing both gram-positive and gram-negative bacteria to a minimum. These are (1) *povidone/iodine* and (2) *chlorhexidine gluconate.* Both these agents meet the criteria for selection of an effective antimicrobial agent.[10] They

- are rapid acting
- are not dependent on cumulative action
- have a broad spectrum of activity in reducing transient/resident flora
- have minimal harsh effects on the skin
- inhibit rapid rebound growth of microbes
- have a contact time based on documentation in scientific literature
- are economical to use

Perioperative Nursing Considerations

Before beginning the surgical skin prep, the perioperative nurse should be mindful of the following considerations:

1. No known patient allergies to planned solution
   - Review patient admission assessment for sensitivity or allergies to iodine or seafood

- For those patients who have demonstrated skin sensitivities to either agent, another broad-spectrum antimicrobial agent, *parachlorometaxylenol,* may be substituted after consultation with the surgeon.
2. Chlorhexidine gluconate should not be used for or near the eyes, ears, or mouth.
3. Alcohol is *not* recommended for use as a primary prepping agent. If it is used, the skin *must* be completely dried before using electrosurgery and/or laser.
4. Sponges need not be saturated (dripping) with the agent in order to be effective. The combination of the chemical and mechanical friction creates an acceptable mechanism for preparing the patient's skin.

Supplies and Set-Up

The supplies needed to perform the surgical skin preparation should be arranged on a separate surface a safe distance from the sterile field. Most prep trays are preassembled and disposable, with contents varying according to manufacturer; some contain individual bottles of prep solution, while others are "dry," to add the solution of choice.

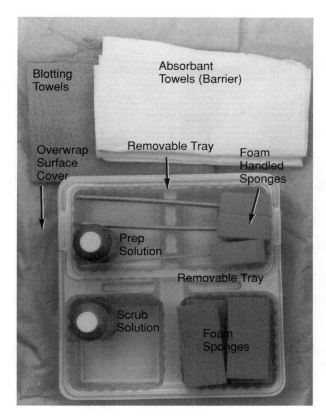

Contents of a surgical skin prep tray

If additional procedures (e.g., insertion of a Foley catheter) are to be performed, they should be done prior to the prep, using a completely separate set-up to avoid accidental contamination of the aseptically prepared area.

Special Areas of Consideration

Eyes

The eyes should be washed with cotton balls and a nonirritating solution (surgeon's preference). Prep should begin at the nose and continue outward toward the cheeks. Prep solution should be rinsed with warm sterile water.

Traumatic/Open Wounds

Large amounts of detergent–irrigating solution combination may be used prior to the prep and/or in addition to the prep, to remove gross dirt from the wound, depending on the condition of the traumatized area. Once the wound has been initially cleansed, handle the prep as if it was a stoma or contaminated area prep.

Stomas

The external stoma (orifice) of a colostomy or ileostomy may be (1) sealed off from the operative site with a detergent-soaked sponge, and the area surrounding it (considered clean) prepped first, or (2) cleaned from the outer boundary of the stoma area outward, then coming back to the stoma with a new sponge. Since the area has been aseptically prepared, the paint sequence is started from the incision site outward, including the stoma area.

Limb Preparation

A circumferential prep should be performed on all extremities, which usually will require an assistant to extend and hold up the extremity. Persons should have sterile gloves so as not to interfere with the aseptic area involved.

Tumors, Aneurysms, Ovarian Cysts

1. Tumors/biopsy: carcinoma cells can become disseminated with vigorous scrubbing; therefore, use gentle yet comprehensive scrubbing technique
2. Aortic aneurysms: aneurysms could rupture during the prepping sequence; thus, work quickly yet gently
3. Ovarian cyst: large ones could rupture as a result of a vigorous scrub

Fractures

Fractures must be stabilized during the prep (e.g., with an additional person holding the affected extremity), and gentle scrubbing should be used to avoid further complications. A circumferential prep should be used. If the fracture is comminuted, solution may be poured over the area instead of painted.

Genitalia

This area is considered dirty; therefore, it should be done last when incorporated with an abdominal prep. Internal vaginal preps should be performed with solution only, since detergent may cause a reaction (itching, burning, etc.).

Dirty/Contaminated Areas (Colostomy, Infections, and so on)

1. Umbilicus: cleaned separately with cotton-tipped applicator
2. Perineal prep: vagina and anus prepped last and with separate sponge
3. Shoulder: axilla is prepped last
4. Draining sinuses, skin ulcers: scrub last—*clean to*

Procedure for Surgical Skin Preparation

PURPOSE

To decrease the number of bacteria on the patient's skin, thus reducing the possibility of postoperative wound infections due to invasion of microorganisms.

PREREQUISITE

1. Patient is in correct position, and anatomical alignment for proposed surgical procedure is correct
2. Prep tray is open on a separate surface
3. Operative site is exposed while maintaining patient's dignity and privacy

PROFICIENCY

One hundred percent accuracy at time of performance

PROCEDURAL STEPS

A. PREPARATION
   1. Apply sterile gloves (open glove technique) and arrange prep tray, maintaining sterile technique. Verify completeness (possible components may include):
      a. Sterile glove packet (1)
      b. Utility drapes (2)
      c. Blotting towels (2)
      d. Winged sponges (for scrubbing sequence)
      e. Paint applicators ("lolly-pop" sticks)
      f. Cotton-tipped applicator sticks (for umbilicus)
      g. Individual scrub and paint solutions (optional)
   2. Place utility towels (absorbent towels) on either side of the patient, near area to be prepped, placing the farthest towel first.
B. SCRUBBING SEQUENCE
   1. Pour scrub and paint solutions into appropriate compartments.
   2. Immerse a winged sponge into the scrub solution, and squeeze out the excess solution.
   3. Beginning at the incision site, and using small circular motions, scrub the area in a "bulls-eye" formation, working from the point of incision outward to the periphery (Fig. A).
   4. Upon reaching outer boundary, discard first sponge, and immerse another sponge. Repeat Step 2 until all sponges have been used.

NOTE: Never use a contaminated sponge to go over an area that has already been prepped.

C. BLOTTING SEQUENCE
   1. Using the sterile towel(s) provided, blot the prepped area, soaking up the scrub solution. (Two towels may be needed, depending on the area.)
   2. Remove the towel(s) by grasping the two far corners and peeling backward and upward toward you, being careful not to drag the towel across the prepped area.
D. PAINTING SEQUENCE
   1. Immerse the applicator sponge stick in the "paint" solution; squeeze out the excess.

2. Starting at the incision site, paint to the periphery, using a "bulls-eye" format (see Fig. A).
3. When the periphery is reached, discard sponge stick, and using a new applicator stick, repeat step 2 until all sponge sticks are used.

NOTE: Avoid contacting prepped area with contaminated sponge.

E. TERMINATION OF PROCEDURE
   1. At the conclusion of the painting sequence, remove the two utility towels from either side of the patient **(do not reach over the prepped area).**
   2. Push the prep stand away from the operating table, discard it in an appropriate receptable, and remove gloves (skin to skin, glove to glove).

POINTS TO REMEMBER

1. Maintain aseptic technique throughout the procedure.
2. Avoid "pooling" of solutions under the patient, which can result in irritation/chemical burns to the skin.
3. The duration of the scrub sequence is usually 5 minutes, unless a longer prep is requested by the surgeon.
4. The outer boundaries should be at least 12 inches from the proposed incision site.
5. When prepping an infected area, the prep should begin at the outer (clean) boundary, and work towards the dirty area (scrub sequence only). Painting sequence is from incision site to periphery.
6. Inserting an indwelling catheter should always precede the prepping procedure. If "straight" catheterizing (D&C; laparoscopy, etc.), the catheter is inserted between the scrub and paint sequence.
7. Work quickly but with accuracy, maintaining an aseptic field at all times.

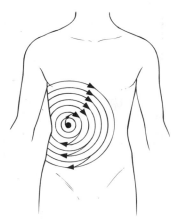

1. Abdominal

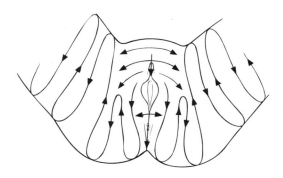

2. Perineal / Vaginal

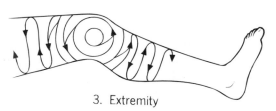

3. Extremity

Fig. A. Diagram of skin prep technique

PERFORMANCE CHECK SHEET

NAME:	TASK # _____11-2_____
	RATING: A Acceptable
	N/I Needs Improvement
PROCEDURE: Incisional Site Preparation (Skin Prep)	

PROCEDURAL STEPS	A	N/I
A. PREPARATION 1. Prepares for prep using proper opening technique 2. Dons sterile gloves correctly 3. Prepares the field using utility towels in proper manner **B. SCRUBBING SEQUENCE** 1. Uses soaped sponges in circular motion, squeezing out excess 2. Uses new sponge each time process is repeated 3. Avoids going over prepped area with contaminated sponge **C. BLOTTING SEQUENCE** 1. Blot drys the area with sterile towel 2. Removes towel in proper manner **D. PAINTING SEQUENCE** 1. Uses solution starting from incision site working to outside borders 2. Uses new sponge for each cycle 3. Avoids going over areas with a contaminated sponge **E. CONCLUSION OF PROCEDURE** 1. Removes utility towels in proper manner 2. Disposes of supplies and equipment in proper container		

COMMENTS: _____

_____

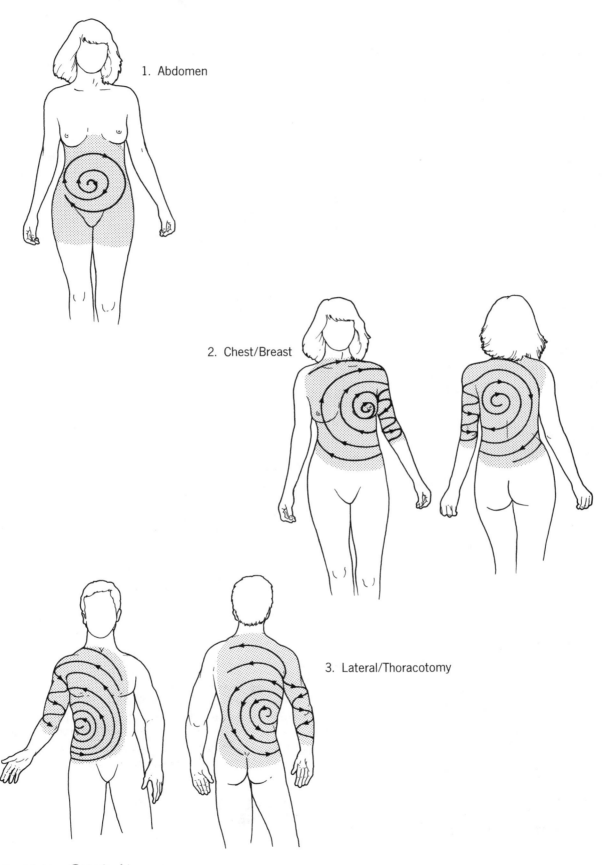

1. Abdomen

2. Chest/Breast

3. Lateral/Thoracotomy

Fig. 11-17. Generic skin prep areas

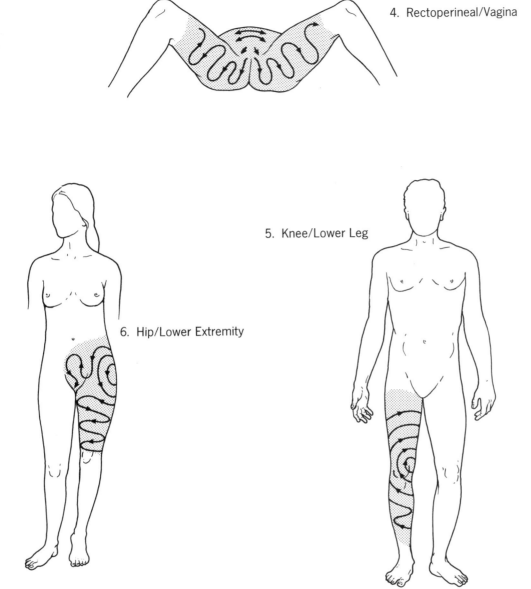

4. Rectoperineal/Vagina

5. Knee/Lower Leg

6. Hip/Lower Extremity

Fig. 11-17. *(continued)*

dirty principle applies to all aseptic skin preps, regardless of the area involved

Grafts

A separate set-up for donor and recipient site should be used. The donor site is prepped first. Two nurses may be required to do a simultaneous prep. The donor site should be prepped with a colorless antiseptic solution to allow postoperative visibility of the vascularity of the graft. The donor site is covered with a sterile towel if not dressed immediately.

Emergency Preps

There are occasions when the urgency to begin the surgery overrides the need for a full surgical prep (e.g., leaking aortic aneurysm, emergency cesarean section, traumatic hemorrhage). The surgical scrub may be omitted and the solution used alone.

SURGICAL PREPARATION GUIDELINES

Surgical preparation guidelines are illustrated in Figure 11-17.

NOTE: For specific procedures, refer to the institutional reference manual or the Physician's Preference Card.

Abdomen

The area should include breastline to upper third of thighs; table-line to table-line, when in supine position.

Chest/Breast

This area should include shoulders, upper arm to elbow, axilla, and chest wall to table-line and 2 inches beyond the sternum to the opposite shoulder. (Lateral or supine with surgical side slightly elevated.)

Lateral/Thoracotomy

The lateral/thoracoabdominal area includes axilla, chest, and abdomen from neck to crest of ilium. Area should extend beyond the midline, anteriorly and posteriorly.

Rectoperineal/Vaginal

Area includes pubis, vulva, labia, perineum, anus, and adjacent areas, including inner aspects of upper third of thighs.

Abdominal/Vaginal

Abdomen to above the umbilicus to pubis area, including vaginal area as previously described.

Knee/Lower Leg

Area includes the entire circumference of affected leg and extends from the foot to the upper part of the thigh.

Hip/Lower Extremity

This area includes the abdomen on the affected side, thigh to knee, buttocks to table-line, groin, and pubis. Prep must be circumferential.

Self-assessment Exercise 4

Directions: Complete the following exercises. The answers are given at the end of this module.

1. As a general rule, the surgical prep is started at the site of the incision and continues outward toward the periphery.

   True   False

2. The information regarding the surgical prep should be documented, including

   _____.

3. An _____ incision is used when performing an appendectomy.

4. Another name for a *transverse suprapubic* incision is a *Pfannensteil.*

   True   False

5. During the prepping procedure, it is acceptable to use a two-handed, side-to-side prepping motion.

   True   False

6. Match the following:
   ___ 1. Right subcostal   a. Laparoscopy
   ___ 2. Oblique   b. Open heart
          (inguinal)   surgery
   ___ 3. Infraumbilical   c. Cholecystectomy
   ___ 4. Sternal split   d. Herniorrhaphy

INTRAOPERATIVE EQUIPMENT AND ACCESSORY ITEMS

Safety: freedom from harm, danger, risk or injury.[11]

This word is associated with every type of business and profession, and should be of primary concern for all those working in the health-care arena. Nowhere else is this more important than in surgery, since the surgical suite uses special equipment and high technology.

In addition to surgical instruments and specialty supplies, there are *standard* pieces of equipment that are used routinely during a variety of surgical procedures.

In order to maintain a safe environment and protect the patient and/or staff from harm, the person handling the equipment must have a thorough knowledge and understanding of the how's and why's of each piece of equipment and accessory item. Additionally, he or she should be familiar with what to do should the equipment fail to function within acceptable guidelines and/or established safety criteria.

POWER EQUIPMENT

Power equipment ranges in type from electrosurgical units to high-technology laser units, and includes equipment such as power drills, saws, tourniquets, and specialized light sources.

They all have one common factor, however techno-logically advanced they may seem: they need a source of power to operate. This power is derived from one of two sources: electrical power or air/gas power, either from a freestanding tank or a supply coming through a wall outlet in the procedure room.

According to AORN's Patient Outcome Standard IV:[12]

The patient is free from injury related to . . . electrical and physical hazards. . . .

This standard can be achieved only by applying safety measures associated with the equipment and thoroughly understanding the equipment to be used.

General Considerations for Safety

The proper handling of any piece of equipment used in surgery is the responsibility of every member of the surgical team. Some general safety guidelines, which can aid in protecting the patient and the staff from harm, include:

1. All electrical equipment should be routinely inspected by qualified personnel.
2. All power equipment should be inspected by the user before and after each use.
3. Power cords should never be crimped or bent; any tears or breaks in the cord should negate the use of the cord until it is repaired.
4. Extension cords should be avoided whenever pos-

sible, and power cords should lie flat on the floor or be suspended to prevent obstruction of traffic areas and/or entrances.

5. Freestanding pressure tanks should be checked before and after each use, replaced immediately when the pressure in the tank is below a safe limit, and monitored during its use.

6. Equipment must be maintained through proper cleaning, lubrication, and sterilization procedures, according to the manufacturer's written recommendations.

7. Verification that the correct attachments for a piece of equipment are in fact being used should be performed by the person using the equipment, including confirmation that the attachments are seated properly before activating the unit.

8. When not in use, equipment should be maintained in a neutral power state, and sharp tips protected to avoid accidental injury.

9. All persons handling power equipment should be educated about their function and proper use.

Electrosurgical Units

The purpose of the electrosurgical unit (ESU) is to (1) control bleeding through the application of heat, and (2) to cut tissue.

The application of heat or fire to sear wounds and stop them from bleeding dates back as far as 3000 B.C. Through the years, many methods have been used to accomplish this task. The discovery of electricity, however, in the middle 1800s led to the development of electrocautery (1875), which is still used today.

In the 1920s, surgical technique began to expand, and the need to control bleeding in a more sophisticated manner became an important factor in the outcome of the surgical procedure. An attempt was made with cold cautery, but it was found to be unacceptable owing to its ineffectiveness in controlling capillary oozing. But with further research, conducted by Dr. William T. Bovie (1925), a physicist at Harvard, a unit was developed that could provide cutting with hemostasis, using heat. The unit was first successfully used during a neurosurgical procedure performed by Dr. Harvey Cushing. This is the origin of electrosurgery and the term *Bovie*.

In the early 1970s, solid-state electrosurgical units were introduced to the surgical setting. These units, unlike their predecessors, were more compact, with new added safety features. Through the years, and with the help of advanced medical technology, changes have intensified the safety features and increased the versatility of the unit. Today, a variety of units are found in most surgical procedure rooms

and in other settings where this technology is required.

Electrosurgery versus Electrocautery

Many people, nurses and technicians alike, use the terms *electrosurgery* and *electrocautery* interchangeably. However, there is a distinct difference.

In *electrosurgery*, heat is generated in tissue by passing a high-frequency current through the tissue.

In *electrocautery*, heat is transferred to the tissues from a preheated object. In other words, tissue is heated by contact with a hot wire (probe), and no electric current flows through the tissue.

Since electrosurgery is the correct term to use when describing the process currently being used in the surgical setting, it will be used in this discussion.

Recommended Practices for Electrosurgery

The following recommended practices have been established by the AORN as guidelines for safely using electrosurgical equipment:[13]

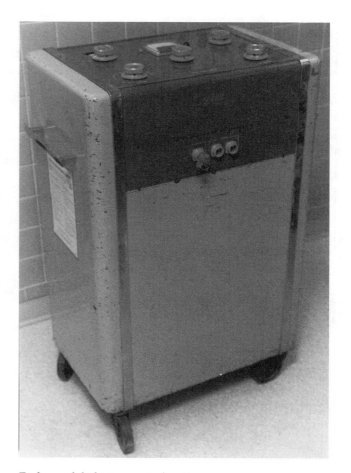

Early model electrosurgical unit

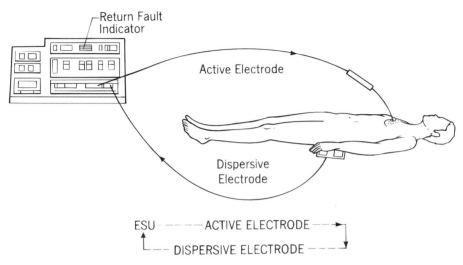

Fig. 11-18. Electrosurgical flow

<hr>

Recommended Practices for Electrosurgery

I. The electrosurgical unit (ESU), dispersive electrode and active electrode selected for use should meet performance and safety criteria established by the practice setting.

II. Perioperative personnel should demonstrate competency in the use of the ESU in the practice setting.

III. The ESU, active electrode, and dispersive electrode should be used in a manner that reduces the potential for injury.

IV. Patients and perioperative personnel should be protected from inhaling the smoke generated during electrosurgery.

Source: AORN. Standards and recommended practices. Denver, CO: The Association, 1995. Pp. 155–159.

<hr>

ESU and Components

To perform electrosurgery, three basic components are required: (1) the power unit, (2) the active electrode, and (3) the dispersive (return) electrode. These, along with the patient, are necessary to complete the electrical circuit.

The Power Unit

The ESU is a high-power generator of high-frequency electrical energy. When applied to tissue with a high current density, this energy causes the desired destruction of tissue cells. High current density is needed at

the *active* electrode, while low current density is desired at the *dispersive* (return) electrode to eliminate adverse heating effects at the dispersive electrode site.

The amount of heat (tissue destruction) generated depends on the power level and duration of application. As the current enters the surgical site via the active electrode, it dissipates through the body, causing heat and tissue destruction, and exits over a large dispersive electrode returning the current to the unit (Fig. 11-18).

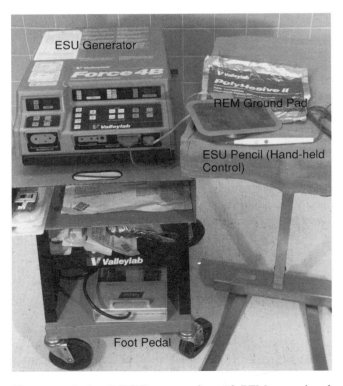

Electrosurgical unit (ESU): monopolar with REM ground pad

Active and Dispersive Electrodes

An ESU has output connections for both the active and dispersive electrodes. The unit should provide a sentry alarm system that will detect incomplete circuits; one for the dispersive electrode–cable contact and one for the dispersive electrode–patient contact. This sentry system can alert the perioperative nurse that the circuit is broken somewhere, which demands immediate action.

Accessory Items

The Active Electrode   The active electrode delivers the power to the operative site, and can be activated by either a hand or foot control.

A variety of tips are available for use in specific areas, and attach at the end of a "pencil-like" control wand. The larger the tip, the greater the tendency to coagulate rather than cut, and the smaller the tip the greater the tendency to cut. The exception to this is the *needle* electrode tip, which is used for pinpoint coagulation.

Most hand pieces are disposable, and come in a variety of shapes other than the traditional pencil wand.

The Dispersive Electrode   The electrosurgical electric circuit requires delivery of the current via the ESU and active electrode, which returns to the ESU via the dispersive electrode, or *patient ground pad*. The functions of a dispersive electrode are to provide a large surface area for the current to leave the patient, maintain low density, and reduce the temperature of the tissue, preventing a surface area burn.

There are five basic criteria for a dispersive electrode:

1. It must provide and assure uniform contact with the patient.
2. It must not cause pressure points to occur.
3. It must be flexible.
4. It must disperse current to ensure low current density.
5. It should contain a built-in monitoring system to warn against a break in the circuit.

To maximize the efficiency and safety of the dispersive electrode, certain general placement/handling guidelines should be followed.

• DO's		• DON'Ts	
DO check all cables for cracks and deterioration. DO follow manufacturer's instructions for checking alarm systems. DO shave (if necessary), clean and dry the site thoroughly before applying the patient plate. DO apply the patient plate in complete contact with well vascularized, muscular tissue. DO apply patient plate before draping patient. DO ensure that a plate supplied without gel is adequately covered with conductive gel before use. DO check the entire surface of a pregelled patient plate for fresh gel before application.	DO check patient plate contact first and cable connections during surgery if abnormal power levels are requested or the surgeon experiences a loss of cutting or coagulation. DO check patient plate for adequate contact if the patient is repositioned during surgery. DO keep active electrode blade clean of tissue buildup. DO use a RF suppressor (RF choke) with the ECG cable. DO keep the active electrode blade from inadvertently touching the patient when not in use. DO remove the patient plate slowly.	DON'T allow fluids to pool at patient plate site. DON'T locate patient plate over bony areas, scar tissue, or implanted prostheses. DON'T use pregelled patient plate with dry or discolored gel. DON'T use gel on capacitive or conductive adhesive patient plates. DON'T cut patient plate smaller to fit patient. DON'T activate the active electrode until it is close to the surgical site.	DON'T pass electrosurgical current through an implanted metal prosthesis (total hip, rod, pacemaker lead, etc.). DON'T wrap patient plate cord or active electrode cord around metal objects. DON'T spark active electrode to ground to check power unit operation. DON'T position the ECG electrodes between the surgical site and the patient plate.

Do's and Don'ts of electrosurgery (Courtesy of the 3M Company)

Monopolar versus Bipolar

The ESU is available as *monopolar* or *bipolar*, and depending on the surgical procedure, one or both may be used.

Monopolar With monopolar electrosurgery, only one pole is *active*, and it carries current to the operative site. The current flows from the monopolar connection output to the electrode, which is applied to the tissue, is dispersed over the dispersive electrode (ground pad), and returned to the ESU via the dispersive electrode cable.

Bipolar A bipolar active electrode has a forceps configuration. In the bipolar electrode, one tip acts as the active pole while the other tip acts as the return (dispersive) pole. With bipolar, a ground pad is not required, since the dispersive electrode is one of the bipolar tips. By using a bipolar electrode, the power is distributed to a very limited area (between the tips only) and the actual wattage power required is reduced, making it safe for use on delicate tissue, such as the brain.

Electrosurgical Safety

Safety measures are intended to minimize the potential for electric hazards. The three most common hazards associated with electricity are fire, electric shock, and burns. These are hazards for both patient and personnel; therefore, the entire staff must make every attempt to maintain a safe environment.

Although fire hazards have been greatly reduced, faulty wiring, poorly maintained equipment, and a lack of regard for safety measures can cause a spark, resulting in a fire.

Contact with 110/120 volt power (common household current) can cause electric shock and/or electrocution. Safety measures that can assist in preventing this hazard should include inspecting electric cords, plugs, and connectors; operating the unit at its lowest acceptable setting; and never operating equipment with wet hands or when standing on a wet surface.

Burns can occur from direct contact with hot electric wires or from items overheating by electric wires. Safety measures that can reduce the possibility of burns include avoiding use of a power unit as an "extra" table surface; not allowing the patient ground cable to contact a hypothermia blanket; never activating the active electrode (hand piece) with wet gloves or gloves with a hole in them; maintaining an awareness of where the active electrode tip is located and/or storing it in an appropriate holder when not in use; checking the equipment before each use, including cords, connectors, and the alarm system; and *never* turning down the volume of the alarm so that it cannot notify the team of a possible problem alert.

The least understood hazard associated with the use of electrosurgery is patient burns. Patient burns usu-

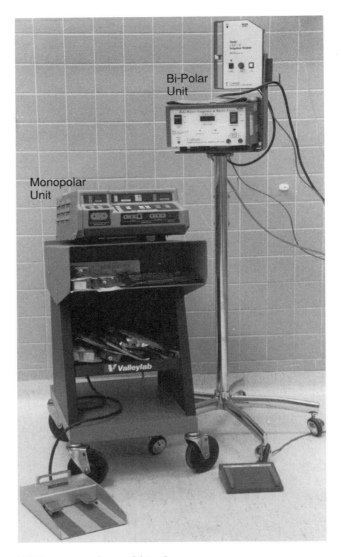

ESUs: monopolar and bipolar

ally result when too much current flows through an inadequate area for too long a time; therefore, the use, placement, and proper connection of the ground pad becomes one of the most important factors associated with safe use of the ESU.

If not properly placed, or if complete contact with the patient is not maintained throughout the procedure, or if the ground pad becomes wet from prepping solutions, the high-frequency current could become concentrated or find an alternative path—the patient—and cause a severe burn. This injury has in fact necessitated plastic and/or reconstructive surgery (at the hospital's expense) in addition to traumatizing the patient.

To avoid this potential problem, the use of an ESU and ground pad with a *return electrode monitoring (REM)* alarm system provides additional safety for the patient by deactivating the system should the dispersive electrode be faulty for whatever reason.

Additionally, electrosurgical burns may result when other electrical equipment is used during a procedure, such as ECG monitoring electrodes or temporary pacing wires. It is recommended that the ECG electrodes be placed on the posterior aspect of the shoulders, away from the dispersive electrode site, thus avoiding any unnecessary hazards when both pieces of equipment are in use.

Since the ESU can interfere with a pacemaker signal, it should not be used in patients with pacemakers if at all possible, to avoid an inadvertent reprogramming of the pacemaker, but if needed, special monitoring of the patient should be intensified.

Electrosurgical Safety Checklist

The creation of an electrosurgical safety checklist should be used for all patients and/or procedure rooms, and should be completed by the person using the ESU.

The following items should be included:

1. ESU alarm activated and audible.
2. Dispersive electrode (ground pad) is the proper size for the corresponding body surface area.
3. The ground pad is properly placed, with postprocedural verification of site.
4. ESU free of extraneous objects anywhere around the unit.
5. Wires, cords, connectors have been checked prior to use/activation.
6. Foot pedal, when used, is covered with clear plastic to keep it dry.
7. If repositioning is required after placement of ground pad, pad is rechecked to assure continuing contact.
8. ESU is operated at lowest effective setting.
9. Use of the ESU is documented on the patient's record, stating: type and ID number of unit, location of ground pad, pre- and postprocedural assessment of contact area, and type and/or manufacturer of active electrode used.

FIBEROPTIC POWER SOURCES

The term *fiberoptic* describes a power source found in a variety of surgical instruments and used for both diagnostic and therapeutic procedures.

A fiberoptic cable is composed of a flexible material, either glass or plastic, which is capable of transmitting light along its fibers by reflecting the light from the side or the wall of the fiber.

To illuminate this cable, a power source is required as the source of light for the cable.

Endoscopic Equipment/Instruments

Fiberoptics are used in endoscopy procedures, performed either in surgery, the GI suite, or the physician's office, through a natural opening in the body (e.g., bronchoscopy, colonoscopy, or cystoscopy) or through an artificial opening created via an incision, such as an arthroscopy or laparoscopy. Additional types of endoscopic procedures can be performed during a surgical procedure—for example, a choledochoscopy during a gallbladder procedure, or a nephroscopy during surgery on the kidney.

Although each piece of equipment is unique and serves a specific purpose, all endoscopic equipment have similar working parts.

Common Components

There are four components associated with endoscopic equipment.

1. Viewing Instrument (Scope)
   The scope is the "eye" of the instrument, and allows the surgeon to view the anatomic structures through the lens or "telescope" or through a lens attached to a flexible instrument. Because of its design, it is the most delicate and expensive component, and can be used with a variety of accessory attachments.

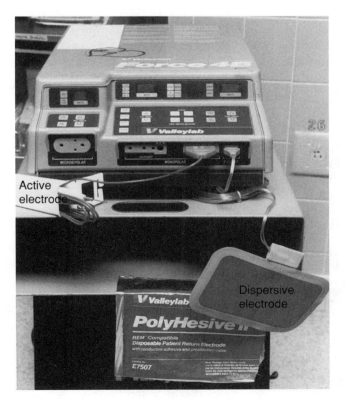

ESU and its parts

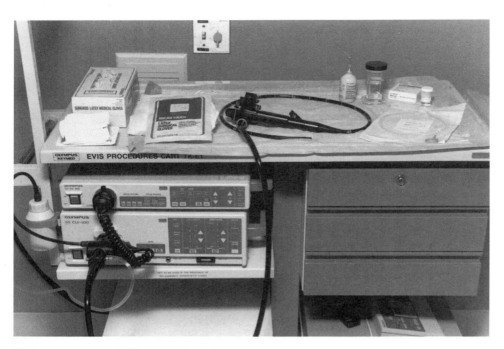

Endoscopy cart with fiberoptic bronchoscope

2. Light Source

The source of light that allows visualization may be emitted by a fiberoptic bundle or from an independent light source housing an incandescent light bulb. The carrier of this light may be part of the instrument (as with rigid or flexible scopes) or a separate light carrier with a bulb attached at the end (for use with hollow rigid scopes).

3. Power Source

The fiberoptic light source is powered by electric current. The power source may be a rechargeable battery or may be electric power cords connected to an appropriate outlet in the procedure room.

4. Projection Lamp Housing/Light Cord

A fiberoptic power cable (*light cord*) transmits the light from the projection lamp to the instrument. Both ends of the cable must have the correct fittings to attach to the lamp housing and the instrument.

Not all fiberoptic cables are interchangeable, and therefore in order to have maximum illumination, the perioperative nurse must make sure that all connections appropriately match before beginning the procedure.

To preserve the efficiency of the light source, the intensity of the light should be lowered before switching the unit on or off, and light cords should be coiled loosely to prevent damage to the fibers. *Never bend the light cord* or the fiberoptic bundles will break, decreasing the amount of projected light.

Today, all surgical specialties benefit from a fiberoptic source of light. Additionally, the optical segment of the instrument may be attached to other pieces of equipment, including a teaching head attachment, laser, or video cameras. The accessory items needed will be determined by the type of endoscope and the purpose of the procedure.

Care and Handling of Endoscopic Equipment

The following recommendations have been created by the AORN as a guide for the care and handling of endoscopic equipment/instruments:[14]

As with any piece of equipment, proper cleaning and maintenance along with gentle handling will save the instrument and/or equipment from costly repairs. Recommendations regarding the sterilization, disinfection, and storage should be known to all persons working with the equipment, and should include, but not be limited to:

- Sterilization rather than disinfection of endoscopes and accessories is preferred to increase patient safety.
- Following cleaning and disinfection, endoscopes should be thoroughly rinsed with sterile water and completely dried before storage.
- The use of damaged instruments could possibly increase the risk of tissue injury, infection, and length of the surgical procedure; therefore, all endoscopes should be inspected and tested prior to each use,

along with power cords and accessory items used during the procedure.

Recommended Practices for the Use and Care of Endoscopes

I. Personnel should be knowledgeable regarding appropriate endoscope selection, proper handling, inspection, testing, and use and processing of endoscopes, endoscopic accessories, and related equipment.

II. Inspection of endoscopes, endoscopic accessories, and related equipment should occur at all stages of handling.

III. Instrumentation, accessories, and equipment should be tested before use, then used and processed according to the manufacturers written instructions.

IV. Cleaning and decontamination of endoscopes should occur immediately after the completion of the procedure.

V. Endoscopes and accessories should be disinfected or sterilized or sterilized according to AORN's "Recommended Practices for Disinfection" and recommended practices for steam and EO sterilization.

VI. Validation and documentation of endoscopic use and processing should occur.

Source: AORN. Standards and recommended practices. Denver, CO: The Association, 1995. Pp. 163–165.

THE OPERATING MICROSCOPE

A microscope was first used clinically for surgery in 1921, when a patient required surgical intervention to correct severe otitis media. The microscope used was very simple: single vision and not very powerful, but it was a beginning.

Approximately 30 years later, using the principles of *binocular magnification* and *stereoscopic vision,* which enabled ophthalmologists to examine the eye in three dimensions, the operating microscope was developed by the Carl Zeiss Company, and the first of the present-day operating microscopes was developed in 1960.

With the advent of this new tool, instrumentation that could be used for this type of surgery followed close behind, and so began the development and clinical use of *microsurgery* techniques in all of the surgical specialties.[15]

Features of the Operating Microscope

The operating microscope has an interchangeable lens that allows for precise visualization of the surgical field. A variety of support systems are available for mounting the microscope, ranging from a floor base to ceiling-mounted brackets, allowing flexibility of use during a procedure.

Autoclavable attachments and/or special microscope drapes allow the surgeon total range of movement during surgery, yet under sterile conditions. The microscope uses an internal fiberoptic light source whose intensity can be adjusted depending on the area being viewed.

Microscope Components

Basically, all operating microscopes consist of the same basic components: (1) an optical lens system with controls for magnification, illumination, and focusing; (2) a mounting system for stability; (3) an electrical system; and (4) accessory items/attachments.

Optical Lens System

The optical lens system, the "eyes" of the microscope, consists of the *body,* which contains the objective lens, and attached to the body the binocular oculars or eye pieces, through which the surgeon views the image. The combination of the lens and the oculars determine the magnification power of the microscope. Depending on the type of surgery, the surgeon will request a specific *objective lens,* which can range from 100 mm to 400 mm, increasing in 25-mm increments. The "mm" is the distance in millimeters between the operative site and the lens when the microscope is in focus (*working distance*). Distances may vary from 6 to 10 inches (15–25 cm); the larger the size of the objective lens, the greater the magnification at the desired working distance.

Magnification

The oculars serve as magnifying glasses that can assist the surgeon in obtaining a sharp, nondistorted image of the surgical site. Since each eye may require different magnification, both oculars can be adjusted separately, until a clear picture is visualized (*stereoscopic vision*).

The magnification of an image is increased by moving the object closer to the eye, and the amount of image increase becomes the magnification value of the microscope and its optical aids.

The magnification changer (dial) is a part of the microscope body, which is attached to a support structure, allowing the instrument to be tilted or positioned as needed.

Light Source

Illumination is the source of light used to view an object. The most common type of microscope illumina-

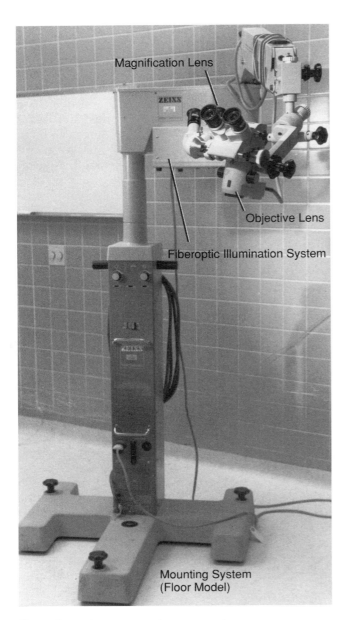

Magnification Lens

Objective Lens

Fiberoptic Illumination System

Mounting System
(Floor Model)

Operating microscope and components

tion used today is referred to as *coaxial* illumination, which is transferred through a fiberoptic cable or from an incandescent bulb housed near the objective lens of the microscope. Fiberoptic illumination increases the diameter of the illuminated field, and the coaxial illumination principles provide a shadow-free circular spot that is uniformly illuminated, even in deep and narrow areas.

Focusing

Focusing can be accomplished manually or by a foot control motor that can raise or lower the body of the microscope to the desired distance from the object to be viewed.

Focus of the ocular lens should start at zero, and adjusted as needed to accommodate his or her individual vision needs.

Mounting Systems

Stability of the microscope is of utmost importance during the surgical procedure. The mounting system allows for portability and flexibility, so that the microscope can be positioned as desired.

Microscopes can be floor mounted, on a movable stand, ceiling mounted on a track, or wall mounted on a bracket. Smaller microscopes, such as those found in physicians' offices, can be table mounted for ease of use and conservation of space.

Power Source

Like all electric equipment, safety and proper maintenance are essential to its optimum usage. Circuits, plugs, and connectors must be protected from overload by breaker relays and fuses. Light controls should be in the "off" position when turning the unit on and off to avoid short circuiting the unit or creating sparks.

Accessory Items

A number of accessory items are currently available to use with the microscope.

Assistant's Binoculars

An additional pair of binoculars can be mounted and used by the assistant/scrub person, so that he or she will see exactly what the surgeon sees. This can only be accomplished, however, with a *beam splitter* attachment and an *observer tube*, which takes the image from the surgeon's oculars and transfers it through the observer tube to the assistant's oculars. The assistant's oculars should be in place prior to the start of the procedure, and the sterile drape should incorporate both the surgeon's and the assistant's viewing apparatus.

Microscope Drape

The entire working mechanisms and support arm should be encased in a sterile drape. Draping the entire microscope allows it to be brought into the sterile field. The drape should be made to accommodate any attachments added to the microscope, and the scrub and circulator should be familiar with its application in order to preserve the sterility of the drape and the operative field.

Camera/Video Adapter

The microscope can accommodate both a still camera and a video camera by using the proper coupling attachments connected to the beam splitter. The camera unit should be in the upright position, and both the video camera and/or still camera should be confined within the drape.

Laser Microadapter

A laser beam can be directed through the microscope for laser microsurgery. The alignment between the microscope and the laser attachment is critical and must be perfect: at a 60-degree angle to the microscope, since it will not usually fire in an upright or horizontal position. Additionally, the microadapter must have the same "mm" lens with focal length as the microscope (200, 300, 400), so that adjustment of the laser beam is exact.

Remote Foot Control

A foot control with motorized functions such as focus, zoom, and tilt capabilities is much more convenient for the surgeon since his or her hands must be free to perform the surgery. The placement of the foot pedal control should be announced to the surgeon so that he or she can easily adjust his or her foot to that location.

If laser or foot control ESU is used, the laser foot pedal should be by itself, with the microscope/ESU pedal on the opposite side.

Sliding Stool/Chair

A comfortable chair with hydraulic foot control and arm rests should be available for both the surgeon and the assistant, since most microsurgery cases are performed in the sitting position. The chair or stool should be draped to allow for greater movement in and around the sterile field.

Special Nursing Considerations

Circulating Nurse's Responsibilities

Know how to care for and position the microscope.

1. Check to see that all knobs are secured after the microscope has been placed in final position
2. Assist the surgeon with attachments of accessory items
3. Take special care of power cables to prevent accidental breakage; position them out of the path of the microscope; be sure they are properly coiled for storage
4. Take special care of lenses to avoid breaking, scratching, or leaving fingerprints; tighten to fingertip tightness only, being careful not to cross-thread during attachment. When attaching the lens, perform the task over a padded surface to prevent accidental breakage if dropped. Cleaning

process should follow manufacturer's recommendations
5. Keep extra lamp bulbs and fuses available and know where to find accessories and anticipate their usage depending on the proposed procedure and/or surgeon's preference
6. When moving microscope, position the viewing portion over the base to add stability; acquire adequate moving help to accommodate the move safely
7. When storing microscope, avoid using a plastic bag or cover; instead, use a cloth pillowcase
8. Cover foot pedal with clear bag to keep it clean and dry, and position it for easy access after surgeon has been seated or has determined desired position to perform the surgery

Scrub Person's Responsibilities

Maintain sterile field and know how to pass instruments when using a microscope.

1. Verify with the circulator the lens and binoculars for a specific surgeon/procedure
2. Make sure lens and oculars are clean
3. Have the proper drape to accommodate microscope accessory items; know how to apply the drape properly, maintaining sterile technique
4. Place Mayo tray and instrument table in convenient location (if assisting) so your eyes do not have to leave the field or look around the microscope
5. Maintain calm atmosphere; know that dissection may be slow and tedious. Do not let attention stray; use video monitor to watch progress of procedure.

The operating microscope has made possible many surgeries requiring delicate and precision work, and can be an important factor in the overall outcome of the surgical procedure. Therefore it must be constantly maintained in an optimal state, and persons working with the microscope should be fully educated about its features and components in order to facilitate a successful outcome.

Additional Light Sources and Magnification Aids

Besides the equipment mentioned earlier in this segment, other accessory aids can provide additional light or magnification during surgery. For example, a *fiberoptic headlight* is used whenever the surgeon requires a highly intense light into a small area, such as the throat, ear, nose, or deep cavities. The headlight has a cord attached to it, and is usually positioned on the surgeon's head prior to the scrub procedure. Once the gowning procedure is finished, the circulator will attach the headlight to the light source and increase the intensity as required.

Magnifying loupes are worn much the same as eyeglasses, and are used to increase an area's size when the use of a microscope is not indicated. Because they are less cumbersome, the loupes are used whenever the surgery does not require the magnification power of the microscope.

Surgical magnifying loupes come in the form of glasses with the magnifying portion attached or in the shape of a visor with magnifying lenses built into the front portion of the unit.

Placing the magnifying loupes in the solution warming cabinet prior to use can reduce the possibility of the glasses fogging.

Before beginning any case requiring delicate surgery in a small area, refer to the Physician's Preference Card for the specific equipment preferred by the surgeon, and confirm its condition for use.

MAINTAINING BODY TEMPERATURE

The skin is the organ that maintains the body's normothermic state. As body temperature increases, superficial blood vessels dilate to allow more blood to circulate near the surface. If the body temperature decreases, owing to prolonged exposure, the body will attempt to self-regulate by decreasing the flow of blood to the surface, thus conserving heat internally. It is obvious, then, that heat loss or heat production can directly affect the patient's physiologic response to surgery.

In the normal course of a surgical event, a loss of heat is primarily the result of exposure to the physical environment, the incision itself, the patient's immobility, and/or coexisting circulatory insufficiency.

Thermal Control Unit

External control of the patient's body temperature can be accomplished through the use of a thermal blanket placed on the operating table. When activated, the thermal blanket will heat or cool the patient through coils filled with water or gel, which circulates through channels in the blanket until the desired, preset temperature is reached.

In emergent situations, such as a malignant hyperthermia crisis, the thermal blanket can be placed on top of the patient to facilitate surface cooling.

Guidelines for Nursing Actions

To ensure effective operation of the thermal blanket, safety guidelines should be followed, since thermal burns, pressure necrosis, or electric shock can occur as a result of incorrect usage.

The AORN recommended practice[16] states that "po-

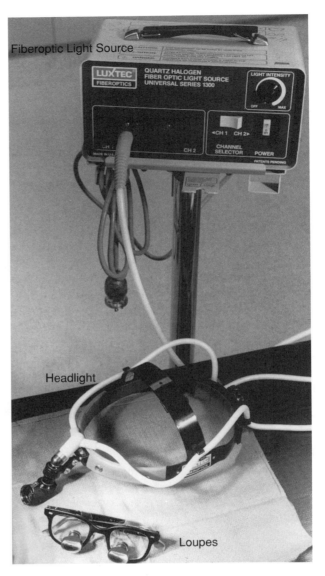

Additional light sources and magnifying aids

tential hazards associated with controlling patient's temperature *should be identified and safe practices established*," which should include preventive measures relating to the safe operational use of the equipment, and monitoring of the patient's response to this intervention.

- Thermal blankets are recommended for any surgical procedure lasting more than 2 hours, and for all pediatric procedures and procedures in patients with impaired circulatory status.
- Direct skin contact with the thermal blanket should be avoided by placing a sheet between the blanket and the patient.
- Folds and/or creases should be avoided so that hot spots or pressure injuries do not occur during its use.

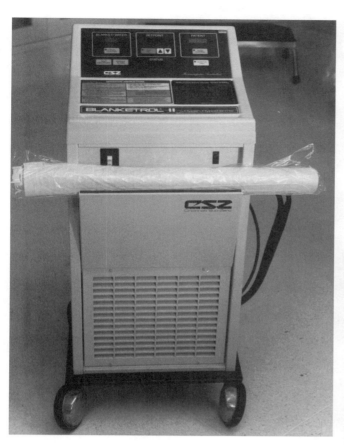

Thermal control unit and blanket

- Observation and monitoring of both the unit and the patient should be constant throughout the procedure.
- Skin integrity should be inspected before and after the procedure with corresponding documentation of assessment findings.
- Power cords and connective lines to the blanket should be checked before and after each use for cracks, breaks, or holes in the cords or blanket that could increase the possibility of electric shock.

When safely used, the thermal blanket can be a major assistance in preventing an adverse response to surgical intervention by maintaining a near-normal physiologic status, and can decrease the possibility of postoperative hypothermia.

Besides the use of a thermal blanket, there are other interventions the perioperative nurse and surgical team can use to maintain body temperature during a surgical procedure.

Some of these include the use of warmed prep solutions and irrigating solutions; providing warm blankets on arrival into the procedure room and before transferring to the postanesthesia area; administering warm blood if transfusions are required; limiting exposure area to the direct operative site; monitoring physiologic parameters, such as skin color, texture, and external/internal temperature throughout the procedure; and providing psychological support, thereby reducing anxiety and fear.

INTRAOPERATIVE AUTOTRANSFUSIONS

Occasionally a patient needs an immediate replacement of blood, or the surgical procedure planned necessitates replacement of several units of blood during the course of the procedure.

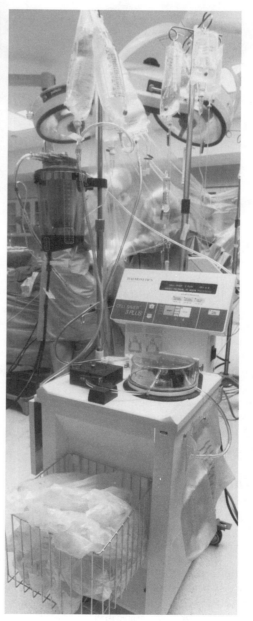

Hemonetics cell saver and autologus transfusion

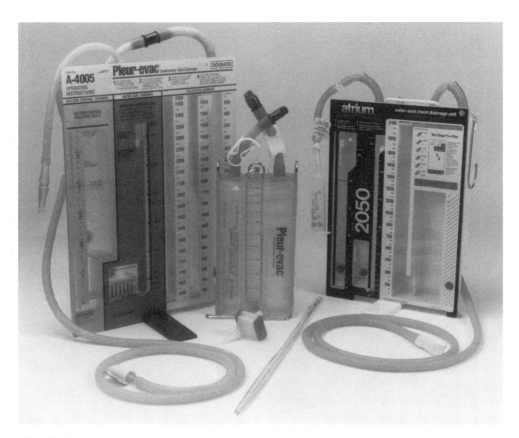

Closed chest drainage systems with ATS system

Autotransfusion is not always applicable; in fact, it is contraindicated if the patient has cancer, if gross contamination from the bowel or stomach contents have occurred, or, in the case of a trauma patient, if the wounds are more than 4 hours old. If these conditions are not present, autotransfusion can be the safest method for replacing lost blood cells.

Autotransfusion can be accomplished before elective surgery, using the patient as his or her own donor. One advantage to autotransfusions is having sufficient blood if there is a blood shortage; it also precludes the danger of receiving contaminated blood from a commercial blood bank, thus increasing the safety factors relating to transfusion therapy.

Cell Saver (Autologous Transfusion System)

The cell saver unit for autologous blood recovery is the next best answer to safe blood replacement during a surgical procedure, since it returns washed, packed cells to the patient via a filtered reinfusion bag. This autotransfusion system provides intraoperative salvage of blood, without the threat of disease transmission, transfusion reactions, or incompatibility testing.

Procedural Overview: Cell Saver

The autologous recovery system works as follows:

1. The shed blood is suctioned from the surgical field and anticoagulated in the collection reservoir.
2. The sterile reservoir filters out tissue, clots, and foreign debris from the blood.
3. Blood from the reservoir is pumped into the centrifuge bowl, which spins and separates the red blood cells (RBC's) from the plasma.
4. The RBC's are washed with normal saline; upon completion of the washing cycle, the cells suspended in saline are spun down, and separated from the solution. The packed RBC's are then pumped from the centrifuge bowel into the reinfusion bag for return to the patient.
5. The plasma and waste fluids overflow from the bowel into a waste bag suspended on the side of the unit, which includes free hemoglobin, irrigation fluids, and activated clotting factors.

Although most units are designed to cycle automatically, a nurse or clinical perfusionist should be assigned to manage the unit while in use, to coordinate the delivery of blood to anesthesia personnel as needed. Full records of the amount of irrigant, numbers of units processed, and so on should be kept during the procedure, and be incorporated with the total amount of infusion solutions administered during the procedure.

The use of this system has created a positive outcome not only for emergency patients, but also for those whose surgery may require extensive replacement (more than 2–3 units) during the course of the procedure.

Examples of surgeries that may require extensive replacement include procedures involving the spleen, liver, chest wall, or heart/pulmonary vessels, or reconstructive orthopedic surgeries such as posterior spinal fusions (Harrington rod insertion) or total hip arthroplasty.

Postoperatively, the autotransfusion system can continue to replace the patient's own blood via an ATS transfusion bag (e.g., open heart procedures with chest drainage devices).

LASER APPLICATION IN SURGERY

The clinical application of lasers is rapidly gaining acceptance as a precision surgical tool primarily owing to its ability to reduce bleeding, reduce swelling, and minimize scar tissue formation.

Laser is acronym for *Light Amplification by Stimulated Emission of Radiation.* A laser beam is created by stimulating photons inside a resonating chamber. As the photons bounce back and forth they gain energy, which is emitted through the delivery system, producing a laser beam that can be used to cut or coagulate tissue.

TYPES OF LASERS

There are a variety of lasers, but three are commonly associated with surgery: the *carbon dioxide laser;* the *ND:Yag laser,* and the *argon laser.* Each has special characteristics, benefits, and disadvantages.

Carbon Dioxide Laser

Molecules of carbon dioxide provide the active lasing medium for the carbon dioxide laser. The carbon dioxide laser is the most versatile laser, since it can perform both coagulation and cutting functions, and can be operated in continuous or pulsed modes. By varying the length and frequency of each pulse, different tissue effects can be produced and thermal effects can be more precisely controlled.

The carbon dioxide laser wavelength is absorbed by water, and since the body is 75 percent to 90 percent water, an extremely precise beam can vaporize even a single cell while avoiding surrounding tissue.

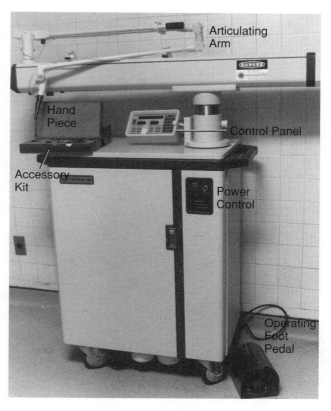

Sharplan carbon dioxide (CO_2) laser

The carbon dioxide beam is regulated by the surgeon, and can be optically controlled to work in three focal positions: focus, defocus, and prefocus. In *focus,* the laser beam vaporizes tissue, and in *defocus,* the reaction on tissue is coagulation; *prefocus* has no practical application.

The precision of the laser beam provides maximum impact on intended tissue with minimal damage to surrounding tissue. In addition, the laser beam causes minimal immediate postoperative pain and allows faster recovery.

Surgical specialties that can benefit from a carbon dioxide laser include general, gynecology, ENT, neurosurgery, and plastic surgery.

ND:Yag Laser

A solid crystal made of *yttrium aluminum garnet* (Yag) covered with *neodymium* (ND) supplies the active medium for the ND:Yag laser.

Electrons are excited, not by electric current as in the carbon dioxide or gas lasers, but by a bright flashing lamp striking the neodymium, causing a mini-explosion. The primary function of this laser is coagulation, and although it provides great penetration depth, the energy is not highly focused. Tissue is

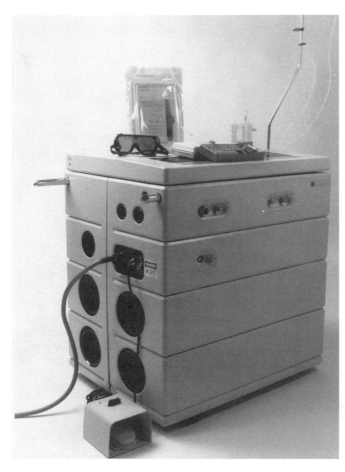

Neodymium (ND) Yag laser

mic surgery, it is the most common form of treatment for diabetic retinopathy, and is well adapted to ambulatory surgery settings and use in an ophthalmologist's office.

Other lasers, and their clinical applications not often seen in surgery, include:[17]

Krypton laser	Ophthalmology
Dye laser	Ophthalmology, plastic surgery, and photoradiation therapy for cancer
Excimer laser	Investigations being conducted in ophthalmology, cardiology, orthopedics, and dermatology
Free-electron laser	Investigations involving photodynamic therapy of tumors, neurosurgery, and treatment of psoriasis and possibly hyperbilirubinemia

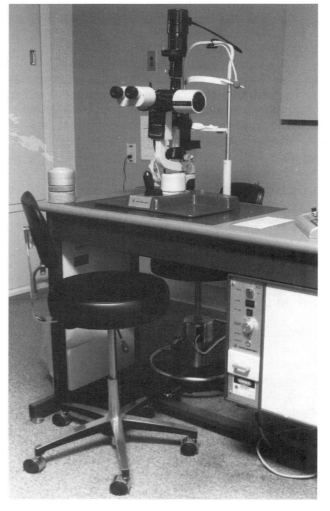

heated to a point of coagulation without vaporization, producing a homogenous coagulative effect.

The special characteristics of this laser medium enables the surgeon to control its impact and judge tissue response during its use. In addition, the surgeon can use this laser through endoscopic instrumentation via a fiber, or by direct contact with the structure using a contact probe (a wand-like instrument). Applications of this laser include gastroenterology, pulmonary, urology, gynecology, and ophthalmology.

Argon Laser

The argon laser also uses gas as its medium; however, it functions at a different wavelength than the carbon dioxide laser. The argon beam is effectively absorbed by pigmented tissue, yet passes through clear structures with minimal effect.

The primary clinical applications include ophthalmology, dermatology, gastroenterology, gynecology, and otology.

Because the argon beam is well suited for ophthal-

Table-mounted argon laser

Credentialing for Lasers

Because of its high technology and specific clinical application, surgeons require specialty certification courses in the various laser mediums before using the laser in clinical application. These courses include laser physics, safety, general operation, and techniques, to provide maximal effectiveness of the equipment and the technology.

By the same token, nurses working with lasers need to attend special education programs so that they too can better understand the energy characteristics of laser light, its clinical application, safety requirements (state, federal, and institutional) regarding both patient and personnel working with the laser, and any specific information related to the medium being used.

PERIOPERATIVE NURSING CONSIDERATIONS

As with any advanced technology, certain hazards are associated with this form of treatment, and the perioperative nurse, as a patient advocate, must ensure a safe environment during its usage.

AORN established recommended practices directly relating to laser safety, which include the following concepts.[18]

1. A warning sign stating the type of laser being used should be pasted on all doors leading in and out of the laser area, to alert all personnel that they must take certain precautionary measures:
   a. Application of special goggles/glasses which are applicable to the medium being used:

CO_2 laser	clear
ND:Yag laser	green tint
Argon laser	orange tint

2. A smoke evacuator system should be used during all laser cases to absorb the plume from the laser.
3. Though the laser beam is invisible, it can ignite flammable materials and be reflected off shiny surfaces. Instruments should be brushed or ebonized and emergency equipment such as sterile water and a halon fire extinguisher should be readily available.
4. Lasers should not be used with alcohol preps, or be kept near combustible solutions or substances.
5. The patient's eyes should be protected, and all sponges used at the field should be damp (for carbon dioxide lasers) to prevent the laser beam from striking any other tissue and/or area or igniting a fire.

6. One nurse who has been instructed in the medium and its safety factors should be assigned to use the laser and should *not* be involved with circulating duties while working with the laser.
7. The laser should be placed in the stand-by mode when not in use.
8. Continuous monitoring and observation of the environment and the patient must be practiced by all persons working with a laser, regardless of the medium.
9. A laser committee, responsible for creating policies, procedures, and protocols, in addition to credentialing physicians wishing to use the laser, should be established within the institution.
10. All personnel should be aware that although the laser is an asset to surgery, it can be a potentially dangerous piece of equipment if not used properly.

Although the discovery and clinical application of lasers in surgery and medicine is not new, each day brings new advances and techniques for clinical application.

AORN Recommended Practices for Laser Safety

I. All health-care workers should be aware of areas of laser use, and controlled access to these areas must be maintained.

II. Eyes of patients and health-care workers should be protected from laser beams.

III. Skin and other tissue of patients and health-care workers should be protected from aberrant and reflected laser beams.

IV. Patients and health-care workers should be protected from inhaling the plume associated with laser use.

V. Patients and health-care workers should be protected from fire hazards associated with laser use.

VI. Patients and health-care workers should be protected from electrical hazards associated with laser use.

VII. A laser team should be available within the practice setting.

VIII. Perioperative personnel working in a laser treatment area should be required to obtain safety training and basic orientation to the technology.

IX. Policies and procedures for laser safety should be developed with regard to the practice setting.

Source: AORN Standards and Recommended Practices. Denver, CO: The Association, 1995. Pp. 211–214.

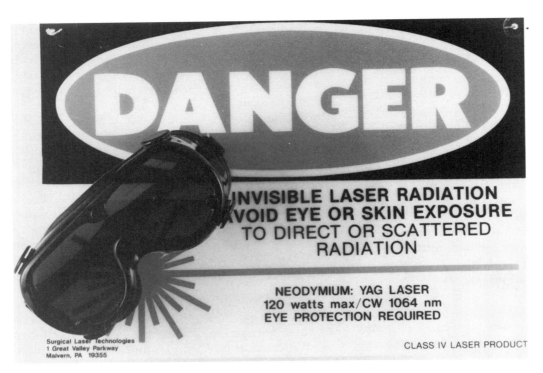

Laser accessory equipment includes warning sign and safety goggles

To provide the patient with a safe, therapeutic environment, the perioperative nurse must maintain current knowledge regarding this form of therapy, and using the nursing process, must assess, plan, implement, and evaluate the environment and the patient throughout the surgical procedure when laser is being used.

AIR-POWER EQUIPMENT

Many power-driven instruments, such as drills, saws, and dermatomes, are used during surgery. Some are electrically powered, as previously mentioned, but others use alternative sources derived from air power

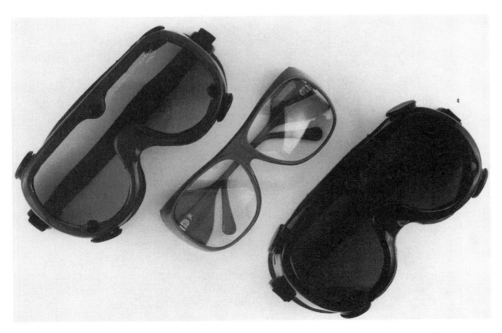

Variety of goggles for laser surgery (type of medium should be indicated on goggles or glasses) (left, Argon; middle, CO$_2$; right, ND: YAG)

in the form of compressed nitrogen or carbon dioxide. The perioperative nurse should be familiar with the tanks, regulators, and power hoses associated with this source of power so that safe connections and usage can be achieved. Most of these pieces of special equipment will be discussed in Chapter 14, as they are associated with specialized surgical procedures, but their general principles of care and handling will be discussed in this chapter since it relates to powered surgical equipment.

The most common piece of equipment associated with air power is the pneumatic tourniquet.

Tourniquets are used during most operations on the extremities when a "bloodless" wound site is desired. They prevent venous oozing, yet do not totally obstruct the arterial blood supply, thereby preserving the circulation through the extremity. In addition to the pneumatic tourniquet, the procedure known as a laparoscopy also requires the use of gas in the form of carbon dioxide. The tank is attached to a gas insufflator unit which assists in establishing the pneumoperitoneum required for a laparoscopic approach.

PNEUMATIC TOURNIQUET

The nonsterile tourniquet is composed of an inner bladder covered with an outer layer of synthetic material, similar to a blood pressure cuff. The tourniquet is connected to a compressed source of air/gas via a regulator attached to a valve extending from near the end of the cuff. Depending on its intended use, the cuff can be single or double, each with its separate gauge.

Application and Nursing Considerations

The tourniquet cuff should be applied far enough away from the incision site so that it will not be in the way, and the area should be prepared with a thin soft cotton sheeting (soft roll), smoothly applied, to prevent the skin from becoming "pinched" during inflation. The cuff chosen must be appropriate in size to the extremity (overlapping of ends by 2–3 inches), allowing for proper expansion of the cuff and constriction of the extremity. Following the application of the cuff, the position should be confirmed by the surgeon, prior to prepping and inflation.

The extremity is prepared by elevating it, with the help of another person, and a circumferential prep is performed up to the tourniquet cuff. On completion of the prep, the surgeon will apply a sterile covering, called a *stockinette*, so that the extremity can be placed onto a sterile surface or held for sterile draping.

To drain the venous blood from the extremity, the limb, still elevated, is wrapped with a wide sterile rub-

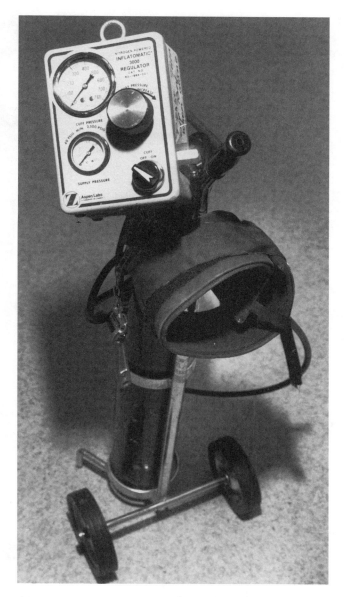

Air-power equipment: tourniquet cuff and tank

ber bandage (*Esmarch* or *Martin*) from the distal to the proximal end, and the tourniquet is then inflated to the desired setting. It is recommended that the setting for an arm be between 250 and 300 mm Hg and for legs, 400–500 mm Hg. Once the setting has been reached, the rubber bandage is removed, and the extremity can be lowered onto the sterile field.

Implications for Safety

Improperly used, the tourniquet can cause serious nerve and vascular damage; therefore, careful planning, application, and monitoring are essential to its safe usage.

Using the AORN recommended practices[19] as a reference guide for safe implementation, the following practices should be employed:

1. Tourniquets should be tested regularly before use, monitored during use, and maintained in proper working order.

 Tourniquet gauges should be checked for accuracy before each application to prevent tourniquet paralysis from occurring. All connectors, the tubing, and the bladder cuff should be checked for cracks and/or leaks, and replaced if not in acceptable working condition. During the procedure, the pressure should be checked and verified at least every 30 minutes to detect any pressure variation, with documentation of the time of inflation, deflation, and location of the cuff.

2. Selection and placement of the cuff should be determined by the patient's age, anatomy, and medical condition.

 The cuff should be applied to the extremity so that underlying shin and tissue are not unduly traumatized. Its use is contraindicated in patients with vascular disease or poor peripheral circulation. The cuff should be positioned at the point of maximum circumference of the extremity. Once inflated it should not be readjusted.

3. Although there is no actual time limit regarding the use of tourniquets, the recommended time limits range from 1 hour for an arm (300 mm) and 1½ hours for a leg (500 mm). If more time is required, the cuff should be deflated for 10 minutes, then reinflated to the desired pressure.

4. Documentation of tourniquet time, position, and the person who applied the cuff should be part of the intraoperative nurse's notes.

5. The tourniquet should be cleaned with an appropriate disinfection solution and stored properly after each use. The remaining air in the tank should be checked, and if low, replaced before storage.

The following pages provide a guide for properly opening, preparing, and closing a freestanding tank, regardless of the size or regulator required.

General Guidelines for Working with Tanks

1. Open tank valve counterclockwise, very slowly, and allow only enough gas to escape to blow out possible debris.
2. Attach appropriate regulator by hand and secure with a wrench. Be sure that regulator is turned off by turning the regulator knob (green) counterclockwise until it stops.
3. Slowly turn tank valve fully open. Tank pressure gauge should read 2000 to 2500 psi on right-hand gauge when full. Listen for air leaks.
4. Scrub person passes off connector end to circulator, who inserts connector to regulator outlet by thrusting upward into the outlet. Check for proper seating of connector.
5. Turn the pressure regulator knob "on" (clockwise) and set pressure on left-handed regulator gauge to desired pressure to effectively operate the instrument.
 NOTE: Pressure setting should be made with instrument running, or operating pressure may not be sufficient.
6. When finished, turn the tank off. Actuate the instrument to "bleed" air in tubing and gauge. Regulator gauge should read "0." Turn off regulator by turning regulator knob counterclockwise until it stops.
7. Turn connector on regulator (clockwise) and pull downward to release connector.
8. If pressure remaining in tank is 500 psi or more, return to storage. If less than 500 psi, remove regulator, replace tank, and reapply regulator.

Surgical power tools and equipment represent a major investment for any institution; therefore, proper care and handling can save costly repairs and extend the working life of the equipment, in addition to providing a safe environment for the patient and personnel working with the equipment.

X-RAY EQUIPMENT IN SURGERY

During the course of a surgical procedure, x-rays may be needed to confirm a location and/or position or to perform diagnostic studies related to the surgical procedure.

Types of Intraoperative X-Rays

The most common types of x-rays, performed during or just prior to the incision, include:

1. X-rays for positioning—KUB, pacemaker, reconstructive orthopedics, tube placement
2. Diagnostic studies—operative cholangiograms, ureteral retrogrades, angiography
3. Emergent procedures—x-ray for trauma, presence of foreign objects (needles, bullets, sponges)

An x-ray procedure can be invasive, in which a dye or radiopaque contrast material is injected into a vein, duct, or passageway within the body, or noninvasive, such as a confirmation x-ray of implantable devices.

Types of X-Ray Equipment

There are three types of x-ray equipment commonly found in today's surgical suite. Although each can be used separately, at times a combination of methods may be used.

Fixed X-Ray Equipment

Predominantly found where orthopedic procedures or closed urologic procedures are performed, this equipment can be ceiling mounted or mounted on a table, and can be placed in the desired position to achieve the right kind of picture.

If ceiling mounted, it is usually placed on tracks, which allows unobstructed movement to the desired site, and then retracted to an out-of-the-way location once the process is completed. In the urologic procedure rooms (cysto rooms), the x-ray machine is incorporated into a specially designed table to accommodate diagnostic studies during the procedure.

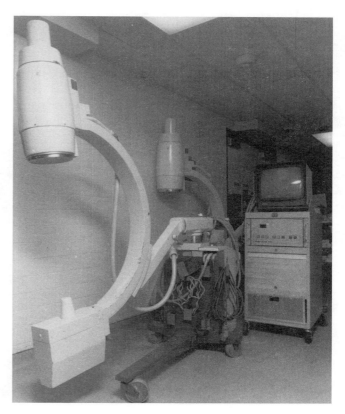

Image intensifier with monitor

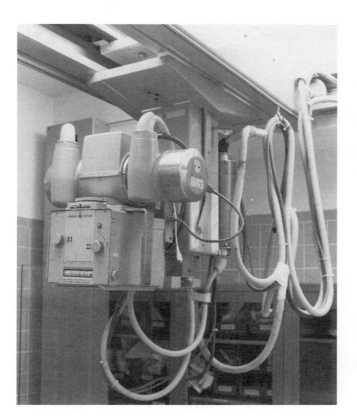

Ceiling mount x-ray unit

Portable X-Ray Equipment

As its name implies, this x-ray unit is mounted on a portable generator and can be moved to any room in the surgical suite. Although it offers flexibility, the disadvantage is the possible contamination of the field when brought in too close to the patient.

If the operating table is not equipped with a special slot designed to hold the x-ray cassette, a sterile cassette cover, similar to a clear plastic pillowcase, must be placed over the cassette so that it can be brought to the field without the risk of contamination. When used in this manner, someone is designated to hold the x-ray cassette in place during the filming.

Image Intensifier

The image intensifier, or "C-Arm," as it has been nicknamed because of its configuration, converts x-ray beams through the body into a fluoroscopic image, which is projected on a TV monitor screen. A special table top, designed for this purpose, must be used to permit the beam to pass through the table and be seen on the monitor. The surgeon can activate the unit with a foot control switch, and a radiologic technician adjusts the position of the x-ray tube as requested so that constant observation by way of the monitor is possible. Still pictures can also be obtained from this unit.

Radiopaque Contrast Media

These agents, composed of nonmetallic compounds or heavy metal salts, permit the visualization of internal structures during an x-ray procedure.

As with many of the contrast media, they contain iodine; therefore, if invasive x-rays are to be taken, it is vitally important that known sensitivities to iodine-related substances such as shellfish or previous problems with invasive studies using iodine be obtained through the preoperative assessment, and the information communicated to the surgeon.

Some of the more commonly used substances for invasive studies include:

Cardiographin	angiography
Hypaque	arteriography, IVP, venography, cholangiography
Renografin	angiography, cystography, pyelography
Cysto/Angio Conray	angiography, arteriography, cystography, retrograde pyelography, ureterography

If contrast media is used during the procedure, it must be dispensed under sterile conditions, and must be administered according to the surgeon's dilution request, using warm sterile saline (usually 50–50 dilution) in a labeled syringe (30–60 mL) with appropriate needle for injection.

Radiation Safety Guidelines

Following the AORN's recommended practices for radiation safety[20] will ensure an optimum environment for the patient and personnel. The following suggestions are based on those guidelines.

1. Sterile technique involving the surgery must be maintained during an x-ray procedure.
2. The x-ray machine or overhead unit should be damp dusted with cleaning solution before use.
3. When using a cassette, the scrub nurse must enclose the cassette in a sterile cassette cover, maintaining aseptic technique, before it can be brought to the sterile field.
4. The sterile members of the team should apply protective "lead aprons" and thyroid shields before the scrub, to facilitate sterile application of the gown while being protected against exposure to x-rays during the procedure.

5. During filming, remove all unnecessary instruments from the field, unless otherwise directed by the surgeon, and cover the incision with sterile towel.
6. An x-ray detector badge, indicating the amount of exposure received in a month, should be worn on the outside of the lead apron (under sterile gown) during all x-ray procedures, by all personnel in the room. Badges should be checked at regularly established intervals.
7. Positioning of the equipment should be done prior to draping and confirmed by a "scout" film, to prevent having to replace the drapes if positioning is not correct.
8. The circulating nurse should assist the x-ray technician in placing the cassette into the cassette table holder by lifting the drapes and sliding the cassette into the desired location.
9. While the film is being developed, the surgical team should not contaminate their gowns/hands by folding arms across chest or under arms, or sit while in sterile attire.
10. Unless absolutely necessary, all nonscrubbed personnel should leave the room during a single-series filming. Those persons who must remain should wear a lead apron or stand behind a protective (lead-lined) screen in the procedure room.
11. Female personnel who are pregnant should be excused from x-ray procedures.
12. For optimum protection during fluoroscopy, persons within 2 meters of the unit should wear a thyroid shield, and leaded sterile gloves should be worn when hands are in direct exposure to fluoroscopy.
13. Leaded protective devices should be routinely checked for cracks or tears, which can significantly reduce the effectiveness of the shield.
14. A qualified radiologic technician (or radiologist) should be in attendance throughout the x-ray/fluoroscopy sequence, and should always be aware of the other members of the team, allowing them time to properly prepare for the x-ray exposure.

As with any potential hazard associated with the environment, the patient, or personnel, added protective measures must be taken to reduce the possibility of harm, and all personnel should be reviewed on safe practices on an on-going basis, including radiation, electrosurgical, laser, and tourniquet use safety, since these are capable of producing dangerous adverse effects both during and after the procedure. Additionally, the department should establish quality monitoring programs to ensure continued safety within the practice setting.

Self-assessment Exercise 5

Directions: Complete the following exercises. The answers are given at the end of this module.

1. Electrosurgery may be used to _____ and/or _____ tissue.

2. The purpose of the "active" electrode is to _____ , while the "dispersive" electrode is used to _____ .

3. A *bipolar* active electrode requires the use of a patient ground pad.

    True   False

4. The ESU can be foot-controlled or hand-controlled.

    True   False

5. List the components associated with all endoscopic equipment, and briefly describe each.

6. _____ is a technique used to increase the patient's temperature, and can be accomplished by the use of a _____ .

7. Briefly describe the nursing actions that can be used to maintain normal body temperature during the intraoperative phase.

8. Laser is an acronym for _____ .

9. List four primary safety requirements when using laser.

10. Describe the circulating nurse's responsibility regarding the use of:
    a. Operating microscope
    b. Pneumatic tourniquet

THE SEQUENCE OF SURGERY

> Be curious always! For knowledge will not acquire you; you must acquire it.
>
> —*Sudie Back*

Although each surgical procedure contains its own special elements, essentially the same sequence of events occurs with each operation. Specific details, relating to a given procedure, involve only the choice of instrumentation, sutures, and other specialized accessory items.

The *art* of intelligent assistance, regardless of the role assumed, requires a working knowledge of the sequential steps for a specific surgical procedure based on four concepts that should be considered for any surgical event. These concepts are the *approach*, the *procedure*, the *possible complications*, and the *closure*.

Effective implementation also depends on six components of knowledge, which include:

1. Understanding the involved anatomy
2. Knowing the surgeon's approach (position and incision)
3. Recognizing accepted techniques for a given institution (counts, usage of equipment, etc.)
4. Capabilities of the nursing staff (scrub, circulator, assistant)
5. General condition of the patient (age, weight, preexisting conditions)

6. Possible complications related to the proposed surgery (intraoperative, postoperative)

As the professional nurse in the procedure room, it is up to the perioperative nurse to create an atmosphere of confidence to assure the procedure is performed using the highest possible quality of standards.

Through assessment, professional judgment, and principles established from educational preparation and experience, the perioperative nurse becomes an important asset to the surgical team, the procedure, and the patient, reaffirming the need for a professional nurse to function as the patient-care manager during the surgical experience.

The Five Phases of Surgery

To provide expert aid to the surgeon and the surgical team, the perioperative nurse should be familiar with the phases of surgery, in order to anticipate the needs of all those involved with the procedure. Each procedure can be broken down into five phases, each phase representing a sequence of events that occurs during a surgical procedure.

A laparotomy procedure will be used to explore each of these phases.

Phase I: Preparation Sequence
1. Selection and preparation of procedure room and supplies

2. Preincisional count—sponges, sharps, and instruments

Phase II: Preincision Sequence
3. Transference of patient to procedure room and positioning
4. Induction of anesthesia
5. Prepping and draping
6. Establishment and verification of suction and electrosurgical capabilities

Phase III: Operative Sequence
7. Incision—The skin and subcutaneous tissue are incised with the skin knife, which is then placed on the back table.
8. Hemostasis—Subcutaneous bleeders are clamped with a curved hemostat and ligated/cauterized according to the surgeon's preference. The area is periodically sponged by the assistant to aid in visualization of further sources of bleeding.
9. Dissection and Exposure—A clean knife, curved cutting scissors (Metzenbaum), or cautery is used to incise the deep fascia and peritoneum. Toothed forceps are used to elevate the peritoneum prior to incising it, as this will prevent inadvertent damage to the underlying bowel.
10. Exploration and Isolation—Before definitive surgery, the entire abdomen is explored, and the pathology isolated for further action. Very often the operative site is obscured by surrounding viscera, making dissection of intended pathology dangerous. In this case, the surgeon will "pack" the abdomen using large moist lap sponges, and insert a self-retaining abdominal retractor (Balfour) to maximize exposure.
11. Surgical Repair: Excision or Revision—Depending on the purpose of the surgery and local anatomy, each surgical procedure will require a certain amount of dissection of surrounding tissue. For most abdominal cases, Metzenbaum scissors, smooth tissue forceps, and sponges are required.

    As the depth increases the length of the instrument should also increase.

    Each surgeon will have a preference as to which instrument, suture, etc. will be used. This choice will be anticipated by the scrub nurse only through experience and familiarity with the surgeon's routine.

    The operation frequently focuses on the removal of an entire organ, resection of a part of an organ, reconstruction of an organ, or both resection and reconstruction. These acts often require specialized instruments designed to accomplish this task.

12. Hemostasis and Irrigation—In preparation for closing, the surgeon will survey the operative site for bleeders, control the bleeding via ligation/cauterization, and irrigate the wound with warmed normal saline (with or without antibiotic). If a drain will be needed, the site is prepared and a drain is inserted.
13. Collection and Verification of Specimen—With permission from the surgeon, specimens for routine analysis are removed from the surgical field and passed off to the circulator for processing.

Phase IV: Closing Sequence
14. Closing Counts—The scrub nurse anticipates the closure and begins the *first* closing count with the circulating nurse. Sponges, sharps, and instruments are counted before closure of the peritoneal cavity.

    In the case of a laparotomy, sponges and retaining instruments are removed, the wound is irrigated, and Kocher clamps used to grasp the edges of the peritoneum. The peritoneum and fascia will be closed serially. Then the *second* closing count is performed; sponges and sharps only, and the skin is closed using either sutures or skin staples.
15. Anesthesia Reversal and Stabilization
16. Application of Dressing/Tape—The dressing is applied by the surgeon and assistant following the surface cleaning of the incision and removal of dried surgical prep solution. The drape sheets are removed, and the tape is applied by the circulating nurse.

Phase V: Postoperative Sequence
17. Preparation for Transfer—The intraoperative records are completed; a warm blanket is placed on the patient; the circulator assists in transferring the patient from the operating table to the recovery bed *only when anesthesia personnel are ready.*
18. Transference to Postanesthesia Area—The circulating nurse accompanies the patient and anesthesia personnel to the postanesthesia care area, and gives verbal report to the nurse who will continue to care for the patient.
19. Postprocedural Routine—The postprocedural routine consists of delivery of specimen and records to designated location by the circulating nurse, and assistance in the clean-up and preparation for the next procedure performed in the room.

As outlined, each phase has specific tasks to be accomplished and specific duties and responsibilities for each member of the surgical team. It takes a great deal of practice and intelligent experience to become proficient in each task, but by understanding the sequence of events, the perioperative nurse can learn to anticipate and to make versatile judgments based on the needs of the patient and the surgical team.

OR nursing is a complicated and highly specialized team effort. The health and life of the patient are in the hands of the surgical team. One break in acceptable practice could spell the difference between a successful surgery and one leaving adverse effects for the patient. Such responsibility cannot be delegated lightly. Only trained and experienced nursing personnel can share in the satisfying work in the OR, and this can be accomplished only through accumulation of knowledge on a continuing basis.

CARE AND HANDLING OF SURGICAL SPECIMENS

Imagine this scenario:

After much planning, expense in time, and many anxious moments waiting with fearful expectations, the surgeon must inform the patient that he or she is still unable to confirm the diagnosis owing to a careless mix-up of specimens obtained during surgery.

This type of problem makes it obvious why the care and handling of surgical specimens is of vital importance to the outcome of the surgical procedure.

During the surgery, the surgeon will hand the specimen, either tissue or fluid, to the scrub person, who then either gives it directly to the circulating nurse for processing or safeguards it on the sterile field (e.g., in a basin) until the end of the procedure. The dispensation will be directly related to the nature of the specimen, and the pathologic examination required.

Types of Surgical Specimens

Two types of specimens are commonly obtained during a surgical procedure:

1. Those collected for routine examination
2. Those collected for diagnostic purposes
   a. frozen section (suspected pathology)
   b. cultures
   c. ERA/PRA examinations

Routine Specimens

These specimens do not require immediate attention by the pathology department, and are collected and placed in a preservation fluid, labeled, and sent to pathology following the conclusion of the procedure.

According to JCAHO recommendations, all tissues removed from a patient should be sent to pathology, with very few exceptions, and these exceptions should be specified in the department's policy and procedures manual, including their methods of collection.

Once the pathologist has reviewed the specimen, a dictated report of the findings will appear on the patient's record to assist the surgeon with further treatment.

Foreign bodies required for forensic identification, such as bullets or a knife used in a homicide case, require additional handling and identification, and therefore an established protocol must be followed for transfer to a law enforcement officer after pathology has made the initial identification of the object.

Proper routine handling of specimens requires some basic guidelines, which should be modified to the institutional requirements.

1. Routine specimens are covered with a preserving fluid, usually 10 percent formalin, unless otherwise directed by the surgeon and/or the pathology department.
2. Both the specimen container and its lid should be properly labeled, using a printed patient label. Additional information should include:

   - Specimen description and analysis to be performed
   - Surgeon's name
   - Date and OR room number

3. A completed *tissue requisition slip* should accompany each specimen container.
4. The scrub nurse should separate like specimens from different locations (e.g., right/left; anterior/posterior) by placing them on a glove wrapper until collected by the circulating nurse.
5. Multiple specimens from the same location should be tagged, if not placed in separate containers, designating side (number) of the specimen (e.g., tonsillectomy—right tonsil tagged).
6. Specimens not immediately passed off the field should be kept moist in saline unless contraindicated or specified by surgeon or pathologist.
7. Calculi should not be placed in formalin, since the preservative could change the chemical composition of stone. They should be placed in a dry container, and labeled as to their source. (Foreign bodies should be sent dry, for example, screws, plates, bullets, etc.)
8. Specimens should *never* be passed off on a counted sponge. The sponge may be taken out of the room, causing possible error during the closing counts.
9. Amputated extremities are wrapped before

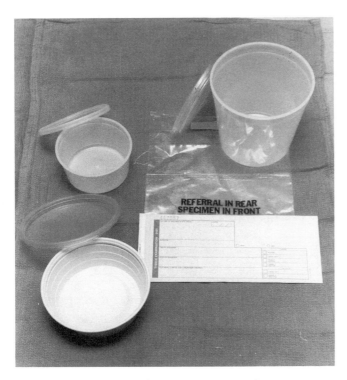

Specimen containers and tissue requisition slip

sending them to the pathology lab/morgue, depending on the specific protocol established by the pathology department.

10. All specimens should be handled with gloved hands *only*.

Diagnostic Specimens

Frozen Section This type of specimen requires special handling and immediate examination by the pathologist, with a verbal report of the findings communicated to the surgeon during the surgical procedure. Examples include a breast biopsy, or biopsy of any organ, tumor, or lesion, for determination of tissue pathology.

The specimen is sent *dry*, in a container or on a towel, properly labeled with a tissue requisition slip and immediately given to the pathologist for microscopic examination. A *fixed*, or permanent, section will follow, reaffirming the preliminary findings. Never send tissue specimens on a counted sponge.

Cultures Wound cultures are taken on a patient who comes to the operating room with a known or suspected infection. Drainage that is cultured may be frank pus or serous fluid.

There are two types of cultures: *aerobic* and *anaerobic*; each collected in a similar fashion, but may require a different medium for growth. Additionally, cultures may be used to determine the antibiotic that will specifically affect the organism (*sensitivity*).

Cultures are obtained under sterile conditions, using an appropriate collection tube consisting of cotton-tipped swab attached to the lid, or the fluid is drawn up into a sterile syringe. The scrub person collects the specimen from the surgeon, and passes it off to the circulator. The exact procedure for collecting cultures for specific tests will vary from each institution, but generally cultures must be sent to the laboratory immediately. If cultures are placed on glass slides (smears), these too must be sent to the laboratory immediately for accurate processing. Each requires an appropriate label and tissue requisition.

The perioperative nurse must be aware of the proper collection procedure for surgical specimens, so that accuracy can be assured during the examination process.

Remember, *both the scrub person and the circulating nurse are legally responsible and accountable for proper handling of tissue specimens*.

MANAGEMENT OF TUBES AND DRAINS

The perioperative nurse is responsible for the proper management of many types of drains, catheters, and other devices used by the surgeon during the course of the surgical procedure. There are a wide variety of devices available, serving several purposes, and the choice will be determined by the surgeon based on the specific need required by the surgical procedure performed.

As a general rule, the terms *tubes* and *catheters* are used interchangeably, but there is a slight difference in the type and materials used.

The primary purpose of all catheters, tubes, and drains is to permit or encourage the escape of body fluids that could be detrimental to the patient's welfare if allowed to remain and/or accumulate within a given area.

Types of Drains

Drains remove fluid or exudate by one of two mechanisms: either by gravity or by mechanical means.

The basic drain used for removing fluid from a cavity via gravity drainage is the *Penrose drain*. This is a soft rubber drain that will not damage nearby organs and causes very little tissue reaction. It is usually placed in a "stab wound" that is made adjacent to the main incision, or may be placed near an intestinal anastomosis. A Penrose drain is considered an "open drain," therefore, it could become a site for possible infection if not monitored properly.

The *Foley catheter*, although usually associated with

urinary drainage, can be used to serve as a gastrostomy tube in addition to draining the gallbladder when a cholecystostomy is indicated. The catheter's balloon acts to prevent accidental extrusion from the gallbladder or stomach. A "T"-tube serves as a drain for the common duct following a cholangiogram or cholecystectomy, when small fragments of stone may need to be evacuated.

A *Salem Sump catheter* is a double-lumen device that prevents adjacent structures from clogging the opening in the suction tube by means of an outer screen of perforated tubing. It is considered a mechanical drainage device, since it is usually attached to low suction (continuous or intermittent), and is particularly appropriate when a large volume of fluid is expected, such as with intestinal fistulae or pancreatitis.

In addition to the drainage tubes mentioned above, there are portable self-contained closed-wound mechanical devices that suction fluid or exudate from a wound after collapsing them and closing the valve, forcing the fluid to be pulled into the collection chamber. Examples of these drains include the *Hemovac* and the *Jackson-Pratt*.

Additional examples of drains commonly used in surgery include the *Pleuro-Vac* and *atrium chest drainage* systems. These systems are used when the thoracic cavity has been entered and the possibility of a tension pneumothorax exists. The *nasogastric tube* (e.g., Levine) is used to decompress the stomach during abdominal surgery. The *Robinson catheter* is used to drain the bladder when an indwelling catheter is not needed, and a variety of urologic catheters used for diagnostic studies, such as a *ureteral olive tip catheter* or a *3-way Foley* are used for continuous irrigation following a transurethral resection of the prostate (TURP).

There are many other catheters and drains, which will be discussed in the chapters dealing with their specific use, but the responsibility of the perioperative nurse for the management of these tubes, catheters, and drains is the same during the intraoperative phase; that is, to record the type and location of the drain(s) in addition to the type and amount of drainage, and to communicate this information to the nurses caring for the patient during the postoperative period.

Possible Complications of Drains

Three basic complications can be associated with the use of drains: hemorrhage, sepsis, and loss of the drain/intraluminal catheter and bowel herniation (when a drain is placed in the abdomen).

Although these complications are rare, any patient with a drainage device should be carefully monitored postoperatively and the surgeon notified immediately for corrective action should a complication develop. An understanding of the basic principles will aid the perioperative nurse in the management of the various drainage devices, regardless of the area of the body. The surgical staff should be properly instructed in the application/insertion techniques, to prepare for use during surgical insertion.

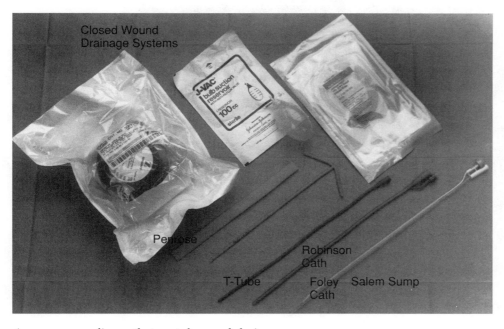

Accessory supplies: catheters, tubes, and drains

APPLICATION OF DRESSINGS AND TAPE

The final step for any surgical procedure is the application of dressings and tape.

Dressings accomplish five basic functions, all of which are important to the final outcome of the surgical intervention.

1. Protect the incision from contamination and/or trauma
2. Absorb drainage
3. Provide support, or splint or immobilize a body part and/or the incision
4. Facilitate hemostasis and minimize edema
5. Enhance the patient's physical, esthetic, and psychological comfort

The choice of the type of dressing used is based on the type of surgery performed, the condition of the wound at time of closure, and the area of the incision.

Under extreme circumstances, the wound may be packed before applying the dressing, to be closed at a later date once an infection has subsided, but most patients will leave the procedure room with a dressing in place.

Postoperative surgical dressings for abdominal procedures are usually applied in three layers, depending on the complexity of the surgery:

First layer (closest to the skin)	nonadherent dressing; most common is Telfa; will not stick to wound, thus decreasing trauma during dressing changes
Second layer	gauze 4 × 4 dressing sponges (Raytec sponges should *never* be used for dressings)
Third layer	absorbent pad, usually an ABD; provides absorbency with protection

Alternative surgical dressings range from an adhesive synthetic permeable membrane, such as Op-Site, for use on a small area, to Montgomery straps, which are applied over a conventional dressing when frequent dressing changes may be required, thus eliminating removal and reapplication of tape.

Application Protocol

1. The wound and surrounding area is cleaned by the scrub person with a sterile sponge and dried with a sterile towel.
2. The sterile dressing material is prepared (cut, fluffed, etc.) and applied in layers using sterile technique. Drain sites require a sterile dressing.
3. The laparotomy drape is removed while the dressings are held in place with sterile gloves.
4. The circulating nurse applies the appropriate tape,

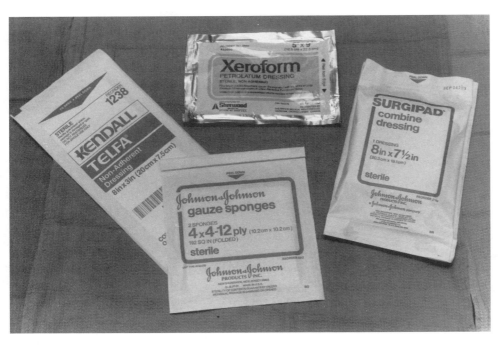

Variety of wound dressings

making sure that all edges are secured and the dressing is sealed.

NOTE: Some patients may have sensitivities to a certain type of tape, and this factor must be taken into account during the application procedure.

Once the dressings are secure, and the patient is relatively stable from the anesthesia and beginning to awaken, the perioperative nurse finalizes the intraoperative paperwork, assists in moving the patient to the recovery bed, and proceeds to transport the patient, with an anesthesiologist/anesthesia clinician, to the Postanesthesia Care Unit (PACU), where the next phase of patient care begins.

Intraoperative Nursing Concepts

Perioperative nurses participate in all three phases of surgical intervention. However, the heaviest of these activities occurs during the intraoperative phase of the surgical experience. Based on professional training and experience, the intraoperative segment requires additional knowledge and understanding of special equipment, accessory items, and concepts relating to specialized skills performed during surgery. Perioperative nurses must function effectively, and in the best interest of the patient, thereby assuring quality management of patient care during the perioperative period.

Self-assessment Exercise 6

Directions: Complete the following exercises. The answers are given at the end of this module.

1. List and identify the five phases of surgery.

2. Applying the principles of basic aseptic technique, state why a clean knife is used to continue the dissection once the skin incision has been made.

3. Briefly explain the role of the circulating nurse during the preincision sequence.

4. According to the sequence of surgery, routine counts are performed three times.

    True   False

5. All surgical specimens should be placed in a specified preservative fluid.

    True   False

6. Since a wound culture is contained in a collection tube, it can be taken to the laboratory at the end of the procedure.

    True   False

7. A Penrose drain uses the principle of mechanical drainage.

    True   False

8. Match the following:

    ___ 1. Chest tube   A. Gastric
                              decompression
    ___ 2. T-tube   B. TURP
    ___ 3. Levine   C. Cholecystectomy
    ___ 4. 3-way Foley   D. Thoracotomy

UNIT 3

Postoperative Phase
Daniel James Little

The *postoperative phase* of the perioperative period begins with the transfer of the patient to the designated postanesthesia area and ends with the resolution of the surgical experience.

POSTPROCEDURAL CHECKLIST

For the perioperative nurse, the care of the surgical patient does not end with the conclusion of the surgical procedure, but continues through to the immediate postoperative phase; that is, transfer of the patient to the PACU or designated postoperative area (e.g., ambulatory surgery unit, surgical nursing unit). Before this transfer is accomplished, however, the following activities should be completed by the perioperative nurse.

This is by no means a comprehensive list, but will provide a guide to efficiency during this transition phase.

1. Intraoperative documentation and charges are completed and reviewed for accuracy.
2. Specimens are properly identified, labeled, and placed in the appropriate container(s).
3. Special equipment for the postanesthesia area, requested by the anesthesiologist or nurse anesthetist, has been communicated to appropriate personnel.
4. Patient is moved to a recovery bed and transported to the PACU.
5. Verbal/written reports are given to the appropriate PACU nurse upon arrival to the unit.

EVALUATING PERIOPERATIVE NURSING CARE

Ideally, the perioperative nurse's role does not end with the admission of the patient to the PACU, but extends to a postoperative evaluation and reassessment phase, in order to obtain information regarding the quality and effectiveness of perioperative nursing care.

Evaluation of patient care may occur not only in the PACU, but in the case of an ambulatory surgery patient, may also be performed through a telephone interview following discharge, or, for the hospitalized patient, a follow-up postoperative visit.

The postoperative evaluation is important for several reasons. For one, it gives the nurse feedback about how successful the care plan was for a particular patient, and can help to determine the quality of care delivered, which is all part of the reassessment process.

The other reason, just as important, is to determine what could have been done differently that would have improved the effectiveness of the nursing care. Therefore, each nurse should ask this question: "Is there something else I could have done to provide better and more efficient nursing care?"

An introspective self-evaluation is sometimes the hardest to accomplish, but through it, the perioperative nurse can continue to develop her or his knowledge and skill levels, which can only strengthen the professional commitment: *to deliver quality patient care throughout the perioperative period.*

POSTANESTHESIA NURSING CARE

> For some must watch while some must sleep
> —*Hamlet, III.ii*

Most modern OR suites are designed with a PACU (recovery room), which is specifically created to manage the postanesthesia patient during the immediate postoperative period.

The nursing staff consists of professional nurses, specifically educated and trained to handle the complex activities that occur with a patient who is recovering from anesthesia.

Postanesthesia care was not always provided by a separate group of nurses; in fact, today in small hospitals and/or during off-shift hours or on-call situations, the perioperative nurse may be responsible for the management of patient care during this phase.

For this reason, and for a better understanding of the perioperative cycle, a brief overview of managing patient care during the immediate postoperative period will be discussed in this unit.

Primary Objectives of Postanesthesia Nursing Care

There are four primary objectives of nursing care in the PACU.

1. Recognize the major potential problems associated with a specific surgical procedure, and the appropriate corresponding actions.
2. Identify and demonstrate the general procedures routinely carried out in the PACU area.
3. Maintain accurate documentation of the patient's progress during the recovery phase.
4. Recognize and use the criteria for discharging a patient from the PACU, using an established scoring guide.

Each institution should have established policies for implementing patient care during the immediate postoperative period, including documentation guidelines and specific tasks and activities that will assist the patient during this critical transition.

Standards of Practice: PACU

In 1986, the American Society of Post Anesthesia Nurses (ASPAN) developed their Standards of Practice to serve as guidelines for providing patient care during the immediate postanesthesia recovery period, and like the perioperative standards of practice, they are based on the nursing process format: *assessment, nursing diagnoses, planning, implementation,* and *evaluation.*[21] These standards were reviewed again in 1992 and state the following principles of practice:

Standards of Practice: ASPAN

1. Health status data is collected. This data is recorded, retrievable, continuous, and communicated.
2. The nursing diagnosis statements are derived from health status data; Goals for nursing care are formulated.
3. The plan for nursing care prescribes nursing actions to achieve the goals.
4. The plan for nursing care is implemented.
5. The plan of care is evaluated.
6. Reassessment of the patient, reconsideration of nursing diagnoses, resetting of goals, and modification and implementation of the care plan are a continuous process.
7. The postanesthesia nurse discharges the patient in accordance with a written policy set forth by the department of anesthesia and by data collected through the nursing process.

Source: ASPAN. Standards of practice. Richmond, VA: The Association, 1992. Pp. 1–49.

Management of Patient Care in the PACU

To ensure the continuity of care from the intraoperative phase to the immediate postoperative phase, the surgical team, consisting of the anesthesia practitioner or nurse anesthetist and the circulating nurse, will give a report to the PACU nurse about the patient's status on admission to the unit. The identity of the patient is verified verbally and visually (the ID bracelet).

This report should include, but not be limited to, the following information:

1. Surgery performed
2. Type/agents of anesthesia administered; time and amount last dose was given
3. Presence and status of drains and dressings
4. Length of procedure/anesthesia
5. Setting for oxygen/administration preference
6. Hemodynamic monitoring lines; peripheral IV lines
7. Status of fluid and electrolyte balance; intraoperative intake and output, including blood and blood products, if used
8. Presence and status of catheters or tubes
9. Potential problems that may occur owing to the patient's physiologic status or surgical procedure

Initial Assessment Activities

The primary goal of immediate postanesthesia nursing care is the safe recovery and arousal of the patient from the effects of anesthesia. The recovery nurse works with the patient, performing specific nursing activities to "stir-up" the patient from the effects of the anesthesia, while providing emotional support through orientation, teaching, and encouragement of specific activities to accomplish this goal.

The patient's well-being is directly related to adequate ventilation and circulation; therefore, the patient's respiratory status, skin color, and cardiovascular status are the first to be evaluated during the initial assessment.

When the recovery nurse is satisfied that the respiratory and cardiac status are adequate, the surgical team members can safely leave the area, and a total assessment of the patient's physiologic status is evaluated according to preestablished protocols and procedures.

Specific nursing activities are based on the patient's individual needs. These activities relate to seven major areas: (1) promoting adequate respiratory function, (2) promoting adequate circulatory function, (3) promoting normal reflex return, (4) promoting safety and com-

```
┌─────────────────────────────────────────────────────────────────────────────┐
│                        Postanesthesia Evaluation                            │
│                                                                             │
│   ACTIVITY:            Ability of patient to move extremities spontaneously or on command │
│   SCORE:          2    Able to move all extremities                         │
│                   1    Able to move two extremities                         │
│                   0    Not able to control extremities                      │
│   CIRCULATION:         Changes of arterial blood pressure from preanesthetic level │
│   SCORE:          2    Systolic arterial pressure ± 20 percent of preanesthetic level │
│                   1    Systolic arterial pressure ± 20 to 50 percent of preanesthetic level │
│                   0    Systolic arterial pressure ± 50 percent or more of preanesthetic level │
│   RESPIRATION:         Respiratory efficiency                               │
│   SCORE:          2    Able to breath deeply and cough                      │
│                   1    Limited respiratory effort (dyspnea or splinting)    │
│                   0    No spontaneous respiratory effort                    │
│   CONSCIOUSNESS:       Determination of patient's conscious level           │
│   SCORE:          2    Full alertness (able to answer questions and respond to simple │
│                        commands)                                            │
│                   1    Aroused when called by name                          │
│                   0    Failure to elicit response upon auditory stimulation │
│   COLOR:               Objective sign denoting tissue perfusion             │
│   SCORE:          2    Normal skin color and appearance                     │
│                   1    Any alterations in skin color                        │
│                   0    Frank cyanosis                                       │
└─────────────────────────────────────────────────────────────────────────────┘
```

Aldrete scoring guide: interpretation and values (Adapted from the Aldrete scoring system. Aldrete JA and Kroulik. A postanesthetic recovery score. *Anesth Analg* 49:924.)

fort, (5) promoting wound healing, (6) promoting fluid and electrolyte balance, and (7) reducing anxiety and providing psychosocial support. These areas will be discussed in the Implementation segment of this unit.

Using the ASPAN Standards of Practice as a guide,[21] the initial assessment of the patient should include, but not be limited to, the following areas:

1. Vital signs
   a. Respiratory status
   b. Circulatory status
   c. Pulses
   d. Temperature
   e. Oxygen saturation level
2. Color and condition of skin and mucous membranes
3. Hemodynamic values
4. Position of the patient (comfort and safety)
5. Type and patency of drainage tubes and catheters
6. Condition of dressings; amount/type of drainage
7. Activity status; extremity movement
8. Level of consciousness; response to stimuli
9. Level of comfort/safety
   a. Pain
   b. Status of protective reflexes
10. IV therapy; patency of catheter

Aldrete Scoring System

The *Aldrete Scoring System* (1970) is used to assess the postoperative patient's status by measuring five physiologic factors: *respiration, circulation, skin color, activity, and level of consciousness.* By using specific, predetermined criteria, values ranging from 0 to 2 are placed on each one of these factors. These assessment factors are usually measured on arrival, then 15 minutes, 30 minutes, 60 minutes, and before discharge from the unit.

Nursing Diagnosis Statements

The postoperative nursing diagnoses for the immediate postanesthesia patient should be incorporated into the overall patient care plan.

Planning

The use of standardized care plans for the postanesthesia area provides continuity of patient care, since more than one recovery nurse may be caring for the patient during the recovery period. The care plan should incorporate all aspects of postanesthesia care, and be modified according to the individual needs of the patient (Fig. 11-19).

TIME PROBLEM IDENTIFIED	NURSING DIAGNOSIS/ PROBLEM	EXPECTED OUTCOME GOALS	PLAN	INITIALS INDICATE IMPLE- MENTATION	EVALUATION		TIME PROBLEM RESOLVED	NOT RESOLVED AT DISCHARGE PAR.
					PLAN MET GOALS	SEE NSG NOTES		
	Altered level of consciousness related to effects of medication.	Resumes normal level of conscious- ness prior to dis- charge from PAR.	Monitor level of consciousness. Stimulate as needed. Medicate as ordered.					
	Gas exchange impaired related to decreased level of consciousness secondary to anesthesia.	Experiences preoperative level of respiratory function.	Monitor respiratory function. Insure airway patency. Encourage deep/ breathing/coughing. Suction as needed. Evaluate muscle tone. Stimulate patient as needed. Position for optimal exchange. ABG's as ordered.					
	Alterations in comfort: □ Related to position □ Related to temperature □ Related to pain □ Related to nausea □ Related to vomiting	Experiences maximal comfort prior to discharge from PAR.	Position of comfort/ safety. Moist sponge for lips. Remove excess covers. Cover w/warm blankets. Reassure patient. Use hyperthermia unit as ordered. Expose patient only as needed. Medications as ordered.					
	Decreased physical mobility related to affects of spinal/epidural anesthesia.	Experiences movement of all extremities to preoperative level.	Explain limitation. Monitor level of anesthesia. Reassure patient. Assist to ascertain highest level of function. Teach alternative methods. Encourage activity within limits.					
	Potential for injury to skin and vascular system due to cast application.	Experiences no tissue damage or compromised circulation.	Ensure that tempera- ture of water is appropriate for cast material. Handle cast without pressure. Support extremity to prevent joint movement. Elevate affected extremity. Wash excess plaster off patient's skin.					
	Sensory-perceptual alteration related to the effects of surgical inter- vention: □ Visual □ Auditory □ Other	Experiences optimal level of function attainable without injury.	Explain limitations. Assist in awareness of impairment. Reassure patient.					
	Other:							

Initials: _____   Initials: _____   Initials: _____
Signature _____   Signature _____   Signature _____

Fig. 11-19.   Generic care plan—adult/client postanesthesia care unit

Implementation

Nursing interventions are based on continued *systems* monitoring that can assist in promoting and maintaining the physical and emotional needs of the patient.

Seven Major Areas of Nursing Intervention

Promotion of Adequate Respiratory Function   Respirations are affected by anesthesia, blood loss, or preexist- ing cardiac or pulmonary disease. The recovery nurse must be observant for changes in rate, rhythm, depth, and quality of respirations, through auscultation of breath sounds at least every 15 minutes, and grade the patient according to the Aldrette score for respiratory status. If supportive respiratory equipment is in place, such as an endotracheal tube or oral airway, it too should be assessed for position and function.

The patient should be positioned so that a patent

airway can be maintained, secretions can be suctioned, and oxygen can be administered, as per protocol/order. Once the patient is breathing adequately and independently, the position can be changed to accommodate comfort. The recovery nurse should encourage the patient to breathe deeply and to move extremities, which will assist in "blowing-off" the inhalation agents and increase circulation. Coughing may or may not be appropriate, depending on the surgical procedure.

Skin Color and Condition   Skin color should be assessed as an indicator of oxygenation, and graded according to the Aldrette scoring system.

A pulse oximeter is now considered the standard of care and should be used with every patient to assess oxygen saturation at tissue level. The condition of the skin should be assessed, especially areas that were subjected to constant pressure because of patient positioning or the use of electrosurgical equipment during surgery.

Promotion of Adequate Circulatory Function   Throughout the immediate postoperative period, circulatory function should be assessed, since it may continue to be compromised owing to the effects of anesthesia, surgical positioning, fluid and blood loss, and general immobility.

The nurse should monitor the patient's vital signs and circulatory status according to protocol, and use the Aldrette score for documenting circulatory status, in addition to obtaining an initial rhythm strip, since all patients should be on a cardiac monitor during the stay in the unit.

Vital Signs   Temperature may be affected by the OR environment, the surgical procedure, or fluid replacement therapy. Lowering the body temperature decreases oxygen demand and therefore, in some surgeries, hypothermia may have been induced. Frequently, the patient's temperature may be lower than normal following surgery. To prevent chill and shivering, which would increase the oxygen demand, the nurse must be aware of the patient's temperature, and take appropriate steps to correct the condition.

Pulse Rate and Rhythm   The pulse may be affected by anesthesia, blood loss, or preexisting cardiac disease. The nurse should note the rate and character of the pulse, and be observant for tachycardia, bradycardia, and/or arrhythmias.

Blood Pressure   As with other vital signs, the blood pressure may also be affected by anesthesia, blood loss, and preexisting cardiovascular or pulmonary disease. The nurse must be observant for hypotension, hypertension, or changes in pulse pressure.

Remember, surgery may produce a great deal of stress on the patient's heart, and even without preexisting disease the heart may not be able to cope with the increased work load, which may be induced by changes in pulse, blood pressure, and respirations.

Promotion of Normal Reflex Return   An indicator of postoperative progress is the patient's level of consciousness. As the patient recovers from anesthesia, he or she should progress from anesthesia-induced unconsciousness, where normal reflexes are absent and respirations must be supported, through semiconsciousness, where normal reflexes are returning and the patient starts breathing on his or her own. Finally, the patient should be awake and oriented with the return of all normal reflexes. The assessment value is entered using the Aldrette score for consciousness.

For the patient who has received spinal or epidural anesthesia, frequent assessment of the lower extremities must be done to determine the return of function. Specific indicators of return of function are mobility, sensation, temperature, and color. The skin must be assessed for signs of pressure or other injuries.

Promotion of Safety and Comfort   Safety factors that should be assessed during the postanesthesia recovery period should include the use of side rails, stretcher safety belts, and wheel locks on stretchers; patient positioning; proper maintenance and grounding of electrical equipment; and availability and proper functioning of emergency equipment (e.g., crash carts, suction devices, tracheostomy trays, etc.).

Although the patient may feel alert and capable of moving, movement may be uncoordinated and residual drowsiness and sedation probably persist.

Pain Management   As the patient recovers from anesthesia, he or she should be assessed for intensity and location of pain or discomfort. How the patient expresses pain (e.g., facial expressions, irritability, restlessness, or verbalization) should be documented.

Do not assume that *pain* refers only to incision pain. General muscular aches and pains may also occur as a consequence of prolonged surgical immobility and positioning, or a sore throat may be present as a residual effect of endotracheal intubation.

Nursing comfort measures to alleviate pain, such as turning, positioning, and distraction, may temporarily lessen the pain, but pain medication should be freely administered as per order, and the response of the patient monitored, evaluated, and recorded.

Pain Management Strategies   Pain management strategies, based on individual patient assessment criteria, should be adaptable to a variety of clinical situations.

Several different methods for managing postoperative pain are available today, including traditional nurse-administered analgesia, patient-controlled analgesia (PCA), and epidural analgesia or local epidural analgesia (LEA).[22]

The last two strategies mentioned are fast becoming important alternatives to the traditional postoperative pain management techniques. The most common agents currently being used, via all three methods, include morphine, fentanyl, and meperidine.

Monitoring for Behavioral Indications of Pain Inadequate analgesia during the immediate postoperative phase is usually the result of fluctuating plasma levels, significant individual variations in pain tolerance, hypothermia, and cultural characteristics. For this reason, as well as others, IM administration is frequently ineffective, promoting the use of other pain management strategies.

Generally, small IV doses of a narcotic analgesic can be titrated to meet the individual patient's needs. The dosage should be determined by the patient's behavior, which includes such actions as

1. Verbalization of pain
2. Agitation (when not related to hypoxia)
3. Crying or "fighting back" tears
4. Changes in vital signs (increase in B/P, HR)
5. Attempting to change positions to find one of comfort
6. Facial expressions (nonverbal language)

Since demand dosing by nurses is not always convenient or effective, strategies that allow patients to medicate themselves under controlled supervision (e.g., the PCA pump) are safe and effective for postoperative pain management.

Documentation of pain and response to analgesia should be made using a visual analog scale (1–10) to quantify and measure change in an otherwise subjective "pain."

Promoting Wound Healing In the immediate postoperative period, observing for hemorrhage is a major responsibility of the nurse caring for the surgical patient. The recovery nurse should assess both the dressings and the drainage tubes.

Incision Dressings Incision dressings should be assessed for signs of postoperative bleeding or other drainage. The dressings should be dry and intact. If the wound can be directly observed, its condition should be assessed, including approximation of wound edges, amount of bleeding, location and function of indwelling drains, and color and amount of drainage.

Drainage Tubes Often during surgery, supportive drainage tubes such as urinary catheters and nasogastric tubes will be inserted to support biologic functions

and prevent possible complications. All drainage tubes should be assessed for patency and appropriate function.

Color and amount of gastrointestinal drainage and thoracic drainage should be noted, in addition to listening for bowel sounds and moist rales in the chest.

Promoting Fluid and Electrolyte Balance The time it takes an anesthetic to wear off depends on several factors, including the amount of saturation of body tissues with the anesthetic. With inhalation anesthesia, recovery may be rapid; however, with intravenous adjuncts, the time may be longer. If the patient is adequately hydrated, and if elimination is adequate (30mL/hr), the body will respond quickly to interventions designed to reverse the effects of the anesthesia agent.

Parenteral Infusions On admission to the postanesthesia area, all infusion lines, central and peripheral, should be assessed for patency. The nurse should also note the type of solution, the prescribed flow rate, the gauge of the needle/catheter, and the type and amount of medication additives.

Reducing Anxiety and Providing Psychosocial Support The postoperative patient who is recovering from anesthesia experiences many anxieties relating to the stress produced by the surgical event. These include physiologic, psychological, environmental, and psychosocial factors. Therefore, nursing interventions should be directed at reducing the patient's anxiety level.

The emotional needs of the patient's family members and significant others must also be considered during this phase. As soon as possible, the patient's family should be contacted and informed of the patient's progress and the anticipated time of arrival back to the surgical unit or designated intermediate postoperative area.

Documentation of Postanesthesia Care

Accurate recording of the patient's progress usually involves the use of a flow sheet, progress note, and standard care plan. Whatever the form, the content should include documentation of all assessment data during the immediate recovery period, in addition to the patient's response to the nursing care provided.

The implementation of the individualized care plan should be documented on the patient's record by denoting:

Standard Care Plan Followed?
Yes ☐ No ☐ If no, list exceptions:

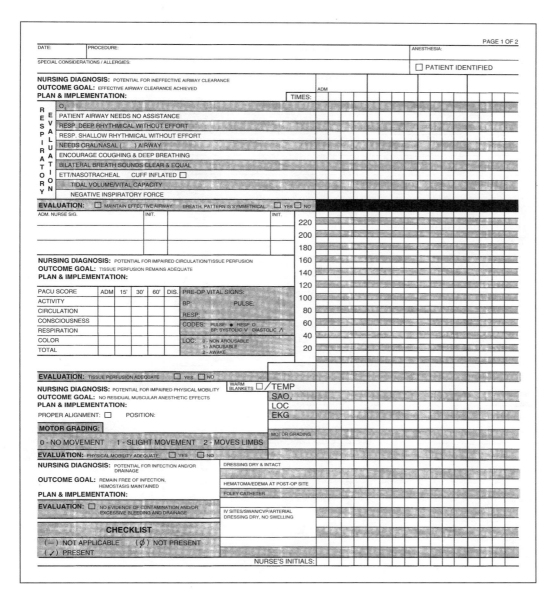

Fig. 11-20. Postanesthesia care unit record (Courtesy of the North Broward Hospital District, Postanesthesia Care Services, Ft. Lauderdale, FL)

Figure 11-20 provides an example of a postanesthesia record, which demonstrates the incorporation of the Nursing Process into the charting mechanism.

Evaluation and Discharge

The recovery nurse must ensure that the patient to be discharged is stable and ready to return to the postoperative area by meeting preestablished criteria for discharge using the Aldrete scoring system and institutional policies for patient discharge. Before discharge, the anesthesia practitioner will assess the patient and

sign the recovery room record, confirming the patient's readiness to leave the unit. Postanesthesia discharge criteria should include the following:

1. Patient is able to maintain a clear airway
2. Vital signs have been stable and/or consistent with preoperative vital signs for at least 30 minutes
3. Protective reflexes are active
4. Patient is conscious and oriented
5. Adequate input and output (urinary output 30mL/hr)
6. Afebrile or condition attended to
7. Dressings are dry and intact; no overt drainage

NURSING DIAGNOSIS: ALTERATION IN FLUID VOLUME DEFICIT/EXCESS   **OUTCOME GOAL:** FLUID VOLUME WITHIN NORMAL LIMITS
PLAN & IMPLEMENTATION:

I.V. FROM OR:

TIME	TYPE	VOLUME	BLOOD NO.	GRP/Rh	CHECKED/HUNG BY	REMARKS

INTAKE		I.V.	BLOOD				OUTPUT		EBL	URINE	NGT		
	O.R.							O.R.					
	PACU							PACU					
	TOTAL							TOTAL					

EVALUATION: FLUID INTAKE/OUTPUT STATUS MAINTAINED   ☐ YES ☐ NO

NURSING DIAGNOSIS: ALTERATION IN COMFORT   **OUTCOME GOAL:** DISCOMFORT MINIMIZED
PLAN & IMPLEMENTATION:

TIME	MEDICATION	GIVEN BY	REMARKS/RESPONSE

EVALUATION: PATIENT COMFORT MAINTAINED   ☐ YES ☐ NO

TIME	OTHER MEDICATIONS, LAB, X-RAYS	GIVEN BY	REMARKS/RESPONSE

NURSE'S NOTES:	NURSE'S NOTES CONT.:

DISCHARGE SUMMARY

CATHETER:	I.V. REMAINING:	DRAINS/PACKS:	PATIENT MAY BE DISCHARGED FROM P.A.C.U.:
DRESSING:			P.A.C.U. SCORE: SIGNATURE:
			M.D.
DESTINATION:	☐ BED DOWN ☐ CALL LIGHT WITHIN REACH ☐ RAILS UP	LOC: ☐ AWAKE ☐ UNRESPONSIVE ☐ DISORIENTED ☐ SEDATED ☐ ORIENTED	REPORT GIVEN TO:
COMMENTS:			TIME AND DATE:
			RN

Fig. 11-20. *(continued)*

An Aldrete score of 8 or higher (out of a possible 10) usually indicates that the patient is ready for transfer to the designated postoperative area. However, individual hospital policies for discharging a patient should be followed.

To provide continuity of care, the recovery nurse should accompany the patient to the designated post-surgical nursing unit, and give a verbal report of the patient's status to the next professional nurse responsible for the continuing postoperative management of the surgical patient.

References

1. Orem D. Nursing: Concepts of practice, 4th ed. St. Louis: Mosby, 1991. P. 24.
2. Ibid
3. Ibid, P. 64.
4. Ibid, P. 22.
5. Maslow AH. Motivation and personality, 2nd ed. New York: Harper & Row, 1970. P. 38.
6. AORN. Standards and recommended practices. Denver, CO: The Association, 1995, P. 125.
7. Ibid, pp. 225–257.
8. Ibid, pp. 108, 126, 235.
9. Ibid, pp. 255–257.
10. Surgical Scrub and Skin Disinfection. Infect Control 5: 23–27, 1984.
11. American Heritage Dictionary, New College Ed. Boston: Houghton-Mifflin, 1988. P. 1142.
12. AORN, 1995. P. 126.
13. Ibid, pp. 155–159.
14. Ibid, pp. 163–165.
15. History of the operating microscope, 1988. Handout used for inservice education. Distributed by Instrument Associates for the Carl Zeiss Co., Germany.
16. AORN, 1995. P. 192.
17. Pfister JF, Kneedler JA, Purcell SK. The nursing spectrum of lasers. Denver: CO, Educational Design Pub., 1988. Pp. 18–19.
18. AORN. Op cit., 211.
19. Ibid, pp. 227–230.
20. AORN, 1995. Pp. 241–245.
21. American Society of Post Anesthesia Nurses (ASPAN). Standards of Practice. Richmond, VA: The Association, 1992. Pp. 1–40.
22. Gilbert HC. Pain relief methods in PACU. Post Anesth Nurs 5:12, 1990.

12 Legal and Ethical Dimensions of Perioperative Nursing Practice

Linda Cruz Agustin Simunek

CAVEAT: Relevant statutes, rules, and regulations are included only to the extent, and in the form, that they are reflected in the court opinions discussed in this chapter. The reader should consult the current status of relevant statutes, rules, regulations, and constitutional provisions.

The practice of perioperative nursing is shaped by scientific, technologic, political, economic, and social forces. A major force impacting on contemporary and emergent perioperative nursing practice is the legal climate of our society. As a jural community, American values are deeply rooted in the respect for the dignity, rights, and freedom of every citizen. Foremost among these rights is the constitutionally protected right to *privacy* and the ethical right to *autonomy* or self-determination.

The goals and values of a profession are stated in a

American Nurses Association Code for Nurses

1. The nurse provides services with respect for human dignity and the uniqueness of the client.
2. The nurse safeguards the client's right to privacy by judiciously protecting information of a confidential nature.
3. The nurse acts to safeguard the client and the public when health care and safety are affected by the incompetent, unethical, or illegal practice by any persons.
4. The nurse assumes responsibility and accountability for individual judgments and actions.
5. The nurse maintains competence in nursing.
6. The nurse exercises informed judgment and uses individual competency and qualifications as criteria in seeking consultation, accepting responsibilities, and delegating nursing activities.
7. The nurse participates in activities that contribute to the ongoing development of the profession's body of knowledge.
8. The nurse participates in the profession's efforts to implement and improve standards of nursing.
9. The nurse participates in the profession's efforts to establish and maintain conditions of employment conductive to high-quality nursing care.
10. The nurse participates in the profession's efforts to protect the public from misinformation and misrepresentation and to maintain the integrity of nursing.
11. The nurse collaborates with members of the health professions and other citizens in promoting community and national efforts to meet the health needs of the public.

Source: American Nurses Association, Kansas City, MO: The Association, 1985. Reprinted with permission from AORN. Standards and recommended practices, Denver, CO: The Association, 1995. Pp. 40–56.

---

code of ethics that professes the moral commitment of that profession to the society it serves. Although not viewed as a legal doctrine, the ANA Code for Nurses (see above) provides the basis for all nursing practice regardless of the setting. To this obligation, the perioperative nurse's actions, on behalf of the patient and family, must reflect the protection, promotion, and res-

toration of health in addition to safeguarding the rights of the patient undergoing an invasive/surgical procedure.

HISTORICAL PROSPECTUS: NURSES AND THE COURTS

Until 1932, nurses were not the object of malpractice suits because of their place in society. In the United States in the mid-nineteenth century, hospitals were a place for the poor who were sick and dying—not a place to seek a cure. There was no anesthesia; whiskey was the drug of choice; and treatments included emetics, purgatives, and bleeding. Nurses were untrained women who could find no other work—the poor, illiterate, and criminal. In fact, in New York City, women arrested for public drunkenness could avoid a sentence to the workhouse if they provided nursing service.[1]

As the new century dawned, and Florence Nightingale's work had its impact on health care, women entered hospital schools of nursing and were trained (not educated) in patient care activities. Women entering nursing had to be over 30 years old and possess good moral character and common sense. Nursing was now more acceptable, but education was not considered necessary to nurse. The students staffed the hospitals, while paternalistic physicians constantly complained that nurses were being overtrained; after all, "a good nurse is born, not made."

In 1932, nursing made it to the courts. In *Byrd v. Marion General Hospital,*[2] Byrd tried to hold a nurse personally liable for burns suffered during a "sweat cabinet" treatment. He lost. But this case was important because for the first time, the court described the legal duty of a nurse. The court said that the nurse must

1. possess the requisite degree of learning, skill, and ability necessary to practice the profession and that others similarly situated ordinarily possess
2. exercise reasonable and ordinary care and diligence in the use of skill and in application of knowledge to a patient's case
3. exert best judgment in treatment and care of the patient

The *Byrd* decision illustrated that in the early twentieth century, nurses were not in a separate profession, but were the "handmaidens" of physicians; if a nurse disobeyed a physician's order, she was excused only if the order was so negligent that an ordinary person would realize its danger.

Additionally, the quality of nursing education, at that time, varied so widely that it was probably in the patient's best interest to restrict the nurse's judgment regarding physician's orders. (At this time any person could practice nursing; only the title of RN was protected.)

The importance of the malpractice case cited above was that the *Byrd* decision laid the foundation for malpractice in nursing by stating that the nurse owed a duty to the patient, a duty to the hospital that employs her, and a duty to the physician whom she assists.

Needless to say, a dilemma occurs when these three duties conflict; however, this dilemma has been resolved.

Privacy and autonomy rights have special application to perioperative nursing. The surgical continuum involves the decisions the patient and his or her family and significant others make regarding what may or may not be done to the surgical patient's body. These decisions pertain to both invasive and/or noninvasive interventions. These decisions are further complicated when the patient is not able to make a decision for herself or himself. In such a situation, others are placed in a position of substituting for the patient in making decisions regarding what "ought" or "ought not" to be done by way of diagnosis, treatment, and surgical intervention.

In this chapter, privacy and autonomy rights are discussed relative to the patient's right to confidentiality and informed consent regarding potential risks and/or collateral hazards imposed by surgical intervention, the availability of alternative therapies, and the like. Informed consent also puts into operation the ethical concepts of *veracity* or *truthfulness.*

The civil right not to be harmed and to be protected from the risks of foreseeable harm is intertwined with the ethical principle of *beneficence*—a concept from the Latin phrase *primo non nocere*, which means "above all do no harm." Further, beneficence grounds the legal branch of law referred to as "torts," on which most lawsuits against nurses, physicians, and other health-care providers are pursued.

In the course of a surgical patient's treatment, both unforeseeable and foreseeable harm could ensue from acts or omissions to act by nurses, physicians, and other health-care providers. The ethical and legal principle of *justice* calls for redress of the harmed or injured patient and others who suffer from the patient's injury. The principle of justice also invokes the protection and preservation of the integrity of health providers to go about their business of providing safe and competent health care.

A basic precept of American law is that for every "wrong" there is a "remedy." This chapter presents the possible "wrongs" (harms) that a patient could potentially incur during the surgical continuum. Through case summaries and analysis, legal causes of action for medical malpractice and remedies accorded as a matter of law and/or through jury verdicts are represented. Cases were chosen to provide representative application of legal and ethical precepts among various jurisdictions (states).

PRECEPTS OF LEGAL ACTIONS IN HEALTH CARE

The "harm" to the patient, his or her family, and significant others could arise from *breach of contract, breach of warranty, assault, negligence, negligent misrepresentation,* or *strict liability for products,* such as experimental or approved drugs and medical devices. Likewise, the health-care provider could be harmed in terms of his or her reputation, standing in the community, economic loss, and ability to innovate and expand the boundaries of his or her professional practice.

In the course of a patient seeking compensation for his or her harm, various issues of who is accountable for such harm (from whom the patient could recover compensation for damages) are often not clear. The legal concepts of *respondeat superior, captain of the ship doctrine, borrowed servant doctrine, apparent and/or ostensible agency* and the like are applied by the judge or the jury in arriving at verdicts regarding causation and compensation for injury to the patient. Further, the concepts of *corporate responsibility doctrine, joint and vicarious liability, contributory negligence, contribution, indemnification,* and *subrogation* among others, facilitate accountability and restitution for harm incurred.

In establishing causal relationships between act(s) and omission(s) of health-care providers, evidentiary concepts such as *foreseeability, res ipsa loquitur, assumption of the risk, contributory negligence,* and *learned intermediary doctrine* are among many legal precepts applied in medical malpractice to establish degree or extent of culpability among many possible defendants, as well as patient/plaintiff's own culpability.

The advent of medical innovations such as use of manufactured artificial body parts, body implants, lasers, and other devices have given rise to numerous individual and class action suits for strict liability for harm caused by products.

Finally, the ethical principles of *loyalty*—fidelity to a cause, ideal, person, office, or position—and accountability made it imperative to include a section on developments spurred by cost containment, such as the increasing acceptance of registered nurse first assistants, unlicensed assistive personnel, prescriptive rights for advanced practice nurses, third-party reimbursements for nursing services rendered, and the legal ramifications of these developments on the perioperative nurse.

OPERATIONAL DEFINITIONS OF LEGAL PRECEPTS: BASIC TO MEDICAL MALPRACTICE ACTIONS

This section presents the foundational concepts necessary to understand the rights of the surgical patient, his or her family and significant others, as well as the countervailing rights of the health-care provider (e.g., the nurse, physician, hospital, and others). The legal process involves the balancing of rights among the surgical patient and those involved in his or her health care, as well as society in general.

This section views the role of the perioperative nurse as a *fiduciary agent* to the surgical patient—someone in a position of trust and confidence. The 1995 AORN Competency Statement requires the perioperative nurse to practice within legal and ethical guidelines.[3] The philosophy statement of AORN asserts that "nurses must be ethical, responsible, and accountable for quality patient care."[4] A surgical patient faces an operation or other invasive procedures and has diminished protective reflexes and/or self-care abilities. As such, the surgical patient is vulnerable and requires a higher degree of care.

Within the framework of this belief, this section will present basic legal precepts underlying a medical malpractice lawsuit.

Basic Legal and Ethical Precepts: "Laws" Defined

Law, in its generic sense, is a body of rules of action or conduct prescribed by controlling authority (legislature, courts) and having binding legal force. Laws may be referred to as statutory law, or, common law.[5]

Statutory law is the body of principles and rules of law laid down in statutes and statutory instruments (legislature-made), as distinct from the common law (case law, judge-made law). *Common law* is the body of principles and rules of law developed and stated by judges in their opinions or derived inductively from examination of various relevant cases.[6]

"The common law derives its authority solely from common use; it originates as courts recognize and affirm and enforce such customs and uses."[7]

Laws may also be classified as civil or criminal law. *Civil law* is concerned with private rights and remedies. *Criminal (penal) law* imposes a penalty, fine, or punishment for certain offenses of a public nature or wrongs committed against the state.[8]

Tort Law, Negligence, and Medical Malpractice

Tort Law

Tort law is the aspect of civil law most applicable to perioperative nurses and other health-care providers.

The word *tort* is used in French to mean "wrong," deriving from the Latin *tortus*, meaning "twisted." A tort is a breach of duty that the law imposes on everyone. A *tortious act* has also been defined as the commission or omission of an act by one, without right, whereby another receives some injury directly or indirectly, in person, property, or reputation.[9]

Negligence Under tort law, the failure to exercise the standard of care that the doer as a reasonable and prudent person should, by law, have exercised in the circumstances is referred to as *negligence*. The theory of negligence is the predominant theory underlying medical malpractice actions. In other words, medical malpractice is a subset of negligence.[10] Negligence is characterized chiefly by inadvertence, thoughtlessness, inattention, and the like, while "wantonness" and "recklessness" are characterized by willfulness.[11]

Malpractice and Medical Malpractice

Malpractice is the term used for the failure of one rendering professional services to exercise that degree of skill and learning commonly applied under all the circumstances in the community by the average prudent reputable member of the profession with the result of injury, loss, or damage to the recipient of these services or to those entitled to rely upon them.

Medical malpractice is an umbrella term specific to the professional misconduct of any health-care provider. As defined by statute, "health-care providers include licensed physicians, hospitals, osteopaths, podiatrists, dentists, chiropractors, naturopaths, nurses, clinical laboratories, physicians' assistants, physical therapists and physical therapy assistants, health maintenance organizations, ambulatory surgical centers, bloodbanks, plasma centers, industrial clinics, renal dialysis facilities, professional associations, partnerships, corporations, joint ventures or other associations for professional activity by health-care providers." Thus, any one of the preceding parties who commit negligence could be liable for medical malpractice.[12]

By statute, *medical malpractice* is defined as an action in tort or in contract for damages because of the death, injury, or monetary loss to any person arising out of any medical, dental, or surgical diagnosis, treatment, or care by any provider of health care.[13]

ELEMENTS OF NEGLIGENCE IN A MEDICAL MALPRACTICE ACTION

Medical malpractice actions against health-care providers may be based on contract, assault, breach of warranty, or negligence. For purposes of this chapter, emphasis will be given to negligence as the most common theory of liability in malpractice actions.

In order to recover for negligent malpractice, the patient/plaintiff must establish the following elements:

1. **the existence of the care provider's legal duty to the patient/plaintiff** within a provider-patient relationship (e.g., nurse-patient relationship; physician-patient relationship);
2. **the violation (breach, departure, deviation) of the applicable standard of care by the health-care provider/defendant** (e.g., noncompliance with nurse practice act, JCAHO standards, standards of care promulgated by ANA, AORN, other nursing organization, hospital policy and procedure manual, and other authoritative sources on standards of care);
3. **a direct or proximate causal connection between the violation or breach of the applicable standard of care;** and
4. **injury to the patient/plaintiff** (e.g., noneconomic, such as pain and suffering, loss of enjoyment of life, disfigurement, loss of consortium, loss of companionship, humiliation, embarrassment; or economic, such as loss of wages, loss of potential earnings, past and future medical expenses).[14]

Reasonable Medical Probability Standard for Medical Malpractice

Under the traditional standard of sufficiency of evidence for submitting a medical malpractice case to the jury, plaintiffs are required to adduce evidence of a *reasonable medical probability* or *reasonable probability* that their injuries were caused by the negligence of one or more defendants, meaning simply that *more likely than not* the ultimate harm or condition resulted from such negligence.

As is true in other types of negligence cases, the ultimate standard of proof on causation in a medical malpractice case is whether, by a preponderance of the evidence, the negligent act or omission is shown to be a substantial factor in bringing about the harm and without which the harm would not have occurred.[15]

PARTIES WHO MAY BE LIABLE IN A MEDICAL MALPRACTICE ACTION

In a medical malpractice action, the obligation to provide competent and ethical care to a surgical patient and to parties who rely on the delivery of such care may rest on one or several members of the health-care team. Thus, the issue of liability is a significant issue in any lawsuit.

Historically and under modern law, the following parties in the health-care arena carry potential liability:

1. the health-care facility, be it a hospital or surgical ambulatory center or a health maintenance organization (HMO)
2. the various members of the health-care team, for example, surgeon, nurse, anesthesiologists, as well as independent contractors
3. the patient himself or herself, and his or her family or significant others who render personal care

LEGAL DOCTRINES AFFECTING PRACTICE

Corporate Liability Doctrine

The liability imposed on the health-care facility (hospital/employer) derives from the corporate liability doctrine. Under this doctrine the hospital owes an independent duty as a corporate entity to render safe care to patients.

Respondeat Superior Doctrine

Respondeat superior means "let the master answer." Under this doctrine the hospital as an employer is the *general master* of its employees or agents,[16] and is answerable for an obligation owed to the patient, including judgment, skill, and capacity of its agents and/or employees, and to repair or otherwise make restitution for any injury it may have caused.[17]

The maxim of *respondeat superior* means that a master is liable in certain cases for the wrongful acts of his servant, and as a principal for those of his agent. Under this doctrine the master is responsible for want of care on the servant's part toward those to whom the master owes a duty to use care, provided failure of servant to use such care occurred in the course of employment.

The doctrine of *respondeat superior* applies only when the relationship of master and servant exists between defendant and wrongdoer at time of injury sued for, in every transaction from whence it arose. Hence, it is inapplicable where injury occurs while servant is acting outside the legitimate scope of authority. Employees or agents for whose negligence a hospital may be liable include nurses, surgeons, physicians, interns, and attendants.[18]

Although under the doctrine of *respondeat superior* a hospital is generally liable for the negligence of a nurse in the performance of the latter's duties, the hospital is not liable if the negligence occurred while the nurse was temporarily under the exclusive control of a treating physician, such as the surgeon in the

OR.[19] When the treating physician's responsibility begins, and the hospital's ends, is usually a question for the jury. Under the *borrowed servant doctrine,* when a patient employs a surgeon and enters a hospital or surgical ambulatory center, public or charitable, and receives the treatment of a nurse furnished by the health-care facility but under the supervision of the surgeon, the nurse is the agent of the doctor, and the hospital is not liable for the nurse's negligence while acting under the surgeon's supervision. Moreover, under *the captain of the ship doctrine* the hospital is *not* responsible for the surgeon's negligence.[20] The important question is not whether the nurse remains the servant of the general employer (the hospital), but whether, in the specific transaction in question, he or she acts in the business of and under the direction of the surgeon or the hospital. Where one person lends particular service he or she is engaged to perform, he or she continues to be liable to the direction and control of his/her master or becomes subject to that party to whom he/she is lent.

Under the *borrowed servant doctrine,* a distinction is recognized in the type of service or act attributed to a hospital nurse assisting in an operation (e.g., scrub nurse, RNFA). Basically, the duties of an assisting nurse that involve professional skill or decisions are regarded as controlled solely by the surgeon or doctor. Thus, when the nurse performs under the direct control and supervision of the surgeon, the surgeon supplants the hospital as the master—the surgeon becomes the *special master* of the nurse.[21] On the other hand, in performing services or acts not involving professional skill or decisions that are ministerial in character, a hospital nurse assisting a surgeon is not regarded as his borrowed servant. For example, a sponge count by an assisting nurse is held to be a ministerial act.[22]

When the nurse's services are simply ministerial in character she is not regarded as the physician's borrowed servant, but rather as a servant of the hospital so that the latter may be *vicariously* liable to the patient.[23] In a malpractice action by parents of a seven-year-old boy who died when his endotracheal tube airway failed, the plaintiffs alleged negligence on the part of the nurses in failing to (1) observe and chart breathing sounds, (2) suction the endotracheal tube as needed to maintain the child's airway, (3) have available the appropriate size catheters for suctioning, and (4) properly complete a specific nursing plan for the child's care consistent with maintaining his airway. Summary judgment for the nurses on the basis of governmental immunity was reversed. The court held that governmental immunity would not shield a nurse from liability where decision making by the nurses is ministerial.

Ministerial decision making includes deciding what size catheter to use in endotracheal tube suctioning and how often suctioning should occur.[24]

In a malpractice suit for negligence in performing transthoracic vagotomy and in rendering inadequate postoperative care, which resulted in serious brain damage to the patient, a ten-year pleading and discovery battle culminated in a jury verdict awarding the plaintiff a substantial amount. The hospital sought to overturn the verdict as excessive. The court stated that "we will not hold a verdict excessive unless it is so grossly excessive as to shock the conscience."

The following factors are relevant in determining whether a particular verdict is excessive: (1) the severity of the injury, (2) whether the plaintiff's injury is manifested by objective physical evidence instead of merely the subjective testimony of the plaintiff, (3) whether the injury will affect the plaintiff permanently, (4) whether the plaintiff can continue with his employment, (5) the size of the plaintiff's out-of-pocket expenses, and (6) the amount the plaintiff demanded in the original complaint.[25]

Independent Contractor: Doctrine of Corporate Negligence

An independent contractor, generally, is one who in exercise of an independent employment, contracts to do a piece of work according to his or her own methods and is subject to his or her employer's control only as to the end-product or final result of the work.

The doctrine of corporate negligence can be traced to *Darling v. Charleston Community Memorial Hospital,*[26] where the Illinois Supreme Court found defendant hospital liable for its failure to review the plaintiff/patient's treatment and require consultation as needed. This established the concept that a hospital had an independent responsibility to patients to supervise the medical treatment provided by its medical staff. Liability for failure to do so was not founded in respondeat superior or vicarious liability, which have been the traditional modes of recovery; rather the court found the hospital liable for its own negligence and not that of the physician.

The doctrine of corporate responsibility imposes a duty of ordinary care on hospitals to ensure that: (1) only competent practitioners are granted staff privileges, and (2) once staff privileges have been granted to a competent practitioner, the hospital takes reasonable steps to ensure patient safety when it knows or should know the staff has engaged in a pattern of incompetent behavior.[27]

Generally, where a nurse follows the instructions and orders given by the attending private physician, the courts have refused to hold the nurse or the hospital employer responsible for resulting injuries.[28]

A nurse's action to "go over the head" of an independent contractor in appropriate situations is defensible. It has been held that nurses have a duty to the patients admitted to the hospitals where they are employed to take appropriate action for the well-being of their patients any time it is obvious that an independent contractor physician is providing negligent or incompetent treatment that falls below acceptable medical standards, or has given an order to the nurse that is so obviously negligent as to lead any reasonable person to anticipate that substantial injury would result to the patient if the order were followed.[29]

Malpractice Actions Based on Corporate Liability Doctrine

The doctrine of corporate negligence reflects the public's perception of the modern hospital as a multifaceted health-care facility responsible for the quality of medical care and treatment rendered. The community hospital has evolved into a corporate institution assuming "the role of a comprehensive health center ultimately responsible for arranging and coordinating total health care." The patient treated in such a facility receives care from a number of individuals of varying capacities and is not merely treated by a physician in isolation.[30]

We also adopt the doctrine of independent corporate responsibility to the extent this doctrine imposes a duty of ordinary care on hospitals to (1) ensure that only competent physicians are granted staff privileges, and (2) take reasonable steps to ensure patient safety when it knows or should know the staff physician has engaged in a pattern of incompetent behavior, once staff privileges are granted to the physician.

Joint or Vicarious Liability

Joint or vicarious liability is liability for which more than one person is responsible.[31] Under the doctrine of *joint and several liability* the tortfeasors are responsible together and in separation. The person who has been harmed can sue and recover from both wrongdoers or from either one of the wrongdoers. (If he goes after both of them, he does not, however, receive double compensation.)[32]

Contributory Negligence of Patient

In some jurisdictions, such as Florida, disobedience by the patient of the physician's instruction may constitute contributory negligence.[33]

Res Ipsa Loquitur

Res ipsa loquitur (the thing speaks for itself) is the rebuttable presumption or inference that defendant was negligent, which arises on proof that the instrumentality causing injury was in defendant's exclusive control and that that the accident was one which ordinarily does not happen without negligence.[34] The doctrine of res ipsa loquitur was applied to establish the negligence of a surgeon who, during the course of a hysterectomy, allowed a needle (used to suture the torn diaphragm) to remain in the patient's body when it disengaged from the needleholder.[35]

In another situation, the doctrine of res ipsa loquitur was applied where a hospital was charged for negligence for failing, subsequent to abdominal surgery for the removal of a kidney stone, to accurately account for scalpel blades, since such a failure could have been a substantial factor in causing a scalpel blade to be left in the bladder of the surgical patient.[36] The hospital supplied the OR with a nursing staff, which was required to set up the room, lay out the instruments, including scalpels with blades attached, to keep count of the number of scalpel blades used, to report any deficiencies. After the operation, no such report was made to either the hospital administration or to the operating surgeon.

A health-care provider is allowed a wide range in the exercise of his or her professional judgment and discretion. Courts recognize that the practice of medicine is not an exact science and any health-care provider is not to be held liable for an honest error in judgment. In order for the health-care provider to be liable for negligence, it must be shown that the course he or she pursued was clearly against that recognized as correct by the profession.[37] He or she will not be held liable where he/she has employed reasonable skill and care in administering proper treatment without negligence, even where the desired results do not ensue.[38]

The standard of care required of a perioperative nurse is an issue that is related to the various roles, responsibilities, and competencies of members of the perioperative nursing team. Thus, the standard of care applicable to unassisted licensed personnel (UAP) would be different from the standard of care applicable to the registered nurse's first assistant (RNFA).

Product Liability

Product liability refers to the legal liability of manufacturers and sellers to compensate buyers, users, and even bystanders for damages or injuries suffered because of defects in goods purchased.[39]

Such a case occurred in a 1991 Alabama products liability case against manufacturers of breast implants.

The plaintiff underwent breast augmentation surgery in 1981 and in 1987 the plaintiff suffered from "capsular contracture."

When the patient first got her implants, the implant manufacturer provided in its literature written warnings including these:

1. that the corporation could not guarantee the structural integrity of its implant should the surgeon elect to treat capsule firmness by forceful external stress;
2. that "the patient should be made aware that any abnormal stress or trauma to the breasts could result in the rupture of the prosthesis";
3. that "should the silicone envelope be ruptured, [the] corporation cannot guarantee reliable gel containment and the prosthesis should be replaced."

Because the implant was an "unreasonably dangerous product" and the manufacturer understated the risks of implant rupture from closed capsullotomies, the jury returned a general verdict of 2 million dollars.[40]

Statute of Limitations

There is a time bar with respect to actions based on tort. An action for medical malpractice must be commenced within 2 years from the time that the incident giving rise to the action occurred, or within 2 years from the time the incident is discovered with the exercise of due diligence.

Damages

Damages may be compensatory or punitive according to whether they are awarded as the measure of actual loss suffered or as punishment for outrageous conduct and to deter future transgressions. Nominal damages are awarded for the vindication of a right where no real loss or injury can be proved. Generally, punitive or exemplary damages are awarded only if compensatory or actual damages have been sustained.[41]

Punitive Damages

In a 1985 Florida case, testimony by recovery room nurses that a physician had the tendency to extubate patients too quickly after surgery was admissible against the hospital on the issue of punitive damages. The case illustrated the nurses' conflicting duties owed to patient, doctor, and hospital/employer.[42]

Confidential relationships are deemed to arise when the circumstances make it certain that the parties do not deal in equal terms, but on one side there is overmastering undue influence, or, on the other, weakness, dependence, or trust, faith, and reliance on the judgment and advice of the other.

Out of such a relationship the law raises the rule that neither party may assert influence or pressure on the other, take selfish advantage of his trust, or deal with the subject matter of the trust in such a way as to benefit himself or prejudice the other except in the exercise of the utmost good faith and with the full consent and knowledge of that other party.[43]

A *deposition* is a discovery device by which one party asks oral questions of the other party or of a witness for the other party. The person who is deposed is called the *deponent*. The deposition is conducted under oath outside of the courtroom, usually in one of the lawyer's offices. A transcript—word-for-word account—is made of the deposition.[44]

Specific Acts of Negligence

Negligence Related to Informed Consent

Lack of informed consent claims combine the legal and ethical content of law. Recovery for negligence related to informed consent may be based on tort, for example, negligent nondisclosure, fraudulent misrepresentation, negligent or intentional infliction of emotional distress, or technical assault and battery.

In a suit against a physician or other health-care provider that is based on the failure of the physician or health-care provider to disclose or adequately disclose the risks and hazards involved in the medical care or surgical procedure rendered by the physician or other health-care provider, the only theory on which recovery may be obtained is negligence in failing to disclose the risks or hazards that could have influenced a reasonable person in making a decision to give or withhold consent. An executed form presents a rebuttable presumption of informed consent.

Technical language will not ordinarily suffice to disclose a risk to an untutored layperson; and abstract or blanket terms may not be adequate to communicate specific damages. In order for a reasonable patient to have awareness of a risk, he or she should be told in lay language the nature and severity of the risk and the likelihood of its occurrence.

For example, in a Louisiana action for lack of informed consent wherein patient/plaintiff acquired a metallic taste post-stapedectomy, and the surgeon wrote "loss of sense of taste" as a risk on the subject consent form, which was explained in great detail to, and signed by, plaintiff, the Louisiana Federal District Court concurred with the surgeon's opinion that the risk of "loss of taste" encompasses risk of "metallic taste."[45]

Because plaintiff was informed of the risk of "loss of sense of taste" and indeed consented to the surgery knowing this risk, the court concluded that a reasonable patient in the plaintiff's position would have still consented to the surgery had the risk of "metallic" taste been specifically disclosed. The court concluded that plaintiff failed to rebut the presumption of informed consent regarding the risk of metallic taste. Judgment will be entered herein in favor of the defendant and against plaintiff, dismissing plaintiff's claim with prejudice.

Exceptions to the Informed Consent Doctrine

Ethical principles of beneficence, autonomy, justice, veracity, and loyalty serve to shape the boundaries of informed consent. The physician's duties to "practice technically sufficient medicine," the duty "to do no harm," and the duty of confidentiality all impose limits on informed consent.

These duties are balanced with the patient's right to self-determination as to what should or should not be done with his or her body. There are various exceptions to the disclosure duty of the physician including (1) the emergency exception, (2) the incompetency of the patient exception (de jure, de facto, general, and specific incompetency), and (3) therapeutic privilege of the physician.

The Emergency Exception to Informed Consent

If a physician determines that the patient needs urgent or emergency treatment, he or she is clearly justified in reducing or suspending his or her disclosure duty. The critical issue is the definition of "emergency." A commentator notes that where the courts have attempted to define the term, the results have varied widely from such strict language as "life or limb" to very loose language such as "suffering or pain [would] be alleviated [by treatment]." There is, therefore, no widely accepted judicial definition of medical emergency.

The Incompetency Exception to Informed Consent

After the doctor's initial act of assessing a patient's medical status, he or she usually evaluates the patient's decision-making ability or competence.

Discussions of incompetency, as it relates to medical treatment, often center on the problem of *who can consent for the incompetent* rather than the substantive question of competency. A group of assistant professors from the University of Pittsburgh's School of Law and Psychiatry have analyzed the subject of incompetency on the basis of de jure (legal) versus de facto (actual) incompetence, and general versus specific incompetence.[46]

In a Hawaii case (one of the few cases which actually turn on the privilege exception to informed consent), the defendant physician had been reluctant to disclose certain information for fear it would add to the patient's hypertension and heart problems. The court agreed with the defendant physician's assertions and very broadly held that "a physician may withhold disclosure of information regarding any untoward consequence of a treatment where full disclosure will be detrimental to the patient's total care and best interest."[47]

Proxy Decision Makers

The President's Commission for the Study of Ethical Problems in Medicine and Biomedical and Behavioral Research has published guidelines concerning who should act as surrogate decision maker in a given situation. Their first guideline is that, although some presumptive priority could be established, the medical practitioner is ultimately responsible for deciding who should act on behalf of the patient.

The commission generally believes the proxy should be a member of the "family" because, among other things, the family is usually concerned about the patient's best interests and is usually the most knowledgeable about the patient's desires and values. Note, however, that the commission's definition of "family" includes "closest relatives and intimate friends, because under some circumstances, particularly when immediate kin are absent, those most concerned for and knowledgeable about the patient may not be actual relatives." The commission further notes that "the appointment of friends may become more common as the numbers of homeless and deserted old persons grow."[48]

When an incompetent patient has no qualified family member available, a legally appointed guardian makes the decision. Other possible surrogate decision makers include the doctor, a state agency, or a (postillness) court-appointed guardian. Each of these proxy decision makers has its own drawback.

Institutional Ethics Committee and Informed Consent

In a 1976 New Jersey landmark decision, In re Quinlan, the New Jersey Supreme Court endorsed a new concept in proxy decision making—the institutional ethics committee. The court noted that the ethics committee has the appealing factor of "the diffusion of professional responsibility for decision, comparable in a way to the value of multi-judge courts in finally resolving on appeal difficult questions of law. Moreover, such a system would be protective to the hospital as well as the doctor in screening out, so to speak, a case which might be contaminated by less than worthy motivations of family or physician."[49]

It is not envisioned however, that ethics committees will become surrogate decision makers. Rather, the committee's function *should involve* "education, development of policies, and guidelines and consultation and review."[50]

The case review function would help patients, families, attending physicians, and other health-care providers face and resolve the ethical dilemmas presented to them by health care. Such direct assistance would have to reduce anxiety, fear, and frustration, as well as reduce the potential for litigation.[51]

In a 1993 Maryland case, at issue was whether a surgeon infected with the AIDS virus has a legal duty to inform patients of that condition before operating on them, and failing that, whether a patient's fear of having contracted the AIDS virus from the infected surgeon constitutes a legally compensable injury where the patient has not shown HIV-positive status.

The physician, an oncologic surgeon specializing in breast cancer, with operative privileges at the Johns Hopkins Hospital in Baltimore, knew himself to be HIV-positive, that is, a carrier of the HIV virus, since 1986. On October 7, 1988, he performed a partial mastectomy and axillary dissection on a patient at a local hospital. He removed an axillary hematoma the following March. On November 14, 1989, at the same institution, the physician surgically excised a benign lump from the breast of another patient. The therapeutic outcome of these operations is not in dispute.

The physician gave up his practice of medicine on March 1, 1990. He terminated his association with the hospital in June of that year. He died of AIDS on November 16, 1990. Both patients learned of their physician's illness for the first time from a local newspaper on or about December 6, 1990, well over a year after the last operation and 20 months after the first patient's last contact with the physician. Both patients immediately underwent blood tests for the AIDS virus which came back negative for both. Nevertheless, by December 11, both patients and the husband of one filed suit against the physician's estate, his state's professional association business entity, and the hospital for compensatory and punitive damages.

The Court of Special Appeals held that the trial court erred in dismissing the negligence complaints against the physician, which were based on his asserted failure to disclose his infected condition, and that the patients alleged facts, which, if proven, indicate that the physi-cian may have breached a legal duty, thereby causing them to suffer legally compensable injuries.

The court commented that negligence is a relative term to be decided on the facts of each particular case, and consequently, it is ordinarily a question of fact to be determined by the fact finder. The court concluded that "where, as here, we must accept as true all well-pleaded factual allegations of the complaints, as well as all favorable factual inferences deducible therefrom, we cannot declare as a matter of law that the physician was not guilty of negligence due to his claimed failure to communicate that he was HIV-positive. We therefore must find as to these negligence counts, that appellants alleged sufficient facts in their complaints to survive the appellees motion to dismiss."[52]

Negligence in Handling Tissue

In a 1974 Florida case, the negligence of a surgeon who removed cysts from each breast of a patient and who allegedly told hospital nurses that cysts could be placed in a single container, and the negligence of hospital pathologists who received tissues and did not keep cysts separated during dissection so as to preserve the identities and integrity of two specimens led to a jury verdict for $100,000, because, although only one cyst was malignant, it was necessary for plaintiff to have both breasts removed.

Negligence in Failing to Remove Sponge

In another case, the plaintiff sought damages from the surgeon and the hospital for negligence in leaving a sponge within her abdomen following a hernia operation. The question presented to the jury was whether the patient's injuries were proximately caused by the negligence of doctor, nurses, or both.

The court held that although the duties of the assisting nurse involving professional skill are generally regarded as controlled by the surgeon, when nurses' services are simply ministerial in character, he or she is not regarded as doctor's borrowed servant, but rather as servant of hospital, so that the latter may be vicariously liable to the patient.

Negligence in Failing to Monitor the Electrocautery Unit

In a 1981 Florida case, a patient entered the hospital to undergo double aortocoronary bypass surgery. The surgical procedure involved removal of some large veins from patient's left upper thigh, which were then grafted onto two of the coronary arteries. Before surgery, patient was placed under general anesthesia. When she regained consciousness after surgery, she discovered the presence of a "full thickness burn" on her left lower leg, which, as noted in the hospital reports, was apparently caused by an electrocautery unit supplied by the hospital and used by the physicians during the surgery.

However, all those present in the OR during the surgery denied knowledge of the cause of the burn. The left lower leg was not involved in the procedure.

The District Court of Appeals held that if the patient could establish that her injury occurred while she was under the complete control of the physicians and/or hospital personnel, that the injury was unrelated to surgical procedures or other medical treatment, and that the injury would not normally occur in absence of negligence, she would be entitled to rely on the doctrine of *res ipsa loquitur*.[53]

TORT ACTION BASED ON BATTERY

Liability for unconsented touching of the body lies in battery. In a 1991 California case, a patient sued a plastic surgeon for professional negligence, lack of informed consent, and battery after she underwent the third of three breast reduction procedures.

Here, the patient testified that she consented to a breast reduction, and her experts testified that the plastic surgeon performed a subcutaneous mastectomy, which, they said, differs substantially from a breast reduction as to the amount and type of breast tissue removed, the reasons each is performed, and expected results.

A jury returned a special verdict and awarded the patient $600,000 in general damages for her pain, suffering, inconvenience, physical impairment or disfigurement, and $17,430 in special damages for the cost of future medical care.[54]

TRENDS WITH LEGAL RAMIFICATIONS ON THE PERIOPERATIVE NURSES' ROLE

The perioperative nurse of the nineties and the twenty-first century is functioning within a rapidly changing health-care environment. Among the many developments impacting on the perioperative nurses' roles are:

1. **Increasing acceptance of the concept of advanced nursing practice as a mechanism to enhance accessible, affordable, culture-sensitive, quality patient care.** The emergence of the role of the RNFA reflects this trend. Issues that are debated nationally and in various jurisdictions pertain to the (a) certification and licensure of advanced practice nurses, (b) educational requirements for certification and licensure, (c) titling of advanced practice nurses, and (d) third-party reimbursement mechanisms for advanced practice nurse services, among others.

2. **Concomitant with the recognition of the role of advanced practice nurses, there is a parallel acceptance of unlicensed assistive personnel as a cost-containment measure.**

The 1995 AORN position statement for the Advanced Practice Nurse (APN) describes the perioperative nursing team as consisting of skilled nursing care providers working in a collaborative partnership to achieve expected patient outcomes and satisfactions.

The Registered Nurse First Assistant

The 1995 AORN official statement on RNFAs describes the RNFA as a qualified RN who ". . . practices under the supervision of the surgeon during the intraoperative phase of the perioperative experience. The RN first assistant does not concurrently function as a scrub nurse. . . ."[55] (1995 AORN Position Statement, AORN Congress Resources 1995.) The observable behaviors of the RNFA are based on an extensive body of scientific knowledge.

The RNFA's nursing behaviors may include (1) handling tissues, (2) providing exposure, (3) using instruments, (4) suturing, and (5) providing hemostasis.

Unlicensed Assistive Persons (UAP)

In the OR, UAPs may assist in the implementation of delegated patient care activities according to the unlicensed individual's education, training, and demonstrated competency in the required skill set. Competency is defined by the policies and procedures of the health care facility/unit. (1995 AORN Congress Resources: Delegate Information.)

The 1995 AORN position statement on UAP proposes that ". . . unlicensed assistive personnel are accountable to and work under the direct or indirect supervision of perioperative registered nurses when performing delegated care activities."[56] Before delegating patient care to UAPs, RNs must consider the following factors: (1) assessment of the patient's condition, (2) complexity of the patient's condition, (3) predictability of patient outcome(s), (4) level of preparation and education of the UAP, (5) competency of the UAP, (6) ratio of RNs to UAPs based on patient need, and (7) amount of supervision RNs will be able to provide.

With the increasing acceptance of the relationship between the UAP and the RN, the doctrine of respondeat superior comes into play. (The ethical principles of beneficence and justice require that personnel policies for the development and retention of UAPs be predicated on ethical guidelines.) Sullivan and Brown propose four guiding questions in the development of such personnel policies:[57]

1. Have all options been explored concerning the acquisition and retention of nurses and other licensed caregivers?
2. How is competence assured in the "delegation of nursing duties" to unlicensed persons in patient care settings?
3. Are the activities, programs, and policies relative to unlicensed persons the result of a participative, manipulative, or coercive style of management?
4. Are underlying values and goals of RNs and unlicensed persons in patient care settings congruent with the standards and codes of ethics of the overall health-care organization and the profession?

LEGAL AND ETHICAL RAMIFICATIONS OF EMERGENT TRENDS ON THE PERIOPERATIVE NURSE

Today's perioperative nurse should take serious notice of developments regarding certification, licensure, titling, and third-party reimbursement mechanisms. The "late entry," "early exit" approaches to hospital care as well as the "curb pick-up" "tuck-in" mind-set regarding surgical patients impose legal and ethical dilemmas for the perioperative nurse.

The legal and ethical issues confronting the contemporary perioperative nurse are reflected in the following self-assessment questions.

1. What is my present level of formal and continuing education preparation in perioperative nursing?
2. What is my present level of technical skills relative to the perioperative nursing setting I am or would like to practice in?
3. Are my present levels of education and clinical preparation adequate to keep me in the mainstream of changing certification and licensure requirements?
4. In my home state, what are the requirements for certification as an advanced practice nurse?
5. Since the ANA certification board requires a master's degree preparation for certification as an advanced practice nurse, is my home state consider-

ing such a requirement? When would such a requirement take effect?
6. As to me personally, what are the benefits and burdens of being an advanced practice nurse?
7. In the face of a legislative licensing requirement change, what are my prospects of being "grandfathered" in?
8. What steps do I need to take to protect my current license?
9. What is the market worth of the services I'm performing?
10. Does my employer recognize the "quantum meruit" of the services I perform?
11. Should I belong to a collective bargaining agreement group (union)? What expectations would I have of a union?
12. Which professional organizations should I belong to?
13. What has my professional organization done for me lately?
14. What have I done for my organization lately?
15. What professional journals do I read?
16. How are research findings in perioperative nursing disseminated in my workplace?
17. What mechanisms are available in my workplace for research participation and research utilization?
18. Do I want prescriptive privileges?
19. Do I want staff privileges in a health-care setting?
20. How do other health-care providers perceive my role as a perioperative nurse?
21. Does my institution have an ethics committee? Are nurses represented in this committee?

The above listing is far from exhaustive. Each reader is strongly encouraged to take stock of his or her own career trajectory and seize control of his or her professional life.

ETHICAL DECISION MAKING AND ANALYSIS

Based on the review of ethical models, frameworks, and issues, Cassals and Redman constructed a set of skills nurses must possess in order to function as ethical agents. The intersection between law and ethics is reflected in the following steps in ethical decision making. Cassals and Redman caution that these skills are not necessarily exclusive or sequential:

1. Identify the moral aspects of nursing care
2. Gather relevant facts related to a moral issue
3. Clarify and apply personal values
4. Understand ethical theories and principles

5. Utilize competent interdisciplinary resources
6. Propose alternative actions
7. Apply nursing code(s) of ethics to help guide actions
8. Choose and act on resolutive action
9. Participate actively in resolving issue
10. Apply state/federal laws governing nursing practice
11. Evaluate the resolutive action to be taken.[58]

TWENTY-FIRST-CENTURY NURSING PRACTICE

There are numerous developments of particular significance for nurses practicing or about to practice as we turn the corner of a new century. Among these are:

1. A push toward master's level of education for certification and/or licensure at the advanced practice level. It is common knowledge that the ANA started requiring master's degree preparation as an eligibility requirement for taking certification exams since 1992. With the introduction by the National Council of State Boards of Nursing of a model advanced practice bill for possible adoption by each state, each nurse is put on notice that, more likely than not, educational requirements for certification and/or licensure at the advanced practice level will continue to escalate.
2. With the advent of use of advanced prepared nurses as well as unlicensed assistive personnel, the boundaries of respondeat superior and the borrowed servant doctrine will continue to change. A certified health-care professional is usually held to the standard of a similar certified health-care professional. For example an RNFA has to show that her or his work is "inextricably bound" to the surgeon's work to avail of the borrowed servant and captain of the ship doctrines.

   The surgeon will not be held liable for ministerial acts of the RNFA or for independent, discretionary judgment within the RNFA's legally recognized competencies.

   On the other hand, RNs responsible for the direct supervision of UAP could be vicariously and jointly liable for negligence of UAPs under their control on the basis of the respondeat superior and borrowed servant doctrines.
3. The expanding body of knowledge of advanced practice nurses, such as in the field of pharmacology and medical devices, will make nurses accountable as learned intermediaries and will have to be vigilant about information given by manufacturers of drugs and other therapeutic devices, to

protect the surgical patient from foreseeable harm.
4. The standard of care expected of the advanced practice nurse is one tailored specifically to the advanced practice nurse who is functioning within a statutorily recognized scope of practice. A nurse who goes beyond her or his scope of practice will be judged based on the standard of the assumed role; for example, a nurse who makes a medical diagnosis will be judged based on the standard of a medical physician.

   As educational requirements are standardized nationally, a national standard of care will be increasingly used as the basis for expert testimony on the standard of care applicable to nurses.
5. The affirmative duty of a nurse to question unclear and confusing orders will continue to be recognized by the courts.
6. The increased body of knowledge of advanced practice nurses will entitle them to greater access to third-party reimbursement mechanisms. The issue for the 1990s and the twenty-first century will focus on the "true" or "real worth" ("quantum meruit") of services rendered by nurses at all levels of educational and clinical preparation.[59]

SUMMARY AND RECOMMENDATIONS

As evident in the medical malpractice cases included in this chapter, the law is a fluid, dynamic force reflective of society's values and beliefs. The perioperative nurse, who functions as a fiduciary agent of the surgical patient as well as the patient's family and significant others, is held to a high degree of legal and ethical conduct. The perioperative nurse has a legal and moral duty to update his or her knowledge and skills relevant to competent, safe, and ethical nursing practice. The nurse could build up his or her repertoire of knowledge in the legal areas through continuing education and on-going independent study.

DOCUMENTING PERIOPERATIVE NURSING CARE

There are other aspects of perioperative nursing care that involve legal ramifications: documentation of perioperative nursing care and counts performed during the surgical procedure.

Documentation in all areas of nursing practice is important. But in the case of a surgical patient undergoing an invasive procedure, it is not only important, but an essential and legal responsibility of the perioperative nurse. In the courtroom, nurses can better meet the burden of proof that they were not negligent if the OR record reflects that the standard of care was met.

Documentation during the perioperative period should meet the AORN Recommended Practices for Documentation, which state

the patient's record should reflect the perioperative plan of care, including assessment, planning, implementation, evaluation, and expected outcomes.[60]

Implementation of Recommended Practices

The most important thing that nurses can do to protect themselves and the hospital is to document everything that is done or not done for the patient, even if it only involves filling out a checklist.

Doing a procedure routinely will not protect the nurse unless it is documented. For example, as part of her or his daily duties, a perioperative nurse routinely checks *all* of the patients' name bands before entering the procedure room.

One day the nurse is in court and states that she or he *always* checks the name band. A lawyer, through questioning, will ask if there is ever a time that the nurse would not do so, such as in an emergency situation where a patient is in critical condition and requires immediate attention. The nurse responds, "If the patient has arrested, the nurse may start the appropriate emergency procedure without checking who the patient is."

This is all the lawyer will need to point out to the nurse, "Oh, then you don't always check the name band; there are times when you do not do this particular task." This action may be enough to cause reasonable doubt and potential legal problems.

An old adage says that "It's not over until the paperwork is done." This is especially true when providing nursing care. Documentation is essential for communication of care to all caregivers. The patient record also serves as legal documentation of care provided to the patient and as such is admissible evidence in a court of law. Additionally, the record can be used as an indicator of the quality of nursing care by hospital quality assurance (surgical audit) committees or the medical records committee.

There are other uses of the patient record. For example, it can be used to gather statistical information for use by the hospital and outside agencies in the planning and evaluation of health care or to provide data for research programs to improve health-care delivery and for the education of students in health-care fields such as nursing and medicine.

The importance of complete and accurate communi-cation through effective documentation between the many individuals providing health care to the surgical patient cannot be overemphasized.

It is the nurse's responsibility to ensure that charting takes place according to institutional policy. The patient record then accompanies the patient throughout the perioperative period, conveying all information gathered regarding assessment, planning, and patient response to treatment and nursing intervention. While the majority of documentation relates specifically to the perioperative nurse, some of the preoperative assessment, planning, and intervention may be conducted and recorded by the office nurse or the nurse on the patient unit, and it needs to be accurately communicated to other members of the health-care team.

In order to be complete, documentation must not only provide the assessment data and planning, but also indicate the patient's response to the care provided and the subsequent modification of nursing care. Documentation can be time consuming, but some institutions are implementing computerized patient records in specialized areas to provide for completeness, accuracy, and legibility, while at the same time decreasing the time spent in recording. This is an area for development in the perioperative setting. However, most hospitals still rely on manual documentation during the intraoperative period.

By documenting assessments, interventions, and evaluation of nursing care provided in a precise manner, the perioperative nurse can show evidence that the standards of patient care have been met, since the court views documentation synonymous with actual care given (Fig. 12-1).

Guidelines for Effective Documentation

Legal standards require the perioperative nurse to record observations accurately and completely, and in a timely manner, reflecting the exact nursing interventions performed during the intraoperative period. As patient care becomes more complex, as in the operating room, accurate documentation is likely to become an even greater legal and professional responsibility.

The most common error made when charting, regardless of the area, is writing value judgments and opinions (subjective data) rather than factual information (objective data). For example, during a preoperative assessment, the nurse may be listening to bowel sounds and may record the following: "Bowel sounds normal." (What is normal?) It would be better to chart "Bowel sounds present in all quadrants. Abdomen flat; N.P.O. since 1201." Now you know the actual status of the patient.

DATE	O.R. ROOM NO.	☐ INPATIENT	☐ OUTPATIENT	☐ EMERGENCY	☐ OVERNIGHT OUTPATIENT/ SHORT STAY PATIENT	☐ TO BE ADMITTED

I. PREOPERATIVE PHASE

NURSING DIAGNOSIS: POTENTIAL ANXIETY RELATED TO KNOWLEDGE DEFICIT **OUTCOME GOAL:** DEMONSTRATES DECREASED ANXIETY

PLAN & IMPLEMENTATION: ☐ SEQUENCE OF EVENTS EXPLAINED ☐ PATIENT CONCERNS COMMUNICATED

ANESTHESIA
☐ GENERAL
☐ BLOCK
☐ EPIDURAL
☐ CAUDAL
☐ SPINAL
☐ MAC
☐ LOCAL
☐ OTHER:

PREOPERATIVE ASSESSMENT (CHECK APPROPRIATE BOXES)

PATIENT IDENTIFIED:
☐ VERBAL ☐ ARMBAND ☐ OTHER (SPECIFY) _____

PRE-OP CHECKLIST COMPLETE AND VERIFIED ☐ YES ☐ NO

UNPLANNED RETURN TO SURGERY ☐ YES ☐ NO

MENTAL / EMOTIONAL STATUS:
☐ ALERT ☐ ORIENTED ☐ DISORIENTED
☐ SEDATED ☐ AGITATED ☐ UNRESPONSIVE

PHYSICAL LIMITATIONS:
☐ NONE ☐ AUDITORY ☐ VISUAL
☐ MOBILITY ☐ LANGUAGE

EVALUATION: VERBALIZES BASIC UNDERSTANDING OF EXPLANATIONS ☐ YES ☐ NO

ALLERGIES:

II. INTRAOPERATIVE PHASE

PATIENT IN	INDUCTION	INCISION	CLOSURE	PATIENT OUT	ANESTHESIA END

SURGEON: ASSISTANT: ANESTHESIOLOGIST:

CIRCULATING NURSE: CIRCULATING NURSE RELIEF: TIME CRNA:

SCRUB NURSE/TECH: SCRUB NURSE/TECH RELIEF: TIME OTHER PERSONNEL:

PREOPERATIVE DIAGNOSIS:

OPERATION:

POST-OPERATIVE DIAGNOSIS:

NURSING DIAGNOSIS: POTENTIAL FOR INJURY **OUTCOME GOAL:** PATIENT REMAINS FREE FROM INJURY

PLAN & IMPLEMENTATION: ☐ REMAINED WITH PATIENT DURING INDUCTION ☐ BONY PROMINENCES PADDED
☐ BODY PROPER ALIGNMENT

SURGICAL POSITION: ☐ FOWLER'S ☐ JACKNIFE ☐ LATERAL ☐ LITHOTOMY ☐ PRONE ☐ SUPINE ☐ OTHER _____

POSITIONAL AIDS: ☐ ABD'S ☐ ARMBOARDS ☐ BLANKETS ☐ BOLSTERS ☐ DONUT ☐ EGG CRATE ☐ EXTREMITY PADS ☐ FOOT EXTENSION ☐ KIDNEY REST ☐ MUSLIN ROLL ☐ NEUROHEADREST ☐ PILLOWS ☐ SAFETY STRAP ☐ SANDBAGS ☐ STIRRUPS ☐ TAPE ☐ VACPAC

TOURNIQUET: ☐ YES ☐ NO LOCATION OF CUFF: _____ TESTED BY ___
PRESSURE _____ mmHg TIME UP _____ DOWN _____

TOURNIQUET: ☐ YES ☐ NO LOCATION OF CUFF: _____ TESTED BY ___
PRESSURE _____ mmHg TIME UP _____ DOWN _____

E.S.U.: ☐ YES ☐ NO MACHINE NO. & TYPE: LOCATION OF PAD:
SKIN CONDITION INTACT: ☐ YES ☐ NO THERMAL BLANKET: ☐ YES ☐ NO

X-RAY: ☐ YES ☐ NO IMAGE INTENSIFIER: ☐ YES ☐ NO

LASER: ☐ YES ☐ NO NO. TYPE: ☐ CO_2 ☐ Nd:Yag

COMMENTS/NURSE'S NOTES

O.R. TABLE: MFG. AND TAG NO.

OTHER EQUIP.: TYPE AND MACH. NO.

EVALUATION: PATIENT SAFETY MAINTAINED INTRAOPERATIVELY ☐ YES ☐ NO

Fig. 12-1. Intraoperative nurse's notes (Courtesy of the North Broward Hospital District, Surgical Services Department, Ft. Lauderdale, FL.)

In another example, the nurse charts "Reddened area, left thigh." What caused this and how much of the area is involved? Was it from an improperly placed dispersive electrode, or was it present prior to the start of surgery? All this information should be noted, giving a factual analysis of the patient's skin condition.

As you can see, the more information, with less conjecture communicated, the less chance for legal problems arising relating to documentation.

Nine Pitfalls of Documentation

According to surveys conducted by lawyers and consultants who review patients' charts, especially those involved with possible litigation, nine common errors (pitfalls) seem to be prominent:

1. Omission of Information: could be misconstrued as a "coverup" or failure to provide care
   Suggestion: Never leave blank spaces, especially on preprinted forms. If nonapplicable signify by N/A.
2. Personal Opinion: use of subjective data
   Suggestion: Document only factual information, and avoid paraphrasing.
3. Generalizations: usage of broad terms, which may mean very little
   Suggestion: Avoid meaningless phrases, such as "apparent absence of foreign bodies" or "skin ap-

NURSING DIAGNOSIS: POTENTIAL FOR RETAINED FOREIGN BODIES   **OUTCOME GOAL:** ABSENCE OF RETAINED FOREIGN BODIES

PLAN & IMPLEMENTATION:

| COUNT STATUS | 1ST PROCEDURE | | | | 2nd PROCEDURE | | | |
COUNTS (IF N/A NOTE)	PRE & INTRA OPERATIVE COUNT	CLOSING COUNTS 1st	2nd	3rd	PRE & INTRA OPERATIVE COUNTS	CLOSING COUNTS 1st	2nd	3rd
COUNTED BY: (NAME & TITLE)								
RAYTEC								
LARGE LAPS								
SMALL TAPES								
INSTRUMENTS								
NEEDLES								
KITTNERS								
NEURO SPONGES								
OTHER								

☐ SURGEON ACKNOWLEDGED COUNTS: ☐ CORRECT ☐ INCORRECT

EVALUATION: APPARENT ABSENCE OF FOREIGN BODIES

NURSING DIAGNOSIS: POTENTIAL FOR INFECTION   **OUTCOME GOAL:** STERILITY MAINTAINED TO PREVENT POTENTIAL INFECTION.

PLAN & IMPLEMENTATION:

SURGICAL SKIN PREP: ☐ NO ☐ IODOPHOR ☐ HIBICLENS ☐ OTHER: _____ AREA: _____

CATHETER: ☐ NO INSERTED BY: _____ TYPE/SIZE: _____ ☐ INDWELLING ON ARRIVAL INITIAL OUTPUT

MEDICATIONS: ☐ NO _____

IRRIGATION: ☐ NO _____

DRAINS: ☐ NO TYPE: ☐ CHEST ☐ N/G ☐ SHIRLEY ☐ T-TUBE ☐ HEMOVAC ☐ PENROSE ☐ SUMP ☐ OTHER: _____ LOCATION: _____

PACKS: ☐ NO TYPE:

DRESSINGS: ☐ NO ☐ ABD ☐ 4X4 ☐ TELFA ☐ ACE BANDAGE ☐ ADAPTIC ☐ BANDAID ☐ BETADINE/VISCOUS ☐ COTTON ROLL ☐ EYE PAD ☐ EYESHIELD ☐ KERLIX ☐ KLING ☐ KNEE BRACE (POST-OP) ☐ OWENS ☐ SCARLET RED ☐ SLING ☐ STERI-STRIPS ☐ VASELINE ☐ XEROFORM ☐ OTHER: _____

TAPE: ☐ NO ☐ ADHESIVE ☐ COVER ROLL ☐ ELASTOPLAST ☐ MONTGOMERY STRAPS ☐ PAPER ☐ SILK ☐ OTHER: _____

SPECIMENS: ☐ NO ☐ ROUTINE ☐ F.S. ☐ C & S OTHER: _____

SOURCE:

IMPLANTS PROSTHESIS GRAFTS ☐ NO	MFG.		SER. NO.	MFG.		SER. NO.
	TYPE/SIZE		LOT NO.	TYPE/SIZE		LOT NO.
	MFG.		SER. NO.	MFG.		SER. NO.
	TYPE/SIZE		LOT NO.	TYPE/SIZE		LOT NO.
	MFG.		SER. NO.	MFG.		SER. NO.
	TYPE/SIZE		LOT NO.	TYPE/SIZE		LOT NO.
	MFG.		SER. NO.	MFG.		SER. NO.
	TYPE/SIZE		LOT NO.	TYPE/SIZE		LOT NO.

EVALUATION: STERILITY MAINTAINED ☐ YES ☐ NO C.D.C. CLASSIFICATION: ☐ I (CLEAN) ☐ II (CLEAN CONTAMINATED) ☐ III (CONTAMINATED) ☐ IV (DIRTY INFECTED)

III. POST-OPERATIVE PHASE DISCHARGED TO: ☐ ACU ☐ ICU ☐ CCU ☐ PACU ☐ PATIENT'S ROOM TRANSPORTED VIA: ☐ STRETCHER ☐ BED ☐ PATIENT'S BED

POST-OP ASSESSMENT: ☐ SATISFACTORY ☐ GUARDED COMMENTS/NURSES NOTES: _____

REPORT GIVEN TO _____ @ _____ CIRCULATING NURSE SIGNATURE _____

Fig. 12-1. *(continued)*

pears to be intact." Definitive statements leave no room for doubt.

4. **Late (Retrospective) Charting:** late entries due to unintentional omissions may be seen as a method to alter a record

   Suggestion: Enter information at time of occurrence; take your time in completing the record. If necessary, consult the medical records department for proper protocol for late entries.

5. **Improper Use of Abbreviations:** arbitrary use of abbreviations, which may not say the same thing you wish to state

   Suggestion: Use only the abbreviations approved by the medical records department, and then only when absolutely necessary; use of abbreviations should be avoided on all consent forms.

6. **Illegibility:** if the court/attorney is unable to read the notes recorded, it may place doubt as to the credibility of the information provided and the caregiver

   Suggestion: Take time when making entries; print if cursive handwriting is illegible.

7. **Incorrect Spelling:** can lead to confusion and/or misinterpretation of the facts

   Suggestion: When in doubt, refer to a dictionary or other reference book.

8. **Improper Error Correction:** could be interpreted as an altered record

   Suggestion: Never use "white-out" or "liquid paper." Errors should be corrected according to hospital policy (single line through error, with initials).

9. Improper Signature: if signature is incomplete, for example, status omitted, questions may arise as to who actually provided care
   Suggestion: Signatures should be standardized within the institution: first initial, last name, and status (including specialty certification, if applicable). Persons licensed or certified by the state hold a legal signature for charting. All others who are allowed to document, by institutional policy, must be cosigned by those legally responsible for documentation.

Points to Remember

1. The intraoperative record is generally in duplicate form that provides a second or third copy; therefore use ballpoint pen for entries (preferably black).
2. There cannot be any erasures or white-out on a legal document. If an error is made, follow the acceptable method for correcting the document.
3. Fill out the record as if you anticipated a court case, since this document can be used as evidence.
4. The preoperative and postoperative diagnosis should be obtained by the surgeon for accuracy and verification with the surgical procedure performed. It is not a safe practice to use the surgery schedule for the operative procedure entry.
5. The operative procedure should correspond with the specimen(s) obtained, and they should be listed on the record.
6. Count status, times of events, and final dispensation of the patient (PCAU outpatient surgery) should be entered on the record.

In addition to the intraoperative nurse's notes, the circulating nurse is responsible for recording the supplies and equipment used during surgery, since the patient is entitled to an itemized accounting of charges incurred during the hospitalization. Since each institution has its own mechanism for charging and charting, it is the responsibility of the perioperative nurse to be familiar with this mechanism.

As the patient advocate, it is the perioperative nurse's responsibility to safeguard the patient against inappropriate use of supplies and equipment. Careful consideration when choosing specific items needed for a case will ensure a safe, cost-effective surgical procedure. If unsure, always consult with the surgeon before the procedure.

Effective documentation of all nursing activities, including the economical usage of supplies, provides a means to ensure that quality patient care was continuous, effective, and conformed to the acceptable standards of care.

In the operating room, documentation reflects the actions of the perioperative nurse. Documentation carries with it the legal and professional accountability for communication of nursing interventions to other members of the health-care team, in addition to ensuring compliance with standards of perioperative nursing practice.

SPONGE, SHARP, AND INSTRUMENT COUNTS

Counting during a surgical procedure is another aspect of the perioperative nurse's legal responsibility. This activity ensures a safe outcome according to the *standards of care for perioperative nursing practice.*

Counting is also a legal responsibility of the surgical team, with complete documentation of the count status entered on the intraoperative record by the circulating nurse.

Counting should include the following:

- Type of count being performed
- Names, titles of persons counting
- Result of the counts
- Action taken, if count is incorrect or if discrepancies occur
- Signature of responsible persons

Counting procedures are not new to surgery, only the standardization involving implementation is. Since 1976, when AORN first published its standards and recommended practices, the counting of sponges, needles, and instruments has been part of the standards of practice for perioperative nurses, as a means of protecting the patient from undue harm. In 1988, the term "needle" was replaced by "sharps," and now includes items such as blades, cautery tips, and hypodermic needles, as well as needles used with suturing materials.

Counts are addressed in the standards of clinical practice (Standard III), in the outcome standards for patient care (Standard IV), and as a recommended practice. The AORN recommended practices state that "Sponges, sharps, and instrument counts should be documented on the patient's intraoperative record."[61] However, in some instances, a patient's emergency condition does not permit time for a count to be taken prior to surgery. When this occurs, it is recommended that the incident be documented, that intraoperative and closing counts be performed, and that an x-ray be performed immediately after surgery.

In the legal climate of today's malpractice arena, a large percentage of all malpractice claims involve foreign objects left in patients during surgery. By adhering to the standards of care, as recommended by AORN, this potential high-risk area need no longer be a factor in malpractice cases brought against nurses and/or institutions.

Criteria for Counts

According to established protocols for sponge, sharp, and instrument counts, it is the responsibility of each institution to develop a well-delineated policy (protocol) and procedure for counts performed in the operating room, which should include 1) the delineation of materials to be counted, 2) the appropriate frequency (intervals) of the counts, 3) the mechanism for performing the count, and 4) the documentation of the count status.

Counting Mechanism and Frequency

Before surgery begins, during the preincision phase, the scrub person and the circulating nurse should count sponges, sharps, and instruments together (and out loud) as each item is separated and identified.

The circulating nurse records the specific amounts of each item, counted by type and units per package, on the appropriate record sheet and/or on a counting board located in a visible spot in the procedure room.

During the operative phase of the procedure, sponges, sharps, and instruments added to the sterile field are simultaneously counted by the scrub person and circulating nurse, and this number is added, per type, to the count record and counting board, maintaining a visible "running" numerical count throughout the procedure.

Sponges

As soiled sponges are discarded from the sterile field, the circulating nurse gathers them according to type and number contained in the original package, and when the designated increment has been reached, the sponges are counted by both scrub and circulator, and then placed in clear plastic bags for future reference.

EXAMPLE: 10 Lap Sponges (requires two plastic bags; 5 sponges in each bag)

10 RayTec Sponges (requires one plastic bag; 10 sponges in the bag)

This mechanism not only provides for quick recounting but provides a technique that maintains the principle of contain and control, advocated by infection control practices.

Surgical Needles

To ensure an accurate needle count, the needles should be passed, and received on a one-to-one basis, between the scrub person and the surgeon. The used needle is placed in a designated and self-closing "needle box" located on the sterile field, and all foil wrappers from

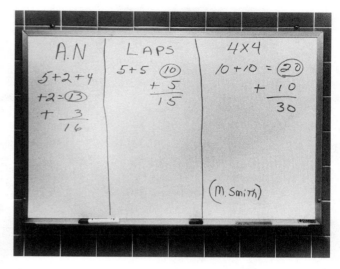

Counting board for intraoperative counts (AN = atraumatic needles; LAPS = laparotomy sponges; 4 × 4 RayTec sponges)

needle packages should be retained by the scrub person until the end of the procedure, until the final count is taken and verified.

If multiple needles are contained in one package, the scrub person should show the circulating nurse each needle during the counting sequence.

Instruments

For instruments, a count sheet, contained inside the instrument tray, will act as the basic reference for the instrument count and is passed to the circulating nurse at the beginning of the procedure. The count sheet can be created by the institution or commercially prepared, as part of a total inventory control system (Figs. 12-2 and 12-3).

The circulating nurse should announce the instrument to be counted, the scrub person counts the specific type of instrument, and the amount is compared to the worksheet total for verification. Should there be a discrepancy during the initial count, the circulator will enter the actual amount next to the instrument type so as not to confuse the numbers during the final count.

Extra instruments, given either at the beginning of the case, or during the case, should be added to the worksheet, specifying type and amount. For example: (1) Gelpi, (2) 9-inch needle holders. The instrument count may or may not be added to the counting board, depending on how the board columns are arranged.

Throughout the procedure, the scrub person keeps a silent count of all sponges, needles, and instruments, since this is her or his area of responsibility: the sterile field.

During the closing phase of the procedure, and prior to the closure of any body cavity and/or incision, the

MAJOR TRAY

Knife Handles

(1) #4
(1) #3
(1) #3 Long

Scissors

(1) Regular Metz
(1) Regular Curved Mayo
(1) Regular Straight Mayo
(1) Long Metz

Needle Holders

(2) 7"

Clamps

(15) Curved hemostats
(10) Kellys
(2) Right-angle clamps
(5) Allis clamps
(5) Babcocks
(5) Short straight knockers
(5) Long straight knockers
(4) Sponge sticks
(5) Towel clips

Retractors

(1) Balfour with blade
(6) Richardsons
(4) Deavers
(3) Ribbons
(1) Probe
(1) Groove director

Tissue Forceps

(2) Short with teeth
(2) Short without teeth
(1) Short Russian
(2) Adson with teeth
(1) Long with teeth
(2) Long without teeth
(1) Long Russian
(2) Long DeBakey

Extras

_____

_____

_____

_____

Prepared by: _____

Date: _____

Fig. 12-2. Instrument count sheet (hospital) (Courtesy of Broward General Medical Center, Ft. Lauderdale, FL)

first closing count is taken and verified by both the scrub person and the circulator, starting at the sterile field, progressing to the instrument table/Mayo tray, and finally to the discarded sponges collected by the circulating nurse. The first closing count involves sponges, needles, and instruments. The status of the count is announced to the surgeon, who verbally confirms that the count has been taken and is correct. This number, per item, is recorded on the intraoperative nurse's notes under the first closing count (actual number of instruments may not be noted, only the status of the count, i.e., "correct").

The second closing count is taken prior to closure of skin/subcutaneous layer, and is taken by both the scrub person and circulator, out loud, and compared with the numbers entered for the first count. Should sponges and/or needles be added between the first and second counts, the numbers are added to the sheet. The count is verified by the circulator, reported to the surgeon, and entered on the intraoperative record under the appropriate column.

If the surgery involves a cavity-within-a-cavity, for example, uterus, lung, or heart, a cavity count must be taken, which becomes the first closing count, making the total number of *closing counts three*, instead of the routine two closing counts.

Guidelines for an Incorrect Count

Although each institution should have its own policies and procedures for an incorrect count, the following

INSTRUMENTS	SET COUNT	FIRST COUNT	ADD	FINAL COUNT	INSTRUMENTS	SET COUNT	FIRST COUNT	ADD	FINAL COUNT
LONG BALFOUR WITH BLADE	1				XLONG RT ANGLES HEAVY	2			
LG. DEAVER	1				XLONG SCHNIDTS	2			
MED. SHARP RAKE	2				PEONS	2			
XLONG DEBAKEY FORCEPS	2				PACKING FORCEP	1			
RIGHT ANGLE DEBAKEY FORCEP	2				STR STONE SEARCHER	1			
GERALD WITHOUT TEETH	2				STR C.V. CLAMPS	2			
GERALD WITH TEETH	1				SATINSKY-DIFFERENT LENGTH	1			
GERALD LG	2				SATINSKY-DIFFERENT LENGTH	1			
VEIN RET	2				SATINSKY-DIFFERENT LENGTH	1			
POTTS SCISSORS	1				ANGLED C.V. CLAMPS	2			
POTTS SCISSORS	2				SLIGHTLY CURVE CV CLAMPS-DIFFERENT	1			
RT. ANGLE SCISSORS	1				SLIGHTLY CURVE CV CLAMPS-DIFFERENT	1			
LONG METZ	1				SLIGHTLY CURVE CV CLAMPS-DIFFERENT	1			
XLONG METZ	1				ST. FOGARTY	1			
#4 PENFIELD	1				ANG FOGARTY	1			
PEDI SUCTION	1				HYPOGASTRIC CLAMPS	2			
BULLDOGS STR.	2				WYLIE CLAMP	3			
BULLDOGS CUR.	2				SUTURE TAGS	4			
FREER ELEVATOR	1				MOSQUITOES	4			
DULL NERVE HOOK	1				POTTS SCISSOR	1			
ANG. X-MAS TREE	1				POTTS SCISSOR	1			
LONG KNIFE HANDLE	1								
CEREBELLA	2								
GELPIES	2								
MED. WEITLANERS	2								
XLONG NEEDLE HOLDERS	2								
G.I. NEEDLE HOLDERS	2								
HEAVY RYDER NEEDLE HOLDERS	2								
MED. NEEDLE HOLDERS	2								
XLONG RT ANGLES FINE	2								

Fig. 12-3. Commercially prepared instrument count sheet (Courtesy of AESCULAP Insta-Count System, 1990)

guidelines should be incorporated into those documents:

1. The circulator should notify the team of the findings and an immediate search for the item should be initiated; at the field, the nonsterile area surrounding the OR table, within the discarded sponge packages, and the receptacles within the room.

2. If the item is not found, the circulator should inform the core desk/supervisor, and make arrangements for an x-ray to be taken to confirm presence/absence of the missing item in the patient.

3. An incident report/unusual occurrence report should be initiated, stating the factual events and activities that occurred, including corrective actions taken and the results.

4. Incorrect count documentation should follow written policy and procedure regarding the intraoperative record.

5. Should the item be found, a recount should be made to reconfirm the presence of the missing

item. X-ray and incident reports are not necessary, since the item was found.

Because of the high level of risk to the patient related to foreign objects left in the wound, a detailed policy and procedure for counts should be known by all members of the surgical staff, including the surgeons, and any deviations from this procedure requires immediate corrective action, according to an established and written protocol.

CRITICAL ELEMENT TASK 12-1

Procedure for Performing Sponge, Sharp, and Instrument Counts

PURPOSE

To provide a means for accounting for any foreign object, used during the surgical procedure, which could be accidentally lost and/or left in the surgical wound once closure has been completed.

PREREQUISITES

1. Knowledge of commercial packaging for sponges and needles
2. Knowledge of proper intervals for counting sequence

PROFICIENCY

One hundred percent accuracy at the time of performance.

PROCEDURAL STEPS

I. SPONGE COUNTS
   A. Preincision Phase
      1. Countable items are arranged according to type.
      2. Scrub person counts individual sponges, by separating each sponge during count.
      3. Circulator and scrub person count together, and out loud, all sponges by type/units.
      4. Number is recorded on appropriate document and count board (if available) in increments of 5 or 10 (depending on item counted).
      5. Preincision number is circled to show initial number.
   B. Operative Phase
      1. Sponges added to the field are counted, out loud, by scrub person and circulator, prior to being used.
      2. Number is added to count sheet and counting board (if available), according to type.
      3. Discarded sponges are collected by circulator according to type/units. When desired increment is obtained, circulator informs scrub person of number collected and places sponges in plastic bag according to type/units.
   C. Closing Phase
      1. Scrub and circulator prepare sponges for final count sequence.
      2. Scrub person and circulator count, out loud, all sponges using a standard sequence of counting: sterile field, then Mayo tray, then instrument table, then discarded sponges.
      3. Count number is compared with accumulated count on appropriate record and count board (if used). Verified numbers are communicated to surgical team.
      4. Circulating nurse documents first closing count status on intraoperative record.
      5. Procedural steps repeated for second closing count and additional count, if required (cavity-within-a-cavity).
II. NEEDLE COUNT (Including Sharps)
   A. Preincision Phase
      1. Scrub person arranges all needles according to type.
         a) Atraumatic needles
         b) Free needles

2. Scrub person and circulating nurse count together and out loud all needles according to type.
3. All sharps are counted (may/may not be entered on count sheet).
4. Circulating nurse records needle count on the appropriate record and count board (if available).
5. Count status is reported to surgical team.

B. Operative Phase
1. Needles added to the sterile field are counted by the scrub person and circulating nurse, according to type.
2. Circulating nurse records count on appropriate record or counting board (if used), according to type.
3. Used needles are maintained in needle box on the sterile field, by scrub person. If needle counter is full, counter is passed to circulating nurse, who confirms count, seals the box, and records the number of needles on the lid of the box.

C. Closing Phase
1. Scrub person and circulating nurse prepare for final count sequence.
2. Scrub person and circulating nurse count all needles according to type, using proper counting sequence: sterile field, then Mayo tray, then instrument table, then discarded needles (if any).
3. Numbers are compared to intraoperative count, verified, and recorded by circulating nurse.
4. Surgical team is notified of count status.

III. INSTRUMENT COUNT
A. Preincision Phase
1. Scrub person arranges instruments according to type.
2. Using the instrument count sheet, the circulating nurse announces the type of instrument, and the scrub person counts the numbers in that group.
3. Circulating nurse compares numbers to instrument count sheet (discrepancies are noted and count sheet is adjusted), and item is checked off.
4. Additional instruments are added to worksheet by type and number.

B. Operative Phase
1. Instruments added to the sterile field are recorded on worksheet according to type.
2. Instruments passed off the field should be cleaned, then kept in one location, in a plastic bag.

C. Closing Phase
1. Scrub person and circulating nurse prepare for closing sequence.
2. Scrub person and circulating nurse count all instruments in proper counting sequence: sterile field, then Mayo tray, then instrument table, then discarded instruments (if any).
3. Count is compared with numbers on worksheet and verified by circulating nurse, and the status of count announced and recorded. (Instrument count sheet should be returned with tray to decontamination area at the conclusion of case for verification of the tray's total content.)

POINTS TO REMEMBER

1. Intervals for Counts (Routine)
   a) Sponges and Needles
      Preincision
      Prior to closure of a cavity
      Prior to closure of skin
   b) Instruments
      Preincision
      Prior to closure of a cavity
2. All counts must be simultaneously counted aloud by both scrub person and circulating nurse.

**CRITICAL ELEMENT
TASK 12-1 *cont.***

3. Discarded sponges are placed in plastic bags in appropriate counting intervals (5s or 10s).
4. If "double procedure" is performed, initial count is performed prior to the changeover and recorded as an additional count.

   EXAMPLE: Dilation and curettage; possible laparotomy
             Count sheet should reflect two procedures, with separate counts for each.

5. Additional counts are required when surgery involves a cavity-within-a-cavity (e.g., uterine count for Cesarean section procedure).
6. An additional count may be requested at any time, by any member of the surgical team, should a question of the status need reconfirmation.
7. **Countable items are never to leave the room once the initial count (preincision) has been taken.**
8. Should incorrect number be found in package, package contents are removed from sterile field, placed in original container, and retained in room for the duration of the procedure; then they are discarded.

PERFORMANCE CHECK SHEET

NAME: _____	TASK # _____12-1_____
	RATING: A Acceptable
	N/I Needs Improvement

PROCEDURE: Sponge, Needle, and Instrument Count

PROCEDURAL STEPS	A	N/I
A. SCRUB NURSE RESPONSIBILITY		
1. Recognizes correct procedural interval for counts		
2. Maintains correct sequential method for counts		
3. Simultaneously counts aloud with the circulator		
4. Notifies circulator of any discrepancies in packaging of counted materials		
5. Discards soiled materials in proper manner		
6. Maintains constant supervision of materials being used		
B. CIRCULATOR RESPONSIBILITY		
1. Recognizes correct procedural interval for counts		
2. Simultaneously counts aloud with the scrub nurse		
3. Handles discarded materials in proper manner		
4. Maintains constant supervision of materials being used		
5. Accurately records counts on the operating room record		
6. Informs surgical team members of the status of the counts		
7. If counts incorrect, initiates prescribed procedure and documents actions taken		

COMMENTS: _____

_____

KEEPING YOUR PRACTICE SAFE

The legal aspects of perioperative nursing practice provide the nurse with a challenge in today's practice setting. It requires that the nurse render safe, quality patient care as evidenced by compliance with preestablished standards of practice.

Although the AORN standards and recommended practices are not a legal document, both the consumer and the legal system will use these statements when comparing the actual care given to what constitutes reasonable and prudent practice by a perioperative nurse, and in this respect, these standards provide the rules and behaviors in conjunction with policy and procedure manuals governing this specialized area of nursing practice.

By incorporating these standards, polices, and procedures into daily practice, the professional registered nurse, practicing during the perioperative period, will continue to provide quality patient care to patients undergoing surgery.

PATIENT CARE MANAGEMENT

The perioperative nurse, practicing in today's complex and technical setting relies on scientific knowledge, technical skill, and a desire to provide the patient with comprehensive nursing care equal to or exceeding the patient's expectations.

If one goal could be stated that incorporates all aspects of perioperative nursing, it should be

to provide safe, efficient, and therapeutic nursing care, through scientific knowledge and technical awareness for patients experiencing surgical intervention based on the individual physiologic, psychological, and psychosocial needs.

Self-assessment Exercise 7

Directions: Complete the following exercises. The answers are given at the end of this module.

1. Nancy Jones, a perioperative nurse, is taking her patient to the holding area. The patient has signed the consent form, but now says she's afraid and doesn't want to go through with the surgery. Ms. Jones informs the surgeon and anesthesiologist of the patient's statement, but the surgeon responds by saying "she is so sedated she doesn't know what she is saying. Let's proceed." Briefly describe how Ms. Jones should handle this situation.

2. A count that is not documented has not legally been performed.

    True   False

3. List the conditions/situations that could probably result in an improper or defective consent.

4. List and describe the correct intervals for performing counts. Are there any exceptions? What corrective action should be taken?

5. Only sponges that contain a(n) _____ strip should be used during an operative procedure.

6. Counts should be done silently so as not to disturb the surgeon.

    True   False

7. List the nine pitfalls frequently associated with documenting nursing care.

8. Abbreviations, if appropriate, can be used on the intraoperative nurse's notes.

    True   False

9. A laparotomy sponge is left in the patient due to an open chest wound, which can only be covered with a translucent dressing, and cannot be closed at the time of surgery. State the perioperative nurse's responsibility in this situation.

10. The proper sequence for counting is as follows: sterile field, then Mayo tray, then instrument table, then discarded items.

    True   False

References

1. Kelly L, Joel L. Dimensions of professional nursing (7th Ed.). New York: McGraw-Hill, 1995.
2. *Byrd v. Marion General Hospital,* 202 N.C. 337, 162 S.E. 738 (1932).
3. AORN, Inc. Competency statement XV (on the nursing actions that demonstrate accountability, standards and recommended practices). Denver, CO: The Association, 1995.
4. AORN. Standards and recommended practices. Denver, CO: The Association, 1995. P. 5.
5. Garner BA. A dictionary of modern usage. New York: Oxford University Press, 1990. P. 330.
6. Ibid.
7. *Kansas v. Colorado,* 206 U.S. 46, 96–97, 27 S. Ct. 655, 657 (1907), as cited in *Lundman v. McKown,* 1995 Minn. App. Lexis 462 @ 25.
8. Black's law dictionary. St. Paul: West Publishing Co., 1979.
9. 74 Am. Jur. 2d, Torts, Section 1; see also Keeton WP. Prosser and Keeton on the law of torts, 5th ed. St. Paul: West Publishing Co., 1984. P. 3.
10. Garner BA, P. 373.
11. Black's, P. 931.
12. Florida Stat. 768.502(b)(5).
13. Florida Stat. 95.11(4)(b).
14. *Kosberg v. Washington Hosp. Med. Ctr,* Inc., 394 F.2d 947, 949. (U.S. App. D.C. 1968).
15. *Hevner v. E-Z Mart,* 85 S.W.2d 456, 459 Tex. 9 (1992).
16. *McFarland v. George,* 316 S.W.2d 662, 671 (Mo. App.).
17. See also Black's law dictionary, P. 1179.
18. *Wilson v. Lee Mem. Hosp.,* 65 So. 2d 40 (Fla. 1953).
19. *Permeter v. Osteopathic Gen. Hosp.,* 196 So. 2d 305 (Fla. App. 1967).
20. *Wilson v. Lee Memo. Hosp.,* 65 So. 2d 40 (Fla. 1953).
21. *Buzan v. Mercy Hosp., Inc.,* 204 So. 2d 11, 29 (Fla. App. 1967).
22. Ibid.
23. *Beaches Hosp. v. Lee,* 384 So. 2d 234, pet. denied, 392 So. 2d 1371 (1980).
24. *Green v. Berrien Gen. Hosp.,* Auxiliary, Inc., 437 Mich. 1, 464 N.W.2d 703 (1990).
25. *Robert v. Chodoff,* 259 Pa. Super. 332, 367, 393 A.2d 853, 871, 1978.

26. *Darling v. Charleston Community Mem. Hosp.*, 33 Ill. 2d 326, 111 N.E.2d 253 (1965).
27. Black's law dictionary, P. 693.
28. *Van Cleeve v. Irby*, 204 Okla. 689, 233 P. 2d 963, 965 (1951).
29. *Blanton v. Moses H. Cone Mem. Hosp., Inc.*, 453 S.E.2d 1984.
30. *Pedroza v. Bryant*, 677 P. 2d 168.
31. Black's law dictionary, P. 823.
32. Ibid.
33. Garner BA. P. 339.
34. *General Hosp. of Greater Miami, Inc. v. Gager*, 160 So. 2d 749 (Fla. 1964).
35. Black's law dictionary, P. 1173.
36. *Somerset v. Hart*, 549 S.W.2d 814 (Ky. 1977).
37. *Bourgeois v. Dade County*, 99 So. 2d 575 (Fla. 1956).
38. *Blackwell v. Southern Florida Sanitarium and Hosp. Corp.*, 174 So. 2d 45 (Fla. App. 1965).
39. Black's law dictionary, P. 1089.
40. *Toole v. McClintock*, 778 F.Supp. 1543 (M.D. Alab. 1991).
41. Ibid.
42. Black's law dictionary.
43. *Fincke v. Peeples*, 476 So. 2d 1319 (Fla. App. Dist. Ct. 1985).
44. Black's law dictionary, P. 854.
45. Fed. R. Civil. P. 26 et seq. as cited in Black's law dictionary, 1979:396.
46. *Houndrulis v. Schumacher*, 612 So. 2d 859, 891 (La. App. 4th Cir. 1992).
47. Roth L, Meisel A, and Lidz CW. Tests of competency to consent to treatment, Am J Pysch 279 (1979); A Meisel, L Roth and CW Lidz. Toward a model of the legal doctrine of informed consent, 134 Am J Psych 134:285, 1979.
48. *Nishi v. Hartwell*, 52 Haw. 191, 473 P.2d 199. 1970.
49. The President's Commission for the Study of Ethical Problems in Biomedical and Behavioral Research: Making Health Care Decisions. Washington, DC, 1982.
50. In re Quinlan, 70 N.J. 50, 355 A.2d 669 (1976).
51. The President's Commission for the Study of Ethical Problems in Biomedical and Behavioral Research: Making Health Care Decisions. Washington, DC, 1982. P. 220.
52. *Faya v. Almaraz*, 329 Md. 435, 620 A.2d 327 (1993).
53. *Borghese and Borghese v. Bartley*, 402 So. 2d 475 (Fla. App. 1981).
54. *Szkorla v. Vecchione*, 8 Cal. App. 4th 1437 (1991).
55. AORN. Standards and recommended practices. Denver, CO: The Association, 1995. P. 17.
56. AORN. "Delegate Information," Congress resource manual. Denver, CO: The Association, 1995. P. 235.
57. Sullivan, Sister PA, and Brown Rev. T. Unlicensed persons in patient care settings: administrative policy and ethical issues. Nurs Clin N Am 24:557, 1989.
58. Cassells JM, and Redman B. Preparing students to be moral agents in clinical nursing practice: report of a national survey. Nurs Clin N Am 4:465, 1989.
59. See *Byrd v. Marion General Hosp.*, 202, N.C. 337, 162 S.E. 337 (1932) see also *Paris v. Kreitz*, 75 N.C. App. 365, 331 S.E.2d 234 N.C. App. (1985).
60. AORN. Standards and recommended practices. Denver, CO: The Association, 1995. P. 151.
61. Ibid, 262–264.

Questions for Review for Module IV

1. Match the following:
   A. Assessment   ___ 1. Prescribes nursing actions
   B. Nursing diagnosis   ___ 2. Includes goals to accomplish
   C. Planning   ___ 3. Reviews nursing actions taken
   D. Implementation   ___ 4. Collection of data
   E. Evaluation   ___ 5. Potential patient problem

2. State the appropriate nursing interventions for "Potential for infection related to the surgical incision."

3. A lower oblique incision in the groin area would be an indication for a (an):
   a. appendectomy
   b. inguinal herniorrhaphy
   c. salpingo-oophorectomy
   d. hiatial hernia

4. In order to prevent damage to the brachial plexus nerve, the arm should never be abducted:
   a. more than 30 degrees
   b. more than 50 degrees
   c. more than 90 degrees
   d. more than 45 degrees

5. During an initial nursing assessment in the Post-anesthesia Care Unit (PACU) area, the _____ and _____ should be assessed first.

6. In supine position, the safety strap should be applied _____ (above/below) the knees.

7. Failure to exercise the degree of skill ordinarily employed under similar circumstances by members of their profession in good standing in the same community or locality, is the legal definition of
   a. default
   b. malpractice
   c. negligence
   d. assault

8. A small, curved, lateral incision above the mons pubis describes a _____ incision.

   a. rectus
   b. pfannenstiel
   c. inguinal
   d. midline

9. A general principle for a surgical skin prep is to begin at the incision site and work toward the periphery.

   True   False

10. When prepping for a colostomy closure, the abdomen is prepped from the incision site to the periphery, using circular motion.

    True   False

11. State the four major principles when performing a sponge, sharp, and instrument count.
    1. _____
    2. _____
    3. _____
    4. _____

12. Safety measures regarding the use of lasers require the use of _____
    _____

13. When preparing to conduct a preoperative teaching program, according to principles of adult education, the perioperative nurse should first:
    a. ask the patient what he or she knows about the planned surgical event
    b. determine the patient's knowledge of his or her current health status
    c. determine the patient's readiness to learn
    d. describe the physical environment

14. When using a pneumatic tourniquet, an essential consideration is that
    a. inflation time should not exceed 3 hours
    b. the cuff should be positioned at the minimal circumference of the limb
    c. the cuff length and width should be appropriate to the size of the extremity
    d. the cuff needs to be placed tightly on the thigh for proper inflation

15. According to AORNs recommended practices, sponges, sharps, and instruments should be counted on all procedures.

    True   False

Glossary

Active Electrode: an electrode that produces the electrosurgical effect, either coagulate or cut

Advocate: a person who argues for a cause; supporter

Aldrete Score: derived from the Apgar Scoring System, a method of determining postanesthesia patient status, using five basic parameters, at predetermined times. These parameters include (1) activity, (2) respirations, (3) circulation, (4) consciousness, and (5) color (skin)

Arbitration: the investigation and settlement of a matter of contention between opposing parties by persons or organizations chosen by the parties

Assault: an intentional act designed to make the victim fearful and that produces a reasonable apprehension; unlawful threat

Assessment: a continuous activity that identifies the existing or potential problems of the patient through the collection of patient-related information

Autologous: related to self; belonging to the same organism

Autotransfusion: reinfusion of patient's own blood

Battery: the touching of one person by another without permission or consent

Bipolar Electrode: electrosurgical accessory with both an active and return electrode in one handpiece. The electrical current flows between the electrode tips, causing tissue coagulation

Borrowed Servant: an employee temporarily under the control of another. For example, a nurse employed by a hospital who is "borrowed" by a surgeon in the OR

Bovie: old nomenclature for an electrosurgical generator, created by William T. Bovie, a Harvard physicist (1925)

Calculi (sing., calculus):   a stone usually composed of mineral salts, occurring within the body (gallstones, renal stones, etc.)

Cause: that which produces or effects a result, even if unintended

Cause of Action: fact(s) that establish or give a right for judicial relief

Cautery: the application of a heated object to cause hemostasis

Civil Law: rights of a nonpolitical kind

Coagulate: to clot; to cause hemostasis; in electrosurgery, to cause tissue desiccation without severing (Antonym: *Cut*)

Consent: a voluntary act by which one person agrees to allow someone else to do something

Corporate Negligence: concept wherein the hospital as an entity is directly liable in a tort action

Dispersive Electrode: pad or contact device that provides a large surface area for patient contact. Large area reduces the concentration of current as it flows from the patient, which should not create an electrosurgical effect at contact point

Evaluation: an appraisal of the nursing activities performed using the patient's outcome goals or standards as criteria for measurement

Fiberoptic: the transmission of an image along flexible bundles of glass or plastic fibers, having special optical properties and orientation

Fluoroscopy: examination by means of visual observation of the form and motion of deep structures by means of x-ray; ability to see movement of joints, organs, or radiopaque materials (catheters, dye, etc.)

Goal: a statement of a desired patient outcome within a specified period, containing conditions or criteria for evaluation

Hierarchy: a body of entities arranged in a graded series, according to rank (either lower to higher or vice versa)

Holistic (Wholistic):   pertaining to totality or to the whole person

Hyperthermia: increased temperature; natural or induced

Hypothermia: low temperature; induced artificially or caused by disorder of temperature regulating mechanism of the body
Induced states:
Light: 37°C to 32°C (98.6°F to 89.6°F)
Moderate: 32°C to 26°C (89.6°F to 78.8°F)
Deep: 26°C to 20°C (78.8°F to 66°F)
Profound: 20°C (66°F) or lower

Implementation: the required nursing actions are carried out in order to accomplish the patient's goals (Synonym: *Intervention*)

Informed Consent: consent given only after full notice (explanation) is given of that which is being consented for

Liability: refers to one's responsibility for his or her own conduct; an obligation or duty to be performed

Malpractice: any professional misconduct, unreasonable lack of skill; an illegal or immoral act or deviation from the professional standards of care

Negligence: lack of care or skill that another person in the same situation would be expected to use; omission or commission based on standards of practice/care

Nursing Diagnoses: a concise statement describing the actual potential problem(s) derived from the assessment data

Nursing Intervention: see *Implementation*

Nursing Process: a systematic, cyclic approach to nursing practice using problem-solving techniques. The major components of the process are (1) assessment, (2) formation of nursing diagnosis statement(s), (3) planning, (4) implementation, and (5) evaluation/reassessment

Outcome Standards: a type of standard that defines results, which are written in the form of patient goals

Patient Outcomes: the intended or realistically expected behavior of the patient following specific nursing intervention

Physiologic: pertaining to the biologic sciences essential and characteristic of the life process

Process Standard: defines the actions and behaviors needed by the nurse and defines what constitutes nursing care given

Protocol: defines the ongoing care and management of patient-care activities involving equipment, diagnostic and therapeutic measures, or physiologic/psychological states and specific nursing diagnosis categories

Psychosocial: a dynamic process that focuses on assessing the social and psychodynamic data gathered from interaction; assessing the patient's difficulties in living

Reassessment: a review of actions previously performed as a method of evaluation and future planning of patient care based on changing data

Res Ipsa Loquitur (Latin): Literally, the thing speaks for itself. The defendant had exclusive control of the thing that caused the harm, and the harm ordinarily could not have occurred without negligent conduct

Respondeat Superior (Latin): literally, let the master answer. Employer is responsible for the legal consequences of the acts of the servant or employee who is acting within the scope of employment

Return Electrode Monitor (REM): a dispersive electrode/unit that can detect improper contact of a ground pad with the patient, causing an alarm and deactivation of the active electrode; built-in safety monitor to avoid electrosurgical burns

Standard: a criterion used by general agreement that determines whether actions are as they should be; an established norm created by opinion, research, and/or theory

Standard of Care (Legal): acts performed or omitted that an ordinary prudent person would have performed under similar circumstances

Standard of Care: defines the predetermined care for a specific group of patients having predictable common problems (surgical procedures)

Standard-care Statements: an alternative style for writing patient-care plans; used for areas considered to be rapid turnover areas

Standards of Practice: a criterion used by general agreement that determines a level of acceptable practice as an established norm for a profession or organization

Statute of Limitations: a legal limit on the time allowed for filing suit in civil matters, usually measured from the time of the wrong or from the time it was discovered. May be different in each state, as determined by legislative act

Tort: a legal wrong committed by a person involving injury to, loss of, or damage to person or property

Bibliography for Module IV

AHA/90 Accreditation Manual for Hospitals. Chicago: Joint Commission of Accreditation of Health Care Organizations, 1990.

Alfaro R. Application of Nursing Process: A Step by Step Guide. Philadelphia: J.B. Lippincott, 1986.

Areen FP, King S, Goldberg A, Capron G. Law, Science and Medicine. New York: Foundation Press, 1985.

AORN. Standards and Recommended Practices for Perioperative Nursing. Denver: The Association, 1995.

Bates B. A Guide to Physical Examination and History Taking. 4th ed. Philadelphia: J.B. Lippincott, 1987.

Beare PG, Rahr VA, Ronshausen CA. Nursing Implications of Diagnostic Tests. Philadelphia: J.B. Lippincott, 1983.

Borg N, ed. AACN Core Curriculum for Critical Care Nursing. 2nd ed. Philadelphia: Saunders, 1981.

Carpenito LJ. Handbook for Nursing Diagnosis. Philadelphia: J.B. Lippincott, 1984.

Creighton H. Law Every Nurse Should Know. 3rd ed. Philadelphia: Saunders, 1982.

Doenges ME, Moorhouse MF, Geissler AC. Nursing Care Plans: Guidelines for Planning Patient Care. 2nd ed. Philadelphia: F.A. Davis, 1989.

Doenges ME, Moorhouse MF. Nursing Diagnoses with Interventions, 3rd ed. Philadelphia: FA Davis, 1990. Pp. 14–16.

Fairchild SS. Perioperative Nursing Practice: Update for the 90's. Hollywood, FL: Educational Design Systems, 1990.

Fiesta J. The Law and Liability: A Guide for Nurses. New York: John Wiley, 1983.

Groah L. Operating Room Nursing: The Perioperative Role. Reston, VA: Reston, 1983.

Gruendemann B. Positioning Plus. Chatsworth, CA: Devon Industries Educational Department, 1987.

Gruendemann B, et al. Alexander's Care of the Patient in Surgery. 8th ed. St. Louis: Mosby, 1987.

Iyer, Taptich, Bernocchi-Losey. Nursing Process and Nursing Diagnosis. Philadelphia: Saunders, 1986.

Jacob JL, et al. Documenting Patient Care in the OR. J AORN 26:659, 1977.

Kleinbeck SVM. Developing Nursing Diagnosis for a Perioperative Care Plan. J AORN, 49:1613, 1989.

Kneedler J, Dodge G. Perioperative Patient Care: The Nursing Prospective. 2nd ed. Boston: Blackwell, 1985.

Kneisl CR, Ames SW. Adult Health Care Nursing: A Biopsychosocial Approach. Reading, MA: Addison-Wesley, 1986.

Knowles M. The Adult Learner: The Neglected Species. 4th ed. Houston: Gulf, 1990.

Knowles M. The Modern Practice of Adult Education. 2nd ed. Chicago: Follett, 1980.

Kozier B, Erb G. Perioperative Nursing. Fundamentals of Nursing: Concepts and Procedures. 3rd ed. Reading, MA: Addison-Wesley, 1987.

Legal Citations: As listed; page 403.

Manual BJ. Documentation Belongs in Patient Record for All to See. J AORN 30:212, 1979.

Marker CS. The Marker Model for Nursing Standards: O.R. Application. Boulder, CO: O.R. Manager, 1988.

Marker CGS. Setting Standards for Professional Nursing: The Marker Model. St. Louis: Mosby, 1988.

Pfister JI, Kneedler JA, Purcell SA. The Nursing Spectrum of Lasers. Denver, CO: Education Design, 1988.

Rothrock J. Perioperative Patient Care Planning. St. Louis: Mosby, 1990.

Spry C. Essentials of Perioperative Nursing: A Self-Learning Guide. Rockville, MD: Aspen, 1988.

Tucker S, et al. Patient Care Standards. 3rd ed. St. Louis: Mosby, 1984.

Wells MP. Decision Making in Perioperative Nursing. Philadelphia: B.C. Decker, 1987.

Zander K, et al. Practice Manual for Patient Teaching. St. Louis: Mosby, 1978.

Answers for Module IV

Self-assessment Exercise 1

1. 1. Chart review
   2. Interview with patient, health-care personnel, family
   3. Observation
2. Outcome standard: The patient's skin integrity will be maintained
   Outcome goal: There will be no alteration in the patient's skin condition during the intraoperative phase
3. 1. D
   2. A
   3. E
   4. B
4. FALSE: medical diagnosis focuses on the pathogenic disease process, while nursing diagnosis focuses on the patient's response to an actual/potential health-care problem
5. Potential loss of dignity related to exposure

Self-assessment Exercise 2

1. To address psychosocial needs as well as physical needs; to reduce the natural fear of the unknown through patient/family education; to allow the patient/family to verbalize fears or concerns
2. Fear of the unknown (death, diagnosis, change in body image)
3. Providing emotional support; simple, truthful responses to questions; creating a therapeutic nurse–patient relationship; using effective communication techniques
4. 1. Assessment of patient's current knowledge
   2. Information regarding sequence of events
   3. Preoperative activities
   4. Postoperative exercises/pain management
   5. Family participation in postoperative regimen
   6. Diet restrictions/physical limitations

5. 1. Identification and verification
      a. Patient
      b. Surgery/surgeon/procedure/anesthesia
   2. Record review
      a. Laboratory data
      b. Diagnostic studies
      c. Consent forms
6. FALSE: a shave prep is not always necessary, depending on the area; it should be performed only if it interferes with incision site

Self-assessment Exercise 3

1. Lower leg is flexed to provide stability and to lift weight off lower leg to facilitate venous drainage
2. At least 2 inches above the knees; provides protection but allows adequate circulation
3. Patient age, weight, activity level
   A. anatomy involved with procedure
   B. optimal exposure/surgeon's preference
   C. patient comfort and safety
   D. respiratory and circulatory freedom
4. FALSE: can be detrimental to lower-extremity circulation
5. Occiput, scapulae, thoracic vertebrae, olecranon, sacrum, coccyx, and calcaneus
6. Sufficient personnel, stretcher and OR bed height equal, stretcher and OR bed locked, move is made as "team" effort.
7. 90; palms down (supinated)
8. TRUE
9. Respiratory
   Cardiovascular
   Muscular
   Skeletal
   Nervous system
10. 1. Egg crate—provides extra padding for bony prominences

2. Bolsters—used in prone position, for back surgery; alleviates pressure on chest and abdomen
3. Sandbags—immobilization/stabilization
4. Doughnut—head rest; replaces small pillow (prone; lateral)

Self-assessment Exercise 4

1. TRUE
2. Solution(s) used; area prepped and skin condition assessed before and after procedure
3. McBurney incision
4. TRUE
5. FALSE: circular motions, starting at incision and toward periphery (bulls-eye)
6. 1. C
   2. D
   3. A
   4. B

Self-assessment Exercise 5

1. Cut; coagulate
2. Perform the task needed; ground the patient
3. FALSE: tips act as both active and dispersive electrodes
4. TRUE
5. Scope—to visualize organs/area
   Light source—provides illumination
   Power source—activation through electricity/battery
   Light cord—projection lamp housing—transmits light
6. Hyperthermia; thermal control unit
7. Warm blankets, warm prepping solutions, warm blood and I.V. solutions, exposure of only operative site, emotional support
8. Light amplification by the stimulated emission of radiation
9. Correct goggles for medium; warning signs on all entry doors; isolation of operative foot pedal; effective smoke evacuator system; one nurse assigned to operate the laser
10. **A.** Knows how to care for and position microscope properly
    B. Knows properly how to place, wrap, and monitor tourniquet; how to work with freestanding tanks; safety measures to employ (time, pressure, etc.)

Self-assessment Exercise 6

1. 1. Preparation sequence: selection/preparation of supplies; preincision count
   2. Preincision: positioning; prepping; equipment verification
   3. Operative phase: incision, isolation, repair/excision/revision; irrigation; specimens
   4. Closing phase: counts; application of dressing
   5. Postoperative phase: transference of patient to Post Anesthesia Care Unit (PACU)
2. Skin cannot be sterilized, therefore the knife cannot be used on deeper tissue
3. 1. Transfer patient from stretcher to OR bed
   2. Assists in positioning
   3. Assists anesthesia personnel as necessary

4. Performs surgical skin prep
5. Connect suction/equipment as needed
4. TRUE
5. FALSE: Frozen section (FS), calculi, and/or foreign bodies are not placed in solution but sent dry
6. FALSE: in order to obtain accurate cultures, it needs to be sent as soon as it is collected and labeled
7. FALSE: Penrose drain works on gravity drainage principle
8. 1. D
   2. C
   3. A
   4. B

Self-assessment Exercise 7

1. Should include the following concepts: inform supervisor and restate patient's request; document conversation (patient's words) and actions taken; try to determine through therapeutic council why patient is feeling anxiety
2. TRUE
3. Signature invalid (age, chemicals, mental confusion); patient does not fully understand nature of consent; not completed within guidelines of hospital policy
4. Preincision
   Before closure of cavity
   Before closure of skin
   YES: Emergency condition of patient; preincision count may be impossible; intraoperative count and closing counts should be taken, with x-ray following procedure; documentation of deviation from policy; unusual occurrence report filed
5. X-ray detectable strip
6. FALSE: counts should be done out loud and simultaneously to verify types/numbers of each countable item
7. 1. Omission of information
   2. Personal opinions versus facts
   3. Generalizations
   4. Late (retrospective) charting
   5. Improper usage of abbreviations
   6. Illegible handwriting
   7. Incorrect spelling
   8. Improper error-correction technique
   9. Improper signature
8. FALSE: abbreviations should be avoided on any intraoperative record to avoid inaccurate accounting/misinterpretation of information
9. Suggest that substitute packing be used. If not successful, document occurrence on intraoperative record, including type, size, and number left in wound and rationale for actions
10. TRUE

Questions for Review

1. 1. D
   2. C
   3. E
   4. A
   5. B

2. Maintain aseptic environment; prepare surgical site with appropriate antimicrobial solution/technique
3. B
4. C
5. Respiratory and circulation
6. Above
7. C
8. B
9. TRUE
10. FALSE: colostomy is considered contaminated; therefore it is prepped last
11. 1. Counts are performed simultaneously by scrub and circulating nurses
    2. Counts are performed out loud
    3. Counts are performed at prescribed intervals
    4. Count status is documented on intraoperative record
12. Appropriate protective eye wear for medium; warning sign on all entrances to room; one nurse managing the laser; smoke evacuator used; emergency fire equipment available
13. C
14. C
15. TRUE

MODULE V — Implementing Perioperative Nursing Care

Chapter Outline

Content Overview

Providing safe and effective nursing care during the intraoperative period requires the nurse to correlate acquired knowledge with skill performance, using sound scientific principles and decision-making processes.

This module is designed to acquaint the reader with information needed to deliver perioperative nursing care safely and efficiently and includes a review of anatomy, terminology, and descriptions of surgical procedures representing a composite of techniques and services.

In addition, the module discusses trends and issues affecting the practice of perioperative nursing in today's practice setting.

Module Objectives

On completion of this module, you will be able to:

1. Identify anatomic structures within the body, and correlate these structures with surgical procedures being performed.
2. Define a variety of terms associated with surgical procedures, supplies, and equipment common to the intraoperative phase.
3. Identify and describe a variety of surgical procedures, including the pathology, surgical sequence, and nursing interventions associated with each procedure.
4. Discuss the changing role of the perioperative nurse in relationship to professional practice, quality assurance programs, and perioperative nursing education, and what impact they have on the practice of OR nursing now and in the future.

411

Anatomic Structures and Terminology

Why Review Anatomy?
Organization of the Body
Cells, Tissues, and Membranes
Organs and Systems
Word Elements
Building Terminology
Standard Abbreviations
Putting It All Together

UNIT 1

Surgical Anatomy Review

WHY REVIEW ANATOMY?

Knowing about and understanding the location and anatomical structures of the body is essential for the perioperative nurse, regardless of the role she or he is performing. Anatomy relates to all aspects of surgery, from the preoperative shave prep to the incision site, and continues throughout the surgical procedure.

This self-study guide offers a means of review to help assess current knowledge and assist in recalling information relating to the human body and all its complex features with the hope of eventual correlation of the anatomic structures to specific surgical procedures being performed.

The exercises are divided into three major areas, and each has a brief overview of the organs and/or system prior to beginning each exercise.

The three major areas include

Organization of the body
Cells, tissues, and membranes
Organs and systems

The reader is urged to consult a reliable anatomy book for reference. However, the answers for each exercise can be found at the end of the module.

ORGANIZATION OF THE BODY

The human body is a well-planned organization. The basic building blocks, the cells, collectively make up the tissues, membranes, and organs, each with its own structures and functions. Together, the organs make up systems responsible for special life-preserving tasks.

In order to give the body direction, and to explain and interpret information referring to those structures, we use imaginary lines, planes, cavities, and regions.

413

Some of the more important of these references refer to the body in anatomical position, that is, the patient is facing you, with arms at the side and palms turned forward.

A. Anatomic directions
1. Superior: above; near the head
   Inferior: below; away from the head
2. Ventral: anterior; front of the body
   Dorsal: posterior; back of the body
3. Cranial: pertaining to the head
   Caudal: pertaining to the "tail" (lower portion of the spine)
4. Medial: middle; near the midsagittal plane
   Lateral: pertaining to the sides
5. Proximal: nearest the origin of a structure
   Distal: furthest from the site of origin
   Peripheral: on the surface; away from the center

B. Body planes
1. Midsagittal: divides the body into left and right portions
2. Frontal: divides the body into front and back
3. Transverse: divides the body top from bottom

C. Body cavities
1. Dorsal: joined together in a continuous area
   a. Cranial
   b. Spinal
2. Ventral: not continuous; separated by the diaphragm
   a. Thoracic
   b. Abdominal
   c. Pelvic

D. Areas and regions of the body
1. Areas
   a. Upper quadrants (left and right); dividing line is the umbilicus region
   b. Lower quadrants (left and right)
2. Regions
   1. Center
      a. Epigastric: located just below the breast bone
      b. Umbilical: at the umbilicus
      c. Suprapubic (hypogastric): just below the ribs
   2. Right and left sides
      a. Hypochondriac: upper region
      b. Lumbar: middle region
      c. Iliac/inguinal: lower region

Exercise 1 Anatomical Directions/Planes

Directions: *Label the directions and planes shown in the figure.*

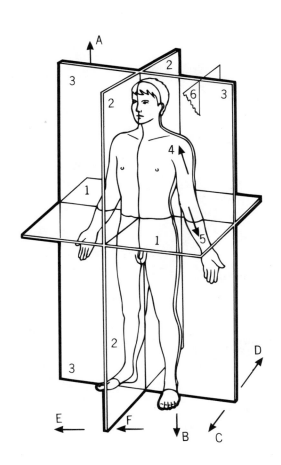

A _____

B _____

C _____

D _____

E _____

F _____

1 _____

2 _____

3 _____

4 _____

5 _____

6 _____

Exercise 2 Body Cavities

Directions: *Label the body cavities shown in the figure.*

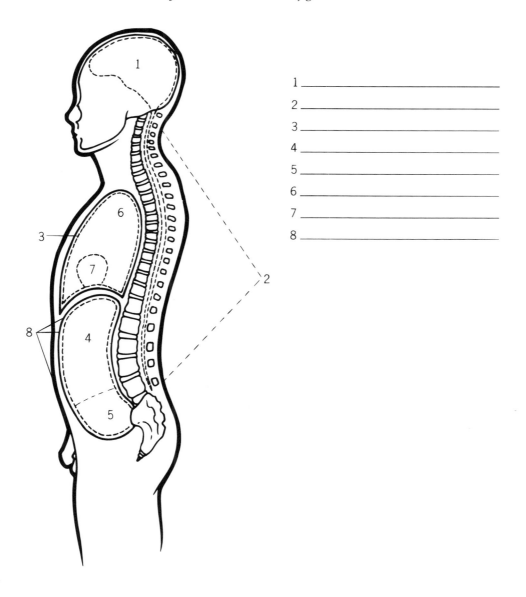

1 _____

2 _____

3 _____

4 _____

5 _____

6 _____

7 _____

8 _____

Exercise 3 Areas and Regions of the Body

Directions: *Label the areas (numbers) and regions (letters) in the figure.*

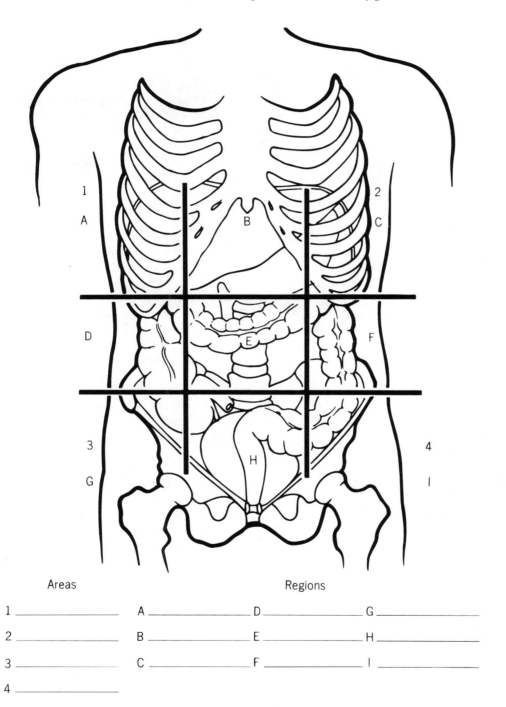

Areas		Regions	
1 _____	A _____	D _____	G _____
2 _____	B _____	E _____	H _____
3 _____	C _____	F _____	I _____
4 _____			

CELLS, TISSUES, AND MEMBRANES

Careful microscopic studies of the cell protoplasm have revealed the presence of tiny structures called organelles that are concerned with a variety of functions. Among these structures are rod-shaped bodies called mitochondria. The mitochondria are responsible for the chemical combinations that result in the release of energy.

A. The cell
   1. Characteristics
      a. Building blocks of all living things
      b. Organelles are responsible for various functions within the cell
      c. Enzymes are catalytic agents
      d. DNA and RNA
      e. Cell reproduces by mitosis
      f. Physical and biological processes bring materials through semipermeable cell membrane (osmosis, diffusion, and filtration)
      g. Chemical action within the cell is called metabolism
   2. Parts of a cell
      a. Cell membrane
      b. Cytoplasm
      c. Nuclear membrane
      d. Nucleus
      e. Nucleolus
      f. Chromatin (chromosomes)
B. Tissues
   1. Characteristics
      a. Group of cells similar in structure and substance
      b. Arranged in a characteristic pattern and specialized for performance of a specific task
   2. Classification
      Four main groups
      a. Epithelium: forms glands, covers surfaces, and lines cavities
      b. Connective: holds all parts of the body in place
      c. Nerve: conducts nerve impulses
      d. Muscle: designed for power-producing contractions. There are three types:
         1. Skeletal: voluntary; provides movement
         2. Cardiac: myocardium
         3. Visceral (smooth): forms the walls of the viscera; organs of the ventral cavity, except the heart
      e. Blood is sometimes considered a type of tissue since it contains cells and performs many of the functions of tissue
C. Membranes
   1. Characteristics
      a. A thin sheet of tissue (material) that separates two groups of substances
         1. May serve as a dividing partition
         2. May line hollow organs and body cavities
      b. Membranes can contain secreting cells that produce lubrication or can anchor various organs together or to a specific surface
   2. Kinds of membranes
      a. Epithelial
         1. Mucous: line tubes and other spaces that open to the outside of the body, for example, digestive, urinary, reproductive
         2. Serous: line closed cavities within the body, for example, pleural, pericardium, peritoneum
      b. Connective (fibrous)
         1. Fascia: serve to anchor and support organs, for example, superficial fascia, deep fascia, meninges
         2. Skeletal: covers bone and cartilage, for example, periosteum, synovium

Exercise 4 The Cell

Directions: *Label the parts of the cell in the diagram.*

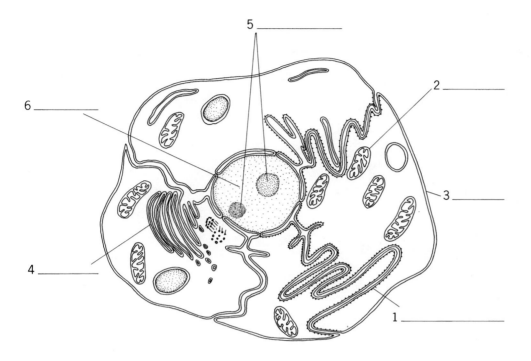

1 _____

2 _____

3 _____

4 _____

5 _____

6 _____

Exercise 5 Tissues and Muscles

Directions: Differentiate the types of muscles and tissues.

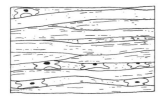

A _____

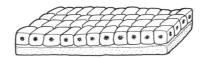

B _____

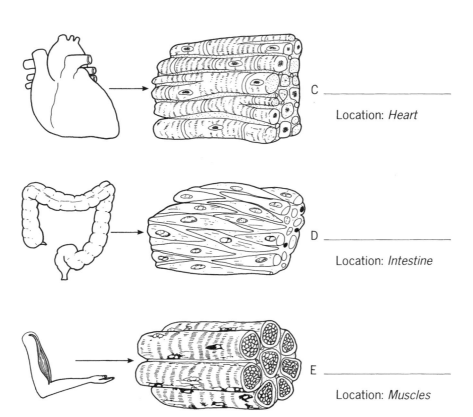

C _____

Location: *Heart*

D _____

Location: *Intestine*

E _____

Location: *Muscles*

ORGANS AND SYSTEMS

Introduction

A. Definitions
   1. Organs: a group of specialized tissue performing similar functions
   2. Systems: a group of organs performing a specific function

B. The ten systems of the body
   1. Integumentary — skin
   2. Muscular-Skeletal — muscles, bones
   3. Cardiovascular (circulatory) — heart, vascular network
   4. Respiratory — lungs
   5. Nervous — brain, spinal cord, nerves

6. Sensory   eyes, ears, nose
7. Digestive   stomach, gastrointestinal
                        tract
8. Endocrine   pancreas, thyroid
9. Urinary   kidneys, urinary bladder
   (excretory)
10. Reproductive   gonads (male and
                        female)

The Integumentary System

The skin is considered the largest organ of the body. It is also considered the first line of defense against invading bacteria.

A. Classification
   The skin can be classified in three different ways:
   1. Enveloping membrane, because it is a thin layer of tissue covering the entire body
   2. An organ, because it contains several kinds of specialized tissues, including epithelial, nerve, and connective tissues
   3. A system (integumentary), because it includes sweat and oil glands as well as other tissues that work together as a system. The word *integumentary* refers to a covering.

B. Layers
   The skin consists of three layers:
   1. Epidermis: outer layer, first layer
   2. Dermis: (true skin) second layer
   3. Subcutaneous: third layer (superficial fascia)

C. Function
   The skin has three important functions:
   1. Protection: of organs and systems
   2. Temperature regulation: maintaining internal environment (homeostasis)
   3. Sensory collector: of environmental information

Exercise 6 Integumentary System

Directions: Label the following diagram of the skin.

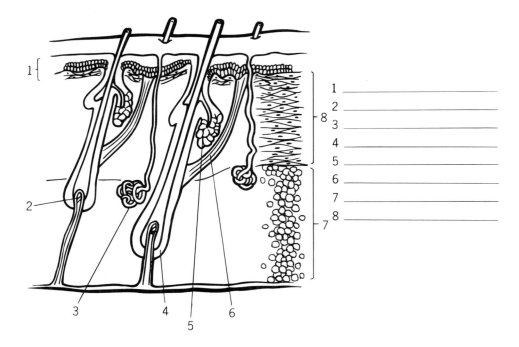

1 _____

2 _____

3 _____

4 _____

5 _____

6 _____

7 _____

8 _____

The Muscular-Skeletal System

Support, movement, and framework are the primary functions of the muscular-skeletal system. Sometimes these systems are handled separately, but for the purpose of this review they have been combined into one system, because their functions are very similar to each other.

Movement not only allows the person to enjoy life, but is essential for maintaining life. Because of constant movement, cells and organs are able to receive the necessary nutrients required to perform specialized tasks.

Muscles and bones, which make up the system, protect vital organs from environmental changes and physical damage and supply the body with energy while maintaining homeostasis.

A. Skeletal system
The skeletal system consists of two divisions:
   1. Appendicular skeleton: bones that are movable
   2. Axial skeleton: bones that are fixed
B. Muscular system
The muscles are frequently named after the bones they are anatomically close to or associated with, and they provide movement by five different mechanisms:
   1. flexion
   2. extension
   3. abduction
   4. adduction
   5. rotation.

Exercise 7 The Skeletal System

Directions: *Name the following bones of the skeleton. Indicate those that are appendicular and those that are axial. Label the areas of the femur (long bone).*

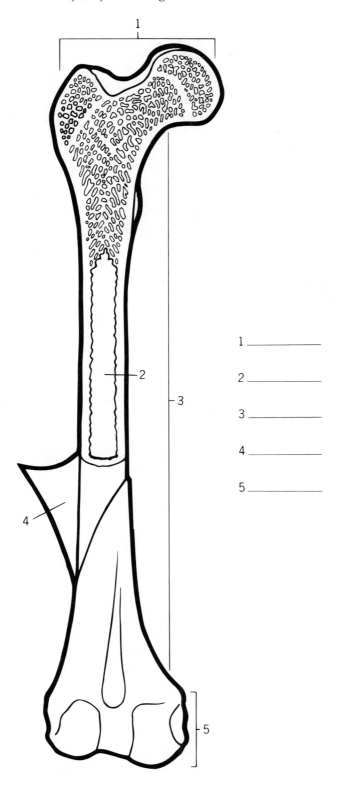

1 _____

2 _____

3 _____

4 _____

5 _____

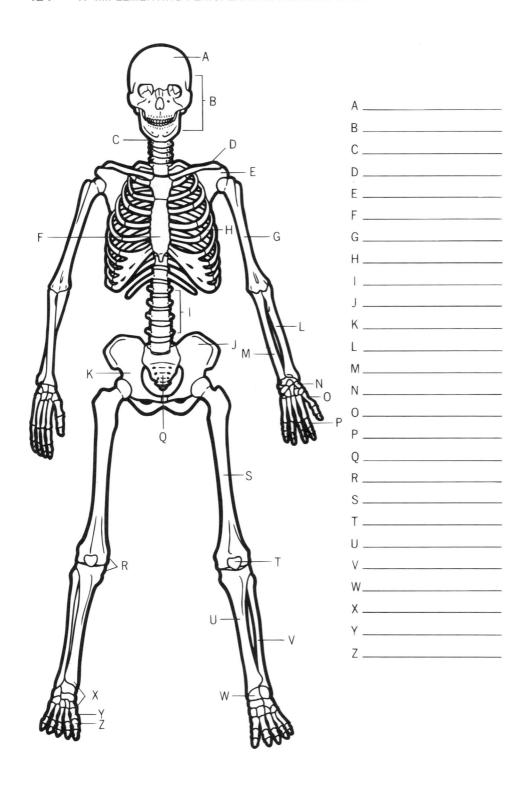

A _____

B _____

C _____

D _____

E _____

F _____

G _____

H _____

I _____

J _____

K _____

L _____

M _____

N _____

O _____

P _____

Q _____

R _____

S _____

T _____

U _____

V _____

W _____

X _____

Y _____

Z _____

Exercise 8 The Skull

Directions: Label the following areas (bone) of the skull.

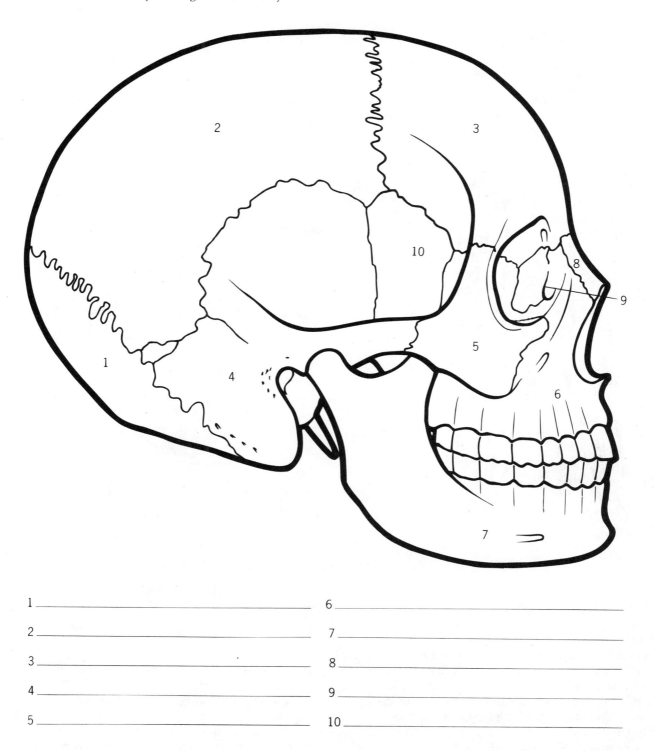

1 _____   6 _____

2 _____   7 _____

3 _____   8 _____

4 _____   9 _____

5 _____   10 _____

Exercise 9 The Muscles

Directions: Label the muscles of the body, both anterior and posterior.

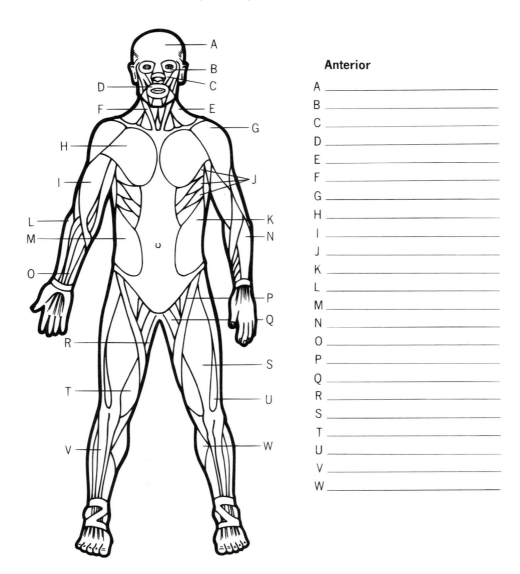

Anterior

A _____
B _____
C _____
D _____
E _____
F _____
G _____
H _____
I _____
J _____
K _____
L _____
M _____
N _____
O _____
P _____
Q _____
R _____
S _____
T _____
U _____
V _____
W _____

The Cardiovascular System

The cardiovascular system, also known as the circulatory system, is composed of the heart and blood vessels. It is a vital transport system, responsible for providing nutrients and oxygen to all body cells, and for removing metabolic waste products from the cells. This closed system consists of a major pump and conduit, and is further divided into the heart, systemic circulation, and pulmonary circulation.

In response to this, the cardiovascular system makes its appearance early in the developmental stages and reaches its full potential before any other major organs or systems.

A. The heart
  1. Muscular pump, enclosed in a tough, fibrous sac (pericardium)
  2. Heart is composed of three layers:
      a. Epicardium: outermost layer
      b. Myocardium: muscle
      c. Endocardium: innermost layer; lines chambers and valves
  3. Composed of four chambers and four valves

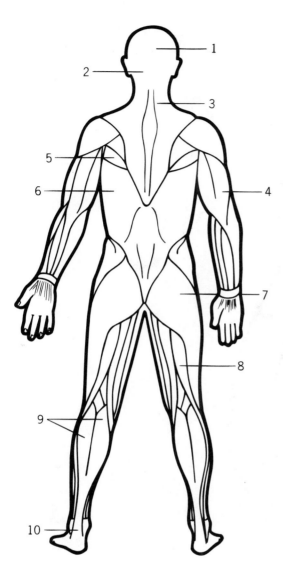

Posterior

1 _____
2 _____
3 _____
4 _____
5 _____
6 _____
7 _____
8 _____
9 _____
10 _____

B. Vascular anatomy
Major vessels
  1. Aorta (systemic circulation)
  2. Pulmonary artery (pulmonic circulation)
  3. Coronary arteries: responsible for nourishment of the heart muscle (right and left coronary arteries)

C. Circulation
The arterial system feeds the body, while the venous system returns the blood to the heart for oxygenation and recirculation.

Exercise 10 The Heart

Directions: *Label the following structures of the heart.*

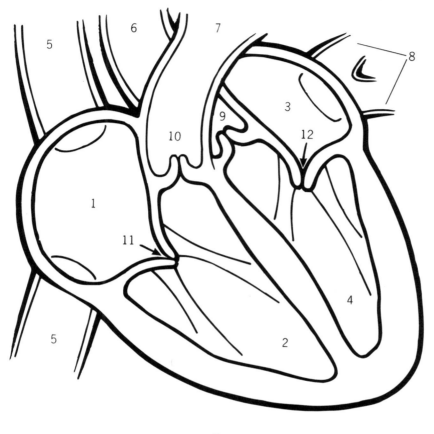

1 _____	7 _____
2 _____	8 _____
3 _____	9 _____
4 _____	10 _____
5 _____	11 _____
6 _____	12 _____

Exercise 11 Systemic Circulation

Directions: Name the following arteries (numbers) and veins (letters).

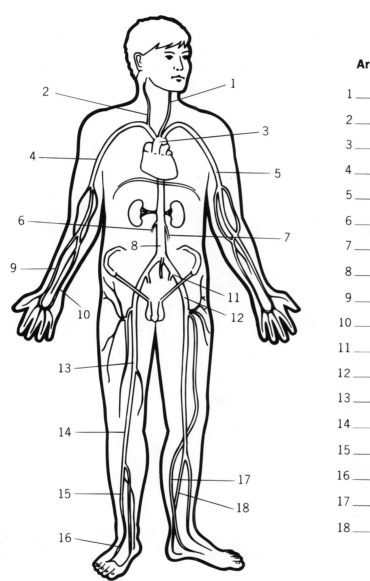

Arterial System

1 _____

2 _____

3 _____

4 _____

5 _____

6 _____

7 _____

8 _____

9 _____

10 _____

11 _____

12 _____

13 _____

14 _____

15 _____

16 _____

17 _____

18 _____

The Respiratory System

The respiratory system functions as the supplier of oxygen to the individual tissue cells and removes their gaseous waste product, carbon dioxide. Since the tissues must receive oxygen in order to survive, the cardiovascular system serves as the pathway, allowing oxygen-rich blood to reach the outlying organs and structures. The levels of carbon dioxide and oxygen in the blood are powerful regulatory agents for controlling activities in both the respiratory and cardiovascular systems.

Specific Organs

All parts of the respiratory system, except its microscopic-sized air sacs, called alveoli, function as the air distributor. Only the alveoli serve as the gas exchanger.

The six organs of the respiratory system include:

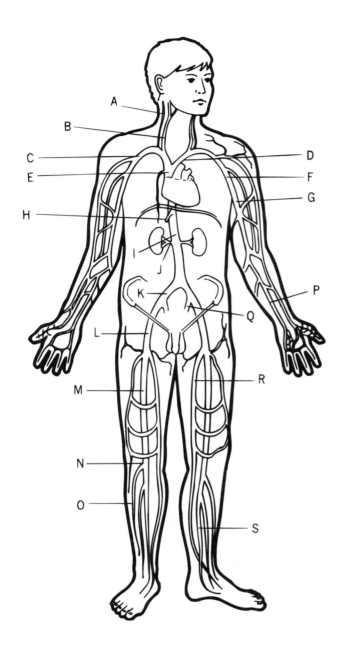

Venous System

A _____

B _____

C _____

D _____

E _____

F _____

G _____

H _____

I _____

J _____

K _____

L _____

M _____

N _____

O _____

P _____

Q _____

R _____

S _____

1. Nose
2. Pharynx
3. Larynx
4. Trachea
5. Bronchi
6. Lungs

Together, they constitute the pathway for air between the atmosphere and the blood.

Exercise 12 The Respiratory System

Directions: Name the following structures.

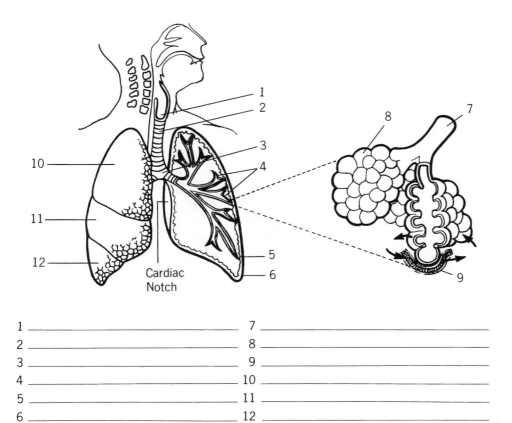

Cardiac
Notch

1 _____   7 _____
2 _____   8 _____
3 _____   9 _____
4 _____   10 _____
5 _____   11 _____
6 _____   12 _____

The Nervous System

The nervous system is the major communication network of the body; coordinating all the systems of the body to function as a whole. Conditions both within and outside the body are always changing, and the nervous system monitors these changes and helps the body to adapt to new conditions.

Structural Classification

The divisions of the nervous system may be grouped according to how they are made (structure) or on the basis of what they do (function). There are two divisions of the nervous system:

1. *Central nervous system* consisting of the brain and spinal cord
2. *Peripheral nervous system* consisting of the cranial and spinal nerves

Through constant communication and coordination of the nervous system, the human body continues to function as one unit, overcoming a variety of obstacles while maintaining life.

Exercise 13 The Brain

Directions: *Name the following structures.*

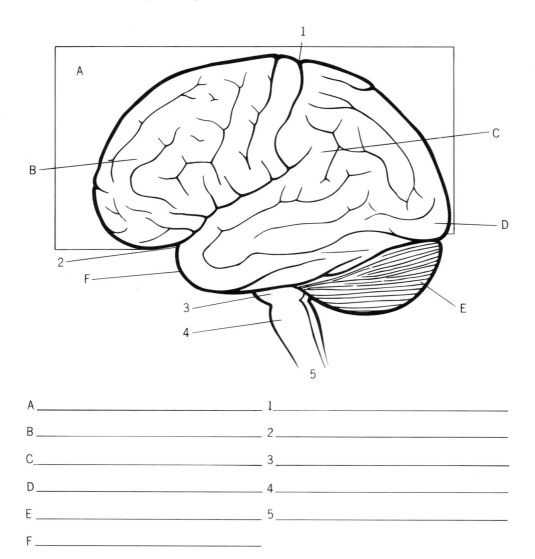

A _____   1 _____

B _____   2 _____

C _____   3 _____

D _____   4 _____

E _____   5 _____

F _____

Exercise 14 The 12 Cranial Nerves

Directions: *Identify the 12 cranial nerves. State if they are sensory or motor.*

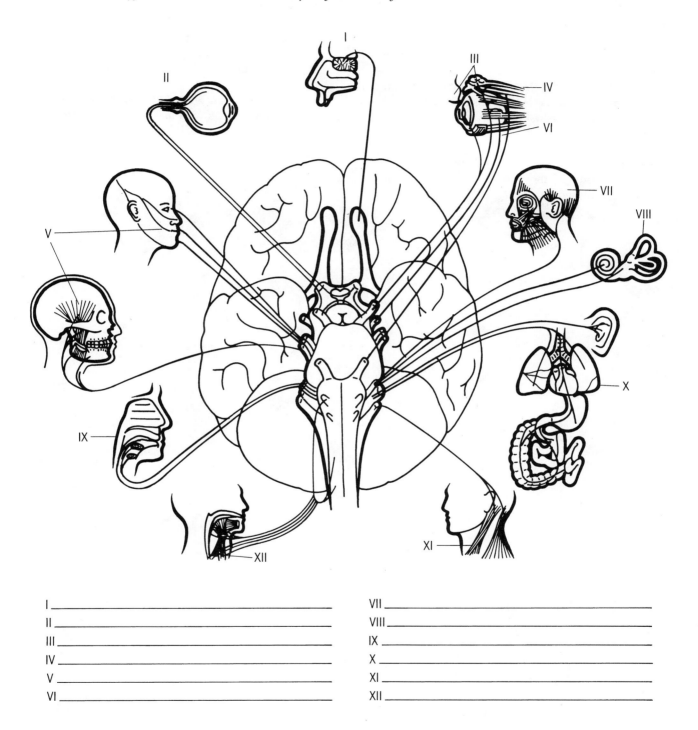

I _____

II _____

III _____

IV _____

V _____

VI _____

VII _____

VIII _____

IX _____

X _____

XI _____

XII _____

The Sensory System

Sensation is the result of processes taking place in the brain in response to nerve impulses from the sensory organs located throughout the body. The sensory receptors consist of the endings of dendrites of afferent neurons.

The proper functioning of these sense organs is a major factor in keeping the body aware of activities, both internal and external. Accurate interpretation of the data from these sense organs assists in making appropriate adjustments to both environmental conditions and bodily needs.

A. Special senses
   Special senses, as they are commonly called, involve the following:
   1. Sight: eye
   2. Hearing: ear
   3. Equilibrium: internal ear
   4. Taste: mouth and tongue
   5. Smell: nose
B. General senses
   General senses consist of:
   1. Touch: cutaneous sensations
   2. Visceral sensations

The sensory system works in close affiliation with the nervous system, as well as the specialty organs.

Exercise 15 The Eye

Directions: Label the following structures.

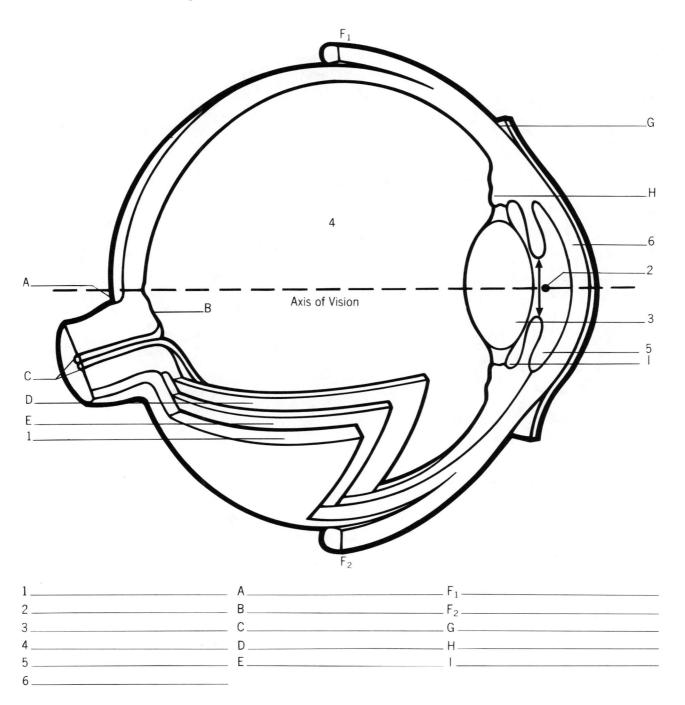

1 _____ A _____ F₁ _____

2 _____ B _____ F₂ _____

3 _____ C _____ G _____

4 _____ D _____ H _____

5 _____ E _____ I _____

6 _____

Exercise 16 The Ear

Directions: Label the following structures.

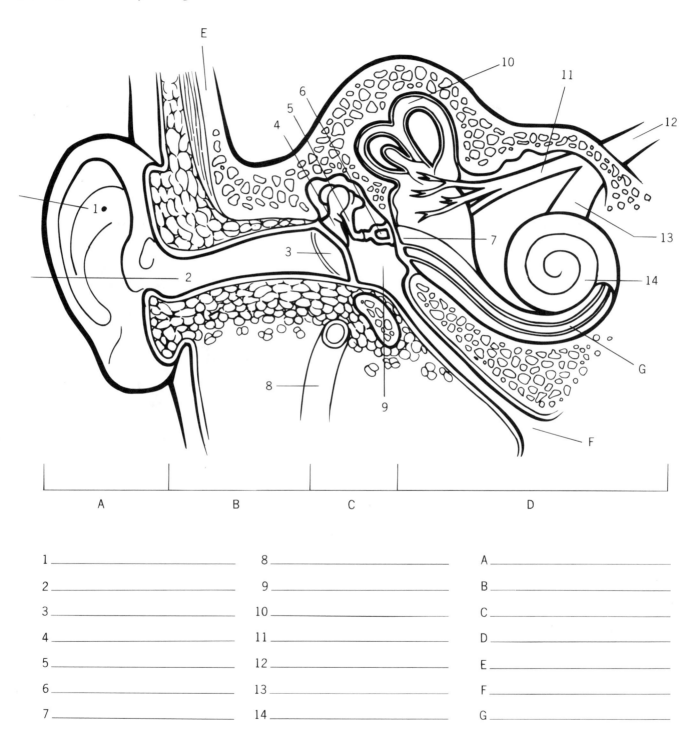

1 _____	8 _____	A _____
2 _____	9 _____	B _____
3 _____	10 _____	C _____
4 _____	11 _____	D _____
5 _____	12 _____	E _____
6 _____	13 _____	F _____
7 _____	14 _____	G _____

The Digestive System

A solitary cell would be baffled if a fragment of food appeared across a lake of tissue and tried to gain admission to the tissues. Therefore, food that is eaten must be converted to substances that the cell can accept. This is the function of the digestive system.

Parts of the digestive system prepare the food for absorption and utilization, while the other sections serve as an organ of elimination, ridding the body of the wastes that result from the digestive process.

Organs of the System

The organs of the digestive system are as follows:

1. Mouth
2. Esophagus
3. Stomach
4. Large intestines
5. Small intestines
6. Biliary circuit; liver and pancreas

Functional Anatomy

For the purpose of study, the digestive system has frequently been divided into two groups of organs:

1. Alimentary canal: a continuous passageway from the mouth to the anus
2. Accessory organs: organs that assist in the digestive processes

Exercise 17 The Alimentary Tract

Directions: *Label the following organs.*

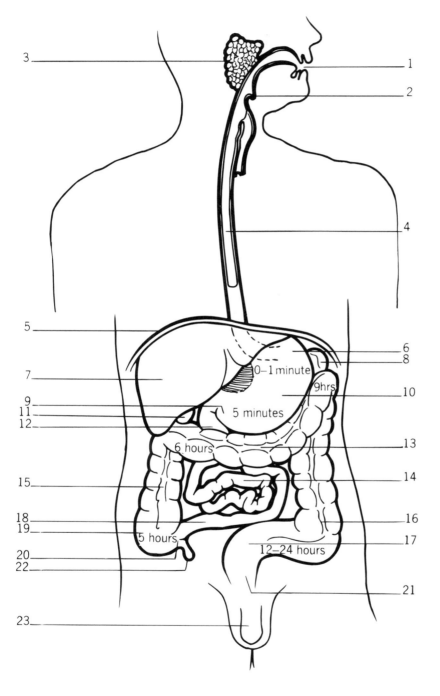

1 _____
2 _____
3 _____
4 _____
5 _____
6 _____
7 _____
8 _____
9 _____
10 _____
11 _____
12 _____
13 _____
14 _____
15 _____
16 _____
17 _____
18 _____
19 _____
20 _____
21 _____
22 _____
23 _____

Exercise 18 The Biliary Circuit

Directions: Label the following structures.

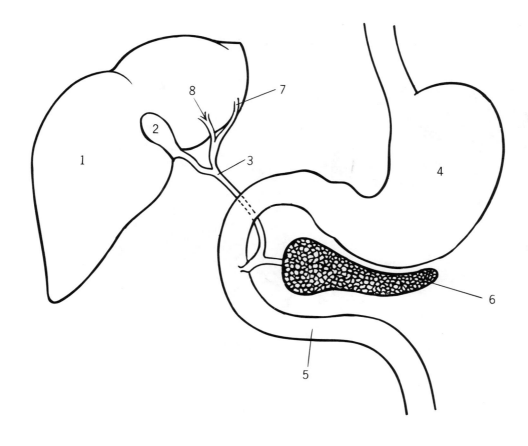

1 _____   5 _____

2 _____   6 _____

3 _____   7 _____

4 _____   8 _____

Exercise 19 The Liver and Surrounding Organs

Directions: Label the diagram.

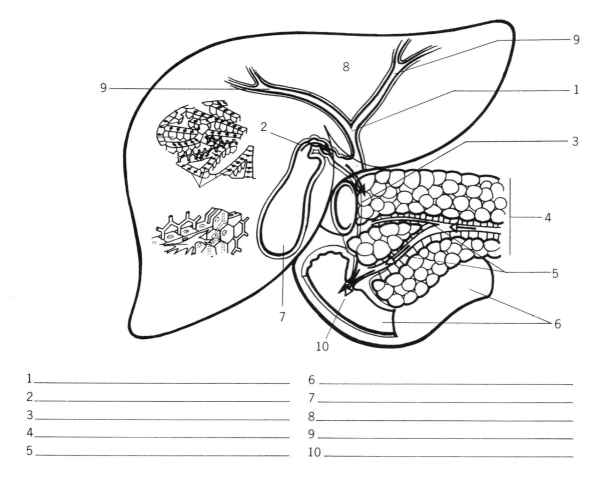

1 _____   6 _____
2 _____   7 _____
3 _____   8 _____
4 _____   9 _____
5 _____   10 _____

The Endocrine System

The endocrine system is made up of specialized glands.

Endocrine glands are ductless and secrete hormones directly into the bloodstream. Hormones are chemical messengers carried from gland cells to nearby organs or body surfaces (external secretions) or carried to all parts of the body by the blood or lymph (internal secretions) systems.

The endocrine and nervous systems both function to achieve and maintain homeostasis of the body. Therefore, they are often cited as a dual-working system (neuroendocrine).

Although they are both responsible for three basic functions—communication, integration, and control—they accomplish these functions through different mechanisms and with somewhat different results and speed.

Organs of the System

The specialized glands of this system consist of

1. Pineal body
2. Pituitary gland
3. Thyroid and parathyroid glands
4. Thymus gland
5. Pancreas (exocrine/endocrine)
6. Ovary and testis

Exercise 20 The Endocrine Glands

Directions: Label the following glands.

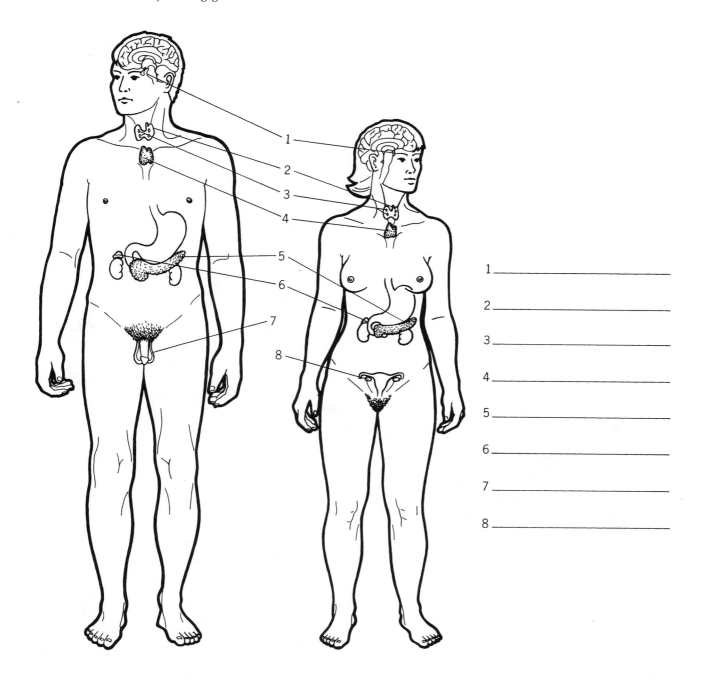

1	_____
2	_____
3	_____
4	_____
5	_____
6	_____
7	_____
8	_____

The Urinary (Excretory) System

The primary function of the urinary system is to remove certain waste products from the blood and eliminate them from the body. Since no system of the body operates independently of the others, in spite of spe-

cialized functions, the elimination of waste materials assists in maintaining homeostasis, thus allowing the body to function effectively.

Organs of the Urinary System

The main parts of the urinary system are

1. Two kidneys, which are glandular organs
2. Two ureters, which conduct the secretion from the kidneys to the urinary bladder
3. The single urinary bladder, a reservoir that receives the urine brought into the two ureters
4. A single urethra, which is the excretory tube for the bladder

The urinary system also serves as a filter system in order to ensure that toxic waste materials are not recirculated into the circulatory system and as a balancing mechanism for fluid and electrolytes.

Exercise 21 The Urinary System

Directions: *Name the following structures.*

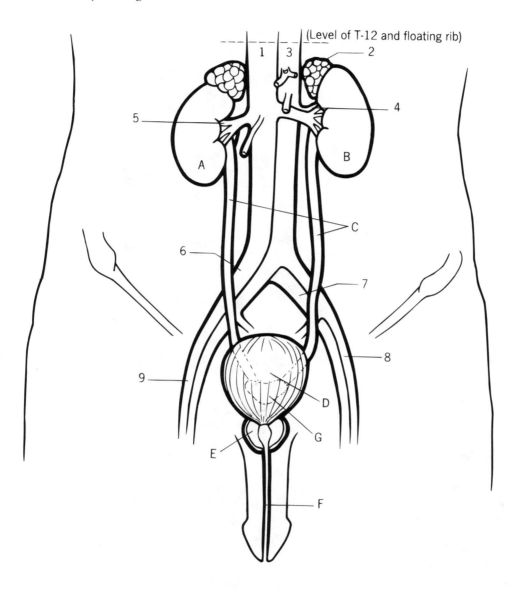

(Level of T-12 and floating rib)

1 _____   A _____
2 _____   B _____
3 _____   C _____
4 _____   D _____
5 _____   E _____
6 _____   F _____
7 _____   G _____
8 _____
9 _____

Exercise 22 The Kidney

Directions: Label the structures of the kidney.

1 _____

2 _____

3 _____

4 _____

5 _____

6 _____

7 _____

8 _____

9 _____

10 _____

The Reproductive System

Cell reproduction is a fundamental process of all living creatures. The creation of all individual organisms and the continuation of the species depends on cell reproduction.

The reproductive system functions to continue life and differs notably from the functions of any other system. Yet it is intricately related to all the systems of the body.

The reproductive system in the male and female have common structures, for example, gonads, passageways for sex cells, and accessory organs, but here the similarity stops.

Organs of Reproduction

In the male:

1. Testes
2. Seminal vesicle
3. Prostate gland
4. Bulbourethreal gland

In the female:

1. Ovaries
2. Fallopian tubes
3. Uterus
4. Vulva
5. Greater vestibular glands

An additional aspect of the female reproductive system is to provide a safe area for growth and development after conception (uterus) and to supply nourishment, through the mammary glands, after birth.

Exercise 23 The Male Reproductive Organs

Directions: *Label the following structures.*

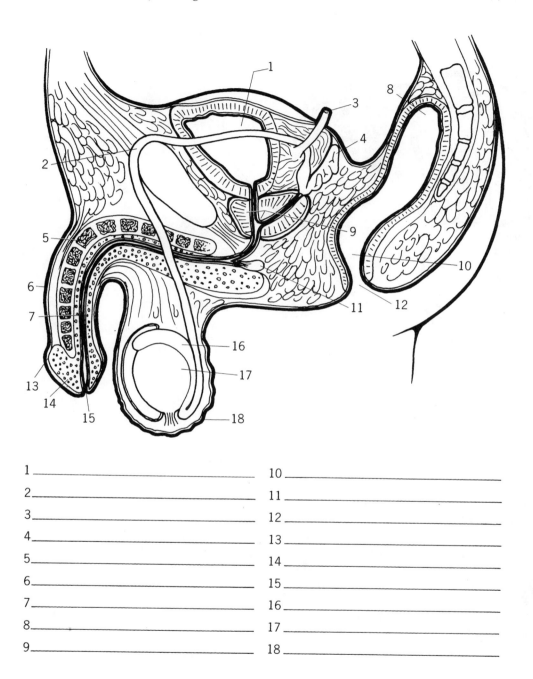

1 _____	10 _____
2 _____	11 _____
3 _____	12 _____
4 _____	13 _____
5 _____	14 _____
6 _____	15 _____
7 _____	16 _____
8 _____	17 _____
9 _____	18 _____

Exercise 24 The Female Reproductive Organs

Directions: *Label the following structures.*

A. Internal Structures

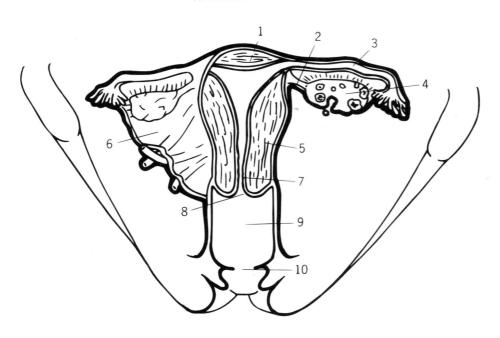

1 _____	6 _____
2 _____	7 _____
3 _____	8 _____
4 _____	9 _____
5 _____	10 _____

B. External Structures

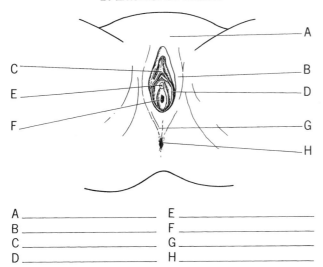

A _____	E _____
B _____	F _____
C _____	G _____
D _____	H _____

Exercise 25 The Breast and Mammary Glands

Directions: Label the following structures.

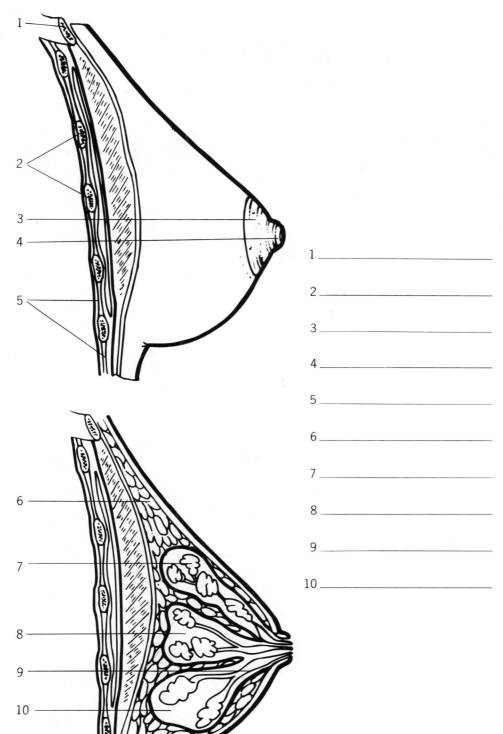

1 _____

2 _____

3 _____

4 _____

5 _____

6 _____

7 _____

8 _____

9 _____

10 _____

UNIT 2
Surgical Terminology

Correct spelling, pronunciation, and definitions of words are the key components for effective communication, regardless of the profession, since they allow us to speak to each other through both the written and spoken word. During the perioperative period, command of medical and surgical terminology is essential, since it can be used to describe a disease process, a procedure, and supplies and/or equipment that will be needed in order to perform the surgery.

This self-study guide was created to help you build your surgical vocabulary; by assessing your current knowledge, building up your current vocabulary, and then applying these terms and phrases to clinical situations frequently encountered during the perioperative period.

The reader is encouraged to use a reliable medical dictionary and to become a "word detective" based on the principles associated with using the five word elements for creating and defining terminology: (1) word root, (2) prefix, (3) suffix, (4) combining vowel, and (5) combining form. The correct answers can be found at the end of this module.

The unit is divided into four sections:

Word elements
Building terminology
Vocabulary
Standard abbreviations

WORD ELEMENTS

There are five word elements that help make up a variety of medical and surgical terms or phrases.

1. *Word root:* This is the meaning of the word. It is usually the main part or body of the word, and it describes a body part or function. It is usually of Greek or Latin origin.
2. *Prefix:* Comes before the word root and can change or add to the meaning of the word root.
3. *Suffix:* Comes after the word root and can change or add to the meaning of the word root.
4. *Combining vowel:* Connects the word root with a suffix (usually the letter "o").
5. *Combining form:* The full word, using prefix, word root, combining vowel, and suffix, or any part of the format.

Examples of each might include:
Prefix: ar-   Word root: -rhythmia
Meaning: variation from normal rhythm

Combining form: hemo-   Suffix: -rrhage
Meaning: excessive bleeding

Prefix: micro-   Word root: scope
Meaning: instrument used to enlarge small objects

Word root: tonsil   Suffix: -ectomy
Meaning: excision of tonsil

Exercise 26 Prefixes and Suffixes

A. Write the suffix that means:

   1. to suture _____

   2. pain _____

   3. pertaining to _____

   4. incision _____

   5. removal of _____

   6. look into _____

   7. (instrument) look into _____

   8. to repair/revise _____

   9. to crush _____

  10. artificial opening _____

B. Write the prefix that means:

   1. within _____

   2. difficult _____

   3. under/below _____

   4. without _____

   5. between _____

   6. above _____

C. Using the medical terms, describe the following:

   1. Inflammation of the colon _____
_____

   2. Plastic repair of the nose _____
_____

   3. A visual examination of the bronchi _____
_____

   4. Removal of the uterus _____
_____

   5. Stones in the gallbladder _____
_____

   6. Surgical repair of a hernia _____
_____

   7. Looking into the urinary bladder _____
_____

   8. Excision of a fallopian tube _____
_____

   9. Incision into the thorax _____
_____

  10. Artificial opening into the colon _____
_____

BUILDING TERMINOLOGY

In many instances, lay terminology must be replaced by medical terms, and vice versa. By knowing the meanings of words, the perioperative nurse can anticipate the supplies and equipment needed, depending on the part of the body the procedure involves.

Using the knowledge of prefixes, suffixes, and root word elements, complete the following exercises.

Exercise 27 Working with Terminology

A.   Match the following directions of the body:

1. ___ cranial
2. ___ proximal
3. ___ peripheral
4. ___ distal
5. ___ external
6. ___ palmer
7. ___ planter
8. ___ sagittal (plane)
9. ___ posterior
10. ___ internal
11. ___ anterior
12. ___ inferior

    a. outside
    b. toward the front
    c. sole of the foot
    d. at or near surface
    e. toward the feet
    f. right and left side of the body
    g. nearest (origin)
    h. inside
    i. palm of hand
    j. toward the back
    k. farthest (origin)
    l. toward the head

B.   Match the following body relationships:

1. ___ toward the bottom
2. ___ located in back of
3. ___ toward the midline
4. ___ side of the body
5. ___ toward the top
6. ___ in front of (belly)

    a. superior
    b. lateral
    c. ventral
    d. dorsal
    e. medial
    f. caudal

C.   Match the following body movements:

1. ___ abduction
2. ___ adduction
3. ___ extension
4. ___ flexion
5. ___ lateral recumbent
6. ___ prone
7. ___ rotation
8. ___ pronation
9. ___ supination
10. ___ circumduction

    a. straightening
    b. toward the midline
    c. draw away from midline
    d. face down
    e. moving on an axis
    f. lying on side
    g. palm down
    h. circular movement
    i. bending
    j. palm up

D.   Match the following terms with their meaning:

1. ___ mandible
2. ___ prosthesis
3. ___ femur
4. ___ occipital bone
5. ___ patella
6. ___ humerus
7. ___ arthralgia
8. ___ frontal bone

    a. knee cap
    b. lower jaw bone
    c. painful joints
    d. upper arm bone
    e. thighbone
    f. artificial part
    g. forehead bone
    h. back of skull

Exercise 28 Applying Medical Terminology

A. Use medical terms to describe the following common terms.

1. belly _____

2. navel _____

3. armpit _____

4. collar bone _____

5. shoulder blade _____

6. finger/toe _____

7. under the tongue _____

Use medical terms to describe the parts of the spine.

8. neck _____

9. chest _____

10. superior/lower _____

11. inferior/lower _____

12. tailbone _____

Use medical terms to describe the anatomic parts.

13. under the rib _____

14. behind the pelvic bone _____

15. eardrum _____

16. windpipe _____

17. bone _____

18. joint _____

19. head (skull) _____

20. stomach and intestines _____

21. ear, nose, and throat _____

22. voice box _____

B. Using medical terms, describe the following:

1. Abnormal fibers that bind one organ to another _____

2. Either half of the brain _____

3. Outermost membrane of the brain and spinal cord _____

4. Herniation of the bladder into the vagina _____

5. A band of fibrous tissue _____

6. Crescent-shaped fibrous cartilage in the knee _____

7. Formation of a new opening to the outside from the colon _____

8. The membrane over the viscera and lining the abdominal cavity _____

9. Joining two parts together (intestine; ducts) when a portion has been removed _____

10. Double mucous membranes that cover the lungs _____

11. Excision of the pituitary gland _____

12. Plastic surgery on an eardrum _____

Exercise 29 Working with Vocabulary

1. Name the five malignant connective or skeletal tissues (tumors):

   Fat _____

   Muscle _____

   Bone _____

   Lymph _____

   Fiber _____

2. Name the instrument used for examining the following areas:

   Eye _____

   Ear _____

   Bronchi _____

   Urinary bladder _____

   Esophagus _____

   Stomach _____

   Larynx _____

   Rectum _____

   Colon _____

   Peritoneal cavity _____

   Mediastinum _____

   Joints _____

   Common bile duct _____

   Ureter and kidney pelvis _____

3. Accurate documentation requires correct spelling of complex, combining-form words.
   Choose the correct spelling and define the word:

   1. (a) oophoro   (b) ophooro   (c) oopohoro
   Definition: _____

   2. (a) rhinito   (b) rhino   (c) rheno
   Definition: _____

   3. (a) salpero   (b) salpingo   (c) salpeno
   Definition: _____

   4. (a) pharango   (b) pharyngo   (c) pragyno
   Definition: _____

   5. (a) urotoro   (b) uritero   (c) uretero
   Definition: _____

   6. (a) chryo   (b) chiro   (c) cryo
   Definition: _____

   7. (a) craino   (b) criano   (c) cranio
   Definition: _____

   8. (a) plegia   (b) plagia   (c) phlagia
   Definition: _____

   9. (a) orhaphy   (b) orrophay   (c) orrhaphy
   Definition: _____

   10. (a) salcro   (b) salpo   (c) sacro
   Definition: _____

4. In common terms, describe the following procedures:

   1. Laparoscopic cholecystectomy _____

   2. Anal fistulectomy _____

   3. Ureterolithotomy _____

   4. Pericardiostomy _____

   5. Embolectomy _____

   6. Dermabrasion _____

   7. Angiography _____

   8. Laminectomy _____

   9. Arthroplasty _____

   10. Esophagogastroscopy _____

   11. Meniscectomy _____

   12. Thoracotomy _____

   13. Rhinoplasty _____

   14. Enucleation _____

15. Hemicolectomy _____

16. Valvulotomy _____

17. Intraoperative cholangiogram _____

18. Portacaval shunt _____

19. Cystourethroscopy _____

20. Antrostomy _____

STANDARD ABBREVIATIONS

Abbreviations are used constantly during a patient's hospitalization. Frequently, when scheduling surgical procedures, the perioperative nurse will write the proposed surgery in abbreviated terms to save time. Standardization of these abbreviated terms will aid in effective communication.

The following exercises represent some of the more common abbreviations related to the perioperative period.

Exercise 30 Common Abbreviations

Directions: Define the following abbreviations.

1. D&C _____
2. 'C'-Arm _____
3. T & A _____
4. AAA _____
5. Cataract Ext. w/IOL _____
6. TOP _____
7. TVC _____
8. Chole. w/CDE _____
9. A & P Repair _____
10. TUR-P _____
11. PTCA _____
12. PCNL _____
13. E-Lap. _____
14. tf _____
15. dx _____
16. ORIF _____
17. F.S. w/Bx _____
18. Fx _____
19. Foley to CBI _____
20. AK/BK amp. _____
21. CR Rt. Wrist _____
22. CABG _____
23. MVR/AVR _____
24. ASD/VSD _____
25. TAH w/BSO _____
26. WNL _____
27. NSR _____
28. CT scan _____
29. IVC _____
30. C & S _____

PUTTING IT ALL TOGETHER

Case Study

Patient: Linda Jones (36)
Admitted: 3/4/90
Surgeon: R. Caldwell, M.D.

Medical History

Admitted to the urological service with a preliminary dx of Rt. Renal Mass; R/O Ca. Rt. Kidney.

Patient was asymptomatic until 2 weeks ago, when FUO, nausea, and vomiting occurred.

Radiologic studies of the abdomen revealed a large mass in the right kidney. An IV pyelogram examination, with nephrotomograms revealed a 16-cm mass in the Rt. Kidney; the other kidney was normal.

Lab/Diag. Values:

CBC: WNL
Hct. WNL
BUN 17 mg/100 ml
ECG NSR
CXR Normal

Proposed Tx.

CT-guided needle biopsy was performed with specimen sent to pathology.

Final Dx: Rt. Renal Mass (renal-cell carcinoma) Scheduled for E-Lap. Poss. Rt. Nephrectomy

Prognosis

Good

Exercise 31

1. Describe the following:

   a. nephrotomogram _____

   b. CT scan _____

   c. intravenous pyelogram _____

   d. biopsy _____

   e. nephrectomy _____

2. Define the following abbreviations:

   a. CBC _____

   b. BUN _____

   c. WNL _____

   d. Hct. _____

   e. Hgb. _____

   f. dx. _____

   g. NSR _____

3. The procedure used to produce images of single layers of tissue is called:
   a. tomography
   b. mammography
   c. angiography
   d. spirometry

4. The instrument used during a percutaneous examination of the kidney would be a
   a. cystoscope
   b. flexible nephroscope
   c. ureteroscope
   d. choledochoscope

5. A small hidden sac usually filled with fluid is called a
   a. bladder
   b. cyst
   c. crypt
   d. tumor

6. Cryosurgery is the medical term for
   a. surgery on the prostate gland
   b. tissue destruction using extreme cold
   c. laser-beam surgery
   d. gallbladder surgery

7. Catgut is a
   a. catheter
   b. congenital deformity
   c. suture
   d. fascia

8. Name the instruments used for visual inspections of the:

   1. Lungs _____

   2. Colon _____

   3. Urinary bladder _____

Surgical Anthology and Nursing Considerations

UNIT 1

Introduction to Surgery

Those who cannot remember the past are condemned to repeat it.
—Santayana

Ancient Egypt, long a fascinating subject to historians and archaeologists, provides examples of some of the earliest known medical and surgical writings. The papyri related to the practice of medicine and surgery have been studied for many years by eminent scholars all over the world in an attempt to discover more about the history of medicine and surgery. The Edwin Smith Papyrus is of greatest interest to the discipline of surgery, and is one of the oldest of the papyri, written in about 1600 B.C. It describes 48 surgical cases, mostly related to wounds, arranged in an order that is referred to in the writing as *capite ad calcem,* or head to toe.[1]

Ancient India also has a rich medical legacy. Susruta, in his book,[2] describes more than 100 surgical instruments, including scalpels, lancets, saws, bone cutters, trocars, and needles as part of the surgeon's tools. The Indian surgeons were best known for their skills as plastic surgeons, especially the restoration of noses and ears, since criminals frequently had them cut off as a form of punishment for their crimes.

In Greek and Roman antiquity, surgeons existed as specialists, and were called on only when medical treatment of the patient had failed. In the treatment of injuries, however, the surgeon would be the "attending" physician, since his knowledge of restoration was greater than that of his medical colleagues.

As science progressed, so too did the practice of surgery, and from as early as A.D. 1200 to the present day, the art and science of surgery have existed as a separate and specialized practice.

THE MODERN ERA OF SURGERY

In 1800, George III of England chartered the Royal College of Surgeons of London; it was changed by Queen Victoria in 1843 to become the Royal College of Surgeons of England. This organization set the acceptable standards for the practice of surgery, and some of its original concepts are still in use today.

In the early 1900s, surgery was still infrequent, and many hospitals in both England and the United States had specific days assigned to surgery during the week, in which two or more procedures were performed. In fact, in many major hospitals, there were fewer operations performed in 1 year than are performed in 2 days in one of our modern surgical suites. Numerous obstacles blocked the advance of surgery, as previously discussed in this book: sepsis, hemorrhage, pain, and shock being the most difficult to overcome. Mortality varied from hospital to hospital, and differed in countries, depending on the conditions, but the highest incidence was on the continent (40–60 percent), varying according to the specific procedure being performed.[3] But as with any science, new technologies, techniques, and patient-care management reforms allowed this specialty to emerge to what it has become today.

The founding of the American Surgical Association (1880), the American College of Surgeons (1913), and the American Board of Surgery (1937) has played a major part in setting and maintaining the quality of patient care and professional standards for the practice of surgery in this country, and through education, specialty groups (societies), and communication among its constituents, today's practitioners have the opportunity to seek continual improvements in their practice, as the art and science of surgery advance into the next century.

CATEGORIES OF SURGICAL PROCEDURES

Surgical procedures, for descriptive purposes, are traditionally classified in groups according to their related anatomic structure or physical system, and/or to

457

the specialist performing the procedure (e.g., general, gynecologist, etc.).

With the incorporation of the nursing process, however, procedures have been reclassified for ease of recognition, according to the reason or reasons for the planned surgical intervention, allowing the perioperative nurse and the surgical team to create a more realistic and effective plan for individualizing patient care.

While the traditional descriptions still exist, the redefining of surgical procedures produced six general categories, which can overlap the traditional descriptions depending on the specific anatomic area(s) involved.

By becoming familiar with these categories, the perioperative nurse can effectively plan for the individual surgical procedure, including supplying accessory items that may not be specifically required, but should be anticipated.

Category I: Surgery Involving the Loss of a Body Part, Organ, or Function

EXAMPLES: include, but are not limited to, hysterectomy; limb amputation; enucleation of an eye; mastectomy

Perioperative Nursing Considerations

A. Patient/Family/Significant Others
  * Recognition of psychic stress, related to
    — Grieving process
    — Loss of positive body image/self-esteem
    — Family/significant other response
  * Support systems/outside agencies to assist with adjustment
  * Patient preparation and education
B. Procedure
  * Selection and preparation of specialty instrumentation, supplies, equipment
  * Positioning, prepping, draping, sequence of surgery

Category II: Surgery Involving the Removal of a Tumor, Cyst, or Foreign Body

EXAMPLES: include, but are not limited to, ovarian cystectomy; craniotomy (for tumor); extraction of a bullet; removal of painful hardware

Perioperative Nursing Considerations

A. Patient/Family/Significant Others
  * Recognition of psychic stress, related to
    — Fear of the unknown

    — Outcome/diagnosis
    — Disfigurement, death
    — Dysfunction of body part
  * Patient preparation and education
B. Procedure
  * Type of procedure, for example, curative, palliative, emergent, elective
  * Trauma/triage activation (personnel)
  * Procedural guidelines/law enforcement protocol
    — Chain of command (bullet, etc.)
  * Selection and preparation of specialty instrumentation
  * Positioning, prepping, draping, sequence of surgery

Category III: Surgery Performed for Diagnostic Purposes

EXAMPLES: include, but are not limited to, mediastinoscopy; frozen section specimens; cystoscopy; cardiac catheterization; endoscopic procedures (colon, stomach, biliary, etc.)

Perioperative Nursing Considerations

A. Patient/Family/Significant Others
  * Recognition of psychic stress, related to
    — Changes in lifestyle, self-esteem, independence, unknown diagnosis
  * Patient preparation
  * Discharge planning and follow-up care
B. Procedure
  * Additional procedures required
  * Additional procedure set-ups as needed
  * Selection and preparation of specialty instrumentation
  * Positioning, prepping, draping, sequence of surgery

Category IV: Surgery for Insertion, Removal, or Application of a Prosthesis, Graft, Transplanted Organ, or Therapeutic Device

EXAMPLES: include, but are not limited to, pacemaker insertion; venous-access graft; kidney transplant; insertion of total hip arthroplasty

Perioperative Nursing Considerations

A. Patient/Family/Significant Others
  * Recognition of psychic stress, related to
    — Acceptance of reconstructed/replaced organ
    — Postoperative effect on current lifestyle

* Patient preparation and education
    — Physical limitations, if any, and for what period of time (dependence)
* Prophylactic antibiotic therapy
* Discharge planning and follow-up care

B. Procedure
* Preparation of implantable devices
* Special set-ups, additional personnel, instrumentation, etc.
* Positioning, prepping, draping, sequence of surgery
* Prevention of postoperative infections

Category V: Surgery for Reconstruction or Cosmetic Revision

EXAMPLES: include, but are not limited to, rhinoplasty; repair of cleft lip; breast reconstruction; skin grafting (post-burn); otoplasty

Perioperative Nursing Considerations

A. Patient/Family/Significant Others
* Recognition of psychic stress, related to
    — Self-image (need for seeking help)
    — Postoperative acceptance (posttrauma)
    — Acceptance (change in image)
* Patient preparation and education
* Discharge planning and follow-up care (sequential surgeries required)

B. Procedure
* Management of patient under local anesthesia
* Alloplastic/autogenous materials (grafting)
* Selection and preparation of instrumentation and specialty supplies
* Positioning, prepping, draping, sequence of surgery

Category VI: Surgery to Establish Drainage or Reestablish a Passageway

EXAMPLES: include, but are not limited to, colostomy; insertion of chest tubes; V-P shunt; colostomy closure; colon resection (with anastomosis); tuboplasty (reestablishment of fallopian tubes)

Perioperative Nursing Considerations

A. Patient/Family/Significant Others
* Recognition of psychic stress, related to
    — Changes in lifestyle; body image
    — Acceptance by family, coworkers, etc.
    — Management of artificial apparatus (e.g., colostomy, ileostomy, etc.)
    — Patient expectations (tuboplasty)
* Patient preparation and education
* Activation of support systems/discharge planning

B. Procedure
* Specialty supplies required
* Special set-ups as required
* Positioning, prepping, draping, sequence of surgery

Knowledge of these categories, and the specific nursing considerations associated with each procedure, can assist the team in preparing and selecting the appropriate equipment and supplies requested by the surgeon, but more important, they can enhance the ability to anticipate the need for special equipment and supplies that may not be specifically requested but by the nature of the surgery may be needed.

The most important factors, regardless of the proposed surgical intervention, are team work and the ability to provide a safe and therapeutic environment for both the patient and the team.

UNIT 2

Systems Approach to Surgical Procedures

Perioperative nursing demands specialized education in anatomy and physiology, in addition to specialized skills and abilities related to the care of the surgical patient. But it also requires a thorough knowledge of operative procedures, including the specific supplies and equipment needed to meet safely and effectively the needs of the patient undergoing surgical intervention.

SUBSPECIALTIES IN SURGERY

The human body is composed of several systems, consisting of closely allied organs and structures that share common concerns for a variety of bodily functions. According to anatomic structure and location, these systems have become the natural subspecialties for the practice of surgery.

Additionally, and because of its uniqueness, pediatric surgery is considered a separate subspecialty, since it is inclusive of all systems as they relate specifically to the pediatric patient.

This collection of surgical procedures (*anthology*) and nursing considerations has been created in an attempt to assist the reader in formulating a basic knowledge of common surgical procedures for each of the subspecialties within the practice of surgery.

The choice of procedures selected was based on three factors: (1) specific principles of surgery, (2) basic principles that could be applied to similar procedures, and (3) the primary services as they relate to surgical intervention.

One of the major difficulties in learning and understanding operative procedures and their varied nursing implications is the wide variations in techniques, supplies, and equipment that are selected by the surgeon based on the specific needs of the patient and the planned surgical intervention.

Unfortunately, a book can never replace actual clinical experience to illustrate these variations, but it can serve as a guideline for the preparation and overview of a selected surgical procedure.

A thorough understanding of the procedure, the patient's needs, and the specific requirements of the surgical team will help your job as a perioperative nurse become a challenging and rewarding experience.

This chapter contains the following subspecialties:

GENERAL SURGERY

General surgery encompasses operations of the digestive system structures, including the gastrointestinal tract, biliary system (spleen, pancreas, and liver), hernias of the abdominal wall, and procedures of the rectum and the breast. Included also in this category are surgeries involving the thyroid gland and associated structures, and the esophagus.

According to the American Board of Surgery, the definition of general surgery encompasses a central core of knowledge and skills common to all surgical procedures. This definition includes knowledge of anatomy, physiology, pathophysiology, immunology, and wound healing, which forms the basis for graduate education and the specialty of general surgery.

General surgery provides the foundation for all surgical procedures. Inherent in all general surgical procedures is:

1. Most procedures require similar instrumentation, as well as special items for rectal, breast, and thyroid procedures. The gastrointestinal instruments can be used interchangeably for various procedures involving the stomach and intestines.
2. A central core of knowledge and skills is common to all surgical specialties, based on similar instrumentation, positioning, prepping, and so on.
3. Diagnosis, preoperative, intraoperative, and postoperative care of the patient with diseases involving organs of the alimentary tract, abdomen and its contents, breast, neck, and immediately adjacent

structures of the endocrine system are involved with general surgical procedures.

4. Employment and knowledge of endoscopic techniques for diagnosis and treatment may also be required, in addition to an understanding of general principles of anesthesiology, pathophysiology, and management of trauma.

5. Laparoscopic procedures, involving a variety of organs (the appendix, gallbladder, etc.), have replaced the open surgical procedure whenever appropriate.

Common Principles and Techniques

Frequently, the surgery to be performed will depend on the results of a biopsy and/or frozen section obtained at the time of surgery.

Although the patient has been informed preoperatively of an anticipated procedure, the fear of the unknown is cause for apprehension and anxiety. The perioperative nurse must convey support and concern for the patient, both physiologically and psychologically.

Operability of malignant tumors may be determined only after a thorough exploration during surgery, and alternative therapy may be decided at this time. The perioperative nurse must be flexible to these situations, and be ready to assist the surgical team should a change in supplies be required.

Frequently, two set-ups must be prepared, depending on the diagnosis and/or anticipated procedures. Two special techniques used with specific procedures, which require special handling, include:

1. *Bowel Technique:* used when the anatomy involves the jejunum or structures below the jejunum, in which instruments coming in contact with this area are isolated from other instruments, and a separate, clean closing set-up is used (new instruments, change of gown and gloves, and reinforcement of drapes around the incision)

2. *No-touch Technique:* not as severe as bowel technique, yet requires isolation of the instruments contacting a contaminated structure (e.g., appendix, gallbladder, lung, cervix)

Positioning and draping for general surgery areas are as varied as the procedure itself, although a general laparotomy pack, with a fenestrated sheet (transverse or horizontal), will usually be appropriate for most procedures. Extra pillows, padding, and positional aides should be available.

Instrumentation is varied and is selected for a specific need, in addition to a generic tray (major laparotomy tray), which can accomplish the initial exploration and closure of the abdomen.

A variety of anesthesia techniques are used during general surgery, depending on the condition of the patient and the type of surgery anticipated.

A number of general surgical procedures are adaptable to an ambulatory surgery setting, while others are extremely extensive and require the patient to be hospitalized following the procedure.

Perioperative Nursing Implications

For procedures performed in the abdominopelvic cavity, the following considerations should be reviewed and applied as necessary, depending on the surgical procedure being performed:

1. The *electrosurgical unit* (ESU) is frequently used, but in some cases, a *laser* may be used, with or without the ESU. The ESU pencil tips may vary, depending on the specific structure/area involved.

2. A *nasogastric tube* (NG tube) is frequently inserted during abdominal surgery by the anesthesiologist, to decompress the stomach during surgery.

3. Following entry into the abdominal cavity, *Raytec* (4 × 4) sponges should be replaced by laparotomy sponges. Raytec's should only be used on a sponge stick for hemostasis or blunt dissection in deep areas.

4. Suction should always be available, even on simple cases. The Poole abdominal tip or the Yankauer tip may be used, depending on the circumstances; therefore, both should be available.

5. Drains can be used as either retractors (e.g., *Penrose*) or for wound drainage. They are either placed along the incision line or used through a stab wound incision. The drain should be moistened first with saline, then passed to the surgeon or placed on an instrument (Kelly clamp) and passed.

6. Before closure, the wound is often irrigated with saline solution. This solution should be warm (not hot) to prevent systemic shock to the system, and may contain antibiotics as per surgeon's preference card. The amount of irrigation must be subtracted from the suction cannister, in order to measure accurately the blood loss during surgery.

7. The insertion of an indwelling Foley catheter is not unusual for involved abdominal procedures, to maintain an accurate record of intake and output during the surgery. Consult with the surgeon and the anesthesiologist before beginning the skin prep for possible insertion.

8. All dyes, medications, and solutions on the back

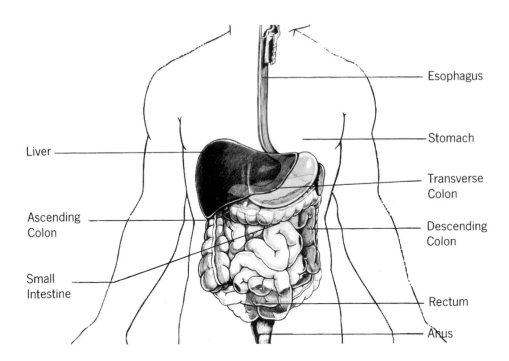

Fig. 14-1. Digestive system structures

table must be labeled with the name and amount of medication. Sterile water should not be on the back table, unless specifically requested by the surgeon (for cancer tumors) and labeled appropriately.

Categories—General Surgery Procedures

The following section has been arranged according to the five common categories associated with general surgery:

Gastrointestinal Surgery
Biliary Surgery
Hernia Repairs
Procedures Involving the Breast
Procedures of the Neck

GASTROINTESTINAL SURGERY

Surgical Anatomy Review

The *gastrointestinal system* is also known as the *digestive system,* and refers to those structures related to the *esophagus, stomach, intestines* (large and small), and accessory structures of the *biliary tract,* since they all aid in the process of digestion.

It is important to remember that the gastrointestinal (GI) tract is one continuous tube. It is a little wider at its upper end, the mouth and pharynx or throat, and narrows for the esophagus, then enlarges again for the stomach. In the small intestines, the continuous tube narrows again, then enlarges for the large intestines, and finally narrows down again to become the anus (Fig. 14-1).

The Esophagus

The esophagus, or gullet, is about 9 inches long, and extends through the neck, behind the trachea, through the mediastinum of the thorax, finally reaching the abdominal cavity after extending through the diaphragm via an opening called the *esophageal hiatus.* There it attaches to the stomach, at a sphincter known as the *cardiac notch* (orifice).

The esophagus is muscular in structure, consisting of skeletal muscles in the upper portion and smooth muscles in the lower portion.

The Stomach

The stomach hangs in the *supracolic* compartment of the abdomen, and is actually an enlarged or dilated section of the alimentary tube. It lies within the partition between the greater and lesser *peritoneal sacs,* and is sandwiched between the two layers of the peritoneum lining both structures. These two layers meet beyond both gastric curvatures, and extend to the liver above and to the diaphragm, spleen, and colon to the left and below.

The stomach has an anterior and a posterior surface. The anterior surface is the one encountered on opening the abdomen. The posterior surface is concealed and is exposed only by opening the lesser peritoneal sac, whose anterior boundary is partially formed by the posterior wall of the stomach.

The stomach has two curvatures: the lesser, which faces the liver, and the greater, which faces the rest of the abdomen. Each curvature has a notch:

1. *Cardiac notch:* lies high up on the greater curvature at its junction with the esophagus
2. *Angular notch:* lies at the junction of the vertical and horizontal portions of the lesser curvature

These two notches help to divide the stomach into its three areas: *fundus, body, and pylorus.* Frequently, the entire pylorus segment is referred to as the *antrium,* which then includes the pylorus vestibule (*pyloric sphincter*).

The Intestines

The *pyloric valve* (or sphincter), a ring-like muscle surrounding the distal end of the stomach, is the anatomic connection between the stomach and the small intestines.

The *small intestine* is by far the longest part of the alimentary canal. More appropriately, it might have been named the long intestine, because it is about 20 feet long (as compared with the large intestine, which measures only 4 or 5 feet), but since it is smaller in diameter, it is true to its name.

The first 10 to 12 inches is called the *duodenum,* which contains two openings for ducts (*pancreatic* and *common bile*). Beyond the duodenum are two more divisions of the small intestines; the *jejunum* and the *ileum.* The ileum joins the large intestine through another muscular valve called the *ileocecal valve* (sphincter).

The *large intestine* begins with a small pouch known as the *cecum,* which is located in the lower right iliac region of the abdomen; attached to the cecum is a blind pouch called the *vermiform appendix.*

The *colon,* the longer portion of the large intestine, extends from the cecum and has four sections: the *ascending* colon, rising up the right side of the abdomen; the *transverse* colon, spreading across the abdomen; the *descending* colon, traveling down the left side of the abdomen; to the *sigmoid* colon, an S-shaped structure, that empties into the *rectum,* to the *anal canal,* and finally to the *anus.*

The Peritoneum

The peritoneum is a serous membrane that covers the surface of most of the abdominal organs to form the

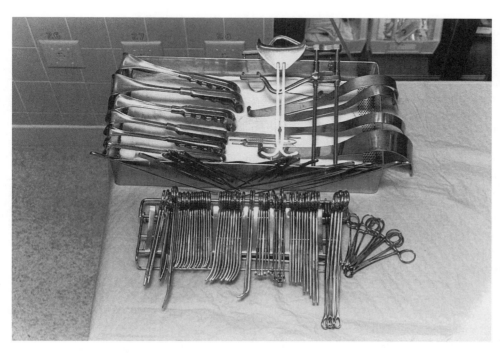

Major laparotomy instrument tray

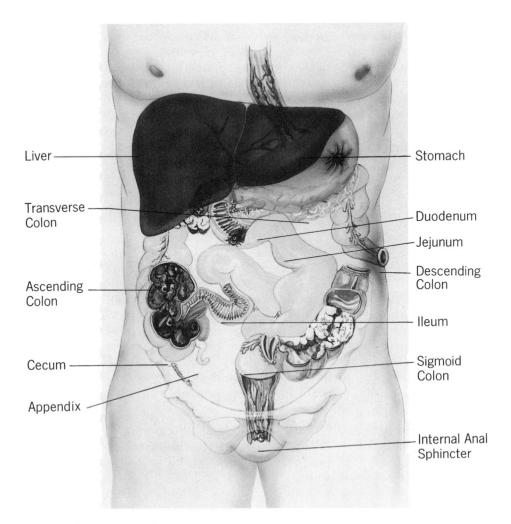

Fig. 14-2. Gastrointestinal structures

visceral serosa, which lines the abdominal wall and forms the *parietal layer.* In addition to these parts of the peritoneum, there are more complex double layers of membranes that separate the abdomen into areas and spaces, and in some cases aid in supporting the organs and holding them in place.

The *mesentery,* for example, is a double-layered peritoneal structure shaped somewhat like a fan, with the handle portion attached to the posterior wall. The expanded long edge is attached to the small intestine. Between the two layers of membrane that form the mesentery are the blood vessels, nerves, and other structures that supply the intestine.

Another double-layered peritoneal structure, called the *greater omentum,* hangs downward from the lower border (greater curvature) of the stomach. This double layer of peritoneum extends into the pelvic portion of the abdomen and then loops back and up to the trans-

verse colon. There is also a peritoneal structure called the *lesser omentum,* which extends between the stomach and the liver.

In addition to the structures just reviewed, several accessory digestive organs are part of the *biliary system: the liver, spleen, pancreas,* and *gallbladder.* They will be reviewed as their surgical procedures are presented (Fig. 14-2).

Procedure
Laparotomy

Definition: A term used to describe an incision made through the abdominal wall in order to perform surgical procedures involving abdominal structures.

CDC Classification: Dependent on procedure being performed

Discussion: When the surgeon performs a laparotomy as a diagnostic procedure, without knowing the exact nature of the patient's disease, it is referred to as an *exploratory laparotomy,* or "E-Lap." Once the abdomen is opened and explored, the specific corrective procedure related to the pathology found is performed.

An exploratory laparotomy may be performed following trauma to the abdomen, or when the patient has undetermined abdominal pain.

Position: Supine, with arms extended on armboards

Incision Site(s): Midline, upper paramedian, lower paramedian (incision site may depend on suspected pathology)

Skin Preparation: (See pp. 337–338)

Packs/Drapes: Laparotomy pack

    Four folded towels

Instrumentation:

    Major procedure (Lap) tray

    Hemoclip/surgiclip appliers (size variety)

    Specialty instruments (if known) (opt.)

Supplies/Equipment:

    Basin set

    Blades—(2) No. 10 or (1) No. 10 and (1) No. 20; (1) No. 15

    Needle counter

    Suction and tip; ESU

    Dressings

Suture—surgeon's preference

Solutions—saline, water

Medications—surgeon's preference

PROCEDURAL OVERVIEW

The surgical sequence outlined for every abdominal procedure is discussed here in order to avoid repetition for each separate procedure.

Opening Sequence

The skin is incised with the "skin knife" (No. 10 or No. 20). The subcutaneous tissue is incised with the second knife or "deep knife" (No. 10) or by the electrosurgical cautery pencil. Blood vessels may be clamped with a hemostat and tied or cauterized.

Fascia is incised and the underlying muscles are retracted or transected. If the incision is on the midline, no muscle tissue is encountered. If, however, the incision lies off the midline (paramedian), there will be a layer of muscle tissue, which will separate manually or with the deep knife (Fig. 14-3).

The surgeon will grasp the peritoneum and incise it with the deep knife and a scissors (usually Metzenbaum, infrequently a curved May) to complete the peritoneal incision (Fig. 14-3).

Exposure and Exploration

In preparation for entrance into the abdomen, the scrub person should have available several laparotomy (Lap)

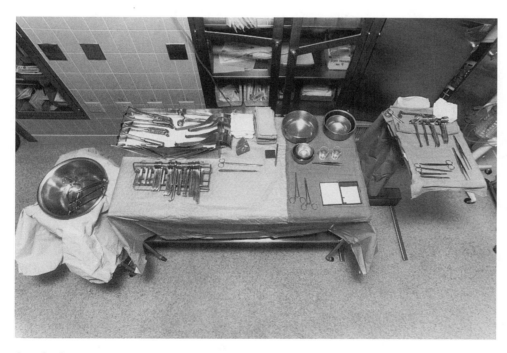

Standard instrument table and Mayo tray set-up

A. Laparotomy incision   B. Subcutaneous layer is incised

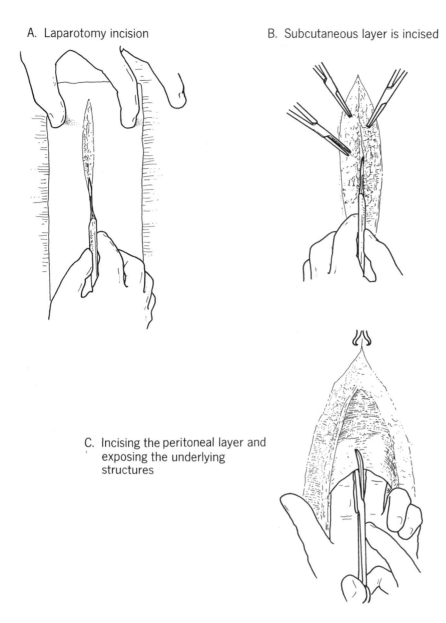

C. Incising the peritoneal layer and exposing the underlying structures

Fig. 14-3. Laparotomy incision into the abdomen

sponges and a self-retaining retractor (usually a Balfour with bladder blade). The Lap sponges may be used dry or moistened with warm saline solution. They are used to protect the wound edges. This procedure is referred to as *packing the abdomen*.

The abdominal contents are explored. If a self-retaining retractor is not used, wound edges may be retracted accordingly by Deaver or Richardson retractors held by the assistant.

Excision, Repair, Revision
When the area of disease has been located, the surgeon will pack the abdominal contents away from the dis-

eased area with several additional moist Laps, and the specific surgical procedure will be performed depending on the nature of the pathology.

Closing Sequence
In preparation for closing the abdomen, many surgeons irrigate the wound with warm saline solution (plain or with antibiotic added), and remove the irrigation fluid by suction. Drains may be used, often through a "stab wound" incision made with the skin knife.

Following the irrigation, the surgeon and assistant remove the sponges and instruments, and the scrub person and circulating nurse prepare for the first closing count.

The peritoneum is usually closed with absorbable sutures with a taper needle (size 0 or 2-0) using a continuous stitch. Two toothed forceps or several Kocher clamps may be used to grasp the peritoneum to assist in its exposure.

Next, the fascia is closed with a variety of materials (silk, Dexon, Vicryl, or staples). Since the fascia is the strongest layer of the abdominal wall, and the integrity of the closure depends on its strength, an interrupted stitch will be used. Size 2-0 is most common; however, size 0 may be used if the patient is muscular or obese. The suture may be mounted on a taper or cutting needle, according to surgeon's preference. During the fascia closure, the assistant retracts the skin and subcutaneous layers with either an Army-Navy, Parker, Eastman, or Richardson retractor (in pairs). On completion of the closure, the second closing count is performed.

The subcutaneous layer is closed next with interrupted sutures (Dexon, chromic, plain) on a fine tapered needle, size 3-0.

The skin edges are approximated using Adson forceps for suture materials or Allis clamps when skin staples are used.

At the completion of the skin closure, the wound and surrounding area are cleaned and sterile dressings are applied. The drapes are removed, while the scrub person protects the dressings, and the circulating nurse applies the preferred tape.

For infected cases, however, the skin and subcutaneous tissue may be left open and either packed or drained.

PERIOPERATIVE NURSING CONSIDERATIONS

- Once the abdomen is entered, the only free sponges used are laparotomy sponges. If Raytec sponges are needed, they should be folded in thirds (blue tape showing) and placed on the end of a sponge stick for blunt dissection and/or blotting deep, yet small, areas.
- Some surgeons may prefer the Lap sponges to be dry. Check the preference card before moistening the sponges.
- All irrigation solution should be warm (not hot) in order to avoid internal chilling and possible hypothermia.
- X-ray–detectable sponges can never be used as dressing sponges; however, if they must be used as packing (for delayed primary closure), they must be accounted for on the intraoperative record, and upon removal be counted with amount documented.
- Specimens collected must be properly labeled and

placed in an approved solution for accurate pathology readings.
- All abdominal cases require two closing counts, to be performed aloud and simultaneously. The result of the count should be reported to the surgeon upon completion.
- All medication, solutions, and so on, on the back table must be labeled, and an accurate record of use must be maintained.

SPECIFIC SURGICAL PROCEDURES

Procedure
Gastrectomy

Definition: Removal of the stomach, and establishment of the continuity of the gastrointestinal tract.
CDC Classification: II, unless gross contamination occurs
Special Technique: Bowel technique (optional, depending on location of anastomosis)
Discussion: Gastrectomy procedures usually are performed one of two ways: as a total gastrectomy or a subtotal (partial) gastrectomy.

Total Gastrectomy
Often performed because of malignancy or uncontrolled gastric bleeding. Continuity of the GI tract is reestablished by anastomosis of the distal esophagus to the proximal jejunum or by replacing the resected stomach with the duodenum or an isolated segment of the colon. When treating malignancies, the lymph nodes, adjacent structures (e.g., spleen), and greater omentum are removed during the procedure.

Subtotal (Partial) Gastrectomy
Refers to the excision of a portion of the stomach, primarily performed for peptic ulcer disease or tumor of the distal stomach. A vagotomy may be included during this procedure. Continuity of the GI tract is reestablished by anastomosis of the gastric remnants to the proximal duodenum (Bilroth I), or to the proximal jejunum (Bilroth II), or a modification of these procedures. As with total gastrectomy, when treating malignancies, the greater omentum, lymph nodes, and adjacent structures are removed.

Position: Supine, with arms extended on armboards
Incision Site(s): Upper median, thoracoabdominal, bilateral subcostal
Skin Preparation: (See pp. 337–338)
Packs/Drapes: Major Lap pack and/or transverse
    Lap sheet
    Four folded towels

Instrumentation:
    Major Lap tray
    Intestinal instruments
    CV instruments (opt.)
    Internal stapling devices (opt.)
    Hemoclip/surgiclip appliers (size variety)
Supplies/Equipment:
    Basin set
    Blades—(2) No. 10 or (1) No. 10 and (1) No. 20; (1) No. 15
    Needle counter
    ESU; suction
    Hemoclip/surgiclips (variety); internal staples
    Solutions—saline, water
    Sutures—surgeon's preference
    Medications—surgeon's preference
    Dressings
    For thoracoabdominal approach:
    Chest tube with drainage unit

PROCEDURAL OVERVIEW

Partial Gastrectomy with Gastroduodenostomy (Bilroth I)

The abdomen is entered through an upper midline approach, and the contents are explored to determine the extent of the disease and to choose a site for the anastomosis. The stomach is mobilized from the ligaments, vessels, and omentum that attach to the greater and lesser curvatures of the stomach. The scrub person should be prepared with Kelly clamps, Metzenbaum scissors, and ligature (silk ties, 2-0 and 3-0). Additional ligature (e.g., 2-0 and 3-0 Dexon or Vicryl), and one or two sutures (silk) on a taper needle should also be available. The ligatures will be used to tie off the large vessels of the stomach.

Once the stomach is mobilized, the duodenum is resected from the stomach. Two intestinal clamps are placed across the duodenum, which is then divided from the stomach by cutting between the two clamps with a knife or cautery pencil. The duodenal stump is then closed. A running suture of silk, chromic, or Dexon on a fine tapered needle is used to close the stump.

Gastroduodenal Anastomosis

The surgeon aligns the stomach and duodenum at the proposed junction site. Silk traction sutures are placed at each end of the site to hold the stomach and duodenum in alignment using a continuous or interrupted suture on a fine tapered needle (3-0 or 4-0) to form the first row of sutures. After completing this row, the surgeon will make two incisions, one at each side of the suture line, to expose the inner surface of the stomach and duodenum; they are joined.

An alternative method is to perform this procedure with internal surgical stapling instruments.

The wound is irrigated with warm saline and closed in layers. Drains (e.g., Hemovac, Jackson-Pratt) are anchored, if used.

PERIOPERATIVE NURSING CONSIDERATIONS

- Check to see whether blood has been ordered and is available.
- Surgeon may request a "clean" closure tray and set-up if bowel technique is required.
- Intestinal clamps should have "rubber shods" to prevent damage to the bowel.
- All instruments coming in contact with the intestine should be isolated and removed with the specimen.
- Specimen should be collected in a basin.
- Maintain an accurate recording of irrigation fluids used.
- Frozen section may be requested.

Related Surgical Procedures:
    Gastrojejunostomy (Bilroth II)
    Esophagogastrostomy
    Gastrostomy feeding tube

Procedure
Appendectomy

Definition: The excision of the appendix, usually performed to remove an acutely inflamed organ.

Many surgeons perform an appendectomy as a prophylactic procedure when operating in the abdomen for other reasons. This procedure is then referred to as an incidental appendectomy.

CDC Classification: II, if nonruptured
Special Technique: No-touch technique
Position: Supine, with arms extended on armboards
Incision Site: McBurney (muscle splitting) incision
Skin Preparation: See pp. 337–338
Packs/Drapes: Laparotomy pack
    Four folded towels
Instrumentation:
    Major Lap tray or minor tray
    Internal stapling device (opt.)
Supplies/Equipment:
    Basin set
    Blades—(1) No. 20, (1) No. 10
    Needle counter
    ESU; suction
    Penrose drain (¼ in. opt.)
    Culture tubes (aerobic/anaerobic)
    Solutions—saline, water
    Sutures—surgeon's preference

Internal stapling instruments (opt.)
Medication—surgeon's preference

PROCEDURAL OVERVIEW

An incision is made in the right lower abdomen, either transversely oblique (McBurney) or vertically (for a primary appendectomy). The surgeon's assistant retracts the wound edges with a Richardson or similar retractor. The appendix is identified and its vascular supply ligated.

The surgeon grasps the appendix with a Babcock clamp, and delivers it into the wound site. The tip of the appendix may then be grasped with a Kelly clamp to hold it up, and a moist Lap sponge is placed around the base of the appendix (stump) to prevent contamination of bowel contents, in case any spill out occurs during the procedure.

The surgeon isolates the appendix from its attachments to the bowel (*mesoappendix*) using a Metzenbaum scissors. Taking small bits of tissue along the appendix, the mesoappendix is double-clamped, and ligated with free ties (absorbable, 3-0).

The base of the appendix is grasped with a straight Kelly clamp, and the appendix is removed. The stump may be inverted into the cecum, using a purse-string suture (silk or cotton, 3-0 or 4-0, on a fine needle), cauterized with chemicals (phenol), or simply left alone after ligation. Another technique is to devascularize the appendix and invert the entire appendix into the cecum.

The appendix, knife, needle holder, and any clamps or scissors that have come in contact with the appendix are delivered in a basin to the circulating nurse.

The wound is irrigated with warm saline, and is closed in layers, except when an abscess has occurred, as with acute appendicitis. A drain may be placed into the abscess cavity, exiting through the incision or a stab wound.

An alternative technique may use the internal stapling device, by placing the stapling instrument around the tissue at the appendiocecum junction.

By using this technique, the possibility of contamination from spillage is greatly reduced.

PERIOPERATIVE NURSING CONSIDERATION

- Instruments used for amputation of the appendix are to be isolated in a basin.
- If ruptured, the case must be considered contaminated, and the surgeon may elect to use antibiotic irrigation before closure of the abdomen with an insertion of a drain.
- There may be no skin closure of the wound if the appendix has ruptured.

Surgery Involving the Intestines

Procedure
Anastomosis of Small Intestine
(Small Bowel Resection)

Definition: Excision of a segment of the small intestine with an anastomosis to a segment of more distal small bowel or colon, thus restoring continuity of the GI tract.

CDC Classification: II

Discussion: This procedure is performed to remove an obstruction, a gangrenous portion of bowel, a perforation, or a source of hemorrhage within the small bowel.

Small bowel resections are infrequently performed as an isolated procedure, except for inflammatory bowel disease, rare primary tumors, or mesenteric infarctions. More often, they are done in conjunction with other procedures because of adhesive obstructive disease, tumors of adjacent organs, diverticulitis, or tuboovarian abscess.

Two techniques frequently used to perform the anastomosis are

1. *End-to-end:* two ends of severed bowel are brought in close approximation, rotated slightly outward, and joined.
2. *Side-to-side:* two surface layers are joined on each side of a suture line, creating an opening on each side, exposing the intestinal mucosa, which is then approximated (Fig. 14-4).

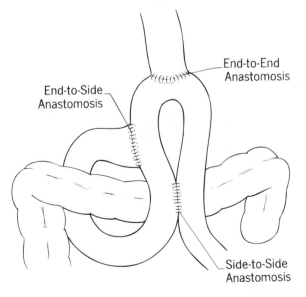

Fig. 14-4. Examples of anastomosis (end-to-end, side-to-side, and end-to-side)

Position: Supine, with arms extended on armboards
Incision Site: Upper midline (isolated procedure)
Skin Preparation: See pp. 337–338
Packs/Drapes: Major Lap pack
    Four folded towels
Instrumentation:
    Major Lap tray
    Intestinal instruments
    Internal stapling instruments (opt.)
    Hemoclips/surgiclip appliers (size variety)
Supplies/Equipment:
    Basin set
    Blades—(2) No. 10, (1) No. 15
    Hemoclip/surgiclips (size variety)
    ESU; suction
    Needle counter
    Internal surgical staples
    Suture—surgeon's preference
    Solutions—saline, water
    Dressings
    Medications—surgeon's preference

PROCEDURAL OVERVIEW

1. **As an Isolated Procedure**
    To identify the diseased portion of the intestines, the surgeon will use an upper midline approach, and then explore the intestines by passing the loops of the intestines through his or her fingers. This technique is called *running the bowel.*

    Once the area has been identified, the section between the proposed site of anastomosis must be isolated from the attached mesentery.

    Using a Metzenbaum scissors, the surgeon makes a small incision into the avascular area of the mesentery. Two Kelly clamps are placed over a section of mesentery, and the section is divided with a knife or cautery pencil between the two clamps; then it is ligated. This process is continued, until the diseased portion and the anastomosis site have been isolated.

    Two intestinal clamps are placed at each end of the isolated segment, and the tissue is divided with a knife or cautery pencil. The affected segment is excised, and continuity of the bowel is restored by either the use of sutures, or the application of internal staples used to both create the anastomosis and restore flow through the bowel. The abdomen is irrigated with warm saline, and closed in layers in a routine fashion.

2. **As Part of Another Procedure**
    Similar steps are taken, leaving the restored segment attached to the adherent organ also resected (e.g., colon, ovary, etc.).

PERIOPERATIVE NURSING CONSIDERATIONS

-   The surgeon may request a clean closure set-up, or may only require the isolation of the instruments, depending on the segment of bowel being repaired.
-   As a general rule, when working with the jejunum or below, bowel technique should be employed, as opposed to a no-touch technique.
-   When part of another procedure, the small bowel segment will be performed following the revision of the diseased area, and appropriate instrumentation for that procedure should be available.
-   If an ileostomy is performed, the ileostomy appliance (e.g., Karaya seal, etc.) may be placed on the patient prior to leaving the operating room.

Related Surgical Procedures:
    Ileostomy   (temporary/permanent opening of the
                ileum, brought out onto the abdomen
                as a stoma)
    Resection of Duodenal Ulcer

Procedure
Resection of the Large Intestine (Right Hemicolectomy Anastomosis)

Definition: Resection of the right half of the colon (a portion of the transverse colon, ascending colon, and the cecum), and a segment of the terminal ileum and their mesenteries. Continuity of the GI tract is reestablished through an anastomosis between the ileum and the transverse colon (ileocolostomy).
CDC Classification: II, unless gross contamination occurs
Special Technique: Bowel technique
Discussion: Indications for a right hemicolectomy include tumors, bleeding, inflammation, or trauma to the large intestine. Obstruction is not often encountered in the right portion of the intestine, but is predominant in the left half of the colon.
Position: Supine, with arms extended on armboards
Incision Site(s): Right paramedian; midline; oblique right midabdominal
Skin Preparation: See pp. 337–338
Packs/Drapes: Laparotomy pack
    Extra drape sheets
    Minor pack (for closure)
Instrumentation:
    Major Lap tray
    Intestinal tray
    Closing tray
    Hemoclip/surgiclip appliers (size variety)
    Internal stapling instruments (opt.)

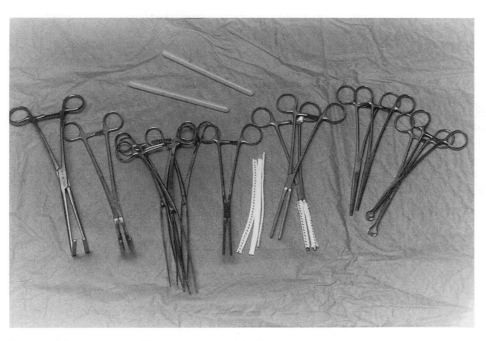

Intestinal instruments with clamp covers (shods)

Supplies/Equipment:
Basin set
Blades—(3) No. 10, (1) No. 15 (extra for closing set-up)
Extra gowns, gloves
ESU; suction (2)
Needle counter (2)
Solutions—saline; water
Sutures—surgeon's preference
Medications—surgeon's preference

PROCEDURAL OVERVIEW

According to the location of the lesion, the surgeon enters the abdomen using the appropriate approach. A midline incision, however, is usually preferred, since it allows for greater exposure of the abdominal contents.

Once the abdomen is entered, the surgeon explores the intestine (runs the bowel), and identifies the diseased portion. If cancerous, a wide margin of intestine, on either side of the lesion, is also removed.

To free the bowel, the scrub person should have available a supply of Kelly clamps (hemostats) and ties (2-0 and 3-0 silk), or surgeon's preference. The surgeon dissects the bowel from its peritoneal and mesenteric attachments using a Metzenbaum scissors. Portions of the mesentery are double-clamped, divided, and ligated. Large vessels and bleeders are controlled with free-ties or a cautery pencil.

The surgeon completes the mobilization procedure along the full length of bowel to be resected.

The appropriate segment of colon is excised between two atraumatic (*intestinal*) clamps or via an internal stapling instrument.

The terminal ileum and midtransverse colon are anastomosed by various suture techniques (fine silk; Vicryl; Controll release needle) or by internal staples. When sutures are used, a second layer of interrupted chromic or Vicryl is used (3-0 on a GI needle) and this technique continues until the two intestinal lumens are joined.

The intestinal clamps are removed and a reinforcing suture layer of interrupted silk is placed. The final step is the closure of the mesentery using an interrupted suture (silk or chromic, 3-0).

The closing instruments and supplies are exchanged (bowel technique), the wound is irrigated with warm saline, and the abdomen is closed in layers in a routine fashion.

PERIOPERATIVE NURSING CONSIDERATIONS

- Bowel technique requires the total changeover of gowns, gloves, instruments, etc. In some institutions, this is performed before irrigation of the abdominal cavity, while in others, it is performed after the irrigation.
- Prior to the changeover, the first closing count should be performed to indicate that the instru-

ments, sponges, and sharps used on the first portion are correct. When the count has been verified, the first table should be covered, but must remain in the room until the final count is verified.

- During the procedure, instruments used on the bowel must be isolated in a basin.
- The scrub person should receive the specimen in a basin to limit further contamination of the field.
- An alternative technique is to use a transfer "sponge stick" to retrieve items from the back table. Then only the Mayo tray need be changed for the closing segment. Institutional policy should dictate the proper procedure to be used.

Related Surgical Procedures: Total Colectomy
Transverse Colectomy

Procedure
Anterior Resection of the Sigmoid Colon and Rectum

Definition: The excision of the sigmoid colon, and when applicable the resection of the rectosigmoid and proximal two thirds of the rectum. Continuity of the GI tract is accomplished by anastomosis of the distal descending or proximal sigmoid colon to the remaining segment of the rectosigmoid or rectum.
CDC Classification: II, unless gross contamination occurs
Special Technique: Bowel technique
Discussion: This procedure is usually performed for benign conditions (e.g., diverticulitis) or malignant tumors.
Position: Supine, with arms extended on armboards
Incision Site: Vertical or transverse abdominal
Skin Preparation: See pp. 337–338
Packs, Drapes, Instrumentation, Supplies, Equipment: See Right Hemicolectomy, p. 470

PROCEDURAL OVERVIEW

The abdomen is opened. The lower descending, sigmoid, and rectosigmoid colon (and proximal rectum) are mobilized by dividing the mesenteric vasculature attachments. In procedures for malignancy, greater portions of the mesentery are excised to include additional lymph node–bearing tissue. The ureters are identified and protected by moist Lap sponges. The appropriate segment of colon is excised, and the bowel is anastomosed with suture or internal staples. Tension is avoided on the anastomosis by mobilizing more proximal colon as necessary.

The set-up is changed, the wound is irrigated with warm saline, and the abdomen is closed in layers in a routine fashion.

PERIOPERATIVE NURSING CONSIDERATIONS

- See Right Hemicolectomy, p. 470.

Procedure
Colostomy

Definition: Formation of an opening into the colon, brought out onto the abdominal wall as a *stoma*. The opening can be either permanent or temporary.
CDC Classification: II, unless gross contamination occurs
Specific Technique: Bowel technique
Discussion: This procedure is usually performed for lesions in the large intestine caused by cancer, diverticulitis, or obstruction of the large intestine in an area close to the cecum.

Types of Colostomy
A colostomy can be permanent or temporary, depending on the pathology and the patient's needs.

1. *Temporary Colostomy:* A temporary colostomy is performed to divert the fecal stream from the distal colon, which may be obstructed by tumor inflammation, or requires being "put-to-rest" because of an anastomosis or a pouch procedure. A temporary colostomy may be created in the transverse colon or sigmoid colon.
2. *Permanent Colostomy:* A permanent colostomy is performed to treat malignancies of the colon. Other indications may include irrevocable rectal strictures, incontinence of bowel, or inflammatory bowel disease. A permanent colostomy can be fashioned similar to a temporary colostomy but most often is an end colostomy.

A colostomy may be performed as part of another procedure or as an isolated surgery.
Position: Supine, with arms extended on armboards
Incision Site: Dependent on the segment of colon to be used
Skin Preparation: Depends on primary area; see pp. 337–338
Packs/Drapes: Laparotomy pack
Four folded towels
Transverse Lap sheet (opt.)
Minor pack (for closing set-up)
Instrumentation:
Major Lap tray
Intestinal tray
Closing tray
Internal surgical staples (opt.)
Supplies/Equipment:
Basin set

Blades—(2) No. 10
Needle counter (2)
ESU; Suction (2)
Penrose drain (1 in. for retraction)
Internal stapling instruments (opt.)
Glass rod and tubing with colostomy pouch (e.g., Karya seal or plastic bridge) and loop colostomy set (e.g., Hollister)
Solutions—saline, water
Sutures—surgeon's preference
Medications
Dressings

PROCEDURAL OVERVIEW

The abdomen is opened in the usual manner and the segment of colon is mobilized. The colon can be brought out through the main incision, or through an adjacent site from which a disk of skin and subcutaneous tissue has been excised. The underlying rectus fascia muscle and peritoneal layers are incised to accommodate the colon. The appropriate segment is excised between two atraumatic (intestinal) clamps or the EEA internal stapling instrument, which is used to prepare and create the stoma.

In a loop colostomy, a rod or bridge may be placed under the colon to avoid retraction.

The abdomen is irrigated with warm saline, and closed in layers in a routine fashion. A colostomy pouch is applied over the stoma.

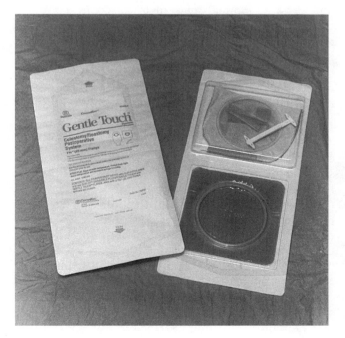

Colostomy supplies

PERIOPERATIVE NURSING CONSIDERATIONS

- See Right Hemicolectomy, p. 470.
- The colostomy pouch may or may not be applied in surgery. A Vaseline gauze may encircle the stoma with a "fluff" type dressing applied. If the institution has an "Ostomy Nurse," the application of the colostomy pouch may be delayed until the clinical specialist can work with the patient and family.

Related Surgical Procedures:
Ileotransverse Colostomy
Loop Colostomy
Double-Barrel Colostomy

Procedure
Closure of Colostomy

Definition: Reestablishment of colonic continuity, and repair of the abdominal wall.
CDC Classification: II
Special Technique: No-touch, unless bowel is reentered
Discussion: The procedure may be simple or complex, depending on the type of colostomy and the area involved.
Position: Supine, with arms extended on armboards
Incision Sites: For end colostomy, incision circumscribes the stoma; for loop or double-barrel colostomy, an elliptical incision is made around the stoma(s)
Skin Preparation: See pp. 337–338
Packs, Drapes, Instrumentation, Supplies, Equipment: See Colostomy, pp. 471–472

PROCEDURAL OVERVIEW

For an end colostomy, the stoma is dissected free from the abdominal wall structures. An appropriate incision is made to enable intraabdominal dissection, permitting reanastomosis at the site of the distal colon. The distal segment is mobilized and anastomosed to the proximal end; an internal stapling device can also facilitate this procedure. The wound is irrigated and closed; subcutaneous tissue and skin may be left open to avoid infection (packing may be used).

For a loop or double-barrel colostomy, the colonic loop is dissected free of scar tissue and skin, and the anastomosis is performed. The proximal and distal segments may need to be resected in order to perform the anastomosis on a well-vascularized bowel of satisfactory diameters. The abdomen is irrigated and closed, often leaving the subcutaneous tissue and skin packed open to prevent wound infection.

PERIOPERATIVE NURSING CONSIDERATIONS

- Instruments used on the bowel must be isolated in a separate basin, and not returned to the sterile field.
- A clean closure tray (e.g., minor tray) may be requested.

Procedure
Abdominoperineal Resection of the Rectum

Definition: Through combined abdominal and perineal incisions, the anus, rectum, and sigmoid colon are removed en bloc.

CDC Classification: II, unless gross contamination occurs

Special Technique: Bowel technique

Discussion: Performed most often for the treatment of rectal malignancy or severe inflammatory bowel disease. An abdominoperineal resection can be performed as two simultaneous procedures, with one team opening the abdomen while the other prepares the perineal area, or as a two-stage procedure, with one team operating. A colostomy is usually performed to facilitate removal of waste products.

Position: When performed with two teams, the patient is usually placed in a modified lithotomy position, with the sacrum elevated on folded towels or a sandbag. If one team is operating, the patient may start in the supine position and later be moved to a modified lithotomy position (or surgeon's preference).

Incision Site: Vertical or transverse abdominal Elliptical sagittal for perianal and perirectal area

Skin Preparation: See pp. 337–338

Packs/Drapes: Laparotomy drape (abdomen)
　Lithotomy pack for perirectal portion

Instrumentation:
　Major Lap tray
　Intestinal tray
　Closing tray
　Basic (minor tray) for perineal approach
　Hemoclips/surgiclip appliers (size variety)
　Large retractor (surgeon's choice)
　Anal retractor; Volkman Rake (4 prong) (opt.)
　Internal stapling instruments (opt.)

Supplies/Equipment:
　Basin set
　Lithotomy stirrups with padding and sandbags
　Blades—(4) No. 10, (1) No. 15
　Needle counter (2 or 3)
　ESU; suction (2 or 3)
　Vessel loops or umbilical tape (retraction)
　Hemoclips/surgiclips (size variety)
　Colostomy supplies

Drainage (Penrose; Hemovac; Jackson-Pratt)
Solutions—saline, water
Medications
Sutures—surgeon's preference

PROCEDURAL OVERVIEW

(To avoid confusion during this discussion, the procedure will be described as if being done by one team.)

The abdomen is entered through a long midline incision. The extent and level of the pathology is determined. The portion of the colon to be removed is mobilized by dividing the mesenteric and vascular attachments to the bowel, carrying the dissection to the rectum. The ureters and other adjacent structures are identified, and otherwise avoided unless they are to be removed. The colon is transected proximally. The distal portion (the transected end which is protected from spillage by the use of moist Lap sponges, clamps, or an intestinal bag secured by umbilical tape) is dissected into the depths of the pelvis, transecting the lateral rectal stalks (middle hemorrhoidal vessels) to the level of the coccyx. As mobilization continues, longer instruments will be needed.

At this point, the abdominal dissection is halted because the depth of the incision is too great for the surgeon to work comfortably.

To prepare the site for the colostomy, the surgeon incises a small circle in the abdomen using the skin knife. The incision is deepened to the inner abdomen, and the small disk of tissue is passed off as a specimen. The proximal end of the bowel is brought through the circular incision, and temporarily clamped in placed, while the abdominal incision is closed in a routine manner. The surgeon then everts the edges of the bowel stoma and sutures the edges to the skin using interrupted suture (3-0 chromic on a fine cutting needle), creating the colostomy stoma. This procedure can be facilitated by using internal stapling instruments.

Perineal Resection

The perineal portion of the surgery begins with the closure of the anus using a purse-string suture of heavy silk, and the perineum is incised using an elliptical sagittal incision, deepened and incising the levator muscles. The pelvis is entered, and the previous dissected distal colon and proximal rectum are passed into the perineal wound. The rectum is excised (avoiding the urethra, prostate, and vagina) and hemostasis is achieved. The wound is irrigated (with an Asepto syringe) and the perineal wound is closed in layers over one or more drains. A bulky abdominal dressing is applied, and a colostomy bag is placed over the stoma or a temporary dressing of Vaseline gauze is applied with a corresponding abdominal dressing.

PERIOPERATIVE NURSING CONSIDERATION

- When a modified lithotomy position is used, the abdominal and perineal approaches should be performed by two teams.
- For a two-stage procedure (one team), the patient is prepared and draped for the second stage after the abdomen has been closed.
- Bowel technique is used, and all instruments contacting the bowel are isolated; the specimen is received in a basin, and is isolated from the field; the abdomen is closed with clean instruments.
- Since there are two separate surgical procedures being performed, even if only one team is operating, additional care must be exercised to avoid confusion during the counting procedures. Documentation should reflect separate counts for each stage.

Rectal Surgery

Procedure
Hemorrhoidectomy

Definition: Excision of painful, distended veins of the anus and rectum

CDC Classification: III

Discussion: Hemorrhoids are classified as internal or external, depending on their location. Hemorrhoids are generally associated with local anal problems such as anal ulcers and fistulas, or they may accompany pregnancy. Anesthesia may be regional, local, or general.

A proctosigmoidoscopy may be performed prior to the open procedure.

Position(s): Lithotomy, modified lateral (Sims), or jackknife

Skin Preparation: The buttocks is taped apart with wide adhesive tape on each side of the anus, attaching the other end to the table frame. Only a minimal prep is usually performed.

Packs/Drapes: Laparotomy pack (jackknife or lateral Sims position)

Lithotomy pack (lithotomy position)

Instrumentation:
Minor tray
Rectal tray with dilators and retractor
Sigmoidoscopy instruments (opt.)

Supplies/Equipment:
Stirrups
Pillows or roll for positioning
ESU; suction
Blades—(1) No. 10, (1) No. 15
Basin set (minor)
Needle counter
Hemostatic agent (Surgicel; Gelfoam)

Lubricant
Pressure dressing (impregnated gauze sponges; 4 × 4's; A.B.D.'s)
Laser (opt.)

PROCEDURAL OVERVIEW

Before beginning the surgical procedure, a sigmoidoscopy may be performed, followed by gentle dilation of the rectum. The rectal specula is lubricated and inserted. The hemorrhoid is grasped with a Pennington, Allis, or Kocher clamp. The proximal portion of the hemorrhoid is excised by scalpel, cautery, or laser. If the anus is stenotic, the distal internal sphincter may be incised.

A mucous membrane flap and/or skin flaps may be used to cover the denuded areas. Bleeders are controlled with ligature ties (3-0 Dexon/chromic) or by cautery. Care is taken not to excise too much skin, anoderm, or mucous membrane and to avoid injury to the sphincter mechanism.

PERIOPERATIVE NURSING CONSIDERATIONS

- Be prepared to perform a sigmoidoscopy prior to the procedure.
- When ESU is used, apply the ground pad after the patient has been placed in the lithotomy position.
- Protect the skin under the adhesive tape with tincture of benzoin.
- Should laser be used, all safety precautions must be in place prior to the patient's entry into the procedure room (CO_2 or ND:Yag).

Related Surgical Procedures:
Excision of Venereal Warts
Rectal Polypectomy

Procedure
Pilonidal Cystectomy and Sinusectomy

Definition: Removal of a cystic mass containing hair, skin, tissue debris, etc., most often located in the sacrococcygeal area. A sinus tract (channel leading to an abscess) is often present. The cyst is usually removed when it causes recurrent infection in the area.

CDC Classification: III

Discussion: The term *pilonidal* refers to any dermoid cyst in a nest formation, and therefore can be found about the perineum. When acutely or chronically infected, surgical treatment is indicated. Such cysts are often caused by a congenital defect that allows epithelial tissue to be trapped below the surface of the skin in the area of the sacrum and coccyx. These cysts may be very extensive with multiple and deep side tracts.

Position: Lithotomy; jackknife; or lateral Sims
Skin Preparation, Packs, Drapes: See Hemorrhoidectomy, p. 475
Instrumentation:
　Rectal tray
　Minor tray
　Extra probes (available)
　Curettes (opt.)
　Rake retractors (opt.)
Supplies/Equipment:
　Basin set
　Blades—(1) No. 10, (2) No. 15
　ESU; suction
　Needle counter
　Methylene blue with blunt needle and syringe (opt.)
　Pressure dressing
　Packing gauze (Iodofor) (opt.)

PROCEDURAL OVERVIEW

The patient is properly positioned, and the buttocks is prepared as for a hemorrhoidectomy.

The surgeon begins by placing a probe into the sinus tract, if one exists. The probe identifies the exact location of the sinus and the cyst itself. Dye may be injected into the tract for further identification.

An incision is made about the cyst or into the cyst directly. Necrotic tissue, hair, debris, etc. are curetted and/or excised, including the cyst wall. Bleeders are controlled with cautery or sutures (3-0 Dexon, chromic).

The wound can be packed open, in the presence of active infection; closed; or completely closed by means of tissue flaps.

PERIOPERATIVE NURSING CONSIDERATIONS

- If purulent drainage is encountered, the CDC classification must change to Class IV.
- As with a hemorrhoidectomy, protect the patient's skin under the tape with tincture of benzoin.
- If using the lithotomy position, apply the ESU ground pad after final positioning.

Related Surgical Procedure: Excision of Anal Fistulas

BILIARY SURGERY

Surgical Anatomy Review

The *liver*, considered an accessory digestive organ, lies under the right side of the diaphragm, and is divided into two major regions: the right and left lobes. The lobes are separated by a fold of parietal peritoneum (*falciform ligament*), which attaches the liver to the anterior abdominal wall. The under surface of the liver is anchored to the lesser curvature of the stomach by the lesser omentum, through which travels the hepatic artery, the hepatic-portal vein, and the common bile duct. The inferior vena cava is partially embedded on the posterior surface of the liver.

The liver receives blood from two sources: the hepatic artery, which supplies it with oxygenated blood from the aorta, and the hepatic portal vein, which carries venous blood from the digestive tract, pancreas, and spleen.

The liver has an external covering (*Glisson's capsule*), which is composed of dense connective tissue, and the peritoneum extends over the entire surface of the liver, except at the point of posterior attachment to the diaphragm.

Another biliary structure is the *gallbladder;* a pear-shaped fibromuscular bag that hangs from the undersurface of the right liver lobe. The gallbladder has two sections: a rounded extremity, the fundus, which commonly projects beyond the liver's edge, and a pointed extremity, the ampulla, or *Hartman's pouch.*

The ampulla leads to a narrow S-curved neck, to which the stem (cystic duct) is attached. The cystic duct connects the gallbladder to the trunk of the biliary tree, and joins with the hepatic duct from the liver to form the common bile duct. The pancreatic duct joins the common bile duct, and the two ducts share a common entrance into the duodenum.

The *pancreas* lies transversely behind the stomach in the upper abdomen. The pancreas, nicknamed "the fish" because of its unusual shape, consists of three segments: the head, the body, and the tail.

The head of the pancreas is fixed to the curve of the duodenum, and shares a blood supply with the duodenum. The body lies across the vertebrae, over the superior mesenteric vasculature. The tail extends to the hilus of the spleen. At the junction of the pancreatic duct and common bile ducts the *ampulla of Vater* enters into the duodenum, allowing digestive enzymes to escape into the GI system for absorption and excretion.

Additionally, the pancreas contains a group of specialized cells, located in the *islets* (island) *of Langerhans.* These cells secrete two hormones into the bloodstream—insulin and glucagon—both of which are associated with carbohydrate metabolism.

The *spleen* is the largest lymphoid organ in the body. It lies in the left *hypochondriac* region, between the fundus of the stomach and the diaphragm. Its size and weight vary with each person, as well as in the same person under a variety of situations.

The spleen has two distinct surfaces: the diaphragmatic surface, which is smooth and convex, and the

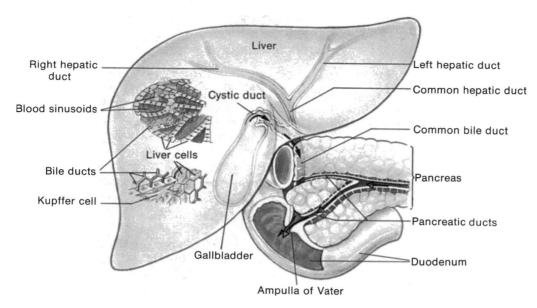

Fig. 14-5. Biliary system: liver and the associated structures

visceral surface, divided into the gastric and renal colic surface, which conforms to the organs adjacent to it. Blood vessels enter and leave the spleen through a region on the visceral surface called the *hilus.*

Like any lymph node, the spleen is covered by a strong fibrous capsule with trabeculae that extend into the organ, dividing it into compartments. The spleen contains two types of tissues: red pulp and white pulp, containing specific types of cells, including lymphocytes, RBCs, and macrophages. Blood enters the spleen via the splenic artery hilus, enters the venous sinuses, and exits through the splenic vein, then travels within the hepatic portal vein network to the liver (Fig. 14-5).

Procedure
Hepatic Resection

Definition: A small wedge biopsy, local excision of tumor, or a major lobectomy.

CDC Classification: II

Discussion: Indications for a hepatic resection include trauma, cysts, or tumors (benign, primary, or secondary). A preoperative CT scan or angiogram can delineate the involved pathology.

Position:

For partial left lobe excision: Supine, with arms extended on armboards

For major lobe resection: Modified lateral position with elevation of hepatic area (Bean-Bag; Vac-Pac)

The position will be determined by the section of the liver to be resected

Incision Site: Thoracoabdominal (right lobe), subcostal; midline abdominal (left lobe)

Skin Preparation: See pp. 337–338

Packs/Drapes: (depending on approach)
  Major Lap pack
  Transverse Lap sheet
  Four folded towels

Instrumentation:
  Major tray
  Chest tray (thoracoabdominal approach)
  Vascular instruments
  Biliary instruments
  Hemoclips/surgiclips (size variety)
  Internal stapling instruments

Supplies/Equipment:
  Basin set
  Blades—(3) No. 10
  ESU; suction (2)
  Hypothermia unit (opt.)
  Cell saver (opt.)
  Dissecting sponges (Kittners)
  Needle counter
  Vessel loops
  Umbilical tape (opt.)
  Hemostatic agents (e.g., Helistat; Gelfoam Thrombostat; Avitine; Cryoprecipitate)
  Sutures—surgeon's preference
  Internal stapling instruments (opt.)
  Hemoclips/surgiclips (variety)
  Solutions—saline; water

For thoracoabdominal approach: Chest tubes with drainage system and ATS (opt.)

PROCEDURAL OVERVIEW

1. Wedge Resection
    a. The abdomen is entered.
    b. A wedge is cut from the edge of the liver, or an automatic stapling device can be used.
    c. Incised edges are closed.
    d. Wound is irrigated and closed.
2. **Hepatic Lobectomy:**
    The incision and feasibility of the resection is determined. If a thoracoabdominal incision is used, the abdominal portion is incised first. The incision is completed through the seventh or eighth interspace, incising the diaphragm. The hepatic artery, portal vein, and major biliary ducts are controlled by vascular forceps or vessel loops. The liver parenchyma is divided, pausing to ligate the major vessels and biliary channels.

    Careful technique is necessary when approaching the posterior surface, since the hepatic veins enter the inferior vena cava at this location. If bleeding is extensive, the vena cava may be controlled by the insertion of a balloon catheter, intracavally.

After hemostasis is obtained, and the bile ducts are ligated, the exposed parenchyma may be covered by the greater omentum or absorbable hemostatic agents. The wound is irrigated with warm saline, the drains are inserted, and the wound is closed in layers.

PERIOPERATIVE NURSING CONSIDERATIONS

*   Confirm with blood bank the number of available units.
*   Consult with the surgeon and the anesthesiologist about using the thermal blanket and cell-saver unit.
*   A ''hotknife'' or ''plasma scalpel'' may be used.
*   For a thoracoabdominal approach, obtain and prepare the chest drainage system.
*   Confirm an ICU bed if requested (lobectomy).

Related Surgical Procedures: Repair of Lacerated Liver

Procedure
Cholecystectomy (Open)

Definition: Removal of a diseased gallbladder
CDC Classification: II, if no spillage is encountered
Specific Technique: No-touch technique
Discussion: In acute cholecystitis, the normally bluish-green gallbladder becomes distended and inflamed due to obstruction by one or more gallstones. In removing the gallbladder, the common duct is left unimpaired so that it becomes a functional passageway for the elimination of bile via the duodenum.

Position: Supine, with arms extended on armboards. A small pad may be placed under the right upper quadrant to facilitate exposure of the gallbladder
Incision Site: Right subcostal, right paramedian, midline
Skin Preparation: See pp. 337–338
Packs/Drapes: Laparotomy pack
    Four folded towels
Instrumentation:
    Major Lap tray
    Biliary instruments
    Hemoclip/surgiclip appliers (size variety)
Supplies/Equipment:
    Positioning aids
    Basin set
    Blades—(1) No. 10, (1) No. 15
    Hemoclips/surgiclips
    ESU; suction
    Needle counter
    Penrose drain (1 inch)
    Dissector sponges (Kittners)
    Culture tubes (aerobic/anaerobic)
    Foley catheter with drainage system (opt.)
    For Intraoperative Cholangiogram:
    Catheter—cholangiocath with radiopaque dye
    Syringes—(2) 30 mL
    X-ray cassette drapes (opt.)
    Special OR table (radiop surface)

PROCEDURAL OVERVIEW

Once the abdomen is entered, the liver is covered with a moist Lap sponge and retracted gently upward (Deaver or Harrington).

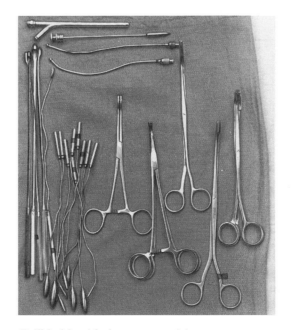

Gallbladder (cholecystectomy) instrument set

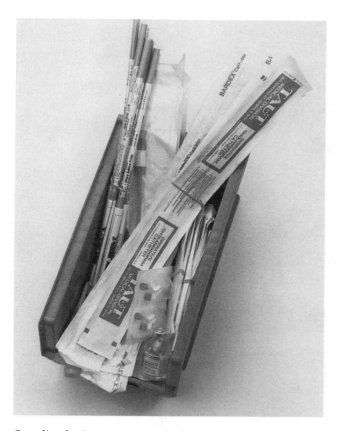

Supplies for intraoperative cholangiogram

If the gallbladder is greatly distended, the surgeon may drain it of bile by the use of a trocar attached to suction. A Kelly clamp is usually placed over the hole made by the trocar to prevent spillage of bile into the abdomen. The trocar should be handed off the field or placed in a separate basin.

The gallbladder is grasped (Kelly or Pean) and the cystic duct, cystic artery, and common bile duct are exposed. The cystic duct is double-clamped (two right-angle clamps) and ligated with 2-0 silk tie or hemoclips/surgiclips. The cystic artery is clamped and ligated in the same manner. The gallbladder is mobilized by incising overlying peritoneum, and is removed. The underlying liver bed may be reperitonealized (3-0 or 4-0 chromic; fine tapered needle). A drain (1-inch Penrose) is inserted via a stab wound.

Intraoperative Cholangiography Common Duct Exploration

This diagnostic procedure is performed prior to the ligation of the cystic duct.

The surgeon will place two traction sutures (3-0 silk) through the wall of the duct. An incision is then made between the sutures with a No. 15 blade or a Potts scissors. The scrub person should have prepared a catheter (cholangiocath), radiopaque dye, and a 30–50-

mL syringe. The dye should be prepared according to the surgeon's preference (usually diluted with saline). Air bubbles must be removed from the syringe, since these may appear as gallstones on the x-ray.

The catheter is passed through the stump of the cystic duct into the common bile duct. A suture or special cystic duct clamp should be placed at the end of the catheter. It may or may not be sutured. Before x-rays are taken, the wound is covered with a sterile towel, and all metal instruments are removed from the field.

Should the x-rays reveal the presence of stones, further exploration of the common duct is indicated; if no stones are present, the catheter is removed and the cystic duct is ligated.

At the close of the procedure, a T-tube is inserted into the common duct via a fine tissue forceps (Cushing). The ductal incision is then closed (3-0 or 4-0 silk; fine tapered needle), and the long end of the tube is brought out of the wound and later will be attached to a special "bile bag" to facilitate drainage while the wound heals.

The wound is irrigated with warm saline, and closed in the routine fashion.

PERIOPERATIVE NURSING CONSIDERATIONS

- Correct positioning is imperative to assure accurate visualization of the biliary tract.
- A scout film should be taken before the procedure.
- Syringes filled with saline and dye must be labeled to avoid confusion and ensure successful x-ray exposures.
- Catheters and drains should be tested for patency with normal saline before use.
- Drains are usually anchored with a skin stitch.
- Instruments coming into contact with the gallbladder and/or bile should be isolated in a basin.

Related Surgical Procedures: Choledochosopy
Cholecystotomy
Choledochotomy

Procedure
Laparoscopic Cholecystectomy
(with or without laser)

Definition: Cannulation of the gallbladder under direct laparoscopic visualization, and removal of the gallbladder
CDC Classification: II
Special Technique: No-touch technique
Discussion: This procedure presents an alternative to formal laparotomy and open cholecystectomy, and has a number of advantages, including reduction of hospital stay and postoperative recovery time. However, if

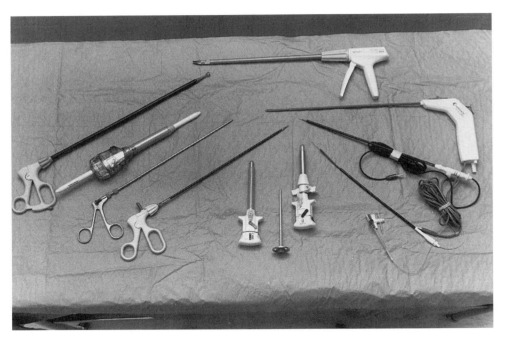

Disposable laparoscopic cholecystectomy instrumentation (Courtesy of Ethicon, Inc., Sommerville, NJ)

needed, following laparoscopic evaluation of the gallbladder and surrounding tissues an open procedure can be performed. Additionally, this procedure can employ the use of a laser via the laparoscope.

Preoperative Evaluation of Candidates
The choice of patient selection for this procedure is based on several factors, including:

1. The results of abdominal ultrasound, to confirm presence of gallstones and detect any dilation of intrahepatic or extrahepatic bile ducts.
2. If suspected gallstones in duct, ERCP (endoscopic retrograde cholangiopancreatography) is advised.
3. Patient should be a candidate for open cholecystectomy, with appropriate preoperative workup, including a biochemical profile.

Contraindications (Absolute)
Contraindications for this mode of treatment include pregnancy, acute cholangitis, septic peritonitis, and severe bleeding disorders, and patients who are not candidates for an open laparotomy because of coexisting medical illness.[4]

Positioning, Skin Preparation, Packs, Drapes: Same as for a cholecystectomy and/or laparoscopy, depending on surgeon's preference

Incision Sites: Umbilicus (laparoscope), anterior axillary, upper midline, midclavicular (operative trocar sites)

Instrumentation:
Endoscopic cholecystectomy instruments
Pneumoperitoneum instruments (disposable or nondisposable trocar and sheath)
Major tray
Biliary tray (available)
Endoclips

Supplies/Equipment:
Insufflation device
Fiberoptic light source
ESU; suction
NG tube
Blades—(1) No. 15 or (1) No. 11
Basin set
Additional equipment/supplies for open cholecystectomy with cholangiogram
Laser (opt.)

PROCEDURAL OVERVIEW

Following positioning, the insufflation needle (Veres or Surgineedle) is placed through a small incision just above the umbilicus, into the peritoneal cavity. A polyethylene tube is connected to the insufflation device and the needle. A pneumoperitoneum is established with approximately 2 to 4 liters of carbon dioxide, until the meter registers 12 to 14 mm Hg of intraabdominal pressure. The pneumoperitoneum is necessary to visualize the abdominal cavity contents with the laparoscope.

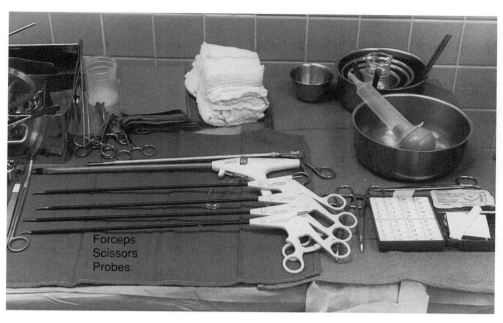

Laparoscopic cholecystectomy instrumentation

The insufflation needle is withdrawn, and the incision is enlarged. The trocar and sleeve (10 or 11 mm) is inserted into the abdomen.

The trocar is withdrawn from the sleeve, and the proper location of the sleeve is confirmed.

An operating laparoscope (10 or 11 mm) with attached camera is inserted through the sleeve to confirm intraperitoneal placement. The carbon dioxide tubing is attached to the sleeve to maintain the inflation of the abdomen.

Accessory Trocar Placement

Two additional puncture wounds are created, and accessory trocars are placed under direct laparoscopic visualization (Fig. 14-6):

1. Ten-mm trocar with cannula is placed between the xiphoid and the umbilicus, to the right of the midline;
2. Five-mm trocars are placed just below the right costal margin; one anterior axillary line and one at the midclavicular line. These two sites can be used for various laparoscopic instruments (including laser), which are inserted to manipulate and dissect the gallbladder and other anatomic structures.

If cholangiograms are required, an endoclip is placed proximately to the cystic duct and a small incision is made just below the clip. A cholangiocatheter is inserted through the midclavicular cannula and directed into the ductal system.

The gallbladder is removed from the liver bed using

electrocautery and/or laser dissection (Fig. 14-7). Occasionally, the presence of very large stones prohibits removal of the gallbladder through the umbilical incision, and in this case, a fascial incision is extended slightly as needed until extraction is complete. The op-

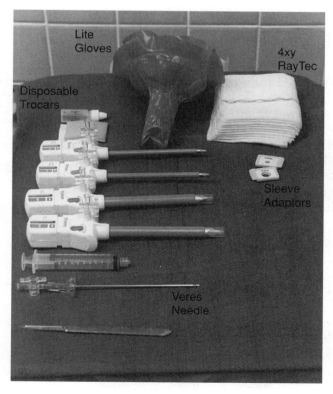

Mayo tray set-up laparoscopic cholecystectomy

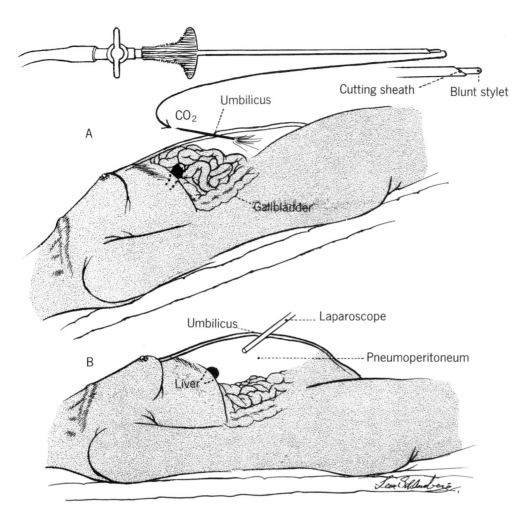

Cutting sheath --- Blunt stylet

Umbilicus

CO₂

A

'Gallbladder'

Umbilicus --------- Laparoscope

B

Liver

Pneumoperitoneum

Fig. 14-6. Laparoscopic cholecystectomy (Copyright © 1991, 1996. United States Surgical Corporation. All rights reserved. Reprinted with the permission of United States Surgical Corporation.)

erative site is irrigated with copious amounts of sterile saline, and the field is observed for possible bleeding sites or bile leakage.

The sheaths are removed after hemostasis has been obtained, and the puncture wounds closed (2-0, 3-0, and 4-0 absorbable sutures).

PERIOPERATIVE NURSING CONSIDERATIONS

- If anticipating the use of the laser, all safety factors must be in place prior to beginning the procedure.
- Check all equipment to promote safety and avoid prolonging anesthesia.
- Heparinized saline solution may be used to irrigate the abdominal cavity and retard clot formation.
- Foley catheter and NG tube should be inserted before beginning the procedure.
- Allow adequate time for room set-up and preparation, owing to amount of extra equipment.

- Patient needs to be prepared (physically and mentally) for the possibility of an open procedure.

Procedure
Pancreatoduodenectomy (Whipple Procedure)

Definition: Removal of the head of the pancreas, the very proximal portion of the jejunum, the distal third of the stomach, and the distal half of the common bile duct, with reestablishment of continuity of the biliary, pancreatic, and gastrointestinal tracts.
CDC Classification: II, unless gross contamination occurs
Specific Technique: No-touch technique
Discussion: This procedure is usually performed for regional malignancy and benign, obstructive, or chronic pancreatitis.

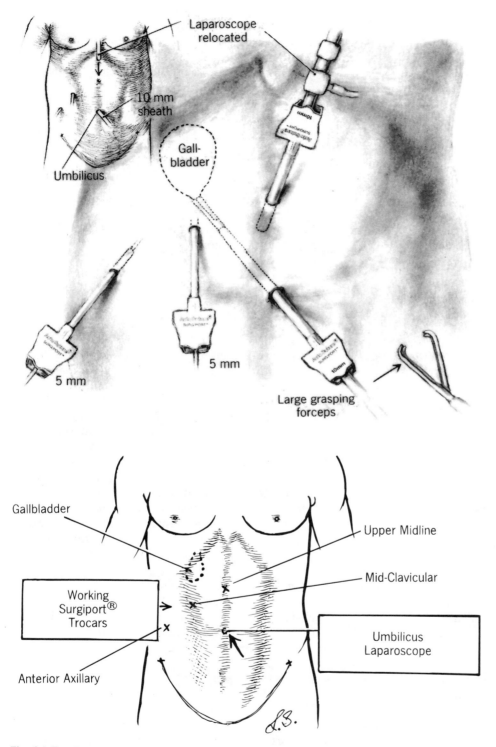

Fig. 14-7. Removal of the gallbladder. (Copyright © 1991, 1996 United States Surgical Corporation. All rights reserved. Reprinted with the permission of United States Surgical Corporation.)

Position: Supine, with arms extended on armboards
Incision Site: Transverse, midline, or paramedian incision
Skin Preparation: See pp. 337–338
Packs/Drapes: Laparotomy pack
    Transverse Lap sheet (opt.)
    Four folded towels
Instrumentation:
    Major Lap tray
    Biliary instruments
    Intestinal tray
    Harrington retractors
    Hemoclip/surgiclip (size variety)
    Internal stapling instruments (opt.)
Supplies/Equipment:
    Basin set
    Blades—(2) No. 10, (1) No. 15
    ESU; suction
    Hemoclips/surgiclips (size variety)
    Dissector sponges (Kittners)
    Needle counter
    Internal staplers (opt.)
    Drains—for retractors: Penrose 1 in. for Drainage: HemoVac, Jackson, Pratt, etc.
    Sutures—surgeon's preference
    Solutions—saline, water
    Medications—hemostatic agents, etc.

PROCEDURAL OVERVIEW

The abdomen is opened and explored; the operability of the findings is assessed. The distal portion of the stomach, extrahepatic biliary tract, head of the pancreas, and entire duodenum are immobilized. (With a total pancreatectomy, a splenectomy and cholecystectomy with vagotomy may be indicated.) If the tumor has invaded the base of the mesocolon, portal vein, aorta, vena cava, or superior mesenteric vessels, this procedure is usually abandoned, and a lesser procedure (usually a bypass of the biliary tree and/or stomach) will be performed.

The proximal end of the jejunum is anastomosed to the distal pancreas. The common bile duct is anastomosed to the jejunum with an end-to-side technique. The distal stomach is anastomosed to the jejunum (also end-to-side). Stapling instruments may be used to mobilize and transect multiple blood vessels and in transection of the stomach and to perform the gastrojejunal anastomosis. Additionally, various plastic stents may be placed in the biliary or pancreatic anastomosis.

The wound is irrigated, drains inserted and secured, and the abdomen is closed in layers.

PERIOPERATIVE NURSING CONSIDERATIONS

- Verify with the blood bank the number of available units.
- Accurate intake and output recording is essential for adequate replacement therapy.
- Instruments that have touched "dirty" areas must be isolated (no-touch technique).
- Scrub person should receive specimens in a basin.
- Have appropriate stents available, unopened.

Related Surgical Procedures:
    Partial Pancreatectomy (removal of the tail of the pancreas)
    Excision of a Pancreatic Cyst
    Pancreatojejunostomy
    Pancreaticocystogastrostomy

Procedure
Splenectomy

Definition: Removal of the spleen
CDC Classification: II, unless gross contamination occurs
Discussion: The most common indication for a splenectomy is accidental traumatic injury. Other indications include hematologic disorders, congenital anemia, splenomegaly (portal hypertension), tumors, or cysts. A splenectomy may also be indicated as the result of trauma during surgery (e.g., gastrectomy; mobilization of splenic flexure of the colon); however, it is repaired rather than removed whenever possible.

If a splenectomy is performed for a hematologic disorder, accessory spleens are also sought and removed.
Positioning: Supine, with arms extended on armboards
Incision Sites: Midline, left subcostal
Skin Preparation: See pp. 337–338
Packs/Drapes: Laparotomy pack or basic pack with transverse Lap universal pack (trauma)
Instrumentation:
    Major Lap tray
    Biliary tray (opt.)
    Intestinal tray
    Hemoclip/surgiclip appliers (size variety)
    Harrington retractor (opt.)
Supplies/Equipment:
    Basin set
    Blades—(2) No. 10, (1) No. 15
    Cell-saver unit (opt.)
    ESU; suction
    Hemoclips/surgiclip appliers (size variety)
    Dissector sponges (e.g., Kittners)

Needle counter
Sutures—surgeon's preference
Solutions—saline, water
Medications—hemostatic agents

PROCEDURAL OVERVIEW

The surgeon enters the abdomen and explores the surrounding area and contents. In situations where the spleen is extremely large, a combined thoracoabdominal incision may be used to allow for greater visualization and manipulation.

The reservoir portion of the cell saver should be set up for immediate suction during trauma, since the abdomen is often filled with blood. Manual removal of clots may be required; therefore, a basin is brought to the incision following entry and exposure.

The spleen is identified, and the splenic hilum is isolated, taking care not to injure the tail of the pancreas. Using sharp dissection (Metzenbaum scissors), the spleen is dissected free from its abdominal attachments.

Once the spleen is mobilized, the splenic artery and veins are identified. Two or three right-angle clamps (vascular clamps) are placed across the structures, and are ligated (2-0 or 3-0 silk ties) separately or together. The vessels are then severed, completely freeing the spleen.

The wound is irrigated with warm saline, and the area further explored for bleeders. When complete hemostasis has been achieved, the abdomen is closed in layers in a routine fashion. If optimal hemostasis cannot be achieved, or there is a question of pancreatic surgery, a closed wound drainage system may be required.

PERIOPERATIVE NURSING CONSIDERATIONS

- The reservoir component of the cell-saver unit should be set up first to accommodate the large amount of blood loss that may occur (trauma surgery).
- Accurate intake and output recording is essential for proper replacement therapy.
- A large number of lap sponges may be needed owing to the vascular nature of the spleen and its components.
- The patient will probably require an ICU bed following surgery, and may leave the procedure room intubated, depending on existing circumstances. The postanesthesia area should be notified of equipment that may be necessary.

HERNIA REPAIRS

Surgical Anatomy Review

The Inguinal Region

The anterior abdominal wall is made up of the muscular fibers and the aponeurostic extensions of the internal and external obliques, the transversus, the rectus abdominis, and occasionally the pyramidalis muscles.

The inguinal portion of these muscles is attached principally to the inguinal ligament and is tunneled through by the inguinal canal. The inguinal canal lies superior to the medial half of the inguinal ligament and supplies communication between the abdominal cavity and the outside. It transmits to the round ligament in the female and the testicle and spermatic cord in the male.

The inguinal ligament is a heavy condensation of the lower most external oblique aponeurosis fibers strung between the anterior superior iliac spine and the pubic tubercle. It is an important anatomic landmark, separating the inguinal from the femoral triangles and establishing the relationships of all the surgically significant structures of both regions.

The ligament is divided into the lateral and medial half. The lateral half serves partly as a line of attachment for the internal oblique and transversus abdominis muscles. The medial half represents the inferior boundary of the inguinal triangle. Its outer two thirds are covered by the insertion of the cremaster muscle and fascia, and only after this veil is detached are the inguinal ligaments barred and the canal clearly visible.

The frequent occurrence of both congenital and acquired herniations through the inguinofemoral quadrants (bilateral) gives this region special surgical significance. While basically the anatomy does not alter much from patient to patient, changes ranging from gross hypertrophy to total atrophy in certain structures give the local anatomy a variable picture, especially in adults.

The Femoral Region

The femoral ring is a rigid aperture between the abdomen and the thigh. It lies beneath the medial insertion of the inguinal ligament and is surrounded by three ligaments and a vessel (femoral vein).

Reduction of a femoral hernia is sometimes difficult because of the rigidity of the femoral ring. Some authorities describe separate femoral and inguinal incisions for the repair of femoral hernias. However, the unpredictability of the findings and the difficulty of reducing the contents usually justify the routine use of an incision that can expose the entire inguinofemoral region.

The Umbilical Region

In fetal life, the umbilicus is a centrally located aperture in the anterior abdominal wall that transmits the umbilical vessels, the urachus, and the oomphalomesenteric duct. Once umbilical circulation is shut off, the aperture becomes obliterated with scar tissue and is covered by corrugated skin.

An umbilical hernia may be congenital or acquired. In children, the congenital variety predominates, while in the adult, it is the opposite. It is very similar to an incision hernia, in that both are due to stretching of a scar. The repair of both, therefore, is essentially the same.

There is one more, less frequently encountered hernia, in the epigastric region, located between the xyphoid process and the umbilicus, on the abdominal wall. If a defect occurs in this region, an epigastric hernia has developed.

Procedure
Herniorrhaphy

Definition: Repair of a herniation (protrusion) of the abdominal contents, caused by a musculofascial defect in the abdominal wall or groin area.
CDC Classification: I, unless incarcerated with bowel
Discussion: In the inguinal/femoral regions, two types of herniation commonly occur: direct or indirect.

1. *Direct Hernia:* Usually resulting from stress, causing the peritoneum to bulge through the fascia in the groin area. The peritoneal bulge (sac) may contain abdominal viscera.
2. *Indirect Hernia:* Caused by a congenital defect in the internal abdominal ring, causing the peritoneum to bulge along the spermatic cord. It may or may not contain abdominal viscera.

In addition, a hernia can occur within an old scar that is usually located in the abdominal (ventral) region, and is referred to as an *incision hernia.*

Hernias are either reducible or irreducible—that is, incarcerated. The contents of an incarcerated hernia may become strangulated, compromising the viability of trapped tissues and thus necessitating their resection in addition to the herniorrhaphy.

For the purpose of this discussion, the inguinal herniorrhaphy will be highlighted. However, the perioperative nurse should be aware of the other surgical techniques related to the specific type of hernia encountered.
Position: Supine, with arms extended on armboards
Incision Site: Groin area, right or left oblique

Skin Preparation: See pp. 337–338
Packs/Drapes: Laparotomy pack or minor (basic) pack
   Four folded towels
Instrumentation:
   Basic (minor) tray
   Self-retaining retractor (e.g., Gelpi, Wietlander) (opt.)
Supplies/Equipment:
   Basin set
   ESU; suction
   Needle counter
   Penrose drain (¼ in. for retraction)
   Dissector sponges (e.g., Kittners)
   Sutures—surgeon's preference
   Solutions—saline, water
   Synthetic mesh (opt.)
   Skin closure strips (e.g., Steri-Strips) for subcuticular closure

PROCEDURAL OVERVIEW

The surgeon begins the procedure by incising the groin. The incision is deepened using the Metzenbaum scissors and cautery is used to control small bleeders. Both blunt and sharp dissection are used to gain access to the hernia. After incising the fascia that lies over the spermatic cord (male), several small hemostats are placed on the edge of the incised fascia (used as retraction).

If direct, the surgeon will begin to suture the defect using interrupted suture (2-0) of varying materials.

If indirect, the surgeon will dissect the sac away from the cord using a Metzenbaum scissors; the sac is opened and the edges grasped with hemostats. The contents of the sac are pushed toward the abdomen (usually with the surgeon's index finger), and if small, the sac may be ligated in place.

For a large sac, a purse-string suture may be used to close the sac. The sac is closed near the abdominal wall, and the edges removed. (*Note: this becomes the specimen.*) The wound is closed in individual layers:
Fascia Layer: 2-0 nonabsorbable suture, with or without a strip of synthetic mesh for extra strength (for recurrent hernias) sewn directly to the fascia edges.
Subcutaneous Layer: 2-0 nonabsorbable suture, with application of Steri-Strips, as a subcuticular closure, or subcutaneous and skin closure performed in a routine manner (skin staples, etc.).

PERIOPERATIVE NURSING CONSIDERATIONS

- The Penrose drain should be moistened with saline before use.
- Synthetic mesh (surgeon's preference) is often used to repair recurrent hernias or large ventral hernias. Follow sterilization instructions.

- A specimen will be collected only during an indirect herniorrhaphy.

Related Surgical Procedures:
Incision Herniorrhaphy
Umbilical Herniorrhaphy
Femoral Herniorrhaphy

PROCEDURES INVOLVING THE BREAST

Surgical Anatomy Review

Although associated with the female reproductive system, breast surgery is performed by a general surgeon, and will therefore be considered in this section.

The breasts lie over the pectoral muscles and are attached to them by a layer of connective tissue (fascia). Laterally, the glands extend over the serratus anterior muscle. *Estrogens* and *progesterone*, two ovarian hormones, control their development during puberty. Breast size is determined more by the amount of fat around the glandular tissue than by hormone production.

Each breast consists of several lobes separated by *septa* of connective tissue. Each lobe consists of several lobules, which in turn are composed of connective tissue in which are embedded the secreting cells (*alveoli*) of the gland, arranged in grapelike clusters around minute ducts. The main ducts converge toward the nipple, and enlarge slightly before reaching the nipple into small reservoirs.

The *mammary gland,* as it is often called, is contained within the two layers of the superficial fascia covering the chest wall, and its size and location vary greatly depending on the age and the functional status at the time of surgery.

Occasionally, the glandular tissue extends beyond the circumference of the breast mass proper, and invades the axilla. When it does, this "axillary tail" perforates the axillary fascia. This axillary tail of the gland may be the site of a primary growth, and frequently is mistaken for lymph nodes.

The mammary gland is supplied by an extensive network of lymphatic vessels, which drain into adjoining and distant lymph nodes, both deep and superficial. The blood supply enters the gland at its lateral and medial aspects (internal mammary and lateral branches of the anterior aortic intercostal arteries).

A knowledge of the lymphatic drainage of the breast is critically important in clinical medicine because cancerous cells from malignant breast tumors often spread to other areas of the body through the lymphatics.

Adipose tissue is deposited around the surface of the gland, just under the skin, and between the lobes. The nipples are bordered by a circular pigmented area (*areola*), which contain numerous sebaceous glands that appear as small nodules under the skin. (See Chap. 13, Exercise 25 for anatomy review.)

Operative Procedures

Breast surgery can be divided into two types, depending on the results desired:

1. *Diagnostic procedures:* Breast biopsy (as a singular procedure, e.g., breast biopsy with frozen section)
2. *Corrective procedures:* Removal of the involved segment of the breast, with an accompanying biopsy (e.g., breast biopsy, possible mastectomy)

Benign or malignant tumors of the breast and infections indicative of a pathologic condition are some of the more common and emotionally distressing health problems confronting women today, although men may also be subject to these conditions.

Procedure
Excision of Breast Mass (or Biopsy)

Definition: The removal of suspected tissue to determine the nature of the mass and/or confirmation of a diagnosis by way of a frozen section tissue examination.
CDC Classification: I, unless abscess/infection is present
Special Technique: If preceding a mastectomy, the biopsy is performed using the no-touch technique
Discussion: For treatment of breast cancer, surgery ranges from the removal of only the tumor (mass) to a radical mastectomy involving the breast and all surrounding tissue. The choice of surgical intervention is dependent on the size, location, and stage of the disease.
Position: Supine, with arms extended on armboards. Affected side may be elevated on towels or sandbag.
Incision Site: The site of the suspected lesion
Skin Preparation: See pp. 337–338
Packs/Drapes: Basic laparotomy pack (single procedure)
Extra Mayo cover, if combined with mastectomy
Four folded towels; one towel bunched in the axillary area
Transverse Lap sheet (for mastectomy only)
Instrumentation:
Minor tray (for biopsy only)

Supplies/Equipment:
Basin set
Blades—(2) No. 10 and/or (1) No. 10 and (1) No. 15
ESU; suction
Needle counter
Small drain (e.g., ¼-in. Penrose)
Sutures—surgeon's preference
Hemoclips/surgiclips (opt.)
Solutions—saline, water
Medications—local anesthesia agent (opt.)

PROCEDURAL OVERVIEW

The incision is generally made over the lesion. For central lesions, a circumferential incision may be used. The incision is deepened with the cautery pencil or dissecting scissors. Using a handheld retractor (Rake; Army-Navy) the underlying tissue is exposed and grasped with an Allis or Kocher clamp, which is used to lift up the mass as dissection continues. Small bleeders are controlled with cautery and/or hemoclip/surgiclip application. When the dissection is complete, the specimen is passed off for a frozen section examination, on a towel or in a basin, never on a counted sponge or instrument.

After hemostasis is obtained, the tissue is approximated with interrupted suture (3-0 Dexon; chromic). A drain may be inserted if the surgical permit does not specify a mastectomy to follow the biopsy. The skin is closed with fine subcuticular suture or fine interrupted skin suture.

PERIOPERATIVE NURSING CONSIDERATIONS

- Circulator should confirm the operative side with the patient.
- Prepping is performed with gentle motion so as not to disturb the cell pattern.
- Exercise extreme caution when handling the specimen to avoid misidentification (multiple biopsies).
- No specimen may leave the procedure room on a counted sponge or instrument. It should be placed in a dry specimen container, and be properly labeled.
- If procedure is being performed under local anesthesia with sedation, tissue requisition should be marked to avoid announcement of the biopsy result to an unprepared patient (e.g., THIS PATIENT IS AWAKE).
- If a mass is suspected, and permit is signed for a possible mastectomy, the patient is prepped and draped for a mastectomy, and all instruments used on the biopsy are isolated. The biopsy segment is considered a separate procedure, requiring separate counts.

Procedure
Mastectomy

Definition: Removal of the breast, with or without surrounding structures
CDC Classification: I, unless abscess/infection is noted
Special Technique: No-touch technique
Discussion: Mastectomies can be performed in four distinct methods, depending on the diagnosis and the extent of the pathologic findings.

1. *Partial Mastectomy:* Excision of breast tumor, leaving appropriate tumor-free margins.
2. *Subcutaneous Mastectomy:* Removal of all breast tissue. Overlying skin and nipple are left intact.
3. *Simple Mastectomy*
4. *Radical Mastectomy*
   a. Modified radical—removal of breast and axillary lymph nodes. Most frequently performed.
   b. Classic radical—includes removal of entire breast, pectoralis muscles, axillary lymph nodes, fat, fascia, and adjunct tissues.
   c. Extended radical—en bloc removal of breast, axillary contents, pectoralis muscles, and internal mammary lymph nodes.

Criteria for Choice of Technique

1. A partial mastectomy, followed by radiation therapy, is now more widely preferred.
2. A subcutaneous mastectomy is recommended for patients with small, centrally located, and noninvasive tumors, or if implants are to be used.
3. A classic radical is infrequently performed unless there is invasion of deeper tissue.
4. A simple mastectomy is preferred for patients who have malignant lesions in which axillary fat and lymphatic tissue are excised. Pectoralis muscles may be removed to encompass more widely any potential tumor recurrence.
5. An extended radical may require resection of the ribs and sternum, with skin graft for closure.

Position: Supine, with arms extended on armboards; folded sheets or sandbag under the affected shoulder
Incision Site: Dependent on the proposed technique
Skin Preparation: See pp. 337–338
Packs/Drapes: Major Lap pack (transverse sheet opt.)
   Impervious stockinette (opt.)
   Extra drape sheet (½ or ¾)
   Extra Mayo tray cover (for biopsy)
   Note: The affected arm, once draped with stockinette, is brought through the fenestration (free draping).

Instrumentation:

> Major Lap tray
> *Additional:*
> Curved Crile hemostats, Gelpi and/or Weitlander
> (self-retaining retractors)
> Hemoclip/surgiclip appliers (size variety)
> Rake retractors (4–6 prong)
> Lahey clamps (8–10)
> Intraductal probes (opt.)
> Minor tray (for biopsy)

Supplies/Equipment:

> Basin set
> Blades—(3) No. 10, (1) No. 20
> ESU; suction
> Needle counter
> Drainage system (e.g., HemoVac; Jackson-Pratt)
> Pressure dressing
> Suture—surgeon's preference
> Solutions—saline, water
> Medications—surgeon's preference

PROCEDURAL OVERVIEW

Partial Mastectomy

The incision is usually made over the lesion. The skin is elevated and the breast mass is excised. Hemostasis is controlled, and the wound is irrigated with warm saline or water. The wound is closed in a routine fashion, and if a drain is used, it is secured.

Simple Mastectomy

The skin is incised using an elliptical incision around the breast. The incision is deepened with the cautery pencil or second knife, and the skin flaps are elevated. Kocher or Allis clamps are placed along the skin edge and retracted upward as the dissection continues.

Once the skin flaps have been raised, the breast is freed from the chest wall at the level of the fascia (entire dissection may be accomplished with the cautery pencil).

If the incision extends into the axilla, sharp dissection is performed (Metzenbaum scissors). If a lymph node is needed for a frozen section examination, the tissue is grasped with an Allis clamp and dissected free.

Once the breast is completely mobilized, it is removed en bloc, and placed in a basin for fixed specimen evaluation.

The wound is irrigated with warm saline (or water if preferred) and the drainage system established. If a HemoVac drain is used, the drainage tubes are brought out of the skin flap through two stab wounds created with the HemoVac trocar. The skin is then closed, and the drains are secured with the surgeon's choice of suture and skin closure material.

Modified Radical

A transverse or longitudinal skin incision is performed. The dissection, as previously discussed, is performed, and the incision is extended well into the axilla.

The axillary contents are dissected free from the vascular and nerve structures, and are carefully removed. Care must be taken to avoid injury to the nerve supply to various muscles. After hemostasis is achieved, the skin flaps are approximated over the drains (Hemo-Vac). The wound is irrigated with warm saline (or water) and closed as described for a simple mastectomy.

PERIOPERATIVE NURSING CONSIDERATIONS

- If a mastectomy is to follow a biopsy, the drape should be reinforced with clean towels; the team should change gloves, and the biopsy instruments removed. This is done to prevent cross-contamination of the wound by cancerous cells released during the biopsy.
- Additional personnel may be needed to hold the arm during a circumferential extremity skin prep.
- Often a great deal of dissection is performed with the electrocautery pencil. Keep the tip clean, and replace it as needed.
- Several knife blades may be needed because of the fibrous nature of the tissue incised. Notify surgeon when changing the blades.
- Irrigation solution may be water in place of saline in order to lessen the survival of the tumor cells. Check with the surgeon as to preference, and label the container accordingly.
- Estrogen and progesterone assays may be requested. Check with the lab manual for proper preparation of the specimen.
- If a skin graft is required, one thigh must be prepared and draped along with the main operative site.

PROCEDURES OF THE NECK

Two structures, commonly associated with procedures of the neck, are the *thyroid gland* and its associate structures, and the *trachea.*

Although performed by general surgeons, procedures involving the trachea will be discussed in association with nose and throat surgery. Surgery involving the thyroid gland will be discussed in this section.

Surgical Anatomy Review

Two fairly large lateral lobes and a connecting portion, the *isthmus,* constitute the thyroid gland. It is located

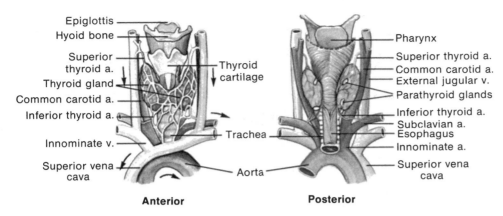

Fig. 14-8. Thyroid and associated structures

in the neck, just behind the larynx. The isthmus lies across the anterior surface of the upper part of the trachea.

Thyroid tissue is made up of several structural units called *follicles,* whose outer cuboidal epithelium is composed largely of an iodine-containing protein, giving the thyroid gland a unique ability to actively take up and concentrate blood iodine.

The *parathyroid glands* are adjacent structures, and consist of small round bodies attached to the posterior surface of the lateral lobes of the thyroid gland. The hormone secreted by these glands—parathyroid hormone—is chiefly responsible for maintaining homeostasis of blood calcium concentration by promoting cal-

cium absorption into the blood, essential for blood clotting, among other functions (Fig. 14-8).

Procedure
Thyroidectomy

Definition: Removal of all or a portion of the thyroid gland

CDC Classification: I

Discussion: This procedure is usually performed to treat various diseases of the thyroid gland (e.g., hyperthyroidism or cancer) that cannot be treated effectively by chemotherapy or medication. A total thyroidec-

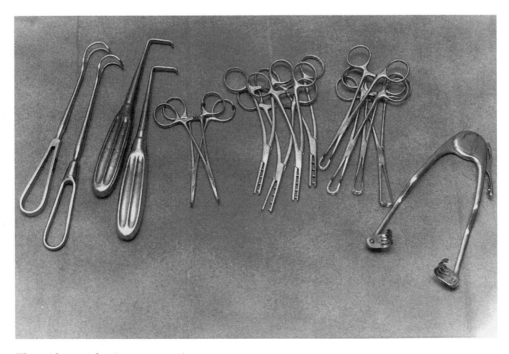

Thyroid specialty instrumentation

tomy is indicated for certain carcinomas and to relieve tracheal or esophageal compression.

Position: Supine, with rolled towel or sandbag between the scapulae, hyperextending the neck. If table is placed in reverse Trendelenberg position, a padded footboard should be used to prevent the patient from slipping down toward the end of the table

Skin Preparation: See pp. 337–338

Packs/Drapes: Laparotomy pack with small fenestrated sheet
    Rolled sheet/towels

Instrumentation:
    Major Lap tray
    Thyroid tray (opt.)
    Lahey clamps (opt.)
    Spring retractor

Supplies/Equipment:
    Basin set
    ESU; suction
    Blades—(2) No. 10, (1) No. 15
    Needle counter
    Dissector sponges (e.g., Kittners)
    Small drain (e.g., ¼-in. Penrose)
    Solutions—saline, water
    Sutures—surgeon's preference

PROCEDURAL OVERVIEW

The incision is made above the sternal notch. The platysma muscle is incised and retracted. The strap muscles are separated or divided, and blunt and sharp dissection are employed until the thyroid is exposed. The gland is then mobilized, and all or part is removed depending on the involved pathology. Hemostasis is obtained, and the wound is irrigated with warm saline. A drain may be inserted, and the incision is closed in layers by an interrupted method.

PERIOPERATIVE NURSING CONSIDERATIONS

*   The surgeon may request a fine silk suture to use to mark the incision line.
*   The dressing is usually secured by a thyroid collar using a towel folded in thirds lengthwise. The towel is placed around the neck and crisscrossed in front, then fastened with tape.
*   The scrub person should maintain the sterility of the back table/Mayo until the patient is extubated and breathing is stabilized (in case of airway problems).
*   In many hospitals, an emergency tracheostomy tray will accompany the patient to the postanesthesia care unit and later to the patient's room until breathing is unlabored and the chance of airway obstruction secondary to edema has passed.

Related Surgical Procedures: Parathyroidectomy
    Thyroglossal Duct Cystectomy

GYNECOLOGIC AND OBSTETRIC SURGERY

Gynecologic and obstetric procedures involve the organs of the reproductive system (see Chap. 13, Exercise 24). Additionally, urological procedures, for female incontinence, are included with gynecologic procedures.

Surgical Anatomy Review

The word root, *gyne,* stems from the Greek word meaning *women.* Therefore, gynecology is the branch of medicine which deals with diseases of the genital tract (reproductive system) in women.

For the purpose of description, the organs involved with the reproductive system can be divided into two areas:

1. Those located within the pelvic cavity.
2. Those associated with the internal and external genitalia.

Structures located within the abdominopelvic cavity consist of the *uterus, fallopian tubes,* and *ovaries.* The structures associated with the internal and external genitalia are collectively called the *vulva* (pudendum), and include the *mons pubis, labia majora* and *minora, clitoris, vestibular glands* (greater and lesser), *hymen,* and the *perineum.* See Chapter 13, Exercise 24 for anatomic insights.

Internal Organs of Reproduction

The Uterus

The uterus (*womb*) is a single, hollow, pear-shaped organ that receives the fallopian (uterine) tubes at its upper lateral angles, and is continuous below with the vagina.

The uterus is divided into three sections. The upper portion is called the *body.* Below the body, the uterus narrows into the *isthmus,* and at the point where it joins with the *vagina,* it forms the cylindrical *cervix.* The opening of the uterus into the vagina is the *ostium* of the uterus. The dome-shaped region of the uterine body, above and between the points of entrance of the fallopian tubes, is called the *fundus.*

The uterus lies in the pelvis, behind the urinary bladder and in front of the sigmoid colon and rectum.

The layers of peritoneum that cover the uterus anteriorly and posteriorly fuse along the lateral margins and extend to the walls and floor of the pelvic cavity. This is known as the *broad ligament,* which somewhat anchors the uterus. Assisting the broad ligament in holding the uterus in place are the *round ligaments,* which are fibrous bands that run within the broad ligament from the lateral margins of the uterus (near the junction with the fallopian tubes), through the inguinal canal, into the labia majora.

These ligaments do not hold the uterus tightly in place, but allow it to have some degree of limited movement. Normally, the uterus is tipped forward, forming a 90-degree angle with the vagina.

The wall of the uterus is covered by a serosa formed by the peritoneum, created from the broad ligament. Beneath this serosa lies a thick muscular layer, the *myometrium.* The uterine cavity is lined with epithelium that, along with an underlying connective tissue, constitutes the *endometrium.* It is this layer that undergoes changes during the menstrual cycle, and if the *ovum* (egg) is not fertilized, this functional layer of the endometrium is sloughed off as menstrual flow.

The Fallopian Tubes

The fallopian tubes, also known as the *ovarian tubes,* extend from the vicinity of the superior lateral angle of the uterus to the *ovaries,* and lie between the layers of the broad ligaments bilaterally.

The fallopian tubes are known as the *site of implantation* (fertilization), specifically in the ampulla, closest to the ovary. The distal end of each tube (*infundibulum*) opens into the abdominopelvic cavity very close to an ovary, and is surrounded by small, ciliated, finger-like projections called *fimbria.*

Note: Since the reproductive tract (in the female only) opens into the peritoneal cavity through the two fallopian tubes and to the exterior of the body through the uterus and vagina, infections of the lower reproductive tract can spread into the body cavity and cause *peritonitis.*

The Ovaries (Female Gonads)

The two ovaries are the primary sex organs of the female in which the eggs (*ova*) are produced. Each ovary is oval and slightly smaller than its male counterpart, the *testis.* The ovaries, like all organs of both male and female, are *retroperitoneal,* and lie against the lateral wall on either side of the uterus. The ovaries are held in place by several ligaments, the largest being the broad ligament, which also supports the fallopian tubes, the uterus, and the vagina. A fibrous band (*ovarian ligament*) lies within the broad ligament and extends from the superior-lateral margins of the uterus to the ovary, while the lateral margins of the broad ligament form

a fold that attaches the ovary to the pelvic wall. This structure is called the *suspensory ligament.*

If one of the ovaries is removed, the menstrual cycle and reproductive capabilities remain intact, as long as the uterus is still present. However, removal of both ovaries will produce *surgical menopause* in younger women of childbearing age, and menstruation will cease.

The Vagina (Birth Canal)

The vagina is the canal that leads from the cervix of the uterus to the exterior of the body. The mucosal lining of the vagina serves as a protective surface layer, composed of stratified squamous epithelium, as is typical of all canals that open onto the body surface. Near the entrance to the vagina, the mucosa usually forms a vascular fold called the *hymen,* which generally blocks only a portion of the vaginal opening, but in some cases completely closes the orifice.

External Genitalia

When considered collectively, the external genitalia are known as the *vulva* or *pudendum.*

Because of the influence of estrogen in the female, fatty tissue is deposited over the *pubic symphysis.* This produces a mound called the *mons pubis.* This area becomes covered with hair following puberty.

Two rounded folds, the *labia majora,* extend posteriorly from the mons; the outer surface is covered with hair and the inner surface is smooth and moist because of the presence of large sebaceous glands.

The *labia minora* are two smaller folds located medial to the labia majora, anteriorly surrounding the *clitoris,* a small elongated structure located at the anterior junction of the labia minora. The labia minora are highly vascular and lack hair. They surround a space, the *vestibule,* into which the vagina and urethra open.

The Vestibular Glands

The vestibular glands, so-called because they lie within the vestibule of the external genitalia, include the *Skene's glands* (the lesser vestibular glands), and the *Bartholin's glands* (the greater vestibular glands).

Skene's glands are two small paired glands that lie beneath the floor of the urethra, while Bartholin's glands lie on either side of the vaginal orifice. Because of their location, they are frequently subject to infection.

The Perineum

The perineum is the skin-covered muscular region between the vaginal orifice and the anus. This area has great clinical importance because of the risk of its being torn during childbirth or other traumatic injuries. If this important support structure is weakened, partial uterine or vaginal prolapse can result.

Gynecologic Surgery Overview

Gynecologic surgery is performed either for diagnostic purposes or as corrective procedures. The diagnostic component includes those that are invasive, such as a biopsy of the cervix, laparoscopy, hysteroscopy, and those that are noninvasive, such as an exam under anesthesia, Pap smear, or pelvic ultrasonography.

Gynecologic procedures can be performed either by an *abdominal* or *vaginal* approach, or by using a combination approach: *abdominovaginal*.

Highlights of the Abdominal Approach

1. The supine position with slight Trendelenberg's is often used for *abdominopelvic* procedures. Preparation of the patient and the packs and drapes used are same as for any abdominal approach.
2. Instrumentation includes a basic laparotomy tray, with the addition of gynecologic instruments, including long instruments for reaching deep inside the pelvic cavity.
3. Instruments coming into contact with the cervix are considered contaminated and should be placed in a separate basin and not brought back to the field (no-touch technique).

Highlights of the Vaginal Approach

1. Usually performed in the lithotomy or modified lithotomy position.
2. Instrumentation includes those sufficient in length for use deep inside the vaginal canal and/or uterine cavity.
3. In addition to the standard instruments, a vaginal set-up may include a *dilation and curettage* tray, since it may be performed prior to the repair/revision procedure.
4. Sponge, sharp, and instrument counts are required on all invasive vaginal procedures.
5. The bladder may or may not be drained, depending on the surgeon's preference. If an indwelling catheter is not required, a straight Robinson catheter may be used for drainage of the bladder.
6. A *D&C* procedure (dilation and curettage) without additional surgery may be set up without a full surgical scrub or the application of a sterile gown by either the scrub person or circulating nurse. Refer to hospital protocol for proper technique.

Highlights of the Abdominovaginal Approach

1. If a combined procedure is performed, the vaginal procedure precedes the abdominal procedure (e.g., D&C, possible abdominal hysterectomy).
2. Separate set-ups are required, and each procedure requires a separate sponge, sharp, and instrument count, which is documented accordingly.
3. Vaginal preps are performed separately from the abdominal prep, except for a laparoscopy, which is performed as one procedure; beginning with the abdominal area and progressing to the vaginal area.
4. If a Foley (indwelling) catheter is required, the insertion procedure is performed as a separate procedure following (or in conjunction with) the vaginal prep.

ABDOMINAL PROCEDURES

During abdominal procedures, a right-handed surgeon usually stands at the patient's left side, thus allowing the best access to pelvic structures. Additionally, the operating table may be placed in a slight reverse Trendelenberg position, to tip the abdominal contents away from the operative area for better visualization.

Procedure
Abdominal Hysterectomy

Definition: Surgical removal of the entire uterus through an abdominal incision.
CDC Classification: II
Special Technique: No-touch technique
Discussion: A hysterectomy is indicated for a variety of conditions, including endometriosis, adnexal disease, postmenopausal bleeding, dysfunctional uterine bleeding, and benign fibromas or malignant tumors. For women in their childbearing years, this surgery, as with a vaginal hysterectomy, can be a devastating blow psychologically, since they may feel they have lost their primary sexual characteristic and therefore can no longer function as women.

Postoperative depression, therefore, is not uncommon following a hysterectomy, and should be approached from a multidisciplinary point of view with the added support from the family.
Positioning: Supine, with arms extended on armboards

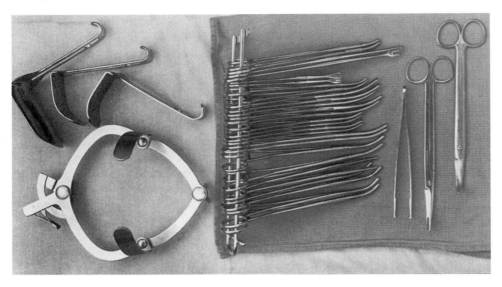

Abdominal hysterectomy instrumentation

Incision Site(s): Lower transverse (Pfannenstiel), vertical, midline, or paramedian (lower)
Skin Preparation: See pp. 337–338
Packs/Drapes: Laparotomy pack and/or transverse Lap sheet
  Four folded towels
Instrumentation:
  Major Laparotomy tray and/or abdominal hysterectomy tray
  Self-retaining retractor (e.g., O'Sullivan-O'Connor; Balfour)
  Internal stapling instruments (opt.)
Supplies/Equipment:
  Basin set
  Blades—(3) No. 10 or (1) No. 20 and (2) No. 10
  Needle counter
  ESU; suction
  Foley catheter with drainage bag
  Solutions—saline, water
  Suture—surgeon's preference
  Internal stapling instruments (opt.)

PROCEDURAL OVERVIEW

Although a lower midline incision can be used for a hysterectomy, the Pfannenstiel approach will be discussed here, since many gynecologic procedures can be performed through this incision.

After incising the skin, the incision is deepened through the subcutaneous tissue with the deep knife or cautery pencil. The next layer (fascia) is nicked with the deep knife and incised using a curved Mayo dissecting scissors. Grasping one edge of the fascial margin with two or more Kocher clamps, blunt dissection separates the fascia from the underlying muscle.

The muscle layer is divided manually. The peritoneum is then knicked with the deep knife, and the incision is lengthened with the Metzenbaum scissors. A self-retaining (e.g., O'Sullivan-O'Connor or Balfour) retractor is placed in the wound, with moist Lap sponges to protect the wound edges; the surgeon will "pack the bowel" away from the uterus with additional moist warm Lap sponges, and the operating table is placed in slight Trendelenberg position.

The uterus is isolated by severing it from the uterine ligaments and adnexa (ovaries and fallopian tubes). The round ligaments of the uterus are ligated, divided, sutured, and tagged with a hemostat. Most surgeons prefer a particular type of clamp, but the most common are Heaney, Ochsner, or Kochers. Absorbable suture is almost always used to ligate the ligaments, mounted on a heavy, tapered needle.

To divide the ligaments, a curved Mayo scissors or scalpel is used. An internal stapling device can be used to free the uterus from the adnexa.

The surgeon mobilizes the uterus to the level of the bladder. At this level, the bladder is continuous with the uterus, since both organs are attached by the peritoneal covering. Using a Metzenbaum scissors and long tissue forceps, the surgeon separates the two structures by dissecting the peritoneal covering away from the bladder. This is called the *bladder flap,* and will be reattached (*reperitonealized*) later. Once the bladder has been separated from the uterus, mobilization is continued as previously described.

At the level of the cervix, long Allis or Kocher clamps are placed around the edge of the cervix, and it is divided from the vagina using a long scissors (pelvic scissors) or a long knife. This can also be accomplished through internal stapling instruments. When using staples, the vaginal vault is closed prior to the resection of the uterus, reducing the possibility of contamination of the peritoneal cavity.

If the ovaries are to be preserved, the ovarian ligament is ligated and divided adjacent to the uterus (avoiding the ureters). The uterosacral ligaments are ligated and divided, along with the cardinal ligaments.

The uterus, now completely free, is passed off as a specimen, along with the instruments that have contacted the cervix or vagina (no-touch technique).

To close the wound, if surgical staples have not been used, the surgeon begins by suturing the vagina (vaginal vault) using an absorbable suture. Following closure, the bladder flap is reperitonealized, using chromic, Dexon, or Vicryl on a fine needle (2-0 or 3-0).

The wound is irrigated with warm saline, and hemostasis is achieved. To close the peritoneum, the surgeon grasps the edges with several Kelly hemostats and the peritoneum is closed with a running suture (0-chromic or Dexon) on a taper needle. The muscle tissue may be loosely approximated (4-0 chromic) and the fascia is closed with a variety of sutures depending on the surgeon's preference. The subcuticular tissue is usually approximated with plain or Dexon suture (3-0; taper needle), and the shin is closed according to surgeon's preference.

PERIOPERATIVE NURSING CONSIDERATIONS

- Foley catheterization is usually performed after the internal vaginal prep is completed but before the abdominal prep is begun.
- A sterilization permit may be required in addition to the operative permit. Consult institutional protocol.
- Instruments that have come in contact with the cervix and/or vagina must be treated as contaminated and discarded into a basin that can be passed off the field (usually with the specimen).
- Once the abdomen is opened, 4 × 4 Raytec sponges should be replaced by Lap sponges. Raytecs should only be used on a sponge stick for blunt dissection and/or hemostasis.
- If a free sponge has been placed in the vagina prior to closing (hemostasis), it is included in the sponge count and must be removed from the vagina before the count is correct and the patient leaves the room.
- Internal staples are usually contraindicated in severe cases of pelvic inflammatory disease or endometriosis. Check with the surgeon prior to the case to obtain the stapling device(s) of choice.

Procedure
Tubal Ligation

Definition: The interruption or ligation of the fallopian tubes, resulting in sterilization.
CDC Classification: II
Discussion: Postpartum tubal ligations are best performed 24 to 36 hours after vaginal delivery, although it can be performed at other times, such as during a cesarean section or as an elective procedure.

Tubal ligations can be performed via a minilaparotomy, a laparoscopy, or, rarely, by a posterior colpotomy, and can either be done with suturing technique, internal stapling, or cauterization of the ends of the tubes, once severed.
Procedural Techniques: Pomeroy/Irving

A.	*Pomeroy:*	Faster, but carries the risk that the ends of the tube may recommunicate at a later date.
B.	*Irving:*	Ensures that the two severed ends of the tube will not rejoin, but takes longer.

Positioning: Minilaparotomy: supine, with arms extended on armboards
  Laparoscopy/colpotomy: lithotomy (modified); arms may be extended on armboards
Incision Site(s): Minilaparotomy: suprapubic
Laparoscopy: See p. 503 for description
Skin Preparation: Dependent on approach
Packs/Drapes: Minilaparotomy: Laparotomy pack
  Folded towels
  Laparoscopy: Laparoscopy pack
Instrumentation:
  Minilaparotomy: Basic or tubal tray
  Hemoclip/surgiclip appliers
  Internal stapling instruments (LDS, opt.)
  Laparoscopy: See p. 503
Supplies/Equipment:
  Minilaparotomy: Basin set
  Blades—(2) No. 15
  Needle counter
  ESU; suction; solutions
  Hemoclips/surgiclips (opt.)
  Laparoscopy: See p. 503
  Fallopian rings (opt.)

PROCEDURAL OVERVIEW

For the purpose of this discussion, a minilaparotomy procedure will be described. The laparoscopic approach will be discussed later in this chapter.

A small incision (lower midline or Pfannenstiel) is made, followed by an opening into the peritoneal cavity. Each tube is grasped with a Babcock clamp, and the tubal procedure is performed (cautery, suture, or internal staple) on a section of the tube. The peritoneum is approximated, irrigated, and closed in layers.

PERIOPERATIVE NURSING CONSIDERATIONS

- Specimens should be placed in separate containers, and labeled right and left.
- A separate sterilization consent form may be required. Consult with institutional protocol concerning the consent form.

Procedure
Tuboplasty of the Fallopian Tubes

Definition: Reestablishment of patency to the fallopian tubes

CDC Classification: II

Discussion: A tuboplasty is usually performed when the patient seeks a reversal of a sterilization procedure. Success depends on the amount of tubal destruction.

Positioning: If dye is to be injected to determine potency, the patient is placed in the lithotomy position, then returned to the supine position.

Incision Site: Pfannenstiel or low midline

Skin Preparation: If a catheter is used for dye insertion, an internal vaginal prep is required, in addition to the abdominal prep

Packs/Drapes: Laparotomy pack with transverse sheet,
   Microscope drape (for microsurgery)

Instrumentation:
   D&C tray
   Major tray
   Microsurgical instruments
   Beaver knife handle
   Mosquito hemostats (curved and straight)
   Frazier suction tips
   Bipolar forceps (cautery)

Supplies/Equipment:
   Stirrups (for initial positioning)
   Basin set
   Blades—(2) No. 10, (1) No. 15, (1) No. 11, Beaver
   ESU; suction; bipolar ESU
   Microscope (check with surgeon as to lens magnification preference)
   Needle counter
   Pediatric catheter or special cannula, syringe extension tubing
   Dye (e.g., methylene blue)
   Solutions—saline, water
   Sutures—surgeon's preference
   Special tubing for tuboplasty (opt.)
   Laser (opt.) to open adhesions

PROCEDURAL OVERVIEW

The peritoneal cavity is entered and a self-retaining retractor is placed in the wound. Tubal patency may be demonstrated by injection of methylene blue through a cervical cannula. The tuboplasty is performed according to the site of the obstruction; for example, cornual resection with reimplantation, tubal resection with anastomosis and fimbrioplasty. The operating microscope is often used, and a laser beam may be directed through the microscope to open adhesions of the fimbria and to lyse lesions within the tubes. The abdomen is closed in layers, and the cervical cannula is removed.

PERIOPERATIVE NURSING CONSIDERATIONS

- Be careful when changing positions (lithotomy to supine), and make sure the stirrups are padded to prevent nerve damage.
- If laser is employed, all safety procedures must be in place prior to the start of the procedure.
- The microscope should be draped prior to the establishment of the sterile field, to save anesthesia personnel time.
- See D&C (p. 498) for additional considerations.

Procedure
Salpingo-Oophorectomy

Description: The removal of one (unilateral) or both (bilateral) fallopian tubes and corresponding ovary.

CDC Classification: II

Discussion: This procedure may be performed in conjunction with a hysterectomy or as a separate procedure. As a separate procedure, it is usually performed for a variety of nonmalignant diseases that include acute and chronic infection, cysts, tumors, and hemorrhage owing to tubal pregnancy. Malignancy of a tube or ovary will usually necessitate a hysterectomy with excision of the opposite adnexae.

Positioning: Supine, with arms extended on armboards

Incision Site, Skin Preparation, Packs, Drapes: See Abdominal Hysterectomy, p. 493

Instrumentation:
   Major tray or abdominal hysterectomy tray
   Internal stapling instruments (opt.)
   Self-retaining retractor

Supplies/Equipment:
   Basin set
   Blades—(2) No. 10, (1) No. 15
   Needle counter
   ESU; suction
   Solutions—saline, water
   Sutures—surgeon's preference

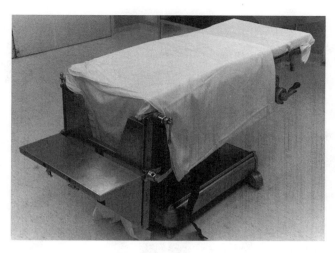

Operating room table with footboard extension used as a Mayo tray while surgeon is seated for vaginal hysterectomy

PROCEDURAL OVERVIEW

The abdomen is entered through a low midline or Pfannenstiel incision, depending on the size of the patient and the known pathologic condition. (If a bilateral procedure is anticipated, a low midline incision is used.)

The peritoneal cavity is entered and a self-retaining retractor is placed in the wound. The operating table is placed in slight Trendelenberg position, and the incision is packed with moist Lap sponges. The uterus is grasped with a tenaculum or uterine elevator, and if adhesions are present, the affected tube and ovary are isolated from surrounding organs.

The tube(s) are grasped with one or two Babcock clamps. Two Kelly or uterine clamps are then placed across the ovarian vessels. The tissue is divided between the clamps with a knife, dissecting scissors, or cautery pencil. Internal staples can also be used to accomplish this task. The infundibulopelvic ligament is ligated and divided, as is the broad ligament attached to the tube and ovary. The tube and ovary are excised.

If internal staples are *not* used, a suture ligature (0-chromic; Dexon) is used to ligate the ovarian vessels. This procedure is repeated on the other side (if bilateral). The raw surface of the ovarian ligaments left by the dissection are reperitonealized using a running suture (0 or 2-0 chromic; taper needle). The wound is irrigated with warm saline, and closed in a routine fashion.

PERIOPERATIVE NURSING CONSIDERATIONS

- For bilateral surgery, a sterilization permit may be required in addition to the operative permit. Consult with institutional protocol.
- When the specimen is collected (if bilateral), each side should be labeled and in separate containers, depending on hospital policy.

VAGINAL PROCEDURES

As discussed earlier, the patient is usually in the lithotomy position for vaginal procedures, and the surgeon is often seated during the surgery.

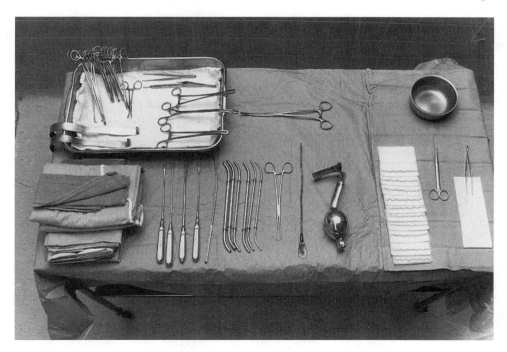

D&C instrumentation supply set-up

Because of this unusual position, a Mayo tray on a stand is often eliminated and the scrub person usually stands to the side of the surgeon. It is important to maintain the sterility of the field, and *not* allow sterile items (instruments/suture) to be passed behind the surgeon. When a Mayo tray is required (e.g., for a vaginal hysterectomy), it is usually placed on the surgeon's lap, over a double-thickness drape, or the footboard of the operating table may be used as a Lap tray extension when placed perpendicular to the lowered portion of the operating table.

Procedure
Dilation and Curettage (D&C)

Definition: The gradual enlargement of the cervical os and the curetting (scraping) of endometrial or endocervical tissue for histologic study.

CDC Classification: II

Discussion: The procedure is usually performed to (1) diagnose cervical or uterine malignancy; (2) control dysfunctional uterine bleeding; (3) complete an incomplete abortion; (4) aid in evaluating infertility; and/or (5) relieve dysmenorrhea. Additionally, *fractional D&C* procedures can assist in differentiating between endocervical and endometrial lesions.

Positioning: Lithotomy; arms may be extended on armboards

Skin Preparation: See pp. 337–338

Packs/Drapes: Gynecologic pack

Instrumentation: D&C tray

Supplies/Equipment:
    Stirrups (padded)
    Telfa (for specimen)
    Perineal pad
    ESU; suction (opt.)
    Lubricant (e.g., K-Y jelly)

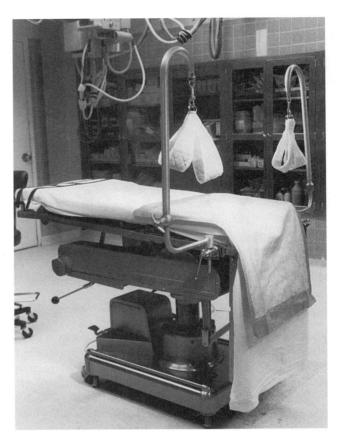

Operating room table with D&C stirrups

PROCEDURAL OVERVIEW

A weighted speculum is placed in the vaginal vault. The cervix is grasped with a tenaculum. A graduated sound is passed through the cervical canal into the uterine cavity to determine its depth and angulation.

Using Hegar or Hank dilators, the surgeon begins to dilate the cervical opening, increasing the size of each dilator. A Telfa sponge is placed over the bill of the weighted speculum, and the uterus is gently curetted, allowing the tissue specimen to collect on the Telfa sponge.

The small serrated curette is used to scrape the uterine walls again or when the D&C is performed to re-

move retained placental tissue, while the large, blunt curette and forceps are used to remove the tissue.

If a fractional D&C is performed, endocervical curettings are obtained before the uterus is sounded, to avoid bringing endometrial cells into the cervical os.

The weighted speculum is removed, and the perineum is dressed with a perineal pad.

PERIOPERATIVE NURSING CONSIDERATIONS

- Stirrups should be padded, and a coccygeal support placed on the table to protect the lower sacral area.
- Raise and lower the legs together and slowly to prevent disturbances caused by rapid alterations in venous return and/or injury to the rotator hip joint.
- Instruments are set up on the back table in order of usage; a scrub person may not be necessary during the procedure.
- If a fractional D&C is performed, multiple specimens may be obtained. They should be placed in separate containers, and labeled accordingly (follow institutional protocol).

Procedure
Conization of the Cervix

Definition: Excision of a cone of tissue surrounding the cervical os.
CDC Classification: II
Discussion: This procedure is usually performed to diagnose and/or treat conditions such as cervicitis, epithelial dysplasia, and carcinoma in situ. Conization can be performed as either a "cold" or a "hot" knife conization.

> *Cold Conization:* A scalpel and scissor dissection of the tissue
> *Hot Conization:* Tissue removal by use of electrosurgical cautery with special tip

If the procedure is performed with a D&C, the D&C is performed first.
Positioning, Skin Preparation, Drapes: See D&C Procedure, p. 498
Instrumentation:
    D&C tray
    Cervical cone biopsy instruments
Supplies/Equipment:
    Same as for D&C, with the addition of:
    Cautery pencil with special tip
    Blade—(1) No. 11
    Shiller's or Lugol's solution (opt.)
    Long cotton-tipped applicators
    Neo-Synephrine (1:200,000) to reduce bleeding with needle, syringe (opt.)
    Hemostatic agent (e.g., Surgicel, Thrombostat)
    Perineal pad
    Sutures—surgeon's preference (opt.)
    Solutions—saline, water

PROCEDURAL OVERVIEW

A D&C is performed first. The cervix may be stained with Shiller's or Lugol's solution (surgeon's preference), and sutures are placed at the 3 o'clock and 9 o'clock positions. The cervix may be injected circumferentially with a phenylephrine (Neo-Synephrine) solution. The uterine canal is carefully sounded. An incision is made circumferentially around the cervix using a scalpel or cautery.

Alternatively, a cervical cyst may be electrodesiccated with a needle electrode. Bleeding is controlled by suture, hemostatic agents, or cautery.

PERIOPERATIVE NURSING CONSIDERATIONS
- See D&C procedure, p. 498
- Dispersive electrode (ground pad) should be placed after final positioning

Related Procedures: Excision of Cervical Cyst

Procedure
Therapeutic Abortion by Suction Curettage

Definition: The termination of a pregnancy by removing the products of conception through the vagina via the vacuum aspiration of the uterine contents.
CDC Classification: II
Discussion: This procedure may also be performed for a missed and/or incomplete abortion, in which placental tissue may still be present.
Positioning, Skin Preparation, Drapes, Instrumentation: See D&C Procedure, p. 498.
    Disposable vacuum curettes (size variety)
Supplies/Equipment:
    Aspiration machine and tubing
    Stirrups
    Perineal pad
    Robinson catheter (for straight bladder drainage)

PROCEDURAL OVERVIEW

A routine D&C is performed, as previously described.
    Sterile suction tubing and specific tip (size determined by the surgeon) are opened, and connections are made (open end is attached to machine) by circulator. The vacuum is activated by the circulating nurse and the uterus is suctioned clean by rotating the curette 360° with a back-and-forth motion, while traction is maintained on the cervix with a tenaculum. The endometrial cavity is curetted with a sharp curette, and a brief suction curettage is repeated. The specimen, trapped in the collection chamber, is sent to pathology for routine examination. A perineal pad is applied.

PERIOPERATIVE NURSING CONSIDERATIONS

- See D&C procedure considerations.
- A gauze tissue bag is contained inside the collection bottle and, depending on the pathologist's instructions, the specimen may be removed from the bag first and placed in the specimen container, or the bag and its contents may be sent to the lab in the routine manner.

Additional Considerations
- This procedure may conflict with ethical, religious, or moral beliefs of personnel assigned to the room. If such is the case, the supervisor should be apprised and a substitute nurse assigned to assist with the procedure.
- It is important to remember that the nurse/technician must *never* allow personal values to interfere with the safe execution of patient care, should the procedure be performed as an elective procedure.

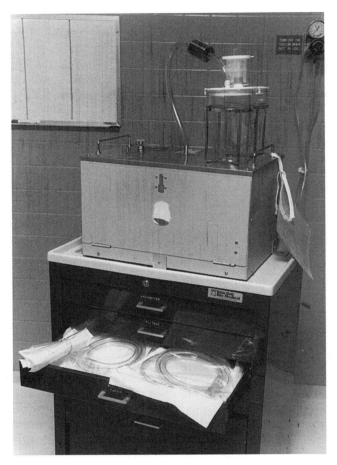

Suction curettage unit

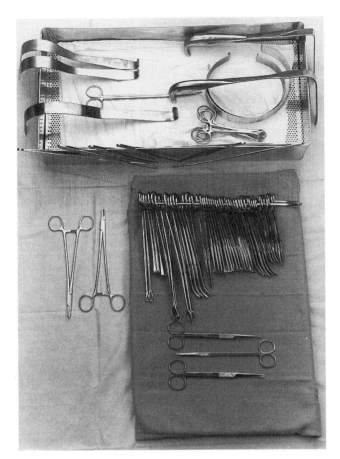

Vaginal hysterectomy instrumentation

Procedure
Vaginal Hysterectomy

Definition: Removal of the uterus via a vaginal approach.

CDC Classification: II

Discussion: Indications for this procedure and/or approach include benign diseases of the uterus in which the uterus is not greatly enlarged. Although a vaginal approach is technically difficult, it is less traumatic for the patient because the abdominal wall remains intact.

Additionally, it may be necessary to perform an anterior and posterior colporrhaphy (discussed on p. 501).

Positioning: Lithotomy with slight Trendelenberg

Skin Preparation: See pp. 337–338

Packs/Drapes: Gyn or lithotomy pack
Sterile Mayo tray (covered)
Extra drape sheets
Folded towels

Instrumentation:
Vaginal hysterectomy tray
Internal stapling instruments (opt.)

Supplies/Equipment:
Basin set
Blades—(2) No. 10
ESU; suction
Stirrups (well padded) or knee support brace
Needle counter
Foley catheter with drainage bag
Sutures—surgeon's preference
Internal staples (opt.)
Solutions—saline, water
Gauze packing (e.g., 1-inch plain) (opt.)
Vaginal cream (surgeon's preference)
Perineal pad

PROCEDURAL OVERVIEW

A major portion of the operation for a vaginal hysterectomy is a series of serial clamping, division, and ligation of ligaments and vessels of the uterus, similar to the abdominal hysterectomy approach. The scrub person should have adequate amounts of Heaney, Kocher, or Ochsner clamps available, depending on the surgeon's preference (both long and regular length).

The surgeon usually sits during the procedure and a Mayo lap tray is prepared for ease of access to instruments during the surgery. If the surgeon prefers to stand, the operating table is raised so that visibility is optimal. However, accommodations must also be made for the anesthesia clinician monitoring the patient.

A weighted vaginal speculum is placed in the vaginal vault, and the cervix is grasped with a tenaculum. Using the knife and/or curved Mayo scissors, a circular incision is made around the cervix, exposing the first set of ligaments. The ligaments are double clamped, divided, and ligated (0-chromic; heavy tapered needle).

Using a toothed forceps, the surgeon picks up the posterior peritoneum and incises it with a knife and/or scissors. With the peritoneal cavity open, the peritoneal attachment to the bladder is detached from the uterus using a Metzenbaum scissors. (Long forceps and scissors should be available as the mobilization process continues.) A Sims or Heaney retractor is used to retract the bladder upward. The cardinal ligaments and uterine arteries are ligated and divided, and the uterus is delivered. If the ovaries are to remain, the ovarian vessels are preserved, and the remaining structures in the broad ligament are ligated and divided. After the specimen is removed (en bloc), the peritoneal cavity is exposed. Before closing the peritoneum, the bladder is reperitonealized with a running suture (2-0 chromic, taper needle).

If an anterior and/or posterior colporrhaphy is required, it is performed at this time.

The peritoneum is closed (0 or 2-0 chromic). The vagina may be packed and perineal dressing is applied.

An alternative technique is the use of internal stapling instruments, to ligate and divide the uterosacral and cardinal ligaments and ligate the adnexa.

PERIOPERATIVE NURSING CONSIDERATIONS

- A sterilization permit may also need to be signed. Check with institutional policy.
- Stirrups should be well padded to avoid nerve damage. A coccygeal support should be used to prevent damage to the sacral area.
- Raise and lower the legs, stopping at the "knee–chest" position, to avoid rapid alterations in venous return and/or damage to the lumbosacral region.
- Instruments for the Lap tray often include weighted speculum, tenaculum, retractors, curved Mayo scissors, and hysterectomy clamps, in addition to long forceps and long dissecting scissors.

Procedure
Colporrhaphy

Definition: Repair and reinforcement of musculofascial support of the bladder, urethra (*cystocele*), and/or distal rectum (*rectocele*), in order to prevent protrusion of the structure(s) through the vaginal wall. *Syn:* Anterior/Posterior Repair [A&P Repair]
CDC Classification: II
Discussion: These conditions may occur simultaneously or independently to varying degrees. Multiparity is the most common cause for these conditions, and may be performed as separate procedures; as an A&P repair or to complete a vaginal hysterectomy.
Positioning: Lithotomy, with slight Trendelenberg; arms supported on armboards
Skin Preparation, Drapes, Instrumentation: See Vaginal Hysterectomy, p. 500
Supplies/Equipment: Same as for a vaginal hysterectomy

PROCEDURAL OVERVIEW

Anterior Colporrhaphy
The anterior vaginal wall is incised. The incised edges are grasped with Allis clamps. A plane of tissue is formed in the vaginal wall up to the bladder. When the surgeon reaches the bladder neck, several sutures (0-chromic) are placed through the fascia, tightening the tissue. The vaginal wall is reconstructed and excess mucosa is excised.

Posterior Colporrhaphy
An incision is made on the posterior vaginal wall. The incision is deepened to the rectum. The levator muscles are brought together with interrupted sutures (2-0 chromic), and the excess vaginal mucosa is excised. The vaginal wall is reconstructed with interrupted suture (2-0 chromic; small needle). A Foley catheter is usually inserted by the surgeon at the close of the procedure, and the vagina is packed with vaginal packing (Iodophor or plain). An antibiotic vaginal cream may also be used.

Internal staples can be substituted for sutures during the ligation and excision of the vaginal mucosa.

PERIOPERATIVE NURSING CONSIDERATIONS
- See Vaginal Hysterectomy, p. 500

Procedure
Marsupialization of a Bartholin Duct Cyst

Definition: Incision and drainage (I&D) of a vulvovaginal cyst, with the suturing of the cyst wall to the edge of the incision.

CDC Classification: II, unless infection or drainage is present

Discussion: The Bartholin gland, which secretes mucus, is a common site of cyst formation. The cyst wall is composed primarily of the duct of the gland, so by not excising the cyst, but only creating a fenestration or window in the gland, the secreting function of the gland may be preserved.

Positioning: Lithotomy

Incision Site: Vertical incision in the vaginal mucosa (outside the hymenal ring)

Skin Preparation: See pp. 337–338

Instrumentation: Cervical cone tray or minor tray

Supplies/Equipment:

   Stirrups
   Basin set
   Blades—(1) No. 15
   ESU; suction
   Culture tubes (2) (anaerobic; aerobic)
   Smear slides (opt.)
   Disposable syringe with long 15- or 18-gauge needle (opt.)
   Suture—surgeon's preference
   Solutions—saline, water
   Sterile Mayo tray (if sitting position is used)
   Drain (e.g., ¼-in. Penrose)
   Vaginal packing (opt.)
   Perineal pad

PROCEDURAL OVERVIEW

With the patient in the lithotomy position, an incision is made in the vaginal mucosa, around the perimeter of the cyst with a No. 15 blade. The cyst is incised and drained. The lining of the cyst is inverted and sutured to the vaginal mucosa with interrupted stitches.

If a cystectomy is necessary, the cyst is mobilized using sharp and blunt dissection. The intact cyst is excised, and the mucosa is approximated (3-0 chromic; small taper needle); a drain may be inserted.

PERIOPERATIVE NURSING CONSIDERATIONS

- See D&C procedure, p. 498.

Procedure
Shirodkar (Cerclage for Incompetent Os)

Definition: The placement of an encircling "tape" ligature at the level of the internal cervical os to maintain the integrity of the cervical canal.

CDC Classification: II

Discussion: The procedure is usually performed to prevent premature dilation and subsequent spontaneous expulsion of the fetus before safe delivery. It is usually recommended for patients who have a history of spontaneous abortion in the first trimester of pregnancy. Incompetency may be related to previous lacerations or a congenital weakness. This procedure has the best results when performed before the cervix actually dilates.

Positioning, Skin Preparation, Drapes: See D&C, p. 498

Instrumentation:

   D&C tray and/or cervical biopsy tray
   Short Haney retractors
   Ligature carrier (for tape)

Supplies/Equipment:

   Stirrups
   ESU; suction (opt.)
   Tape ligature (e.g., 5-mm Mersilene tape)
   Perineal pad
   Solutions—saline, water

PROCEDURAL OVERVIEW

The cervix is excised using a transverse incision in the vaginal mucosa, at the anterior aspect of the cervix. The bladder is retracted away. A similar incision is made posteriorly. The synthetic tape ligature is placed around the internal os; the tape is tightened and secured. The posterior portion of the tape loop may be sutured to the vaginal mucosa, and the cervix is closed.

PERIOPERATIVE NURSING CONSIDERATIONS

- See D&C Procedure, p. 498.

Related Procedures: McDonald Procedure

Procedure
Salpingectomy for Ruptured Ectopic Pregnancy

Definition: Removal of a ruptured fallopian tube and ectopic fetus.

CDC Classification: II

Discussion: An ectopic pregnancy can occur when the fetus lodges in any area other than the uterus. If the fetus lodges in the tube, it soon becomes too large for the tube, causing the tube to rupture.

- *Positioning, Incision Site, Skin Preparation, Packs, Drapes:* See Salpingo-oophorectomy, p. 496

Instrumentation:

   Major tray or tubal tray
   Self-retaining retractor

Supplies/Equipment:

   Same as for a salpingo-oophorectomy

PROCEDURAL OVERVIEW

The abdomen is entered in a routine fashion. Large blood clots, if present, are removed. The fallopian tube is mobilized and removed, and the wound is closed.

This procedure is similar to the salpingo-oophorectomy. It differs primarily in that a ruptured ectopic pregnancy often necessitates emergency surgery. If bleeding vessels are not occluded quickly, the patient may be in extreme danger of hemorrhage.

PERIOPERATIVE NURSING CONSIDERATIONS

- A large basin should be available to receive blood clots.
- If there is significant bleeding, the scrub person should have a Poole abdominal suction tip available, and if necessary, the outer casing should be removed.
- The wound is irrigated with warm saline to remove any remaining clots or tissue debris.

ABDOMINOVAGINAL PROCEDURES

Procedure
Laparoscopy

Definition: The insertion of an endoscope through the anterior abdominal wall following the establishment of a pneumoperitoneum.
CDC Classification: II, due to manipulation of the cervix
Discussion: A laparoscopy permits visualization of the pelvic structures without performing an open laparotomy. It is usually performed as a diagnostic procedure for infertility, pelvic mass identification, ectopic mass, etc., in addition to elective sterilization procedures (Laparoscopic Tubal Ligation).
Positioning: Modified lithotomy (45 degrees) position with knee-brace stirrups; arms may be extended on armboards
Incision Site: Infraumbilical (single puncture), suprapubic (second puncture if needed)
Skin Preparation: See pp. 337–338 (combined abdominal-vaginal)
Packs/Drapes: Laparoscopy pack
Instrumentation:
  Laparoscopy tray with soft tissue instruments
  Disposable trocar and veres needle (opt.)
  Uterine retractor, tenaculum, manipulator
  Laparoscopic telescope (diameter preference)
  For Infertility: Intrauterine cannula (e.g., Cahn)
  For Laser: Laser laparoscopic instruments
Supplies/Equipment:
  Insufflation device (may be a combined unit)
  Fiberoptic light source

ESU (bipolar for tubal ligation); suction
Insufflation tubing
Light cord
Blades—(1) No. 10, (1) No. 15, (1) No. 11
Sutures—surgeon's preference
Solutions—saline, water
For Infertility add: Plastic tubing, syringe, methylene blue dye
For Tubal Ligation add: Cautery forceps

PROCEDURAL OVERVIEW

The vagina is retracted and the anterior tip of the cervix is grasped with a tenaculum. A self-retaining cannula is inserted into the cervix.

Two towel clips (or Allis clamps) are placed on the inferior rim of the umbilicus, and a 2-mm incision is made. Traction is placed on the towel clips (clamps), and a veres needle is inserted through the incision, into the peritoneal cavity. Proper placement is confirmed (via aspiration with syringe), and the polyethylene insufflation tubing is connected to the needle and the insufflation device. The pneumoperitoneum is established using approximately 2 liters of carbon dioxide gas.

The needle is withdrawn and the incision is enlarged to 1 cm. As the towel clips (clamps) provide upward traction, the trocar with its sleeve is inserted (angled toward the pelvis). The trocar is withdrawn, and proper placement of the sleeve is confirmed. The insufflation tubing is attached to the sleeve to maintain the pneumoperitoneum.

The operative telescope (laparoscope) is inserted into the sleeve, and the fiberoptic light cord is attached to the scope and the power source, then illuminated.

If a procedure such as a tubal ligation is performed, a second incision may be required, allowing for insertion of accessory instruments through the initial incision (laser laparoscope), or a single-puncture laparoscope may be used.

At the completion of the procedure, the laparoscope is withdrawn, and the gas is allowed to escape from the sleeve. The sleeve is withdrawn, the incision(s) closed with a subcuticular stitch, and Steri-Strips or a Band-Aid is applied. The vaginal cannula is removed.

PERIOPERATIVE NURSING CONSIDERATIONS

- The laparoscope lens may be warmed in a lens "boat" or warmer, and an antifogging solution may be applied to the eyepiece, then wiped off (e.g., Ultra-Stop).
- The insufflation device gauges should be visible to the surgeon at all times. Place the unit on the opposite side of the surgeon.

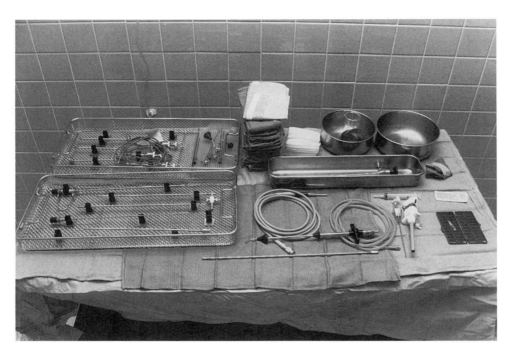

Laparoscopy instruments and set-up

- All gauges and tanks must be checked prior to beginning the case. If the tank pressure registers less than 100 psi, the tank should be changed before use.
- If laser is used, all safety precautions for its use must be in effect (e.g., proper eye wear, danger signs).
- During the examination, the patient is placed in a modified Trendelenberg position.
- An abdominal laparotomy set-up should be available in case an open procedure is required.

Related Procedures: Laser Laparoscopy
   Laparoscopic Tubal Ligation
   Laparoscopic Chromotubation (infertility detection)

OBSTETRIC SURGERY

Procedure
Cesarean (caesarean) Section (*Syn:* C-section)

Definition: The delivery of a viable fetus through abdominal and uterine incisions (in the operating room).
CDC Classification: II
Discussion: The procedure takes its name from the Latin word *caedere,* to cut. Whether it is scheduled or emergent, it is an exciting, fast-paced, and gratifying procedure for all members of the surgical team.

There are numerous indications for this method of delivery, including dystocia (failure to progress); cephalopelvic disproportion; malrotation; and placenta pre-

via. Additionally, uterine fibroids, which may block the vaginal passageway, herpes, and condylomata may also be indications for a cesarean section. Previous C-sections, however, are no longer single indications for this procedure unless the conditions mentioned above are also present.

Emergency C-sections are those performed because of threatening conditions to the mother and/or the baby (e.g., fetal distress, umbilical cord prolapse, or abruptio placentae).
Positioning: Supine, with a small roll under the right hip (to reduce vena cava compression); arms extended on armboards
Incision Sites: Classic Approach: Vertical (low midline)
   Pfannenstiel (low transverse)
Skin Preparation: See pp. 337–338
Packs/Drapes: C-section pack or laparotomy pack
   Extra drape sheet
   Towels
   Receiving pack for baby
Instrumentation:
   C-section tray
   Delivery forceps
   Cord clamp (disposable)
Supplies/Equipment:
   Basin set
   Blades—(2) No. 10 or (1) No. 10 and (1) No. 20
   ESU; suction
   Neonatal receiving unit (e.g., Ohio neonatal unit; self-contained with oxygen, suction, heat, lights, etc.)

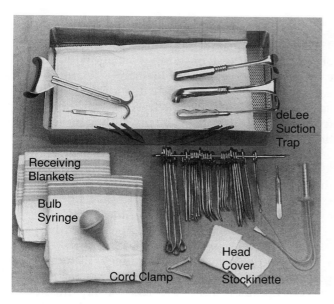

C-section tray with accessories

ID bands (for mother and baby)
Bulb syringe; mucus trap (e.g., DeLee suction)
Solutions—water, saline
Sutures—surgeon's preference

PROCEDURAL OVERVIEW

Using the appropriate incision, consistent with the estimated size of the fetus, the abdomen is opened, the rectus muscles are separated, and the peritoneum incised (similar to an abdominal hysterectomy), exposing the distended uterus. Large vessels are clamped or cauterized, but usually no attempt to control hemostasis is made since it may delay delivery time (3–5 minutes after initial incision is ideal). The scrub person must be ready with suction, dry Laps, and a bulb syringe. The bladder is retracted downward with the bladder blade of the Balfour retractor, and a small incision is made with the second knife and extended with a bandage scissors (blunt tip prevents injury to the baby's head).

The amniotic sac is entered and immediately aspirated of fluid. The bladder blade is removed, and the assistant will push on the patient's upper abdomen while the surgeon simultaneously delivers the infant's head in an upward position. The baby's airways (nose then mouth) are suctioned with the bulb syringe, and the baby is completely delivered and placed upon the mother's abdomen.

The umbilical cord is double-clamped and cut. The baby is wrapped in a sterile receiving blanket and transferred to the warming unit for immediate assessment and care (neonatal or nursery nurses and a pediatrician/neonatologist may be in attendance).

Once the baby has been safely delivered, the emergent phase of the procedure has ended.

The cord blood samples are taken at this time as the team waits for the expulsion of the placenta, which is delivered into an awaiting basin. The uterine cavity is irrigated with warm saline and inspected for any remaining tissue or clots, then wiped dry with a Lap sponge in preparation for the uterine closure.

Using a noncrushing clamp (Pennington, Duval, or ring forces) the uterine wall is grasped for traction during closure. The closure is performed in two layers with a heavy absorbable suture (0-chromic or Vicryl), using a continuous stitch; the second overlapping the first. Following closure of the uterus, the bladder flap is reperitonealized with a running suture (2-0 or 3-0 absorbable, taper needle), and the uterus is pushed back inside the pelvic cavity. The cavity is irrigated with warm saline, and closed in layers. Skin is closed with the surgeon's preference (suture or staples). If a tubal ligation is to be performed, it is done prior to the abdominal closure sequence.

PERIOPERATIVE NURSING CONSIDERATIONS

- In preparation for a C-section, the neonatal warming unit should be turned on and all components checked for proper working order prior to the patient entering the operating room.
- A C-section requires an additional uterine count of sponges, sharps, and instruments prior to its closure.
- Oxytocin should be available for the anesthetist to administer IV.
- Once the uterus is opened, immediate suctioning is necessary.
- Records pertaining to the birth and ID bands are completed by the circulating nurse per hospital protocol, before the infant leaves the operating room.
- The pediatrician and other personnel who will care for the baby should be notified in ample time to complete their required infant set-up.
- Cord blood is sent to the laboratory following hospital protocol with pertinent delivery information on the corresponding laboratory slips.
- After the baby's nose and mouth have been cleared, the bulb syringe should be passed off the field with the baby for continuation of airway clearance measures.
- Two perioperative nurses should be assigned to the room (one to circulate and one to care for the baby) if nursery personnel are not available.
- A warm, portable isolette should be available to transport the infant to the newborn nursery.

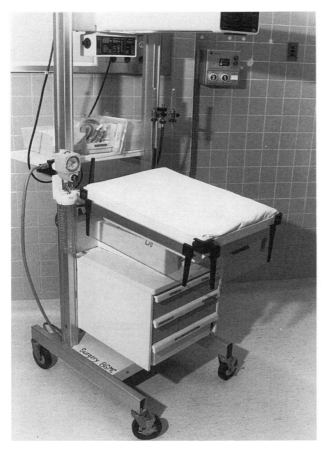

Neonatal surgical unit: self-contained with heat, light, oxygen, and suction

GENITOURINARY SURGERY

Genitourinary (GU) surgery involves procedures of the male and female urinary (*renal*) system. The organs involved with this specialty consist of the *kidney*, the *urinary bladder*, the *urethra*, and the *ureters*.

Because of the close proximity of the urologic and reproductive structures in the male, it is often referred to as the *genitourinary system*, and includes the male reproductive structures. The female reproductive structures and surgeries have already been covered.

Surgical Anatomy Review

The urinary system consists of the *kidneys*, which produce the urine, the *ureters*, which carry the urine to the *urinary bladder*, where it is temporarily stored, and the *urethra*, which transports the urine to the outside of the body.

The Kidney

The kidneys are paired reddish-brown organs situated on the posterior wall of the abdominal cavity, one on each side of the vertebral column.

Each kidney is capped by an endocrine gland (*adrenal gland*), and is approximately 11 cm long, extending from the level of the eleventh or twelfth thoracic vertebrae to the third lumbar vertebra. Because of the presence of the liver, the right kidney is generally slightly lower than the left. The kidneys are located between the muscles of the back and the peritoneal cavity. This *retroperitoneal* location makes it possible for surgical exposure without opening the peritoneal cavity.

Each kidney is surrounded by three layers: the *renal capsule*, the *fibrous capsule*, and the *renal fascia*.

The internal structures of the kidneys include three general regions: (1) the *cortex*, (2) the *medulla*, and (3) the *pelvis* (kidney basin). The *renal tubules*, the nephrons are the functioning unit of the kidneys and there are over 1 million nephrons in each kidney. The vascular network associated with the kidney is unusual, since blood flows through a series of two sequential capillary beds: the *glomerulus* and *peritubular* structures. From the aorta, blood enters the kidney via the *renal artery*; it exits the kidney to the systemic circulation by way of the *renal veins* into the inferior vena cava.

The Ureters

From the renal pelvis in the kidney, urine is transported to the urinary bladder by ureters from each kidney. The ureters descend between the parietal peritoneum and the body wall to the pelvic cavity, where they turn medially and enter the urinary bladder on its posterior lateral surface. The ureter wall consists of three layers: the inner *mucosal lining*, a middle *muscular layer*, and an outer *fibrous layer*. The muscular layer is capable of undergoing *peristaltic contractions*, thereby propelling the urine into the bladder.

The Urinary Bladder

The urinary bladder is a hollow, muscular organ that rests on the floor of the pelvic cavity. Like other urinary structures, it is *retroperitoneal*, and the anterior surface lies just behind the *pubic symphysis*. In the male, it is located in front of the rectum, while in the female, it lies anterior to the uterus and the superior portion of the vagina. It is lined with a mucous membrane (*transitional epithelium*), and its covering consists of three layers of smooth muscle. There is a smooth muscular section caller the *trigone* of the bladder, which is marked by the internal openings of the two ureters laterally, indicating the corners of this triangular area. The bladder, which acts as a reservoir for the urine, can hold approximately 600 to 800 mL of urine, but it generally empties before reaching this capacity.

The Urethra

The urethra is a muscular tube, lined with mucous membrane, that exits from the inferior surface of the urinary bladder.

In the female, the urethra is short (approximately 4 cm), and runs along the anterior surface of the vagina to an opening (*external urinary meatus*) located between the clitoris and the vaginal orifice.

The male urethra is about 20 cm long. It extends to the external urinary meatus at the tip of the penis, and is divided into three sections: the *prostatic, membranous,* and *spongy urethra,* named according to the regions through which it passes. A short distance below the *urogenital diaphragm* or pelvic floor, the spongy urethra receives the ducts of the *bulbourethral glands (Cowper's gland)* of the reproductive system.

Male Reproductive Structures

The male reproductive structures, which are usually treated along with the urinary structures, include the *testes,* a number of *ducts,* several accessory *glands,* and the *penis.*

The male peritoneum includes all the structures that are located between the *pubic symphysis* anteriorly, the *coccyx* posteriorly, and the *ischiopubic rami* and *sacrotuberous ligaments* laterally. The portion of the sacrotuberous ligament that binds the peritoneum runs from the lateral margin of the sacrum and coccyx to the *ischial tuberosity.*

The Testes and Scrotum

The testes are the organs of sperm production. They are located in a skin-covered pouch called the *scrotum.* The scrotum consists of an outer layer of skin and a thin layer of smooth muscle (*dartos tunic*). Each testis is an oval organ surrounded by a connective tissue capsule (*tunica albuginea*). As the testes descend into the scrotum from their original position in the abdominopelvic cavity, their blood supply travels with them. The *testicular arteries* leave the aorta, and the *testicular veins* join the inferior vena cava in the region of the kidneys.

Epididymis

The epididymis, located in the scrotum, is the first portion of the *duct* system that transports sperm from the testes to the exterior of the body. There are smooth muscles in the wall of the *epididymal tube* that contract during ejaculation, moving the sperm into the *ductus deferens* and then out of the body.

Ductus (Vas) Deferens

The vas deferens is a continuation of the duct of the epididymis. As it enters the abdominopelvic cavity, it lies next to the vessels and nerves supplying the testis. All these structures are enclosed in a sheath of fascia known as the *spermatic cord.* On reaching the inferior surface of the urinary bladder, each vas deferens is joined by a duct of the *seminal vesicles,* a membranous pouch, to form the *ejaculatory duct,* which passes through the *prostate gland.*

The Prostate Gland

The prostate gland is a single organ that encompasses the urethra just below the bladder and directly in front of the rectum. Because of its location, the gland can be manually palpated by means of a rectal examination. The prostate tends to enlarge in older men and may cause difficulty in urination by compressing the prostatic portion of the urethra. This condition is known as *benign prostatic hypertrophy,* and necessitates surgical removal (resection) of the gland.

The Penis

The penis is the major sexual organ of the male, in addition to its role in the elimination of urine from the body via the urethra. It consists of a shaft covered with loosely attached skin and an expanded tip (*glans*). The skin continues over the glans as the *prepuce* or *foreskin,* which is often surgically removed (circumcision) shortly after birth (Fig. 14-9).

General Considerations

Genitourinary procedures are classified in two areas or techniques: *open* or *closed.*

An *open* procedure is performed through an incision, while a *closed* procedure is performed through direct visualization with the aid of a *cystourethroscope* inserted into the urethra and bladder. Closed procedures are primarily performed for diagnostic examination and selected corrective procedures, while open procedures are usually performed for repair or revision of urinary structures.

Closed Genitourinary Procedures

Closed genitourinary procedures involve the urethra, bladder, ureters, and prostate gland. These procedures

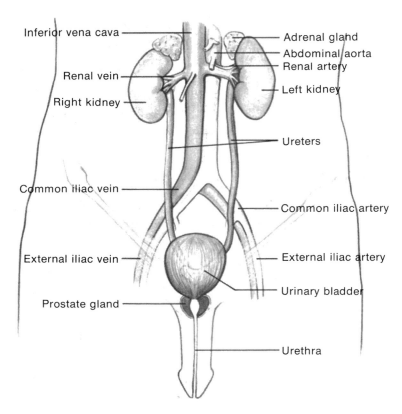

Fig. 14-9. Urinary system with blood vessels

are performed in a special room—the *cysto room*—that is equipped with a special cysto table, overhead x-ray equipment, and storage area for the special instruments, supplies, and equipment. Because of the nature of the procedure, and the anatomic areas, these procedures are usually performed under aseptic, rather than sterile, technique, and a mask is not always worn by members of the team during these procedures, depending on specific written hospital protocol.

Special Equipment and Supplies To perform a cystoscopic examination, special equipment and supplies must be available to the *urologist* performing the procedure. The following list of supplies is considered generic for all cysto rooms:

1. Cysto table with x-ray unit
2. Instrumentation
3. Fiberoptic light cord and cysto irrigation tubing
4. Irrigation solutions
5. Cysto packs; drapes, gowns, and gloves

1. *Cysto Table:* The cysto table is specifically manufactured to accommodate closed urologic procedures. It differs from any other operating table in that it is designed to (1) maintain a patient in the lithotomy position, (2) receive an x-ray cassette in a holder located within the table itself, and (3) allow for drainage of irrigation fluid. Additionally, the stirrups of the table are removable, and differ in design according to the table manufacturer.

2. *Instrumentation:* The *cystoscope* is a delicate fiberoptic tool that allows the surgeon to visualize, make a diagnosis, and perform selected corrective procedures on the urinary structures. There are different types of cystoscopes, varying according to the manufacturer, yet they all have similar components and accessories. The major components for all cystoscopes are the *telescope* and the *sheath and obturator*.

• *The Telescope:* The telescope is the optical system of the cystoscope. It offers the urologist an unimpaired view of the bladder, urethra, and distal ureters. There are a variety of telescopes, each offering a specific angle or view: forward angle scope, foroblique right-angle scope, lateral scope, and a retrospective scope. All telescopes are stainless steel with a *Bakelite* ocular. The telescope has an adapter that, when connected to a fiberoptic light cord and power source, allows for illumination of the internal structures.

The telescope must be handled gently; in particular, care must be taken to avoid scratching the lens or bending the shaft of the scope.

• *Sheath and Obturator:* The sheath is a hollow tube constructed of either a *Bakelite* (fiber-glass) or stain-

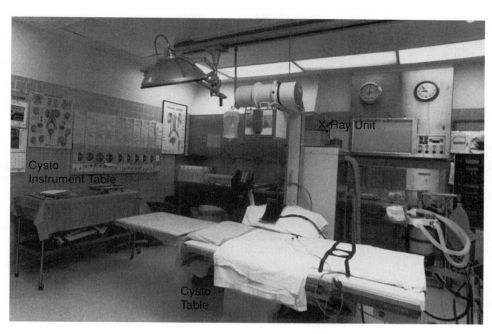

Cystoscopy room set-up

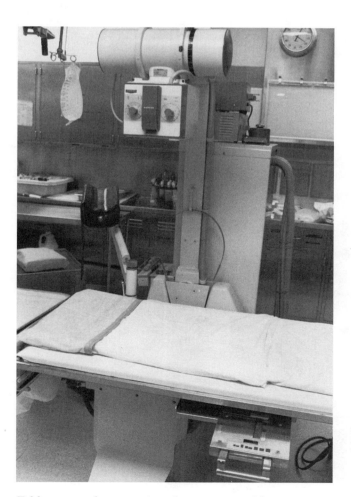

Table mounted x-ray unit and cystoscopy table

less steel material. The sheath provides a passageway for instruments used during a cystoscopy and/or a resection procedure, and contains the light carrier. Sheaths range in size from 14 to 30 French. The sheath has a stopcock adapter that allows it to connect to the irrigation fluid necessary during a closed urinary procedure. Insertion of the sheath into the urethra is aided by an obturator.

The obturator is a metal rod with a rounded (blunt) tip that is inserted into the sheath and advanced so that the tip is in line with the tip of the sheath. This prevents the end of the sheath from injuring the mucosal lining of the urethra during insertion. The obturator may be straight or deflecting. Each sheath and obturator comes in specific French sizes, and must be matched with its appropriate counterpart before usage. The most commonly used urologic endoscopes are the *Brown-Buerger Cystoscope*, the *McCarthy Panendoscope*, and the *Wappler Cystourethroscope*.

The telescope, sheath, and obturator may be soaked in a high disinfectant solution prior to beginning the procedure, and, after the appropriate interval, be removed and rinsed with sterile water before being placed on the instrument table.

3. *Fiberoptic Light Cord and Cysto Tubing:* The fiberoptic light cable is similar to the one discussed with the laparoscope in gynecologic surgery. It connects to a fiberoptic light source that is adjustable in intensity. The cable should never be tightly coiled or twisted since the fiberoptic fibers might break and destroy the illumination capabilities of the cord and the telescope.

The water cord, known as *cysto tubing,* is designed to accommodate up to four bags of irrigation solution. It is a commercially prepared, presterilized, disposable item, and connects to the instrument by an adapter, permitting the irrigation fluid to distend the bladder, which is a vital technique whenever a cystoscopic examination and/or resection procedure is performed.

4. *Irrigation Solutions:* For a cystoscopic examination or a cysto with a retrograde examination or simple bladder fulguration, a 1000- or 3000-mL bag of sterile water is used to assist the urologist with visualization through continuous irrigation. For procedures requiring the use of electrocautery, an isotonic, non-hemolytic solution, 1.5% sterile glycine, may be used in place of the water. Commercially prepared sterile irrigation solutions with the appropriate closed administration set (cysto tubing) prevent the possible inherent risk of cross-contamination during the procedure.

The fluid is evacuated from the bladder by the urologist by rotating the stopcock on the sheath to an open position, or the instrument may be equipped with a suction apparatus, depending on its design.

5. *Cysto Pack, Drape, and Gown:* A specially designed cysto pack is used during a closed urologic procedure. It is similar to a gynecologic pack, with the major difference being that the abdominal drape sheet has a screen built into the perineal portion of the sheet. The leggings may be preattached as one continuous drape with side wings, or supplied as separate leggings.

The surgeon's gown is usually reinforced with a waterproof front to prevent strike-through of irrigation solution.

The instrument table is prepared under strict aseptic technique by either the circulating nurse or a scrub technician assigned to the room; however, a surgical scrub is not required to set up the back table.

Ancillary Equipment and Supplies

1. *The ESU:* During specific cystoscopic procedures (e.g., transurethral resection of a bladder tumor or the prostate), the electrosurgical unit may be required. The patient should be prepared with the dispersive electrode (ground pad) in place, so that manipulation of sterile drapes is not necessary if the unit is needed (see pp. 344–345 for a review of electrosurgical safety).

2. *Special Catheters:* Urinary catheters are used for a variety of reasons, including short-term urinary drainage, long-term urinary drainage, hemostasis, evacuation of blood clots or blood, diagnosis, and maintenance of urethral continuity. Most operating suites maintain a supply of sterile catheters, designed for single use only. They are made of flexible, nonirritating materials (e.g., Latex, Teflon, and plastic), and are available in a variety of sizes and with special features.

- *Urethral Catheters*
  1. *Straight catheters*—lack a retention balloon, and are used for diagnostic purposes or immediate drainage of the bladder prior to a procedure. (Example: red Robinson catheter.) Straight

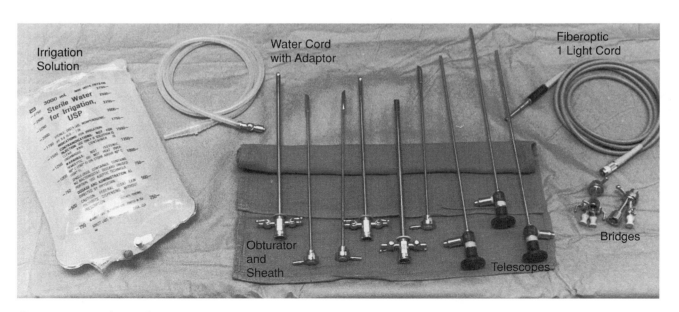

Cystoscopy supplies and equipment

catheters are also referred to as a *utility* catheter.

2. *Foley (retention) catheters*—the most commonly used retention catheter with an inflatable balloon (5 mL or 30 mL) that remains inside the bladder for continuous bladder drainage via a closed system. Foley catheters can also be used as a means to continually irrigate the bladder, via an extra port allowing for the connection of an irrigation solution (3-way Foley). Other retention catheters include a Phillips, Coude Gibbons, and Malecott, each with a specific tip to provide for specific needs of the patient.

- *Ureteral Catheters*—chiefly used for *retrograde pyelography* and/or collection of urinary specimens directly from the kidney. They are available in a variety of sizes and tip shapes, and are selected by the urologist for a specific need.

3. *Resection Instrumentation:* To perform a resection procedure, a special instrument—a *resectoscope*—is required. The resectoscope is the instrument used to cut and coagulate tissue during a transurethral resection. It consists of a *telescope, cutting electrodes* (cutting loops), a *working element,* and a specially treated *sheath and obturator.* The resectoscope uses electrical current generated by the electrosurgical unit to remove tissue piece by piece.

Several types of working elements vary according to the way in which the cutting electrode operates. These include the *McCarthy, Nesbit, Iglesias, Stern-McCarthy,* and *Brummrucker;* the choice is determined by the urologist's preference.

CLOSED UROLOGIC PROCEDURES

Procedure
Cystourethroscopy (Cystoscopy)

Definition: An endoscopic examination of the interior of the urethra, bladder, and ureteral orifices.
CDC Classification: II, unless urine cultures are positive
Discussion: A simple cystoscopic examination is indicated for diagnosing urinary tract symptoms (e.g., hematuria, pyuria, or urinary tract infections), to catheterize the ureters, to obtain a biopsy specimen, and for follow-up examination of an operative or endoscopic procedure. These procedures can be performed as outpatient surgery, in the urologist's office, or in the OR, under local or general anesthesia.
Position: Lithotomy
Skin Preparation: See pp. 337–338
Packs/Drapes: Cysto pack with reinforced gown

Instrumentation:
Cystoscope, including telescope (Foroblique), sheath, obturator, and short bridge
Urethral sounds (opt.)
Stopcocks and water cord adapter
Supplies/Equipment:
Fiberoptic light cord and power source
Cysto tubing
Albarran bridge with rubber catheter "nipples" or adapters (opt.)
Test tubes (specimen container) for urine sample
Ureteral catheters (opt.)
Lubricant
Irrigation solution—water (1000 or 3000 mL)
Foley catheter with syringe (5 or 30 mL) (opt.)

PROCEDURAL OVERVIEW

A well-lubricated sheath and obturator are inserted into the urethra, which may be initially dilated by urethral sounds (e.g., Van Buren). In the presence of a stricture, the urethra is usually dilated with *Phillips filiforms and followers.*

The obturator is withdrawn, a urine specimen is collected, and the telescope is inserted into the sheath and locked in place. The light cord and water cord are attached and the examination is performed.

The urethra is inspected as the cystoscope is advanced into the bladder. The bladder is dilated with irrigation fluid, and under direct visualization the bladder, ureteral orifices, bladder neck and urethra are examined (Fig. 14-10).

If an additional procedure is required, a panendoscope or resectoscope or a ureteral catheter adapter (Albarran bridge) may be used.

When the examination is complete, the sheath and telescope are removed. A Foley catheter may be in-

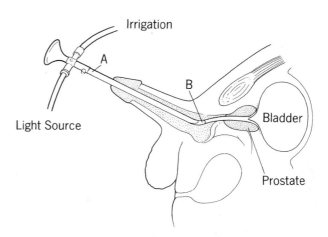

Fig. 14-10. Cystoscopy (A) obturator; (B) cystoscope tip

serted by the urologist and attached to a closed drainage system.

PERIOPERATIVE NURSING CONSIDERATIONS

- The sheath and obturator must be of the same diameter.
- Place telescopes on a towel, to act as a padding, to protect them from damage by hard surfaces.
- The circulating nurse should have the ancillary equipment and/or supplies in the room.
- All cystoscopic instruments and accessories may be disinfected with a 2% aqueous gluteraldehyde solution (e.g., Cidex; Sporicidin), then rinsed with copious amounts of sterile water in between procedures. Soaking time depends on the solution being used.
- Cysto stirrups should be well padded to avoid pressure on the neurovascular structures in the popliteal space.
- For bladder fulguration, a resectoscope and flexible-stem electrodes are needed. For retrograde ureteral catheterizations and pyelography examinations, the Albarran bridge, dye (30% Renographin or 50% Hypaque), and x-ray are required, in addition to ureteral catheters. A positioning x-ray (KUB) may be taken prior to beginning the procedure.
- Maintain adequate irrigation solution at all times, avoiding the possibility of air bubbles in the system. When the bag needs to be changed, notify the surgeon of the change, to avoid leakage of fluid.
- Irrigation solutions should be used at body temperature and stored at not more than 65°C (149°F).
- Apply the ground pad after positioning the patient (lateral aspect of upper thigh is a safe distance to avoid the possibility of fluid interference).
- At the end of the procedure, the instruments must be thoroughly cleaned before immersing them in the disinfectant solution. Place a towel on the bottom of the tray to protect the telescopic lens from damage. Cover the disinfecting pan (tray) at all times to prevent noxious fumes from irritating your eyes and nose.

Related Procedures: Transurethral Resection of a Bladder Tumor
Retrograde Pyelography

Procedure
Transurethral Resection of the Prostate Gland (TUR-P)

Definition: The *piecemeal* removal of the prostatic tissue and/or lesions transcystoscopically (transurethrally).

CDC Classification: II

Discussion: The procedure is particularly desirable when the patient is a poor surgical risk, as it eliminates the need for an open prostectomy. If carcinoma is found during histologic studies of the resected specimen, an open prostectomy may be indicated in an otherwise healthy (good-risk) patient. Regional or general anesthesia may be used.

Irrigation Solution for a TUR-P

The irrigation solution of choice for a TUR-P is 1.5% glycine solution. For this procedure, the irrigation solution must be isotonic, non-hemolytic since H_2O or saline may cause the dissipation of electricity when the electrosurgical unit is used. Water must never be used because the irrigation solution, if absorbed into the venous system during the procedure, could cause hemolysis, a breakdown of the red blood cells. Glycine neither conducts electricity nor is harmful if it is absorbed by the body during a resection procedure. Additional solutions include sorbitol, Urogate, and Uromatic.

Position: Lithotomy, with sacral support

Skin Preparation: See pp. 337–338

Packs/Drapes: Cysto pack
   Extra drape sheet (opt.)
   Urologic drape with rectal sheath

Instrumentation:
   Cystourethroscope, with components
   Resectoscope (e.g., McCarthy, Nesbit, Iglesias, Brummrucker), complete with foroblique telescope, post-resectoscope (Bakelite) and obturator (24 to 28 French); cutting loops
   Urethral sounds (opt.)
   Stopcock and water cord adapter
   Electrosurgical cord

Supplies/Equipment:
   Cysto tubing (2- or 4-prong)
   Fiberoptic light cord and power source
   ESU cable and ground pad
   Toomey syringe
   Ellick evacuator (for manual irrigation of fragments)
   Lubricant
   Strainer or metal screen (opt.)
   Irrigation solution (Glycine—3000-mL bags)
   Foley 3-way catheter with drainage bag (CBI Setup)

PROCEDURAL OVERVIEW

A cystourethroscopy is performed, which may include a urethral dilation. A cystoscope is always performed to help in assessing the hypertrophy and inspect the bladder. The resectoscope, complete with sheath and obturator, is passed through the urethra. The irrigation tubing, fiberoptic light cord, and cautery cable are connected. The obturator is removed and the operating element with the foroblique telescope and cutting loop

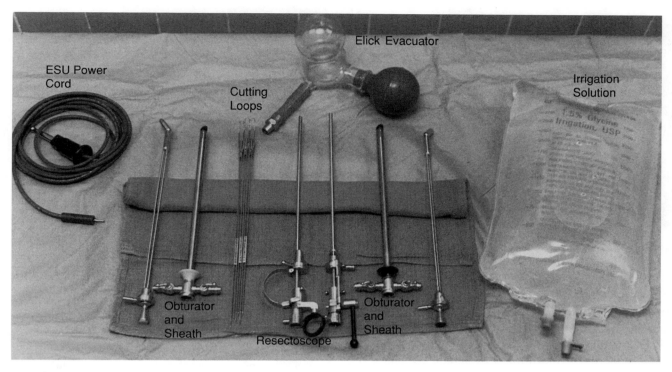

TUR set-up: instruments, supplies, and equipment

is inserted through the sheath. The urethra and bladder trigone are reexamined, and electrodissection is used to remove pieces of the hypertrophied prostate.

Periodically, the fragments of tissue and blood clots are washed out of the bladder using the Ellick evacuator and Toomey syringe. Total removal of all fragments of tissue is required to prevent postoperative bleeding and/or complications.

When the resection is complete, the bladder and prostatic fossa are examined for residual unattached fragments of tissue. Adequate hemostasis is ensured, and the resectoscope sheath is removed. A 3-way Foley catheter (30-mL balloon) is inserted, and attached to a continuous bladder irrigation set-up for postoperative management (normal saline is used as the irrigation solution).

PERIOPERATIVE NURSING CONSIDERATIONS

- Position the dispersive electrode (ground pad) on the lateral aspect of the thigh after the patient has been positioned.
- Irrigation solution must be nonelectrolytic isotonic nonhemolytic. Usually three or four bags are required per procedure.
- See Cystourethroscopy, p. 511, for additional considerations.

OPEN GENITOURINARY PROCEDURES

General Considerations

The instruments used for open genitourinary procedures are similar to those used in general surgery, with the addition of longer instruments (e.g., right-angle, Allis, and Babcock clamps), prostatic retractors, stone-grasping forceps, and kidney pedicle clamps.

Since the approach to most urinary structures often crosses highly vascularized muscle tissue, ample sponges, hemostatic clamps, and hemostatic agents may be required. Natural and synthetic absorbable sutures are commonly used when the surgeon is repairing structures in and around the tissues of the urinary tract, since nonabsorbable sutures can cause the formation of stones (*calculi*).

The patient is usually placed in the lateral position for procedures involving the bladder and reproductive structures.

Procedure
Nephrectomy

Definition: The surgical removal of a kidney (partial or total)

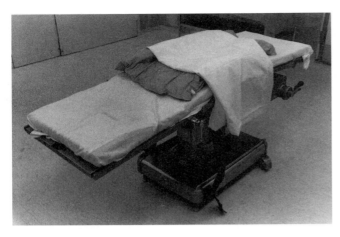

Vac-pack used for positioning clients for nephrectomy

CDC Classification: II

Discussion: A nephrectomy may be performed for many reasons, including hydronephrosis, pyelonephritis, renal atrophy, renal artery stenosis, trauma, and tumors of the kidney and ureters. If a major portion of the ureter is also excised, the procedure is termed a *Nephroureterectomy.*

Positioning: Lateral (lumbar flank or transthoracic), with affected side up

Incision Site: Flank (posterior axillary line, beneath the twelfth rib to suprapubic area)

Skin Preparation: See pp. 337–338

Packs/Drapes: Laparotomy pack with transverse
    Lap sheet
    Extra drape sheets
    Towels (opt.)

Instrumentation:
    Major procedure tray
    Kidney tray
    Thoracotomy tray with vascular clamps (opt.)
    Hemoclips/surgiclips (size variety)
    Internal stapling instruments (opt.)

Supplies/Equipment:
    Positioning aids (e.g., Vac-Pack; kidney rests)
    Basin set
    Blades—(2) No. 10, (1) No. 15, (1) No. 11
    ESU (long tip extra); suction
    Needle counter
    Asepto syringe
    Hemoclips/surgiclips (size variety)
    Dissector sponges (e.g., Kittners)
    Penrose drains (2) (for retraction and drainage)
    Closed-wound drainage (opt.)
    Chest tube and drainage unit (opt.)
    Suprapubic catheter (for nephroureterectomy)
    Solutions—saline, water

Medications—hemostatic agents (opt.), surgeon's preference
Sutures—surgeon's preference

PROCEDURAL OVERVIEW

A curved incision is made across the flank (for benign disease), and the fascia and muscle tissues are divided with a dissecting scissors and/or cautery. Occasionally a rib must be sacrificed to gain access to the retroperitoneal space. If a rib is to be taken, periosteal elevators and rib shears should be available.

The kidney and ureters are mobilized. The ureter is divided and the distal end ligated. For malignant disease, a radical nephrectomy is performed. On the right side, the duodenum is protected with moist Lap sponges. The vascular pedicle is transected and lymph node–bearing tissue is excised. Gerota's fascia is dissected from surrounding tissue; the ureter is divided and the kidney and surrounding fat, adrenal gland, and fascia are removed en bloc (radical).

If a flank incision is being used, a second lower flank or inguinal incision is used to expose the distal ureter extraperitoneally. The distal ureter is dissected free of surrounding tissues and a small cuff of bladder is excised with the intramural portion of the ureter. The bladder incision is repaired; a suprapubic cystostomy catheter may be placed, and the distal ureter and bladder cuff are delivered into the flank wound and removed with the kidney.

The flank incision may be closed with or without drainage, in separate layers: peritoneum (0-chromic); muscle (surgeon's preference); fascia (Dexon or synthetic sutures); subcuticular (3-0 absorbable); and skin (surgeon's preference). The wound is dressed in the normal manner.

For trauma and some presentations of calculus disease involving only a portion of the kidney, a partial nephrectomy may be performed.

PERIOPERATIVE NURSING CONSIDERATIONS

- The surgeon or anesthesiologist may request hypothermia measures during the procedure.
- Have all x-rays in the room.
- Verify with the blood bank the number of available units. If trauma, cell-saver unit may be used for blood salvage.
- Chest tube and drainage unit will be needed for a transthoracic approach.
- A suprapubic catheter (e.g., Pezzer, Malecott) and drainage unit may be used if nephroureterectomy is performed.

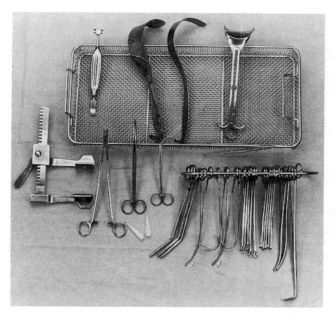

Kidney instrument tray

- When two incisions are used, the patient is repositioned, reprepared, and redraped; an additional instrument tray is necessary.

Related Procedures: Kidney Harvesting (cadaver donor) for Transplantation

Procedure
Kidney Transplantation

Definition: The implantation of a kidney from a living donor or cadaver donor (kidney harvesting) to a tissue-matched recipient.

CDC Classifications: II

Discussion: A kidney transplantation is usually performed on an otherwise healthy patient who suffers from renal failure.

Ideally, the donor should be a close family member (twin, sibling, parent). However, with today's technology involving tissue typing, and the establishment of a National Transplantation Clearing House that is fully equipped to provide computerized tissue matching, obtaining a donor kidney is not the difficult problem it was in the past. However, more public information and education are greatly needed to make the program successful and available to all patients in need of this intervention.

Two surgical teams may work simultaneously if the procedure involves a living donor. If the transplant is from a cadaver donor, a team from the transplant cen-

ter removes the cadaver donor's kidney for external perfusion prior to implantation, to minimize the time that elapses between the recipient's nephrectomy and the implantation of the donor kidney (4–6 hours after removal, with a maximum time of 72 hours).

Contraindications for kidney transplantation include

1. Systemic disease that precludes major surgery
2. Active cancer
3. Oxalosis (an autosomal-recessive hereditary disease)
4. Fabry's disease (an inherited metabolic disease resulting in excessive amounts of glycolipids in the kidney)

For the purpose of this discussion, the procedure will be described in two stages: Stage I, the nephrectomy, and Stage II, the transplantation.

STAGE I: NEPHRECTOMY

Positioning, Incision Site, Skin Preparation, Packs, Drapes, Instrumentation, Supplies, Equipment: See Nephrectomy, pp. 513–514

PROCEDURAL OVERVIEW

The donor is placed in the lateral position (living donor) or supine position (cadaver donor). Following a routine prep and draping, a flank nephrectomy is performed. Careful attention is given to preserving the renal vein, artery, and ureter. Before applying clamps to the renal vessels, the patient is systemically heparinized to prevent coagulation.

If a cadaver kidney is used, the patient must be on life support up to and during the procedure until the moment of extraction, to preserve the kidney.

Perfusion of the Kidney
Once the kidney has been removed from the donor, it must be perfused with cold (4°C) electrolyte solution prior to its transfer to the recipient. This is usually performed by the transplant team, with the solution infused into the kidney through an IV catheter or a portable kidney perfusion unit. The kidney should be flushed for at least 5 minutes before placement in the recipient.

STAGE II: TRANSPLANTATION OF THE KIDNEY

Positioning: Supine

Packs/Drapes: Laparotomy pack
    Basic pack (for perfusion set-up table)

Instrumentation:
    See Nephrectomy, p. 513

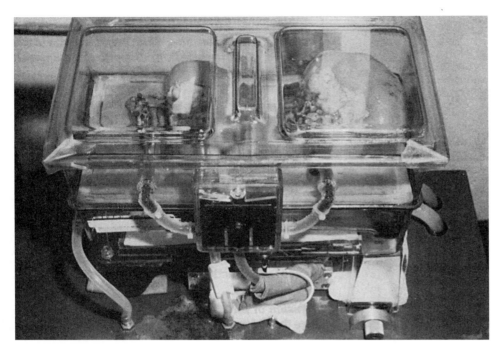

Kidney perfusion unit can maintain kidneys for up to 3 days by perfusion solution and oxygenation (Courtesy of the University of Miami Organ Procurement and Transplantation Program)

Minor tray may be added to the perfusion table set-up

Supplies/Equipment:
Basin sets
Blades—(2) No. 10, (1) No. 15
Foley catheter with drainage unit
ESU; suction
Needle counter
Drain (e.g., Penrose)
Solutions—saline, water
Sutures—surgeon's preference
Medication—heparinized saline

PROCEDURAL OVERVIEW

The kidney is brought to the recipient team by the donor's surgeon or designee. The recipient's surgeon makes a long inguinal incision that is carried down to the iliac fossa by blunt and sharp dissection. (The kidney is usually placed in the patient's iliac fossa to avoid peritonitis.) The surgeon identifies the external iliac vein and hypogastric artery. Anastomoses are then performed between the renal artery and hypogastric artery and between the renal vein and external iliac vein (4-0 or 5-0 nonabsorbable vascular suture). Before the anastomoses, the patient is given a systemic dose of IV heparin by the anesthesiologist.

The surgeon will implant the donor ureter into the bladder. The bladder is grasped with two or more Allis clamps, and then incised. A separate incision is made to accommodate the ureter. The surgeon sutures the ureter through the first incision (3-0 or 4-0 chromic; Dexon). A Penrose drain is placed near the bladder wall, and the first incision is closed in three layers 2-0 or 3-0 chromic; Dexon).

This completes the procedure, and the wound is closed in three layers (as for an inguinal hernia repair).

PERIOPERATIVE NURSING CONSIDERATIONS

- Permission to harvest the donor kidney must be obtained from the family and the medical examiner, only after the patient has been declared *legally dead* according to state statutes. It is advisable to be aware of existing state legislation and transplantation protocol in this complex area.
- Support systems for the families of both the donor family (especially following a traumatic death), the recipient family, and the patient should be activated since psychologic changes may develop that need professional intervention.
- A harvesting procedure (cadaver donor), especially on a young patient, may be traumatic on the participating nursing staff, since once the kidney is out, the need for life support from anesthesia is no longer required. Ample support should be available to assist the staff in overcoming any potential

psychologic problems that could interfere with the efficient execution of care required.

- Following the harvesting procedure, postmortem care is performed according to hospital protocol.

Procedure
Open Prostectomy

Definition: Excision and removal of the prostate gland via a surgical excision.

CDC Classification: II

Discussion: Although 90 percent of prostectomies are performed via the transurethral approach, there are occasions when a surgical incision and removal is required (e.g., due to the size or coexisting circumstances).

Four approaches can be used to excise the prostate gland:

1. *Transurethral Prostectomy*—see TUR-P, pp. 512–513.
2. *Suprapubic Prostectomy*—performed after incising the bladder, which permits correction of associated conditions, such as calculi and diverticula. However, it is not used for malignancy.
3. *Retropubic Prostectomy*—avoids entry into the bladder and allows for good visualization of the field. Limited malignancies may be treated by this approach.
4. *Perineal Prostectomy*—affords excellent visualization and access to the prostate and seminal vesicles. Useful for radical excision of the prostate, including the capsule, seminal vesicles, and portions of the vas.

A bilateral vasectomy may be performed in conjunction with a prostectomy to avoid retrograde infections.

Positioning:
  Suprapubic and retropubic: Supine with slight Trendelenberg
  Perineal: Exaggerated lithotomy with slight Trendelenberg

Incision Site: All approaches use the same incision site: transverse or longitudinal, above the pubis

Skin Preparation: See pp. 337–338

Packs/Drapes:
  Suprapubic: Laparotomy pack
    Extra drape sheets
    Transverse Lap sheet (opt.)
  Retropubic: Laparotomy pack
    Impervious sheet (for scrotal area)
    Folded towel over scrotum and penis
  Perineal: Cysto pack
    Towels around the perineal area
    Fenestrated sheet

Instrumentation:
  Major tray
  Long instruments (open prostectomy tray)
  Heaney needle holders (2)
  Lahey clamps (4)
  Prostatic urethral sounds
  Hemoclips/surgiclips appliers (size variety)
  For suprapubic add:
  Self-retaining retractor (e.g., Judd-Mason)
  For retropubic add:
  Retropubic bladder retractor (e.g., Millin)
  For perineal add:
  Perineal prostectomy retractor (e.g., Denis-Brown; Lowsley, etc.)

Supplies/Equipment:
  Basin set
  Blades—(2) No. 10, (1) No. 15, (1) No. 11
  Needle counter
  ESU; suction
  Dissector sponges (e.g., Kittners)
  Irrigation syringe (30 mL with cone tip)
  Solutions—saline, water
  Lubricant
  Sutures—surgeon's preference
  Suprapubic catheter (e.g., Malecot; Pezzer) (opt.)
  Drain (e.g., 1-in. Penrose)
  Foley catheter with 30-mL balloon (for postop hemostasis)

PROCEDURAL OVERVIEW

For the purpose of this discussion, a suprapubic prostectomy will be outlined.

The surgeon makes the appropriate incision, and after access is gained into the *space of Retzius*, a self-retaining retractor is placed into the wound.

Before the bladder is opened, the surgeon places two traction sutures (0-chromic) on either side of the incision. The bladder may be grasped with an Allis clamp and pulled upward. A short incision is made into the bladder, and suction is applied to drain its contents. (The tip should be changed after this process.) After draining the bladder, the surgeon places a bladder retractor (Judd-Mason or Deaver) in the bladder wound. The surgeon incises the prostatic mucosa by either knife or cautery, and the bladder retractor(s) are removed.

Using finger dissection, the surgeon enucleates the diseased prostate from its fossa (cavity), and the specimen is delivered and passed off to the scrub person.

The cavity is inspected for bleeders. Many surgeons prefer to pack the cavity with a sponge for a few minutes to maintain hemostasis. Large bleeding vessels are ligated with suture (0 or 2-0 chromic) or ligiclips. Oozing surfaces may be covered with a hemostatic agent (e.g., Surgicel; Avitine). A Foley catheter (30-mL balloon) is placed into the bladder neck. Some surgeons prefer to drain the bladder through a suprapubic catheter (e.g., Malecot; Pezzer), which is placed in the wound at this time through a small incision (stab wound) near the suprapubic incision.

The bladder is then closed with two layers of 0 or 2-0 chromic interrupted sutures. A large Penrose drain is placed into the space of Retzius; and the wound is closed in a routine manner.

PERIOPERATIVE NURSING CONSIDERATIONS

- If a retropubic prostectomy is performed, a suprapubic incision is used, exposing the prostate and bladder neck.
- Continuous bladder irrigation fluid should be isotonic and at body temperature (postoperative).
- If stirrups (knee brace) are used in positioning, they should be well padded, with a sacral support to prevent nerve injury or pressure.

Related Procedures: Retropubic Prostectomy
Perineal Prostectomy

Procedure
Upper Tract Urolithotomy

Definition: Removal of *calculi* (stones) from the ureter, renal pelvis, and/or kidney.
CDC Classification: II
Discussion: If a *lithotriptic* procedure (e.g., ESWL, ultrasonic, or other nephroscopic and transcystoscopic modality) is unsuccessful or unavailable, or these procedures are contraindicated, open surgery is required for the extraction of the stone(s).
Positioning: Lateral, if stone is in the kidney or proximal ureter (see Nephrectomy, p. 513)
Supine, for stones in the distal ureter
Incision Site: Flank (proximal calculi), lower midline abdominal or transverse oblique (distal calculi)
Skin Preparation: See pp. 337–338
Packs/Drapes:
Laparotomy pack
Transverse Lap sheet (opt.)
Folded towels
Instrumentation:
Major tray
Kidney tray
Thoracotomy tray (available)
Hemoclips/surgiclips (size variety)
Supplies/Equipment:
Positioning aids
Basin set
Blades—(2) No. 10, (1) No. 15, (1) No. 11
ESU; suction

Needle counter
Asepto syringe (opt.)
Hemoclips/surgiclips (size variety)
Vessel loops and umbilical tape
Dissecting sponges (e.g., Kittners)
Drain (e.g., ¼-in. Penrose for retraction; 1 in. for drainage [2])
Ureteral catheter
Solutions—saline, water
Sutures—surgeon's preference
Note: Have nephroscope and fiberoptic light source available.

PROCEDURAL OVERVIEW

For the purpose of this discussion, a *pyelolithotomy* will be outlined.

With the patient in the lateral position, the surgeon enters the retroperitoneal space through a flank incision (simple nephrectomy). The ureter is mobilized with blunt and sharp dissection, and a small Penrose drain is placed around the ureter for traction and to prevent the stone from traveling down the ureter.

Before incising the renal pelvis the surgeon may place two or three traction sutures (3-0 chromic) on either side of the incision. The kidney is incised with a knife (or cautery) and the stone is lifted out with a tissue forceps and passed off as a specimen.

A ureteral catheter is passed down the ureter and into the bladder to make sure no other stones are present or have migrated down into the ureter.

The incision in the renal pelvis is closed with interrupted suture (4-0 or 5-0 on a fine tapered needle). The wound is irrigated with warm saline. A large Penrose drain (one or two) may be placed near the renal pelvis, and the wound is closed in a routine fashion.

PERIOPERATIVE NURSING CONSIDERATIONS

- Have all the patient's x-rays in the room.
- Calcium chloride, thrombin, and cryoprecipitate may be injected to form a clot around the stone, preventing migration.
- A gastrointestinal and vascular instrument tray should be available.
- See Nephrectomy, p. 513, for additional considerations.

Related Procedures: Ureterolithotomy
Nephrolithotomy

Procedure
Vasectomy (Bilateral)

Definition: Excision of a segment of the vas deferens with ligation of distal and proximal ends.

CDC Classification: II

Discussion: This procedure is performed as an elective sterilization procedure or to prevent orchitis prior to a prostectomy. It can be performed under local, regional, or general anesthesia and as an outpatient procedure.

Positioning: Supine, with legs slightly apart

Incision Site: Scrotum

Skin Preparation: See pp. 337–338

Packs/Drapes: Laparotomy pack or basic pack with transverse Lap sheet

Instrumentation:

Vasectomy tray (if available) or minor (very fine) tray

Supplies/Equipment:

Basin set

Blades—(1) No. 10, (1) No. 15

ESU; suction

Solutions—saline, water

Sutures—surgeon's preference

Scrotal support (opt.)

PROCEDURAL OVERVIEW

The vas deferens is palpated through the scrotum before anesthesia (local) is administered. A small incision is made in the scrotum. The vas is seized with an Allis or Babcock clamp and is freed of surrounding tissue. A segment of the vas is excised and the ends ligated or cauterized. The ends may be buried within the scrotal fascia with one or two sutures (3-0 chromic/Dexon). The procedure is repeated on the other side, and the incision is closed in layers (3-0 or 4-0 Dexon, interrupted on a cutting needle).

PERIOPERATIVE NURSING CONSIDERATIONS

- Local anesthesia is frequently used.
- An ice pack may be applied to the scrotum immediately after surgery.
- A sterilization permit may be needed in addition to the operative consent. Check hospital protocol.

Related Procedure:

Vasovasostomy: The reestablishment of the severed ends of the vas deferens (usually requires microsurgery)

Cutaneous Vasostomy: An opening of the vas onto the scrotal skin (for drainage)

Procedure
Circumcision

Definition: The excision of the foreskin (*prepuce*).

CDC Classification: I

Discussion: Circumcisions are commonly performed on the male infant at birth or shortly thereafter. However, the uncircumcised adult may experience difficulty in retracting the prepuce from the glans of the penis because of a stricture (*phimosis*), which requires surgical intervention, or circumcision may be performed to treat recurrent balanitis or as a religious rite.

If performed on an infant, the procedure may take place in a separate part of the newborn nursery, aseptically suited for the procedure.

Positioning: Supine, with legs slightly apart, or lithotomy

Children and infants may be placed in a frog-leg position or on a specially designed board (circumcision board)

Incision Site: Circumferentially around the glans penis

Skin Preparation: See pp. 337–338

Packs/Drapes:

Child: Pediatric Lap sheet

Adult: Laparotomy pack

Folded towels around the perineal area

Infant: Pediatric Lap sheet or folded towels

Instrumentation:

Infants and Children: Pediatric Lap tray

Circumcision clamp (e.g., Gomco)

Adults: Minor/very fine tray

Probe and groove director (opt.)

Supplies/Equipment:

Basin set

ESU; suction (opt.)

Blades—(2) No. 15

Needle counter

Catheter (e.g., Foley [adult surgery])

Gauze roll and impregnated gauze strips

Solutions—saline, water

PROCEDURAL OVERVIEW

If phimosis is present, a dorsal slit is made. Adhesions are lysed. A circumferential incision is made at the reflection of the foreskin, which is then excised. Hemostasis is achieved, and the wound edges are approximated using absorbable suture.

For a very young infant, the skin edges are usually not approximated.

A strip of nonadherent gauze (e.g., Vaseline; Adaptic; Xeroform) is placed around the incision and is covered with a gauze roll dressing. A piece of umbilical tape may hold the gauze roll in place. No other dressing is usually necessary.

PERIOPERATIVE NURSING CONSIDERATIONS

- Consider the special needs of the Jewish patient for a ritual circumcision. All female surgical team members may be asked to leave the room during the procedure. Therefore, staff accordingly if male personnel are available to assist.

Procedure
Hypospadias Repair

Definition: Correction of a condition in which the anterior urethra terminates on the undersurface of the penis.

CDC Classification: I

Discussion: Hypospadias is a congenital defect that interferes with normal urination and fertilization of the female. Hypospadias can be noted distally, midpenile, perineal, or penoscrotal.

It should be noted that circumcisions should not be performed on infants with hypospadias, in order to preserve the skin that may be used in correcting the deformity. Correction may be delayed until full penile growth has occurred.

Incision Site: Ventral aspect of the penis

Positioning, Skin Preparation, Packs, Drapes, Supplies, Equipment: See Circumcision, p. 519

Instrumentation:

> *Adults:* Minor/very fine tray
> Urethral sounds (graduated sizes)
> *Children:* Pediatric Lap tray (small infant/child) or very fine tray (toddler size or larger)
> Lacrimal duct probes

PROCEDURAL OVERVIEW

The *chordee* (downward curvature of the penis) is repaired by lysing the fibrous tissue on the ventral aspect of the penis. The absent portion of the urethra is reconstructed out of foreskin. If the patient has been circumcised, other tissue may be used.

An incision is made on the ventral aspect of the penis. The reconstructed urethra, splinted from within by a catheter, is placed in a tunnel over which the remaining foreskin is grafted.

A variety of procedural steps can be used according to the severity of the defect, and some may require a second stage for complete repair.

PERIOPERATIVE NURSING CONSIDERATIONS

- When very distal, the deformity is minimal, and may not require correction. Continence of urine is not usually affected because the urinary sphincters are not involved.
- Proximal locations necessitate correction to avoid dysuria and difficulty in intercourse.
- The adult may feel extremely self-conscious. Male personnel (if available) may be more appropriate.
- Care must be taken to adequately secure the child while preventing trauma to skin and pressure points.

Related Procedures: Espadias Repair (urethral opening on the dorsal aspect of the penis)

Procedure
Urinary Diversion, Ileal Conduit

Definition: The use of an isolated segment of the ileum into which the ureters are implanted, exiting as a urostomy stoma on the abdominal wall.

CDC Classification: II

Discussion: There are many different types of urinary diversion procedures that use a segment of the bowel to replace the bladder (e.g., ureterosigmoidostomy, cutaneous ureterostomy). The creation of an ileal conduit has superseded these procedures, however, avoiding the potential of ascending urinary tract infection, diarrhea, skin problems, and so on. This procedure is usually performed for malignancy of the bladder, severe strictures of the distal ureters, or other conditions that may require urinary diversion (e.g., following a cystectomy).

Positioning: Supine, with arms extended on armboards

Incision Site: Cystectomy incision (midline or low transverse)

Skin Preparation: See pp. 337–338

Packs/Drapes: Laparotomy pack

Instrumentation:

> Major tray
> Intestinal tray
> Hemoclip/surgiclip appliers
> Internal stapling device (opt.)

Supplies/Equipment:

> Basin set
> Blades—(2) No. 10, (1) No. 15, (1) No. 11
> Needle counter
> ESU; suction
> Dissector sponges (e.g., Kittners)
> Ureteral stent (e.g., silastic ureteral catheter)
> Urostomy pouch
> Internal staples (opt.)
> Drains (e.g., Penrose) (opt.)
> Solutions—water, saline
> Sutures—surgeon's preference

PROCEDURAL OVERVIEW

The abdomen is entered and a portion of the colon and ileum is mobilized. The distal ileum is exposed and a segment (15 cm) is divided from the ileum, maintaining the mesentery.

The continuity of the proximal and distal ileum is reestablished, and the mesentery is closed over the intervening mesentery of the isolated loop, to prevent herniation. The proximal end of isolated loop is closed with a double layer of suture (3-0 chromic; taper needle). The ureters are dissected and anastomosed to the ileal loop (end-to-side; 4-0 chromic) (Fig. 14-11).

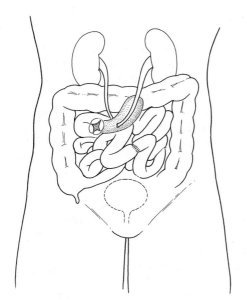

Fig. 14-11.   Ileal conduit: Urine is diverted into a portion of intestine. Skin stoma requires a pouch.

Internal staples may be used to perform the intestinal anastomosis and closure of the proximal end of the isolated loop. The wound is irrigated and closed in the routine manner.

PERIOPERATIVE NURSING CONSIDERATIONS

- The ileal conduit may be constructed before or after the bladder is excised.
- In selected cases, when urinary sphincter function remains intact, the ileal segment may be anastomosed as a bladder substitute to the proximal urethra, preserving urinary function.
- Verify with the blood bank for available units.
- If a colonic conduit is necessary, no-touch technique must be used.

Related Procedures: Ureterosigmoidostomy
　　Ureteroenterocutaneous Diversion
　　Sigmoid Conduit Diversion
　　Ureterojejunal Cutaneous Diversion

Procedure
Nephroscopic Extraction of a Stone via Percutaneous Nephroureterolithotomy (PCNL)

Definition: Removal or disintegration of kidney stones (*litholapaxy*) using a percutaneous approach via a flexible or rigid nephroscope.

CDC Classification: I

Discussion: Numerous techniques are available for removing calculi from the urinary tract and/or the kidney without the need for an open nephrolithotomy if the calculi are no larger than 1 cm and are free-floating, radiopaque, and solid.

Accessory instrumentation, such as the ultrasound wand (sonotrode) or the electrohydrolic lithotripter probe, can be passed through the lumen of the nephroscope to achieve the desired results.

The patient may be scheduled for a cystoscopic examination first to try to remove the stone. If this is unsuccessful, the anesthetized patient is moved to an open procedure room for the second stage of the procedure.

Positioning: Supine, with affected side up

Incision Site: Area of the kidney pelvis (site is confirmed by x-ray before start of procedure)

Packs/Drapes:
　　Major pack
　　PCNL drape sheet
　　C-Arm drape
　　Basic pack (PCNL set-up for radiology)

Instrumentation:
　　Nephroscope (flexible or rigid)
　　PCNL tray
　　Major tray
　　Kidney tray (available)

Supplies/Equipment:
　　Positioning aids
　　Carousel suction (multiple cannister set-up)
　　IV pole
　　Cysto tubing (four spikes)
　　Fiberoptic light source
　　C-Arm (fluoroscopy with camera)
　　PCNL accessory cart (opt.)
　　Blades—(2) No. 10, (1) No. 15, (1) No. 11
　　Drainage tube (e.g., nephrostomy; Penrose)
　　Solutions—saline for bladder irrigation warmed (to avoid fogging of lens), saline, water
　　Sutures—surgeon's preference

PROCEDURAL OVERVIEW

Using fluoroscopy, a small incision is made and a guidewire is introduced inside a transluminal angioplasty catheter. Dilators are placed over the guidewires to enlarge the entrance. (The radiologist and urologist work as a team to achieve proper placement.) The nephroscope is inserted into the opening, and the lithotriptor is passed through the scope. The stones are fragmented and suctioned out.

A drainage tube is left in place for continuous irrigation, and the percutaneous incision site is closed and dressed.

PERIOPERATIVE NURSING CONSIDERATIONS

- The basic concern during the procedure is the proper position and the type of anesthesia to be administered.
- Irrigation solution, unlike with the cysto set-up, must be monitored and changed as solution containers become low. Because of the large amount of solution, and the lack of drainage set-up as in the cysto room, a multicannister set-up (carousel) is required.
- The procedure may be a continuation of a cysto procedure, in which the patient is transported to the open room, asleep. The perioperative nurse caring for the patient during the cysto portion should give a verbal report to the nurse assigned to the PCNL procedure to maintain continuity of care. Documentation is recorded as two separate procedures (two records). Follow hospital protocol.
- The PCNL room is set up on a stand-by basis during the cysto procedure to minimize anesthesia time following transfer from the cysto room.
- For a two-stage procedure, the nephrostomy tract is established with the patient under local anesthesia. The patient is discharged the following day with a 22 or 24 French nephrostomy tube connected to drainage. The patient is readmitted 5 to 7 days later for the percutaneous removal of the calculi under general anesthesia.

Noninvasive Therapy for Renal Calculi

Procedure
Extracorporeal Shockwave Lithotripsy (ESWL)

Definition: Disintegration of upper urinary tract calculi by means of precisely directed shock waves delivered to the patient either immersed in a water bath or lying on a special table.

Discussion: The ESWL unit makes possible the removal of most upper urinary tract calculi without surgery. Multiple shock waves produced by an electrode beneath the immersed patient pass from the water into the body, pulverizing the calculus into sandlike particles that are eliminated in the urine.

A modular lithotriptor, developed by the manufacturer of the currently used ESWL system, has made the availability of this procedure possible even if the hospital does not have its own unit.

The ESWL procedure may be performed under general, spinal, or epidural anesthesia. Following the administration of anesthesia the patient is transferred to the gantry stretcher and strapped in for safety and to counter the effects of buoyancy.

PERIOPERATIVE NURSING CONSIDERATIONS

- A lithotriptor supervisor is essential to the well-run lithotripsy unit. He or she is responsible for checking and preparing the equipment and assisting the physician and anesthesia personnel.
- It is absolutely essential for the circulator working with the lithotripsy patient to be thoroughly familiar with the ESWL unit.
- ESWL is frequently used in conjunction with PCNL, open surgery, and transurethral ureteropyeloscopy if the patient does not pass the "gravel."
- For the majority of circumstances, the perioperative nurse, working in surgery, will not be involved with the ESWL procedure, but knowledge of this alternative technique should be acquired should the need for assistance arise.
- ESWL may be performed in a special water tub or on a special table depending on the facility and surgeon's preference.

Self-assessment Exercise 32

Directions: Complete the following exercises. The answers can be found at the end of this module.

1. Place the following layers of the abdominal wall in proper sequence for a laparotomy closure.
    1. subcutaneous tissue
    2. muscle
    3. peritoneum
    4. extraperitoneal fat
    5. transversalis fascia
    6. skin
    7. deep fascia
       a. 4, 3, 7, 2, 5, 1, 6
       b. 3, 7, 2, 5, 4, 1, 6
       c. 3, 4, 5, 2, 7, 1, 6
       d. 4, 3, 5, 2, 7, 1, 6

2. A hernia that passes through the inguinal ring into the inguinal canal is called an *indirect hernia.*

    True   False

3. An anastomosis between the stomach and the jejunal portion of the small intestines is called

    a _____.

4. List the common types of catheters related to urologic procedures.

5. The operative procedure that could cause "surgical menopause" is a bilateral salpingo-oophorectomy.

    True   False

6. The incision site for an appendectomy is called

    a _____.

7. A percutaneous approach to isolating and crushing a kidney stone is called a _____

    _____.

8. A direct inguinal hernia (*would/would not*) have a specimen.

9. A right hemicolectomy is performed to remove pathology involving the _____

    _____ portion of the colon.

10. What two anatomical structures are identified and ligated to effect a cholecystectomy? _____

    _____.

11. List the four approaches that could be used to remove an enlarged prostate gland.

12. List the instrumentation required to perform a cysto with TUR bladder tumor.

13. A C-section requires _____ counts. They are performed at specific intervals. List them.

14. The specimen usually obtained during a D&C procedure is a(an):
    a. myometrial curetting
    b. cervical curetting
    c. endometrial curetting
    d. perimetrial curetting

15. A 22-year-old primagravida, in the first trimester, is admitted with sudden intense, knife-like abdominal pain, vaginal bleeding, and symptoms of shock. She is scheduled for surgery.
    a. The preoperative diagnosis would most likely be:

       _____.

    b. The surgical procedure would most likely

       be: _____.

ORTHOPEDIC SURGERY

Orthopedics is derived from the Greek words meaning "straight" and "child," and was originally concerned with the treatment of deformities in children using braces, limiting activity and exercises. According to the American Board of Orthopaedic Surgery, the contemporary definition of this specialty service states it is the "branch of surgery especially concerned with the preservation and restoration of the functions of the skeletal system, its articulations and associated structures."

Orthopedic surgery is performed to (1) repair a fractured bone, (2) reconstruct a joint, (3) repair or correct deformities in bone and/or soft tissue, and (4) perform diagnostic examinations to determine the extent of damage to a joint.

As with many of the surgical specialties, changes have been rapid as new technology and equipment become available. Because of the dynamic nature of this service, and because of continuing changes in technology and equipment, this unit will focus on the "foundation" procedures, techniques, and equipment that apply to the major types of orthopedic procedures.

The selected surgical procedures have been placed in the following divisions for ease of reference:

Repair and Management of Fractures
Revision/Reconstruction of Joints
Correction of Deformities (Soft Tissue or Bone)
Arthroscopic Surgery

Surgical Anatomy Review

The *musculoskeletal system* provides support and movement, and it consists of bones, articulations (joints between bones), and skeletal muscles.

The Skeleton

Divisions of the Skeleton   The human skeleton consists of two main divisions.

1. *Axial Skeleton*—made up of 80 bones that form the upright axis of the body and six tiny middle-ear bones. These bones do not move, and they form the rigid support for the body
2. *Appendicular Skeleton*—consists of 126 bones that form the appendages that move and articulate with the axial skeleton

Components of the Skeleton   Bones perform five basic functions:

1. Support—framework of the body
2. Protection—for delicate structures and major organs
3. Movement—mobility through muscular attachment
4. Reservoir—for calcium deposits
5. Hemopoiesis—formation of blood cells

Classification/Types of Bones   There are four types of bones. Their names suggest their shape and primary location:

1. *Long Bones*—upper and lower extremities
   Examples: humerus, femur, tibia, phalanges
2. *Short Bones*—wrist and ankle
   Examples: carpals, tarsals
3. *Flat Bones*—certain bones of the cranium and the shoulder
   Examples: frontal cranium, ribs, scapula
4. *Irregular Bones*—spinal column and certain bones of the cranium
   Examples: vertebrae, coccyx, sphenoid, mandible

Reference Landmarks   Various points on bones, used as reference landmarks, are labeled according to the nature of their structure. They are used to assist in locating other structures, such as muscles, blood vessels, and nerves.

For example, the ulna has the following landmarks: (1) the olecranon process, (2) the semilunar notch, and (3) the radial notch. The cranium has such markings as (1) the frontal tuberosities, (2) the supraorbital notch, (3) the foramen magnum, and (4) the sutures and fontanels.

In addition to the bone markings, there are openings and depressions that also serve as anatomical landmarks, such as a fossa (hollow depression), a sinus (cavity or space in a bone), a foramen (a hole), or a meatus (a tube-shaped opening).

Projections and processes are also a part of bone structure; some enter into the formation of joints, such as a condyle or head, while others—such as the trochanter or crest, spinous process, tuberosity, and tubercle—are attachments for muscles.

Articulations of the Skeletal System

Articulations are actually joints between the bones that hold bones together while permitting movement.

Classification of Joints and Structures   There are three basic kinds of joints, each serving a specific purpose:

1. *Fibrous Joints*—found attaching two bone surfaces and made up of fibrous connective tissue that bind them together
2. *Cartilaginous Joints*—Cartilage joins one bone to another. There are two types: (1) symphysis and (2) synchondrosis. Symphyses are located in the middle of the body (e.g., symphysis pubis), while the synchondroses are joints between the ribs and the sternum.
3. *Synovial Joints*—the most mobile and make up the larger portion of joints. These permit a variety of movement and are found at most hinged joints in the body.

Because synovial joints differ somewhat in structure and the kind of movement they permit, they have been subdivided into six types (Fig. 14-12):

1. *Ball and Socket*—hip, shoulder
2. *Hinge*—knee, elbow
3. *Pivot*—first and second cervical vertebrae
4. *Ellipsoidal*—radius and carpal bones
5. *Saddle*—joints between the metacarpal bone of the thumb and carpal bone
6. *Gliding*—most joints of the wrist and ankle and between articular processes of the vertebrae

Bursa, Tendons, and Ligaments   Bursa are small connective tissue sacs lined with synovial membrane and containing synovial fluid. Bursa act as a cushion, re-

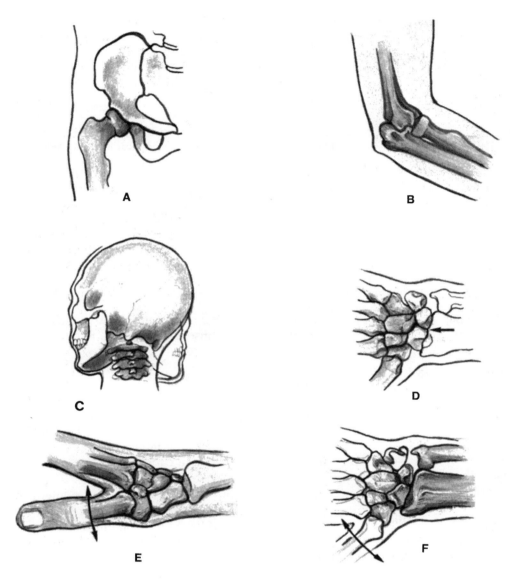

Fig. 14-12. Types of synovial joints: (A) ball and socket; (B) hinge; (C) pivot; (D) ellipsoidal; (E) gliding; (F) saddle

lieving pressure on the joints. They are located wherever pressure is exerted over moving parts (bone and skin, tendons and bones; or muscles, ligaments, and bone), and can become inflamed if the lining becomes thin or worn by age or consistent use.

Tendons are a group of connective tissue that aid in attaching the muscle to the bone. Such an extension may take the form of a cord or may be in the form of a sheet (fascia). The purpose of tendons is to furnish a means of power for movement.

Ligaments are strong cords of dense white fibrous tissue at most synovial joints, holding the bones together. They are predominantly found in connection with all the freely movable joints, and many of the less movable articulations.

The Muscular System

Types/Locations   There are three major muscle types in the human body:

1. *Smooth*—activated involuntarily, that is, we have no direct ability to cause their contraction
2. *Cardiac*—the muscles of the heart; also involuntary but represent a separate group because they are different in structure and mechanism
3. *Striated*—under voluntary control, such as those classified as skeletal muscles

Skeletal Muscle Group   The human body contains more than 400 skeletal muscles, constituting between

35 and 40 percent of body weight. A large number of skeletal muscles are arranged in pairs and/or groups, according to their location:

1. Muscles of the Head
2. Muscles of the Neck
3. Muscles of the Upper Extremities
4. Muscles of the Abdomen
5. Muscles of the Lower Extremities

Characteristics of Skeletal Muscles   Bones and joints cannot move by themselves. They must be helped by muscles, which give the skeleton movement. Muscle tissue, because of its irritability, contractility, and elasticity, is suited to this function.

Skeletal muscles serve three general functions:

1. *Movement*—Skeletal muscle contractions produce movements either of the body as a whole (locomotion) or its parts.
2. *Heat Production*—Muscle cells, like all cells, produce heat by a process known as catabolism. Because skeletal muscle cells are both highly active and numerous, they produce a major share of the total body heat.
3. *Posture*—The continued partial contraction of many skeletal muscles makes possible standing, sitting, or other maintained positions of the body.

Origin, Insertion, and Movement   Most muscles have two or more attachments to the skeleton, one of which is more freely movable than the other. The less movable (fixed) attachment is called the origin, while the part of the body that the muscle activates is called the insertion.

General Discussion

Instrumentation

Orthopedic procedure requires specific instrumentation for a particular procedure or specific piece of hardware that will be used. Using the five general categories of instrumentation (Chap. 9), orthopedic instruments can be classified into the same categories, but this is where the similarity ends. The following is a descriptive listing of some of the more commonly used orthopedic instruments.

Cutting Instruments

Description: used to remove soft tissue around bone or to cut apart or cut out portions of bone, or to smooth jagged edges of bone

Examples: include, but are not limited to, osteotomes, rasps, curettes, rongeurs and special knives; power or manual saw/drills

Grasping/Holding Instruments

Description: are required to hold, manipulate, and provide traction of bone or bone fragments

Examples: include, but are not limited to, bone clamps, bone hooks, bone holding forceps, and cartilage clamps

Exposing/Retracting Instruments

Description: used to expose a bone or joint, retract soft tissue away from the bone, or elevate tissue away from bone

Examples: include, but are not limited to, hand-held retractors—Rakes, Hibbs, Bennett; self-retaining—laminar spreaders, Adson cerebellum retractors; elevators—Langenbeck, Freer, Key

Suturing Instruments

Description: used to approximate bone and/or soft tissue

Examples: include, but are not limited to, Wagensteen needle holders, Johnson, Crile-Wood, Ryder needle holders

Miscellaneous Instruments

Description: used to assist in applying specialty devices, cut wire/pins, or to measure depth

Examples: include, but are not limited to, calipers, screw depth gauges, acetabular gauges, needle pliers, screwdrivers, pin cutters, wrenches

In addition to the specialty instruments required to perform a specific procedure, a basic instrument tray (for soft tissue) is added to the bone instruments. In some hospitals, they may be combined, creating a *Basic Orthopedic Tray* (for bone and soft tissue), with the specialized instruments associated with a specific device selected in addition to the basic orthopedic tray.

Accessory Supplies/Equipment

1. **Power-Driven Equipment/Instruments**

Frequently, orthopedic procedures require a variety of power-driven drills and saws to accomplish a specific job related to the surgery. This equipment offers precision in drilling, cutting, shaping, and beveling bone and may have a variety of attachments depending on the immediate need.

In addition to power-driven saws and drills, hand drills or braces may also be used to accomplish a similar task.

2. **Implant-Related Instruments**

Specific clamps, drivers, and retractors are used for inserting and securing implanted devices. Each type of implant demands its own instrumentation.

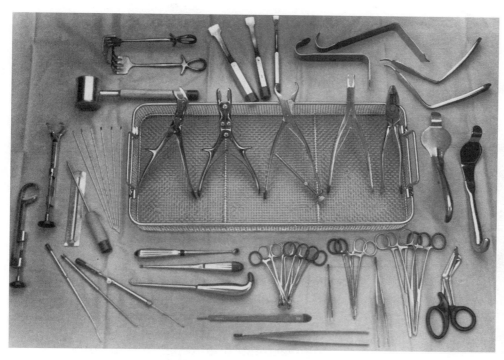

Major (basic) orthopedic instrument tray

3. Casting Materials

In order to help stabilize a limb following surgery, a cast may be applied made of either fiberglass or plaster, depending on the preference of the surgeon. Casting materials are available in either rolls or strips of various widths and, depending on the type of material, either hot or cold water will be used to help apply the cast to the extremity. The limb is first wrapped in a soft material (e.g., Webrill, Soft Roll) and the casting material is applied and shaped to fit the extremity. After the limb has been casted, a pillow should be placed under it, preventing the plaster from becoming indented or misshaped. Until it dries, the cast should be handled as little as possible.

4. Bone Cement

Bone cement (methylmethacrylate) is often used to hold a metal or synthetic prosthesis in place, as in a total joint replacement. Because of the fumes from the cement, a closed mixing system with suction should be used any time a cementing procedure is indicated. The cement begins as a powdery substance, and when solution is added it begins to harden, forming a pastelike substance. When the cement takes on a doughy consistency (which sticks to gloves), it is ready for use. Many scrub persons will don two pairs of gloves during the preparation phase, removing the outer pair once the cement is ready for usage.

5. Orthopedic Hardware

Plates, pins, screws, and nails form the backbone for a majority of orthopedic procedures. Plates are available in a wide variety of sizes and shapes. Pins and nails are inserted with special impactors or driving instruments. In order to insert a screw or nail into a bone, a hole must be created first with a drill bit specifically sized to accommodate the size of the screw or nail. A depth gauge and guide wire are used (1) to measure the depth of the hole created by the drill bit so that the screw or nail of the proper length is used, and (2) to guide the screw or nail into the proper position to accomplish correct placement.

6. Bone Grafts

When it becomes necessary to remove a piece of bone from one part of the skeleton to replace or reinforce another bone, a bone graft is needed. This process can either be accomplished by taking the piece of bone from the patient (autogenous), or it may be ordered from a professional bone bank (allograft), which specializes in procuring and preserving bone for future application.

Perioperative Nursing Considerations

Transport, Moving, and Lifting

Orthopedic patients require special handling since they may arrive in surgery in severe pain, wearing splints or in traction, and/or may have gaping wounds. Moving and lifting must be accomplished

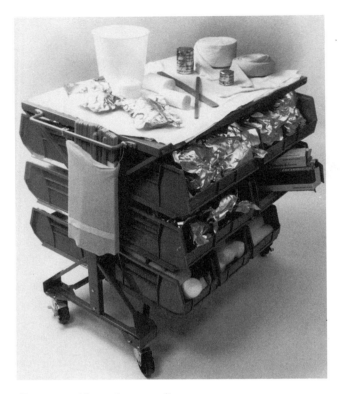

Cast cart with casting supplies

with utmost care, immobilizing the affected part, and with adequate help during the transfer and moving phase. For example, a patient with a fractured hip should not be moved from the bed to a stretcher to be taken to the OR, but should be transported in the bed to avoid unnecessary pain and movement while awake.

Before the patient is moved, the site and type of injury should be well known by all members of the team and the area protected from accidental reinjury. If the patient arrives with splints or traction in place, the surgeon should be available to supervise its removal.

Preliminary Room Preparation

The surgical team must be able to manage an abnormal amount of instrumentation, supplies, equipment, and additional furniture while maintaining an aseptic environment.

X-rays have an important role in enabling the surgeon to determine the location, size, deflection, and repair route for the planned surgical intervention. All of the patient's x-rays should be in the room before starting the procedure, and if needed, the x-ray technician should be notified that films may be required during the procedure.

Special operating tables and/or positioning aids may be needed to accommodate specific types of sur-

gery, for example, fracture table, side (hand table), Wilson frame, and Vac-Pack.

Positioning aids, such as gauze, tape, ABDs, Webrill, should also be available to assist in securing the patient in the proper position without additional discomfort. Usually, the patient will be put to sleep on the bed and then moved and properly positioned.

Power equipment, frequently used during an orthopedic procedure, should be checked prior to use, and suctioning equipment should be adequate to handle the extra fluid/blood loss.

A pneumatic tourniquet is usually used for operations on or below the elbow and knee, providing better visualization during the procedure. The cuff is applied before the prep; however, it is not inflated until the draping is completed.

The successful management of an active orthopedic operating room depends on the maintenance of adequate supplies and the teamwork employed during the surgical procedure.

Management and Repair of Fractures

Classification of Fractures

Fractures are classified by their type, location, and direction. Figure 14-13A on the following page illustrates the most common types of fractures.

1. *Closed-nondisplaced*—Fracture that does not extend through mucous membrane or skin
2. *Open; Compound*—Bone is broken and an external wound leads down to site of fracture. Trauma graded I–III depending on extent of injury
3. *Comminuted*—A fracture causing the bone to splinter/shatter into several small pieces; usually more than one fracture line

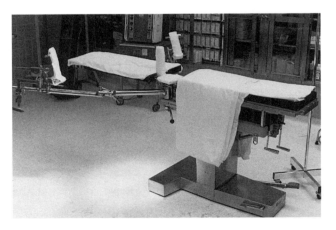

Fracture table with accessories

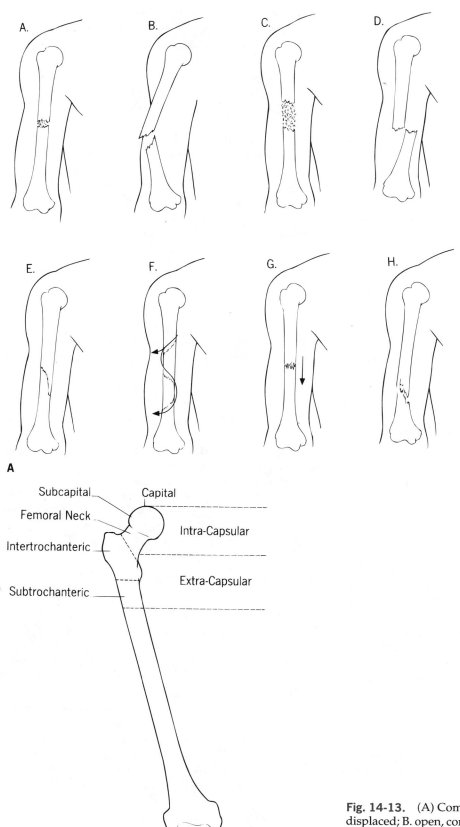

Fig. 14-13. (A) Common types of fractures: A. closed-non-displaced; B. open, compound; C. comminuted; D. displaced; E. oblique; F. spiral; G. impacted; H. greenstick. (B) Location (types) of hip fractures

4. *Displaced*—A fracture where fragments are misaligned at the fracture site
5. *Oblique*—Fracture line runs at a 45-degree angle across the bone's longitudinal axis
6. *Spiral*—Caused by torsional force or twisting; fracture line twists around bone shaft
7. *Impacted*—A fracture in which one fragment is driven or telescoped into the other
8. *Greenstick*—An incomplete fracture where one side of bone is broken but other side is intact, yet bent. More common in children than adults

Additional types of fractures include *articular*, involving both articulating surfaces; *pathological* fractures, caused by a slight degree of trauma on weakened bone due to a pathologic process; *intracapsular* fractures (Fig. 14-13B) occurring within the joint capsule (i.e., femoral head or neck); and *extracapsular* fractures (Fig. 14-13B) occurring outside the joint capsule (i.e., intertrochanteric).

Directions of Fracture Lines

Fractures can occur in several directions or lines, as illustrated in Fig. 14-13B.

In addition, fractures in adults usually sever both the periosteum and cortical tissue, completely splitting the bone. This is referred to as a complete fracture. Children, on the other hand, frequently experience incomplete fractures, which only partially break the bone (greenstick).

Any of these classifications and/or descriptions can be used in combination to describe better the location and severity of the break.

Treatment of Fractures

Fractures are treated by several surgical methods, but first the bone must be reduced by bringing the bone together in alignment. Reduction can be accomplished by one of two methods: (1) open reduction, which requires surgery to correct the fracture, and (2) closed reduction, reducing the fracture without making an incision. Once this has been accomplished, some method of stabilization is necessary until the bone heals. This term is referred to as *fixation*, and it can be accomplished internally by the use of screws, plates, pins, or rods, or externally by using casting materials or external fixation devices, which are placed through the skin to the bone, and anchored as a means for temporary stabilization. External fixation does not require surgery, although in some cases it may require general anesthesia and is therefore performed in the operating room.

Orthopedic procedures, involving fractures, may be listed on the operating schedule as:

1. ORIF (Open reduction—internal fixation)
2. CRIF (Closed reduction—internal fixation)
3. CRExtF (Closed reduction—external fixation)

Open reduction—internal fixation: The surgeon makes an incision to expose the fracture site and uses the implant to hold the bone fragments together.
Closed reduction—internal fixation: The fracture is reduced manually by the surgeon, guided by x-ray films, who then inserts an internal fixation device through the skin and into the bone fragments. Traction is commonly used with this method.
Closed reduction—external fixation: The fracture is reduced manually with the application of an external fixation device such as a cast.

Internal Fixation Devices The treatment of fractures will vary according to the type of fracture and its location. Specific orthopedic hardware is required to facilitate the stabilization of the fracture, and can include plates, pins, screws, and nails.

Occasionally, because of a severe breakage, the bone will need to be totally replaced. This is accomplished by a metal implant or endoprosthesis. This device is usually associated with a joint fracture (e.g., hip, knee, or shoulder). Most implants are manufactured from stainless steel or from a stainless steel alloy such as vitallium, and require special instrumentation to prepare the area and insert the prosthesis (see Total Hip Arthroplasty, pp. 535–536).

Because the endoprostheses are very expensive, special handling is required, since once it has been scratched or damaged in any way, it can no longer be used. Certain general considerations, therefore, should be followed when working with these items, as described below.

General Principles—Prosthesis

1. Handle the implant as little as possible with a soft sterile cloth or towel.
2. Avoid contact between metal surfaces during storage and/or preparation.
3. Avoid mixing different metals in the body, for example, plate and screws, as different metals may react and weaken each other.
4. When an implant (endoprosthesis) is used, trialers or sizers will be used first to determine the correct size of the prosthesis to be inserted. If necessary, these may be flash sterilized before the procedure. The **endoprosthesis may never be flash sterilized.** It should be supplied sterile from the manufacturer.
5. If the implant is the type that requires force to drive it into its location, the driver must not come in direct contact with the implant since this could

cause damage to the prosthesis. A Teflon-coated mallet/driver should be used.

REPAIR OF FRACTURES

Surgeries Involving the Upper Extremities

Procedure
Open Reduction of the Humerus

Definition: Realignment and fixation of a fracture of the arm necessitating an operative incision.

CDC Classification: II (unless compound fracture exists)

Discussion: A variety of fractures of the humerus may occur. If closed reduction and immobilization are unsatisfactory or when there is nonunion, fixation may be achieved by using a number of internal fixation devices, including screws, rods, and compression plates (Fig. 14-14).

Positioning: Supine, affected arm in a comfortable position, unaffected arm extended on an armboard

Skin Preparation: See pp. 337–338

Packs/Drapes:
Extremity pack with fenestrated sheet
Impervious stockinette

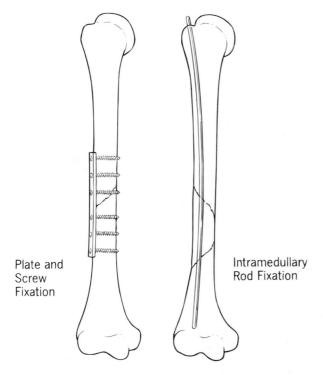

Plate and Screw Fixation

Intramedullary Rod Fixation

Fig. 14-14. ORIF—fractured humerus (Adapted from *The Nurse and Orthopedic Surgery*. The Orthopedic Nurses' Association, 1980.)

Eshmarch bandage, towels
Split sheet (optional)

Instrumentation:
Basic orthopedic tray
Soft tissue tray (optional)
Drill bits, retractors
Fixation device (e.g., Rush rods, Steinman pins, screws/plates, compression set)
Power drill/cord

Supplies/Equipment:
Basin set
ESU/suction
Power source for drill
Tourniquet and insufflator (for distal fractures) (optional)
Sheet wadding/casting materials
Blades—(2) No. 10
Needle counter
Sutures—surgeon's preference
Solutions—saline, water
Medications—antibiotic (for irrigation)

PROCEDURAL OVERVIEW

An appropriate incision is made over the fracture site, avoiding neurovascular structures. If malunion has occurred, an osteotomy (cutting through a bone) is performed to restore alignment. Generally, fixation is performed with screws and a compression plate. For condylar fractures, threaded Kirschner (K) wires or screws may be used. The wound is irrigated and closed; the arm is immobilized.

PERIOPERATIVE NURSING CONSIDERATIONS

- Have x-ray capabilities in the room
- For management of tourniquet, see Chapter 11, pp. 357–358.
- Be prepared to assist the surgeon in applying a cast or splint
- Check tank levels for power equipment before beginning the procedure
- Have adequate help to hold up and stabilize arm during prepping and draping procedure
- If distal fracture (near wrist), a hand table (side extension table) may be used

Related Procedures ORIF—supracondylar fixation—humerus

Procedure
Open Reduction of the Radius and/or Ulna

Definition: Realignment and fixation of a fracture occurring in the forearm necessitating a surgical incision.

CDC Classification: II (unless compound fracture exists)

Discussion: The open method is used when a closed reduction is unsatisfactory or when a nonunion exists. Fixation may be achieved with a variety of devices, including rods, intramedullary nails, and long screws.

Positioning: Supine, the affected arm is positioned across the chest or on an extended hand table. The other arm may be extended on an armboard.

Skin Preparation: See pp. 337–338

Packs/Drapes: see Open Reduction—Humerus

Instrumentation:
    Basic orthopedic tray
    Small bone holders, nail set, drill bits, awl
    Power drill/cord
    Fixation devices (e.g., Steinman pins, K-wires, long screws, intramedullary nails, Rush rods)

Supplies/Equipment:
    See Open Reduction—Humerus
    Additional: hand table (optional)

PROCEDURAL OVERVIEW

An appropriate incision is made depending on the location of the fracture. Neurovascular structures are identified and protected.

Plate/Screw Fixation

A bone plate with bone screws is applied over the fracture site. A bone graft may or may not be used, depending on the extent of the fracture or length of time since the injury.

Intramedullary Rod

Sage, Rush, or Steinman pins may be used in the medullary canal of the radius or ulna. The fracture line is exposed and held in reduction. In ulnar fractures, the pin is driven down from the olecranon; in radial fractures, the pin is driven up from the radial styloid.

For fixation of a distal wrist fracture, screws, K-wires or specifically shaped plates (e.g., T-plate) may be used. A splint or bivalve cast is applied.

PERIOPERATIVE NURSING CONSIDERATIONS

- A long arm cast, with elbow in 90 degrees of flexion and the arm in neutral position, is applied.
- See Open Reduction—Humerus for additional information.

Related Procedure: ORIF—Wrist, Elbow

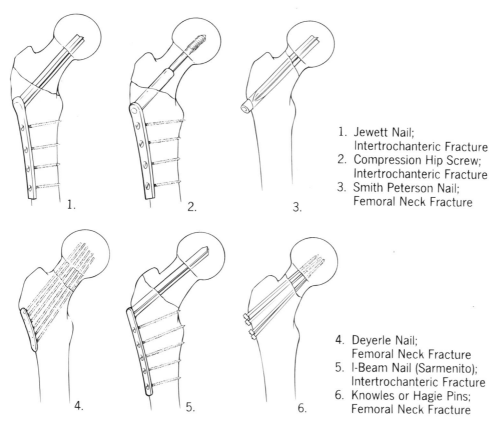

1. Jewett Nail;
   Intertrochanteric Fracture
2. Compression Hip Screw;
   Intertrochanteric Fracture
3. Smith Peterson Nail;
   Femoral Neck Fracture
4. Deyerle Nail;
   Femoral Neck Fracture
5. I-Beam Nail (Sarmenito);
   Intertrochanteric Fracture
6. Knowles or Hagie Pins;
   Femoral Neck Fracture

Fig. 14-15. ORIF—femoral neck/intertrochanteric fx (Adapted from *The Nurse and Orthopedic Surgery.* The Orthopedic Nurses' Association, 1980.)

Surgeries Involving the Lower Extremities

Procedure
ORIF—Fracture of the Femoral Shaft

Definition: Realignment and fixation of a fracture of the femur through an operative incision

CDC Classification: II (unless compound fracture exists)

Discussion: Surgical intervention may be indicated in certain fractures of the femur (in adults). Fractures of the femur, in children and young adults, are treated with traction followed by immobilization. Fractures of the femoral shaft are treated with intramedullary rods (nails) (e.g., Hansen-Street; K-wires, Lottes, Rush, Schneider, Enders, and Zickle), depending on the surgeon's preference. Compression plates that reduce the fracture mechanically are commonly employed, but must have at least three holes above and three below the fracture site for proper stabilization (Fig. 14-15).

Positioning: Supine on a fracture table, with the table slightly rotated to a lateral position. The fracture is reduced by manipulation of the foot extension. The arm on the unaffected side is extended on an armboard, and the other arm is flexed across the chest. If the fracture table is not used, the patient is placed in the lateral position with the unaffected leg extended and the affected leg flexed over it, with a pillow placed between the legs.

Skin Preparation: See pp. 337–338

Packs/Drapes: Hip pack
Plastic adhesive drape sheet (optional)
If fracture table not used, fenestrated sheet with adhesive plastic drape
Towels, extra drape sheets

Instrumentation:
Basic orthopedic tray
Drill bits, power drill/cord
Fixation device and tools specific to the device

Supplies/Equipment:
Basin set
ESU/suction
Fracture table (e.g., Striker, Chick, Amsco, and positioning aids)
Power source for drill
Needle counter
Blades—(2) No. 10
Sutures—surgeon's preference
Solutions—saline, water
Impervious stockinette (if fracture table not used)
Medications—antibiotics for irrigation

PROCEDURAL OVERVIEW

A posterolateral incision is made over the fracture site. The medullary canal is reamed with special medullary reamers. A guide pin is driven from the fracture site proximally to emerge subcutaneously just proximal to the greater trochanter. The position of the guide pin in relation to the fracture is visualized by fluoroscopy. The internal fixation device (surgeon's preference) is used to stabilize the fracture. A postpositional x-ray is taken, and the device is securely seated once proper positioning has been determined. If the fracture site is comminuted, wire loops are placed around the fragments. The wound is irrigated and closed.

PERIOPERATIVE NURSING CONSIDERATIONS

- Have x-ray capabilities in the room.
- Notify x-ray department when patient is being positioned on the table. Observe radiologic precautions, see pp. 357–358.
- The extremity may be supported postoperatively in a cast, depending on the location/severity of the fracture.
- Some surgeons prefer to double glove during draping procedure and remove outer gloves following the draping segment.

Related Procedures: Femoral neck fractures
Femoral head fractures

Procedure
Internal Fixation of the Hip

Definition: Stabilization of an intracapsular fracture of the femoral neck or an extracapsular fracture of the intertrochanteric region.

CDC Classification: II

Discussion: This procedure is indicated for the patient when early postoperative mobilization may not be feasible (e.g., in poor-risk patients). The procedure could be performed under local anesthesia if necessary because of poor physiologic status. Fixation can be achieved with a variety of fixation devices, including nails (Jewett, Smith—Petersen), pins (Knowles, Deyerle, Hagie), or compression screws (Richards) across the fracture site, or sometimes in conjunction with a plate along the femoral shaft (Fig. 14-15).

Position: Supine, either on a fracture table or regular operating table that can accommodate fluoroscopy

Incision Site: Lateral over the fracture site

Skin Preparation: See pp. 337–338

Packs/Drapes: Total hip/extremity pack
Folded towels
Stockinette cuff (optional)
Image intensifier drape

If a regular OR table is used, the affected extremity is draped with a stockinette then brought through a large fenestrated sheet. If the fracture table is used, a sterile plastic adhesive drape may be part of the draping system

Instruments:
　Basic orthopedic tray
　Power drill, cord, drill bits
　Fixation device, guide pins (surgeon's preference)

Supplies/Equipment:
　Basin set
　ESU/suction
　Blades—(4) No. 10
　Power source for drills
　Asepto syringe
　Stockinette (impervious) if regular table is used
　Solutions—saline, water
　Medications—antibiotics for irrigation
　Sutures—surgeon's preference

PROCEDURAL OVERVIEW

After the patient is asleep, the fracture is reduced and checked by x-ray film. The incision is made, exposing the fracture site, and the appropriate fixation device is placed after guide wires are inserted temporarily to check alignment. A drill is used to assist in placement of fixation device, and an x-ray film is taken to reaffirm placement. The wound is irrigated with antibiotic solution and closed.

PERIOPERATIVE NURSING CONSIDERATIONS

- See ORIF—Femoral Shaft, p. 533.

Procedure
Amputation of a Lower Extremity

Definition: Severance of a thigh, leg, foot, or portion thereof.

CDC Classification: III or IV (depending on pathology and underlying causes)

Discussion: Amputations of the lower extremity are classified as (1) above the knee (AK), (2) below the knee (BK), or (3) transmetatarsal (TM). The level of amputation is determined by the patient's general health status, vascular status of the limb, and/or rehabilitation potential. Amputations may be indicated for gangrene secondary to diabetes, vascular insufficiency, malignancy, or severe trauma. The procedure may also be performed by a general or vascular surgeon, under general or regional anesthesia.

Positioning: Supine, arms extended on armboards, safety strap applied over unaffected leg

Skin Preparation: See pp. 337–338

Packs/Drapes: Extra Mayo stand cover or intestinal pouch (for confinement of amputated limb)
　Impervious stockinette

Laparotomy pack
Extra drape sheets, towels

Instrumentation:
　Basic orthopedic tray
　Amputation knife, saw
　Oscillating power saw/cord (optional)

Supplies/Equipment:
　Basin set
　ESU/suction
　Blades—(2 to 4) No. 10
　Needle counter
　Culture tubes—aerobic, anaerobic
　Medication—antibiotic for irrigation
　Solutions—saline, water
　Sutures—surgeon's preference
　Closed wound drainage system (e.g., Hemovac)

PROCEDURAL OVERVIEW—AK Amputation

The incision is made so that a musculocutaneous flap can be created for better coverage of the femoral stump (circular incision over the distal femur, transecting fascia and muscle). Vessels and nerves are ligated and severed. The femoral periosteum is incised, and bone edges of the stump are smoothed with a rasp. Hemostasis is achieved, and the wound is irrigated. A closed wound drainage system is placed in the wound and the wound edges are closed.

PERIOPERATIVE NURSING CONSIDERATIONS

- A bulky dressing may be used or a cast or temporary prosthesis may be employed to reduce postoperative edema and to prepare the stump for a permanent prosthesis at a later date.
- Follow hospital policy and/or patient request for disposal of the limb.
- If procedure is performed under regional anesthesia, ensure that the specimen is **never** within the sight of the patient.
- Dispatch cultures immediately.
- Confirm with surgeon the preference for dressing material and/or the need for the temporary prosthesis.

REVISION/RECONSTRUCTION OF JOINTS

Joint Replacement Procedures

Procedure
Replacement of Femoral Head

Definition: Substitution of the femoral head with a prosthesis made of vitallium or similar inert metal

CDC Classification: I (if nontraumatic injury)

Discussion: This procedure is indicated for nonunion of femoral neck fractures, avascular necrosis of the femoral head, degenerative changes of the hip post-fracture, or from severely limiting arthritis.

A femoral head prosthesis is designed to replace only the head of the femur and is snapped into a rotating polyethylene-lined cup placed into the acetabulum, which can then act as the ball and socket joint of the hip. Examples of these prostheses include Universal Head Replacement, Gilberty II, Bateman Universal Proximal Femur, Moore, and Muller. The femoral cup is not usually cemented, but the femoral stem can be secured with or without cement, depending on the type.

One advantage of this procedure is that immediate weight-bearing is permitted; it is more extensive and entails more risk than procedures retaining the femoral head.

Positioning: Lateral position with sandbags, Vac-Pack, or kidney rests supporting the torso. Arm on affected side-armboard, the other arm across the chest; pillow between the arms. Unaffected leg is extended with affected leg flexed over it. Pillow is placed between the legs.

Skin Preparation: See pp. 337–338

Packs/Drapes: Hip pack w/fenestrated sheet
   Impervious stockinette
   Towels
   Extra drape sheets (optional)

Instrumentation:
   Basic bone tray
   Prosthesis tray
   Special instrumentation for prosthesis
   Drill bits, guide pins
   Power saw and cord
   Femoral head extractor tray
   Prostheses (sterile)

Supplies/Equipment:
   Basin set
   ESU/suction
   Blades—(3) No. 10
   Needle counter
   Adhesive drape (e.g., Vi-Drape, Ioban Drape) (optional)
   Solutions—saline, water
   Sutures—surgeon's preference
   Medications—antibiotic for irrigation
   Positioning aids—Vac-Pack, pillows, etc.
   Bone cement kit with evacuator (optional)
   Closed wound drainage system (optional)

PROCEDURAL OVERVIEW

Several incisions and approaches can be employed. A posterior incision may be made over the gluteus max-

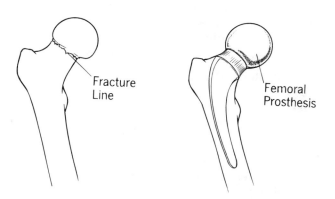

Fig. 14-16. Femoral head prosthesis (Adapted from *The Nurse and Orthopedic Surgery*. The Orthopedic Nurses' Association 1980.)

imus (superiorly) paralleling the proximal femur. The muscle fibers are split, and the external rotators of the hip are freed from the femur. The joint capsule is then incised. The femoral head is excised and measured. The size of the actual acetabulum is determined with the use of the trial-sizers, and the appropriate prosthesis is selected. The medullary canal is reamed with a special rasp, and the neck is shaped to receive the prosthesis.

The prosthesis is then seated using special driving instruments, and excess bone fragments are trimmed. The prosthesis may or may not be cemented into place, depending on the type being used. The hip is reduced; the wound is irrigated and closed (Fig. 14-16).

PERIOPERATIVE NURSING CONSIDERATIONS

- Have all x-ray films taken in the room.
- Notify radiology department of times films need to be taken. Observe radiologic precautions (see Chap. 11, pp. 357–358).
- Some surgeons may prefer to double glove during the draping procedure.
- Record all information regarding prosthesis according to hospital protocol.
- For additional considerations, see p. 530 regarding the handling of endoprostheses.

Procedure
Total Hip Replacement (Arthroplasty)

Definition: Substitution of the femoral head with a prosthesis and reconstruction of the acetabulum with replacement of an acetabular cup, which may or may not be fixed using methylmethacrylate bone cement.

CDC Classification: I (unless traumatic injury)

Discussion: This procedure is usually associated with the following disorders:

1. Rheumatoid arthritis
2. Degenerative diseases
3. Avascular necrosis (postinfection or as a result of failed reconstruction [nonunion])

A variety of prostheses are available, such as a porous coating, ceramic, various alloys, or a bipolar cup. Some will require bone cement to seat the prosthesis (Charnley, Bechtol, Aufranc-Turner, Harris/Precoat, porous coated anatomic [PCA]) while others, like the hybrid arthroplasty, involve the cementing of the femoral stem and not cementing the acetabular cup. The noncementing technique may be preferred when the prosthesis can be tightly fitted into healthy strong bone. The "press-fit" (AML, Osteolock), porous metal (Harris/Galante), bipolar cup (Precision, Bateman), and ceramic (Mittlmeir) are varieties of noncemented prostheses. The Charnley-type cemented total hip cup prosthesis remains the standard; however, the Hybrid design is becoming more popular.

It is important to note that no one prosthesis is suitable for every patient; therefore, a variety of types, designs, and insertion procedures are available from which the surgeon may choose, depending on the pathophysiologic needs of the patient.

Positioning, Skin Preparation, Packs, and Drapes:
   See Femoral Head Prosthesis

Instrumentation:
   Basic orthopedic tray
   Osteotomes, curettes, extra guide wires
   Hip prosthesis tray (specific to type used)
   Trial prosthesis (sizers)
   Specific instrumentation for prosthesis
   Prosthesis (sterile)
   Power drill with reamers, power saw with blades (optional)

Supplies/Equipment:
   Basin set
   ESU/suction (e.g., Simpulse Suction Irrigator)
   Positioning aids (Vac-Pac, pillows, etc.)
   Power source for drills, blades (optional)
   Blades—(3) No. 10
   Needle counter
   Impervious stockinette
   Sterile plastic adhesive drape
   Sutures—surgeon's preference
   Solutions—saline, water
   Medications—antibiotics, hemostatic agents
   Closed drainage system (e.g., Hemovac)
   Bone cement kit with evacuator (optional)

PROCEDURAL OVERVIEW

One of several techniques and prostheses may be employed when performing this procedure. In the lateral approach, a longitudinal incision is made proximal to the greater trochanter and distally along the proximal femoral shaft. The hip joint capsule is exposed; the femoral head is excised, the femoral neck is osteomotized, and the femoral canal is reamed slightly larger and deeper than the stem of the proposed femoral component.

A capsulotomy is performed, and the acetabulum is reamed slightly larger than the prostatic cup size. Anchoring holes are drilled into the acetabulum. The proper positioning and angulation of the cup is determined.

The bone cement is prepared and applied, then the cup is positioned. The femoral component is inserted, and the surgeon performs a test relocation, making any positioning adjustments at this time. The femoral component is removed, the cement is applied, and the femoral component is reinserted and seated into the canal. Once the cement has set (10 to 12 minutes), the hip is relocated. The soft tissue is approximated; the wound is closed after insertion of a closed wound drainage device. An abduction pillow is placed between the legs postoperatively to maintain proper alignment (Fig. 14-17).

PERIOPERATIVE NURSING CONSIDERATIONS

- The operative leg must be kept in abduction and slight external rotation.
- Check all equipment/power sources prior to use.
- Have all x-ray films taken in the room. Observe all radiologic precautions.
- Keep conversation and traffic in the room to a minimum to reduce microorganisms.
- Have all prosthesis sizers and special instrumentation sterile. This may require the use of a separate draped table.
- Check blood bank for available units. Cell saver may be employed.
- Follow hospital policy for recording prosthesis information (intraoperative record).
- Be prepared to change suction tubing and canister if it gets clogged.
- If the greater trochanter is not removed, partial to full weight bearing may be allowed using crutches or a walker. If removed, however, only partial weight bearing is allowed (surgeon's preference).
- Instruments and hardware are counted according to institutional protocol.

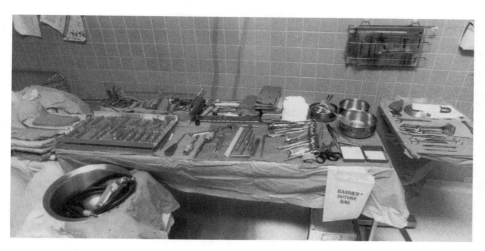

Orthopedic set-up for hip surgery

Procedure
Total Knee Arthroplasty

Definition: The replacement of the articular surfaces of the knee joint by a prosthesis

CDC Classification: I (except for traumatic injury)

Discussion: This procedure is usually indicated for severe destruction of the knee joint due to degenerative, rheumatoid, or traumatic arthritis. The prostheses are secured to the bone with bone cement. When indicated, a single component of the knee's articular surface may be replaced (unicompartmental), but more commonly the entire or total surface requires replacement.

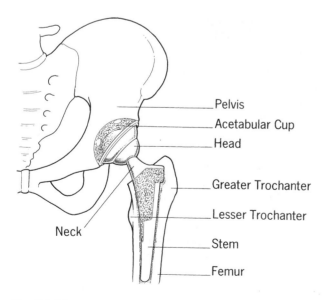

Fig. 14-17. Total hip prosthesis—porous coated (Adapted from *Core Curriculum for Orthopedic Nursing* [2nd ed.]. NAON.)

A variety of prostheses are available; they belong to one of four systems:

1. Constrained (hinged)
2. Nonhinged constrained—nearly duplicate normal knee
3. Nonconstrained
4. Partially constrained

Examples include, but are not limited to, PCA, Microlock, Kneematic II, Richards Maximum Contact (RMC).

Positioning: Supine; knees over the lower break in the table, arms extended on armboards. A tourniquet cuff is applied to the top of the thigh of affected leg

Skin Preparation: See pp. 337–338

Packs/Drapes: Extremity pack
  Impervious stockinette
  Split sheet/extra drape sheets (optional)
  Towels

Instrumentation:
  Basic orthopedic tray
  Knee arthrotomy tray
  Trial prosthesis tray, prosthesis, and special instruments
  Power drill/cord, oscillating saw, template, and cord

Supplies/Equipment:
  Basin set
  ESU/suction
  Blades—(3) No. 10, (1) No. 15
  Eshmarch, tourniquet cuff, and insufflator
  Needle counter
  Solutions—saline, water
  Sutures—surgeon's preference
  Medications—antibiotics for irrigation
  Bone cement kit with evacuator
  Closed wound drainage system (optional)

PROCEDURAL OVERVIEW

A longitudinal incision extending from over the patella to the tibial tuberosity is usually performed, and the knee is opened. The synovial membrane is removed. The distal femoral and proximal tibial joint surfaces are excised. Any varus or valgus deformity is corrected with osteotomes. The femoral joint surface is replaced with a metal implant, and the tibial surface is replaced with a high density polyethylene implant. Both are set in place with bone cement.

With some versions, the undersurface of the patella is also replaced with a polyethylene component in order to reduce patellofemoral pain. A closed wound drainage system is inserted, and the incision is closed.

PERIOPERATIVE NURSING CONSIDERATIONS

- Follow hospital policy for recording the prosthesis.
- Progressive range of motion may begin approximately 3 to 7 days postoperatively, or an automatic motion device may be employed.
- Have all x-ray films taken in the room.
- Have prosthesis and all necessary instrumentation sterile (on separate table if necessary).
- For tourniquet precaution, see Chapter 11, pp. 357–358.
- Keep conversation and traffic flow to a minimum.

Related Procedures: In addition to the hip and knee arthroplasty procedures just outlined, there are other joints in the body that can be replaced when disease or injury prevents the joint from performing.
These include:

1. *Metatarsal/Metacarpal Arthroplasty*—using a Silastic implant (fingers, toes)
2. *Total Ankle Arthroplasty*—using a high-density polyethylene and metal component implant fixed with cement
3. *Total Elbow Arthroplasty*—using metal and polyethylene components, seated with cement
4. *Humeral Head (Shoulder) Arthroplasty*—using a Neer Humeral Head prosthesis, usually indicated primarily with comminuted fractures of the humeral head.

Dislocation of a Joint

Dislocation of one or more bones at a joint may occur with or without an associated fracture. In most instances tendons, ligaments, and muscles are deranged and the articular surfaces of the bone are displaced from the joint capsule.

Closed reduction, with or without skeletal traction, may be necessary at the time of the acute injury. However, if the closed reduction fails to stabilize the joint, an open procedure with internal fixation may be necessary. The most common internal fixation is usually performed on the shoulder.

Procedure
Open Reduction for Recurrent Anterior Shoulder Dislocation

Definition: Strengthening of the anterior joint capsule and musculotendinous support of the shoulder
CDC Classification: I
Discussion: There are a variety of procedures and modifications, including (1) Bankart, (2) Bristow, and (3) Putti–Platt. The Putti–Platt technique will be outlined here.
Positioning: Supine, the affected shoulder elevated (sandbags or folded sheet), and flexed over the chest
Skin Preparation: See pp. 337–338
Packs/Drapes:
  Extremity pack/split sheet
  Impervious stockinette
  Towels, extra drape sheets
Instrumentation:
  Basic orthopedic tray/osteotomes
  Steinman pins, power drills/cord/drill bits
  Fixation devices (e.g., screws, staples) and instrumentation
Supplies/Equipment:
  Basin set
  Positioning aids
  ESU/suction
  Blades—(2) No. 10, (1) No. 15
  Needle counter
  Sutures—surgeon's preference
  Solutions—saline, water
  Medications—antibiotic for irrigation
  Dressing (e.g., sling/velpeau)
  Power source—drills

PROCEDURAL OVERVIEW

An anterior incision is made over the pectoral groove. The joint capsule is exposed, and the damage is assessed. The subscapularis is divided approximately 1 inch medially to its insertion on the lesser tuberosity. The free edge of the lateral part of the subscapularis is taken across the joint and sutured to the soft structures along the anterior rim of the glenoid cavity. The free edge of the medial part of the subscapularis is taken across laterally to the area of the greater tuberosity and sutured to the rotator cuff. This overlapping and shortening of the subscapularis limits external rotation, thus preventing dislocation. The wound is irrigated and closed.

PERIOPERATIVE NURSING CONSIDERATIONS

- Have x-ray films taken in the room.
- Check levels of power source before procedure.
- Care should be taken during the procedure to avoid pooling of solution under the shoulder.
- Confirm with the surgeon what equipment will be needed for immobilization following surgery. (Immobilization is usually maintained for 3 to 4 weeks, with gradual pendulum and active exercises performed.)

Arthrodesis

In addition to procedures reviewed in this section, another type of procedure involving a joint is called an *arthrodesis*: the fusion of a joint for the purpose of stabilization and/or repair of an injured joint. This procedure is accomplished by removing the articular surface and securing the bony union or by inserting a fixation implant that inhibits movement. The procedure is usually indicated following resection of a recurrent benign, potentially malignant or malignant lesion/tumor that involves the ends of the bones and joint. Following the resection, the joint may be stabilized with a bone graft or an intramedullary fixation device. Because this technique limits motion, other joint reconstructive procedures are usually attempted first.

CORRECTION OF DEFORMITIES (BONE AND SOFT TISSUE)

Tendons and Ligaments

Tendons and ligaments may be severed, torn, or ruptured. These injuries are seen mostly in athletes. Total or partial avulsion of major ligaments and tendons torn from their attachments in or around an extremity joint requires repair to stabilize the joint.

Tendons can be lengthened, shortened, or transferred depending on the nature of the injury or deformity. This type of surgery is a meticulous procedure, and may or may not require microsurgery depending on the location. Although this surgery is well within the realm of orthopedic procedures, many plastic surgeons and neurosurgeons may be involved with hand reconstruction, including repair or transfer.

Soft Tissue and Bone Deformities: Foot and Spine

Conditions such as hallux valgus, excisions of neuromas, correction of hammer toe deformity, excision of popliteal (Baker's) cyst, and corrections of spinal deformities, such as scoliosis, are procedures that are frequently performed by the orthopedic surgeon. In recent years, the specialty of podiatric medicine has developed, and many of the procedures involving both bone and soft tissue of the feet and toes are now being performed by a Podiatrist, a physician who specializes in correcting deformities of the feet.

Correction of Foot Deformities

Procedure
Bunionectomy

Definition: Excision of a scar tissue and/or bony mass of the first metatarsophalangeal joint and medial exostosis of the first metatarsal head.

CDC Classification: I

Discussion: The procedure is performed to relieve pain and correct the deformity. A variety of procedures may be employed specific to the nature of the problem, including (1) metatarsal osteotomy, (2) McBride operation, and (3) Keller arthroplasty.

Although different in their end result, the preparation, supplies, instrumentation, and equipment required to perform the procedures are very similar. The procedures can be performed under general or regional anesthesia on an inpatient or outpatient basis.

Positioning: Supine, arms may be extended on armboards. A leg holder may be used during the skin preparation procedure.

Skin Preparation: See pp. 337–338

Packs/Drapes: Extremity or laparotomy pack
　Impervious stockinette
　Extra drape sheets, split sheet (optional)

Instrumentation:
　Minor orthopedic tray or specific podiatric tray
　Hooke osteotomes, small power drill and blades (e.g., minidriver with oscillating blades)
　Kirschner wires and pin cutter
　Silastic implant (optional)

Supplies/Equipment:
　Leg holder (optional)
　Tourniquet and insufflator unit
　Power source for drill/saw
　ESU/suction
　Basin set (minor)
　Blades—(2) No. 10, (1) No. 15
　Needle counter
　Esmarch bandage
　Medications—local, antibiotics (optional)
　Solutions—saline, water
　Sutures—surgeon's preference

PROCEDURAL OVERVIEW—*Keller Arthroplasty*

A curved incision is made dorsally along the medial aspect of the first metatarsophalangeal joint. Care is taken to preserve the cutaneous nerves. The capsule and periosteum at the base of the proximal phalanx are incised and retracted and the metatarsal head dislocated. The proximal half of the phalanx is resected. The exostosis and osteophytes are excised. A Kirschner wire is inserted, aligning the toe and the metatarsal head. In addition, the resected joint surface may be replaced by a Silastic prosthesis by reaming the medullary canal of the proximal phalanx in order to insert the stem of the implant. The wound is irrigated and closed.

PERIOPERATIVE NURSING CONSIDERATIONS

- If regional anesthesia is used, conversation should be kept to a minimum, since the patient may be awake or lightly sedated.
- The surgeon may inject a local anesthetic, after the procedure, to reduce incision pain.
- Have x-ray films taken in the room.
- Check pressure levels of tanks prior to use.
- For tourniquet precaution, see Chapter 11, pp. 357–358.
- A plaster toe spica or slipper is usually applied, and special shoes may be needed for 3 to 4 months. If a K-wire is used it is removed in 3 to 4 months.

Related Procedures:

1. *Metatarsal Osteotomy*—metatarsal alignment is corrected by moving the metatarsal head slightly
2. *McBride Operation*—abductor tendon is fixed to lateral portion of metatarsal neck and sesmoid bone is excised
3. *Silastic Great Toe Implant: Swanson Design*—Silastic implant replaces the metatarsal head, providing a smooth articular surface

Correction of Deformities: Spinal Column

Procedure
Correction of Scoliosis

Definition: The insertion of various rods, frames, or other fixation devices that act as internal splints until the vertebrae involved in the curvature fuse, correcting the deformity.

CDC Classification: I

Discussion: Scoliosis is described as a lateral "S" or "C" deviation of the spine, which may include a rotation or deformity of the vertebrae. Scoliosis can be idiopathic or congenital, and may result from muscular or neurologic disease.

Surgical treatment is usually performed when musculoskeletal and respiratory functions become compromised or for cosmetic purposes. Indications may also include an increase of the spinal curvature in a growing child or pain from the curvature (in adults), uncontrolled by conservative methods.

Several systems and techniques are available, each requiring its own instrumentation, and using compression and distraction rods, hooks, spring hooks, etc. The systems include (1) Harrington rods, (2) Cotrel-Du-Bouset (a variation of the Harrington rod system), (3) Luque system, (4) Wisconsin segmental system, employing the use of Keene hooks, and (5) Dwyer instrumentation. A posterior spinal fusion is frequently performed in adolescence since the curvature is still flexible. The Dwyer system is used for an anterior approach for a thoracolumbar deformity.

For the purpose of this discussion, the Harrington rod procedure for posterior spinal fusion will be outlined.

Positioning: Prone, on a Wilson frame or chest bolsters with arms placed on armboards, angled toward the head; hands pronated

Skin Preparation: See pp. 337–338

Packs/Drapes:
Laparotomy pack
Sterile adhesive drape (e.g., Vi-Drape, Ioban)
Extra drape sheets
Towels
Minor pack (Harrington rod instrumentation table) (optional)

Instrumentation:
Laminectomy tray
Kerrison and pituitary tray
Spinal fixation device tray with specific instrumentation
Steinman pins and protractor
Self-retaining retractor (e.g., Beckman, Weitlander)

Supplies/Equipment:
Special frame; positioning aids
ESU/suction
Fiberoptic headlight and light source (optional)
Cell saver (optional)
Cast cart
Basin set
Blades—(2) No. 10, (1) No. 15
Needle counter
Bone wax, sutures, neuro sponges (cottonoids)
Medications—hemostatic agents, antibiotics
Solution—saline, water
Closed drainage system (e.g., Hemovac)

PROCEDURAL OVERVIEW—Harrington Rod with Fusion

The appropriate incision is made, and the vertebral levels are identified. Muscular and ligamentous structures are denuded from the spinous processes laterally to the transverse processes on both sides before placement of the rods. Distractor hooks are placed on the concave side, and the distraction rod is then placed. Hooks for the compression rod are also applied. Large amounts of cortical and cancellous bone are placed over the rods (on the concave side) and the denuded area. Suction drains are placed and the wound is closed (Fig. 14-18).

PERIOPERATIVE NURSING CONSIDERATIONS

- The individual is placed in a posterior plaster shell or Rizer jacket for approximately 6 to 12 months, or until fusion is solid.

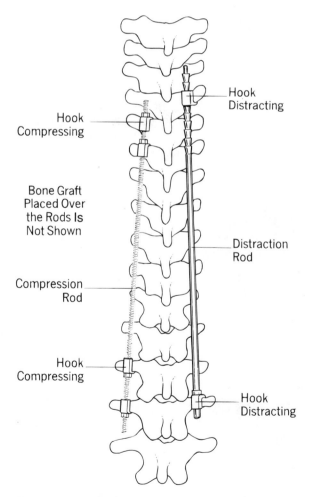

Fig. 14-18. Harrington rod and fusion (Adapted from *The Nurse and Orthopedic Surgery.* The Orthopedic Nurses' Association, 1980.)

- Have x-rays taken in the room.
- Check with blood bank for available units. Measure blood loss accurately.
- Have additional suction available if cell saver is not used.
- If skin and subcutaneous tissue is injected with a vasoconstricting agent (e.g., epinepherine), notify anesthesia personnel.

ARTHROSCOPIC SURGERY

Arthroscopic surgery can be performed on any joint and can be diagnostic or operative depending on the immediate need of the patient and the condition.

Diagnostic arthroscopy is indicated for patients whose diagnosis cannot be determined by history, physical examination, or radiologic studies (e.g., arthrogram). An operative arthroscopy, on the other hand, is performed on patients who show an intraarticular abnormality or ligamentous injury. The procedures may be performed together or separately.

General indications for arthroscopic surgery include

1. Synovial biopsies
2. Removal of loose bodies (trauma)
3. Resection of plicae or shaving of the patella
4. Removal of torn meniscus (trauma)

Arthroscopic surgery may be performed under general or regional anesthesia on an outpatient or inpatient basis. It is most frequently performed on the knee.

General Discussion

Instrumentation

Arthroscopy requires the visualization of a joint through a fiberoptic telescope.

Fiberoptic arthroscopes have diameters ranging from 1.7 to 6 mm, with viewing lenses varying from 30- to 90-degree angles. The operating arthroscope may have a separate channel for passage of manually operated scissors, probes, shaving knives, or biopsy forceps. These tools can also be manipulated through separate puncture holes into the joint under direct visualization.

Care and Handling of Equipment

Like any fiberoptic scope, care must be used in cleaning, sterilizing, storing, and general handling of the

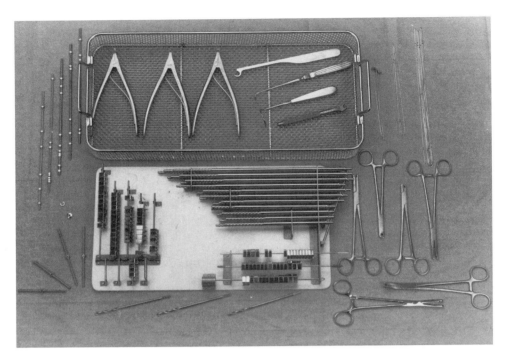

Harrington rod instrumentation with fixation devices

instrument in order to prevent damage of the fiberoptic filaments that pass through the scope. Some of the newer scopes may be steam sterilized; however, the majority still require gas sterilization. Most equipment used with the scopes can be steam sterilized.

Although sterilization is optimal, and should be encouraged, the disinfection of the telescopic lens in a high-level disinfectant solution is the standard of practice among some of the surgeons specializing in arthroscopic surgery.

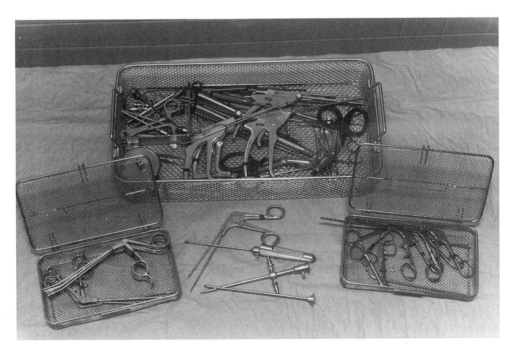

Arthroscopy instrumentation

Equipment and Supplies

Irrigation Solution Sterile irrigation solution, such as normal saline or lactated Ringer's solution, at room temperature, is necessary to distend the joint, allowing for visualization of the structures. The irrigation solution, usually in 1000- or 3000-mL bags, should be placed on an IV pole, and elevated at least 3 feet above the joint to ensure adequate hydrostatic pressure. Two to four bags may be required; however, extra solution should be available to avoid the possibility of air in the tubing from an empty bag. Cystoscopy tubing can serve as the water cord for the arthroscopic procedure, since the solution bag has the same receiving port.

Accessory Items Power-driven shavers, carbon dioxide lasers, and video cameras can be adapted for arthroscopic procedures. Because of the large amount of irrigation fluid used throughout the procedure, a multicanister suction apparatus (Carosel) may be used to remove the fluid without necessitating frequent changes in suction collection canisters.

A fiberoptic light source, similar to those used for laparoscopy and/or cystoscopy procedures, with an appropriate fiberoptic light cord, illuminates the arthroscope allowing for direct visualization of the involved anatomy.

A pneumatic tourniquet is applied to produce a fluid-free field, except for the irrigation solution, and all tourniquet precautions must be employed (see pp. 357–358).

Procedural Overview— Knee Arthroscopy

The patient is placed in a supine position, with knees over the lower break in the table. A tourniquet is applied to the affected leg, and the leg is placed in a "knee holder" apparatus. The knee joint is distended with the appropriate solution via the insertion of a large-bore needle into the suprapatellar pouch near the superior pole of the patella. A trocar and sheath are inserted through a stab wound at a point predetermined according to the known pathology. When the trocar penetrates the capsule, the capsule and synovium form a tight seal around the sheath. The trocar is removed and is replaced by an obturator, which is advanced into the joint. The obturator is removed and replaced by the arthroscopic telescope for direct visualization of the knee joint (Fig. 14-19). The inflow and outflow irrigation tubes are attached to the sheath, and the knee joint is thoroughly examined. Following completion of the examination and/or corrective procedure, the irrigation solution is aspirated; the scope is withdrawn and

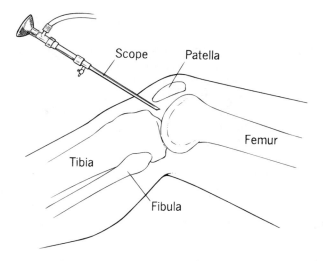

Fig. 14-19. Arthroscopy of the knee (Adapted from *The Nurse and Orthopedic Surgery.* The Orthopedic Nurses' Association, 1980.)

the wound is closed. A Band-Aid or gauze dressing is applied.

Perioperative Nursing Considerations

- If sterilization is not feasible, a high-level disinfectant solution may be used. Copious rinsing of the scope must be performed prior to use in order to remove all traces of the disinfection solution.
- Check all equipment (power sources) before the start of the procedure.
- Have x-ray films taken in the room.
- Room lights are usually dimmed for better visualization.
- A self-contained unit housing all the equipment (e.g., monitor, IV poles, leg holder, etc.) may be used; this is placed over the patient at thigh level following the draping procedure.
- If an arthrotomy is to follow, the patient should be redraped, and gowns and gloves changed. New instruments should be brought to the field for the open procedure.

Related Procedures Arthroscopy of the Elbow, Wrist, or Shoulder

NEUROSURGERY

Neurosurgical procedures are performed on the brain, spinal cord and nerves, and peripheral nerves.

They are performed for a variety of reasons, including to (1) resect pathologic lesions, (2) relieve pressure on the brain or spinal cord related to disease or injury, and (3) repair injured or diseased peripheral nerves and structures.

Because of the changing technologic advancements in both procedures and equipment associated with neurosurgical procedures, communication between the surgeon and the surgical team is essential for intelligent and effective planning and implementation of neurosurgical procedures. Therefore, basic general information that can assist the perioperative nurse in performing safely and effectively during a neurosurgical procedure will be outlined in this unit.

Classification of Neurosurgical Procedures

For the purpose of discussion and clarification, neurosurgical procedures can be placed into three major groups. These groups are

Group I: Cranial Surgery (Brain and Accessory Structures)
  Example: craniotomy for tumor, aneurysm
Group II: Spinal Surgery (including Cord and Nerves)
  Example: laminectomy, anterior cervical fusion
Group III: Peripheral Nerve Surgery
  Example: carpal tunnel release, neurorrhaphy

This unit will outline the procedures that are commonly associated with each of these groups.

Surgical Anatomy Review

The nervous system is structurally divided into two main groups:

1. *Central Nervous System* (CNS)—consisting of the brain and spinal cord
2. *Peripheral Nervous System* (PNS)—consisting of cranial and spinal nerves. Within this system lies another group, frequently separated, the autonomic nervous system (ANS), separating the structures that control automatic and voluntary functions of this highly complex group of organs.

Central Nervous System

Brain and Cord Coverings Because the brain and spinal cord are both delicate and vital to the existence of the human organism, nature has provided them with two protective coverings. The outer covering consists of bone: 26 cranial bones, each connected by a membranous substance known as a suture, and the vertebrae, which encase the cord. The vertebrae are divided into three sections, cervical, thoracic, and lumbar, and consist of 26 irregularly shaped bones (in adults).

The inner coverings, called the meninges, are formed in three distinct membranous layers: the dura mater (outer meningeal layer), the arachnoid (between the dura mater and the interior covering), and the pia mater (the innermost meningeal covering). The pia mater adheres to the outer surface of the brain and cord and is highly vascularized. Between the dura mater and the arachnoid membrane lies a small space called the subdural space, while between the arachnoid and the pia mater another space exists—the subarachnoid space.

The meninges of the spinal cord continue down inside the spinal cavity for a short distance below the end of the cord. At the level of the third segment of the sacrum, a slender band of the pia mater joins the dura mater to form a fibrous cord, which disappears into the periosteum of the coccyx. This extension of the meninges beyond the cord is convenient for performing lumbar punctures (L-3, -4, -5) without endangering the spinal cord itself.

Brain and Cord Fluid Spaces Besides the bony structures and meninges, which act as a protective shield to sudden impact, nature has further fortified the brain and cord with an additional protection; a cushion of fluid both in and around each structure. This fluid is known as cerebrospinal fluid (CSF), and it is contained within the following structures:

1. *Subarachnoid Space*—surrounding the brain and cord
2. *Ventricles and Aqueducts*—inside the brain
3. *Central Canal*—inside the cord

The Ventricles The ventricles are cavities (spaces) located within the brain. They number four: the first two on either side (hemispheres) of the cerebrum, the third located beneath the midportion of the corpus callosum and longitudinal fissures, and the fourth ventricle is between the cerebellum (posteriorly) and the medulla and pons (anteriorly).

Cerebrospinal fluid acts not only as a protective cushion, but as a carrier of substances needed to vitalize the nervous system structures. For example, changes in the carbon dioxide content of cerebrospinal fluid can affect neurons (nerve cells) of the respiratory center in the medulla, thereby helping to control respirations and acid–base balance.

The Brain The brain is one of the largest organs in the adult, weighing about 3 pounds. It attains its full size in about the 18th year of life, but grows rapidly during the first nine years, then slows down over the remaining years. The brain has six major sections/divisions:

1. *Cerebrum*—hemispheres, fissures, and lobes, with the longitudinal fissure dividing the cerebrum into two hemispheres. Each hemisphere contains five lobes: frontal, parietal, temporal, occipital, and the island of Reil. The cerebrum is responsible for co-ordinating sensory, motor, and integrative functions.
2. *Cerebellum*—the center portion, which performs synergistic control of skeletal muscles and mediates posture and equilibrium reflexes.
3. *Diencephalon*—containing the thalamus, hypothalamus, and posterior pituitary gland. Tracts within the diencephalon connect the cerebral cortex, basal ganglia, brainstem, and cord.
4. *Medulla Oblongata*—a portion of the brainstem, which is formed by an enlargement of the cord as it enters the cranial cavity through the foramen magnum. It functions as a two-way connection between the cord and the brain (autonomic nerve functions, e.g., cardiac, respiratory, and vasomotor centers).
5. *Pons*—another segment of the brainstem, it lies above the medulla, and houses the centers for cranial nerves V through VIII.
6. *Mesencephalon* (*Midbrain*)—the last segment of the brainstem, it is located just above the pons, below the diencephalon and cerebrum. It connects the pons to the cerebrum and the cerebral aqueduct, the fluid space of the midbrain. It houses the center for cranial nerves III and IV.

The Spinal Cord   The spinal cord lies within the spinal cavity, extending from the foramen magnum to the lower border of the first lumbar vertebrae. The cord does not completely fill the cavity since the cavity also contains the meninges, spinal fluid, a cushion of adipose tissue, and blood vessels.

The spinal cord is oval in shape and tapers slightly toward its termination point; it has two distinct bulges: one in the cervical region and the other in the lumbar region. There are two deep grooves (fissures), anterior and posterior, which serve as a landmark when determining the specific sections of the cord, since the anterior fissure is deeper and wider than the posterior fissure.

The spinal cord performs sensory, motor reflex functions, both transmitting and receiving involuntary responses.

Peripheral Nervous System (PNS)

The PNS is composed of cranial and spinal nerves and their tributary branches.

Cranial Nerves   There are 12 pairs of cranial nerves that arise from the undersurface of the brain, mostly from the brainstem. After leaving the cranial cavity, by way of a small foramen in the skull, they extend to their respective destinations. Both names and numbers identify the cranial nerves. Their names suggest their distribution or function, while the numbers indicate the order in which they emerge, from front to back. Cranial nerve functions are classified as sensory (afferent), motor (efferent), or both.

See Chapter 13, Exercise 14 for anatomic insights.

Spinal Nerves and Dermatomes   Thirty-one pairs of spinal nerves are connected to the spinal cord. They have no special names, as do the cranial nerves; however, they are numbered according to the level of the spinal column at which they emerge from the spinal cavity. There are 8 cervical, 12 thoracic, 5 lumbar, and 1 coccygeal pairs of spinal nerves.

Each spinal nerve, instead of attaching directly to the cord, attaches indirectly by means of two short roots: the dorsal root and the ventral root. The dorsal roots generally lead nerve fibers from the sensory receptors to various areas of the body, while the ventral roots are a combination of motor nerve fibers, supplying voluntary muscles, involuntary muscles, and glands.

Each spinal nerve contains large branches that form a network called plexuses, which then distribute branches to the body parts. There are three main plexuses:

1. *Cervical Plexuses*—supply motor impulses to the muscles of the neck and receive sensory impulses from the neck and back of the head.
2. *Brachial Plexuses*—send numerous branches to the shoulder, arm, forearm, wrist, and hand.
3. *Lumbosacral Plexuses*—supply nerves to the lower extremities; the largest of these branches being the sciatic nerve.

Dermatomes   When first reviewing the spinal nerve distribution, it does not seem to follow an orderly arrangement, but through a detailed mapping of the skin surface, a close relationship between the source on the cord of each nerve and the vertical position of the body it innervates with becomes more apparent. This mapping is referred to as dermatomes, and the knowledge of this segmental arrangement of spinal nerves has proven to be invaluable for physicians, especially when trying to locate the exact point of interruption of pain or a loss of sensations (Fig. 14-20).

The normal function of the nervous system may be altered by metabolic disorders, chromosomal defects, a disease process, or traumatic injury, interrupting the transmission of vital sensations or actions to the body. Assessment of neurologic deficits or changes in the

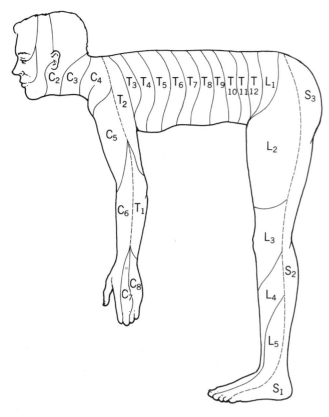

Fig. 14-20. Dermatomes of the body

functional activity of this system establishes the indication for neurosurgical intervention.

General Considerations

There is a unique body of knowledge that is considered essential in order to manage the intraoperative nursing care of the patient requiring neurosurgical intervention.

Neurosurgical procedures have been performed, according to ancient writings, as early as the Egyptian civilization, when the skull was opened (trephination) to release "evil spirits." With the development of specialized instrumentation and growing technologic advancements, the depth of neurosurgery continues to advance in order to alleviate the problems that can be treated through modern neurosurgical intervention.

Regardless of the new technology, however, certain general principles and nursing considerations are essential for every neurosurgical procedure.

Positioning, Skin Preparation, and Draping

Depending on the location of the involved pathology, the patient may be placed in one of several positions.

In most instances, the surgeon will be present during this phase to direct and assist in properly positioning the patient, especially if a special headrest or alignment of the head is indicated.

The supine position may be used for many craniotomy and anterior cervical spine procedures, and for repair of peripheral nerves. A modified Fowler's position may be used for selected craniotomy procedures involving the posterior aspect of the skull/brain, and for posterior cervical spine operations. Selected laminectomies are performed in the prone position with the use of a special frame used to elevate the vertebral column or chest bolsters or rolls, Vac-Pac or other positioning aids used to elevate the thoracic cavity. At all cost, the patient's safety and comfort must be of primary concern to avoid postoperative complications that could be associated with improper positioning.

When preparing the surgical site for a craniotomy, the hair is first shaved with electric clippers and then shaved with a razor (see pp. 310–311 for details). The patient's hair should be saved, properly labeled, and returned to the patient, since it is considered personal property. Some surgeons may prefer to perform their own shaves; therefore, the perioperative nurse should assemble the necessary equipment for this procedure, and be prepared to assist with it.

Draping procedures can be complex, especially if a microscope, video camera, and/or laser must be included in the draping process. A craniotomy incise drape sheet is available to assist in the process, creating a continuous sterile field while providing a pouch for the immediate suctioning of fluids that can accumulate during the procedure. For a procedure involving the spine, for example, laminectomy, a laparotomy pack is usually sufficient to cover the patient adequately. However, many neurosurgeons prefer to add a plastic adhesive drape, either plain or impregnated with iodine (e.g., Ioban Drape) over the proposed incision site for extra protection against possible contamination of the wound.

Special Equipment and Supplies Neurosurgical procedures, especially involving the brain, require special equipment according to the needs for the procedure and the surgeon's preference.

The operative microscope, for example, is frequently used during cranial, spinal, and/or peripheral nerve procedures. When less magnification is required, however, special magnifying loops may be used, along with a fiberoptic headlight for added visibility.

The electrosurgical unit (ESU) and/or the bipolar cautery unit are frequently used concurrently during a neurosurgical procedure. In order to avoid injury to brain tissue, once the skin flap has been created the cutting selection of the ESU should be turned off. The bipolar forceps will be used exclusively on delicate structures, and the settings will be determined by the surgeon, depending on the involved anatomy (see Chap. 11 for electrosurgical safety).

A special overhead instrument table, known as a Mayfield table, can be used either as a substitute for the Mayo tray or as an instrument table during a craniotomy procedure. With the surgeon standing at the patient's head, the table can be positioned over the patient's chest or at the side of the table, and raised or lowered to provide an ideal location for the instruments and supplies. The Mayfield table is usually draped continuously with the patient to provide one large sterile field.

Drills and perforators (e.g., Craniotome; Midas Rex) are common power tools used to penetrate the skull for a craniotomy. The use of these power tools varies according to the manufacturer's specifications, and all personnel involved with the equipment should be thoroughly familiar with their handling and usage.

Special neurosurgical headrests, varying in shape and application (e.g., Mayfield Pin; Horseshoe; Gardner Pin), are used to stabilize the head and cervical spine. They may either attach to the table, or be placed as a positioning aide at the head of the table. Some headrests are designed with detachable pins which should be sterilized prior to use since they penetrate both the skin and skull.

Suction and irrigation are essential to every surgical procedure. During neurosurgery, the wound must be

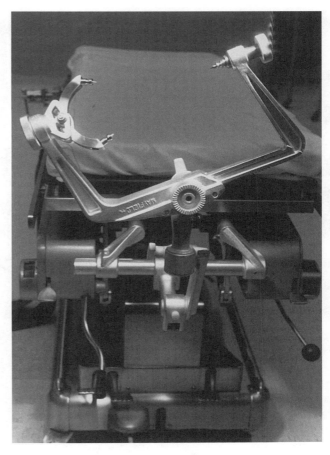

Mayfield pin headrest attached to operating room table

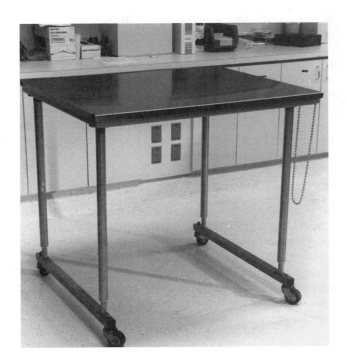

Mayfield instrument table

kept free of bleeders and debris, and since the skull cannot accommodate the accumulation of fluid or blood, suction must be available at all times. A Frazier tip (disposable or nondisposable) is commonly used, since it is smaller in diameter, and can be used effectively without injury to brain tissue.

Irrigation solutions are used primarily with an Asepto syringe, and the temperature should be warm, but never hot, since fluid that exceeds 120°F can cause cell damage to the cortex. When drilling bone, the scrub person should keep the field moist by dropping solution onto the surface, thereby avoiding a buildup of heat as the drill perforates the bone.

Additionally, a combination suction/irrigation unit (the CUSA) may be used to facilitate this process in a more precise manner.

Special radiopaque neurosurgical sponges (Cottonoids) are used during cranial and spinal surgeries. They are available in a variety of sizes ranging from very small flat squares (¼ in. × ¼ in.), to large rectangular sponges (3 in. × 3 in.). A string is attached to each sponge to facilitate identification in the wound, and they should be moistened with saline prior to ap-

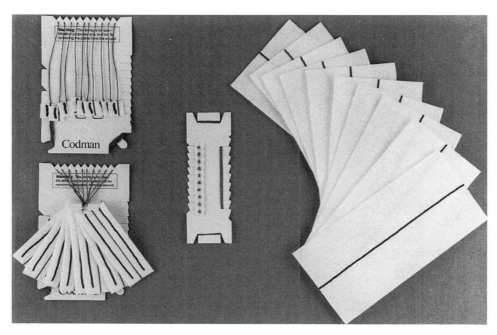

Variety of neurologic (cottonoid) sponges

plication. All sponges, Raytex, and cottonoids are counted in the appropriate manner. Raytex should be restricted to the opening and closing sequences, since the gauze fabric may be too coarse for brain or cord tissue.

Hemostasis is a critical factor for all procedures. During a neurosurgical procedure hemostatic agents such as bone wax, Gelfoam, Thrombin, Oxycel, or Surgicel are commonly used. The Gelfoam should be cut into strips or squares, and according to the surgeon's preference, should be either soaked in saline or Thrombin or used dry. Avoid handling the wet substance by either passing it on a smooth forceps or on the back of a gloved hand.

In addition to the pharmacologic methods, ligating clips may be used where electrocautery would be hazardous to tissue or vessels.

Most neurosurgeons use an antibiotic solution for wound irrigation before closure. If a bone flap is created, the flap should be placed in the antibiotic solution during the procedure until it is used to close the cranium.

The laser (carbon dioxide or neodynamic yag) is selectively used in conjunction with the operating microscope for precise management of hemostasis and/or vaporization of tumor cells. The laser provides minimal damage to vital structures during resection of tumors of the brain or spinal cord. All laser precautions must be maintained before and during the procedure, even if the use of the laser is only a possibility.

A thermal blanket should be placed on the operating table to help prevent a hypothermic episode resulting from a possibly prolonged procedure. Consult with the anesthesiologist and/or the surgeon for recommended settings. Good body alignment and adequate protection of bony prominences are also required.

Instrumentation

Neurosurgical instruments range from the standard soft tissue instrument tray to the specialty trays needed for a specific procedure. The instruments may be combined to produce specialty trays—for example, a brain tray, a neurologic dissecting tray, a burr hole/emergency tray, a peripheral neurologic tray, depending on the size and need of the service, preferences of the surgeons, or institutional categorizing of instruments according to like procedures (for example, laminectomy tray, craniotomy tray, etc.).

Diagnostic Procedures

Most diagnostic procedures are performed before the patient is brought to surgery. The variety of radiologic studies and scans provide an accurate means for visualizing the location of the defect/injury, and these films/scans should always be available to the neurosurgeon to review before or during the procedure.

Examples of the more commonly performed diagnostic studies include

1. computerized tomography (CT scan)
2. cerebral angiography

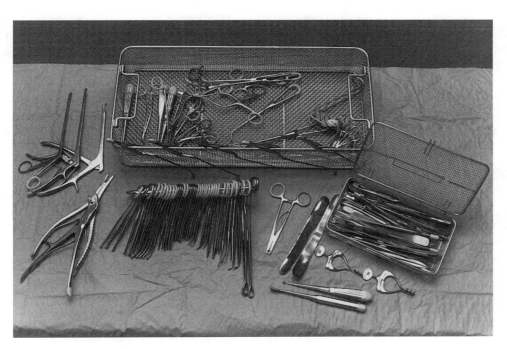

Major neurologic (brain) instrument tray

3. nuclear magnetic resonance imaging (NMRI)
4. pneumoencephalography, myelography, arteriography

Recently, a procedure usually performed in the radiology department, a Stereotaxis procedure, has been added to the diagnostic and operative procedures that can provide a less destructive technique for pinpoint location of tumors and/or sites of injuries. Brain biopsies and coagulation of vessels can now be performed with minimal trauma or damage to brain tissue, and without the necessity to perform a craniotomy procedure. (See p. 550 for further details.)

CRANIAL SURGERY

Cranial surgery is performed to (1) relieve pressure on the brain due to injury or disease, (2) remove pathologic lesions/tumors, or (3) create cerebrospinal diversions in order to reduce CSF accumulation in the cranial cavity.

Neurosurgical Emergencies Related to Trauma

Head injuries are often the most frequent cause of neurosurgical emergencies and can be as simple as a lacerated scalp or may involve the evacuation of a clot (hematoma) which has accumulated in or on brain tissue.

Intracranial Hematomas

Intracranial hematomas are classified as epidural, subdural, or intercerebral, depending on the nature of the injury and/or the location of the involved pathology/injury.

1. *Epidural Hematomas*—Bleeding is due to a rupture or tear of the middle meningeal artery or its branches, which forms a hematoma between the cranium and the dura. This condition is a severe surgical emergency and requires immediate intervention (evacuation of clot/clipping of artery).
2. *Subdural Hematoma*—The bleed occurs between the dura and the arachnoid space and is usually caused by a laceration of a vein that crosses the subdural space. The treatment may necessitate only a burr hole procedure and is subdivided into acute (arterial bleed), subacute (venous bleed), or chronic (occurs 6 months or more after injury). If arterial, immediate intervention is usually required.
3. *Intercerebral Hematoma*—This condition involves a tear in the brain tissue at the point of greatest impact (or injury). Although it usually absorbs, the hematoma may require evacuation and debridement of necrotic tissue if the patient's condition or level of consciousness changes, indicating a possible increase in intracranial pressure or ICP (pressure on the brain tissue).

Procedure
Craniotomy

Definition: Opening of the skull to expose the brain and intracranial structures.

CDC Classification: I (unless a crushed skull exists)

Discussion: Burr holes, the most basic form of a craniotomy, are made to remove localized fluid collection beneath the dura mater and/or to tap a lateral ventricle to relieve pressure.

Burr holes may also be used as a preliminary step to other cranial procedures, creating connecting points during the creation of a bone flap.

Numerous neurologic conditions can be treated by a craniotomy, including intracranial aneurysm, arteriovenous malformations, occluded intercranial vessels, pituitary tumors, acoustic neuromas, hydrocephalus, and congenital abnormalities such as premature closure of sutures, in addition to the neurosurgical emergencies mentioned earlier.

Craniotomies are classified according to their locations: anterior, middle, or posterior fossa, or according to the specific location of entry on the cranial bone.

Positioning: Supine, sitting, or prone depending on the pathology

Skin Preparation: See discussion on p. 310–311 and Module IV, p. 337. In addition, eyes and internal ear should be protected from solution.

Packs/Drapes: Craniotomy pack or Laparotomy pack with craniotomy incise sheet

    Plastic adherent sheet (plain or Ioban)

    Towels, extra drape sheets

    Microscope drape/laser drape (optional)

Instrumentation: Craniotomy tray and/or Microsurgical instruments (optional)

    Power saw/drill (for example, Craniotome, Midas Rex)

    Hemoclips/surgiclips, Raney scalp clips

    Specialty tray (e.g., aneurysm clips and appliers)

Supplies/Equipment:

    Basin set

    Blades—(2) No. 10, (1) No. 15, (1) No. 11

    Needle counter

    ESU/bipolar unit/suction

    Cottonoids—variety

    Bone wax, sutures—surgeon's preference

    Medications—hemostatic agents, antibiotics

    Microscope and/or magnifying loops

    Fiberoptic headlight (optional)

    Thermal blanket with controls

    Laser/video camera with monitor (optional)

    Mayfield overhead table (optional)

    Neurologic headrest—surgeon's preference

    Solutions—saline, water, Asepto syringe (2)

    Power source for drill

    Cell saver (available)

    CUSA unit (optional)

PROCEDURAL OVERVIEW—General

The first step in performing a craniotomy is the creation of a bone flap, which may be left attached to muscle and turned back with soft tissue to which it is attached, or it may be totally removed (free bone flap).

The surgeon may mark the incision site with a needle, scalpel blade, or marking pen and then incise the skin. Once the incising process has begun, Raney scalp clips are applied to the tissue edge, forming a circle around the proposed site of injury/disease. The pericranium is elevated from the skull so it can be drilled. Two or more burr holes are made in the skull and a power saw is used to separate the skull between the holes in order to gain entry to the cranial cavity. If the bone flap is removed totally, burr holes are usually placed in the periphery of the skull for easy reattachment.

Bleeding is controlled with the ESU, bipolar forceps and/or bone wax. The dura mater is incised, vessels are coagulated or ligated and the dura mater may be tacked up to the pericranium. Moist cottonoids are placed as necessary; the brain is continuously moistened by saline irrigation through an Asepto syringe to prevent injury due to cortical drying.

The repair, revision, evacuation/ligation, or excision of a lesion/tumor is performed, depending on the pathology.

When the procedure is completed, the wound is irrigated, hemostasis is confirmed, and the dural flap is closed, making the suture line watertight. If the dural flap is too large to be closed, a dural graft may need to be inserted.

The bone flap is reset and wired back into place (No. 28 wire). Burr holes may be covered with a variety of materials, including autogenous bone chips. As the scalp is closed, the skin clips are removed, and should be accounted for as part of the instrument count. The wound is dressed according to the surgeon's preference.

PERIOPERATIVE NURSING CONSIDERATIONS

- Planning prior to bringing the patient to the operating room is essential. Consider placement of furniture and equipment in relation to maintaining a sterile field.
- Headrest clamps attach to the table headrest attachment slots. Head is secured in proper position by two or three sterile fixation pins. Insertion site should be prepared with Betadine ointment or solution. Prep is performed with patient in headrest.
- Have CT scans and x-rays in the room.

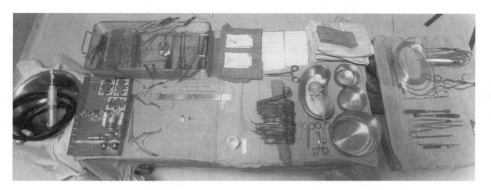

Basic set-up craniotomy

- Ensure that all bony prominences are well padded and the body is in as close to normal alignment as possible for that position.
- Have all equipment tested and ready prior to patient's arrival in the room.
- Keep both Asepto syringes filled and ready. Moistened cottonoids and bone wax should be kept within easy reach of the surgeon.
- Cords from equipment should be positioned to avoid an accident (tripping over cords), especially away from entrances to the room.

Specific Surgical Interventions

1. *Intracranial Aneurysm*—The aneurysm is approached through a standard suboccipital or subfrontal craniotomy. Once the arachnoid tissues have been freed, the base of the aneurysm and often its "parent" or subbranches are occluded using an aneurysm clip applied with a special clip applicator.
2. *Excision of Brain Tumor*—Laser or suction-irrigation system (e.g., CUSA) may be used to remove the tumor or other pathologic lesions following the routine opening for a craniotomy procedure.
3. *Correction of Arteriovenous Malformation*—A standard supratentorial or infratentorial craniotomy is performed; the feeding arteries are exposed and occluded (clipping, coagulation, ligation, or laser-beam coagulation). The malformation is dissected. The wound is closed in a routine craniotomy fashion.

Stereotaxic Procedures

Stereotaxic procedures use a complex mechanism to locate and destroy target structures in the brain with the aid of a computer, radiologic equipment (imaging units), and a special head-fixation device. Common target areas include tumors of the basal ganglia, thalamus, and hypophysis and aneurysms and lesions of the anterolateral spinal tracts. A biopsy is usually performed first, using the stereotaxic approach for pinpoint accuracy, and if feasible, the pathology could be destroyed by chemical or mechanical means or the disease corrected by electrical stimulation to control

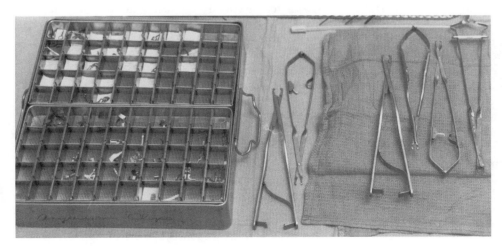

Aneurysm clips and appliers

intractable pain without necessitating an open procedure.

The patient's head is placed in a special head holder and the probe is introduced into the brain through a burr hole created along one axis of the head holder. With the probe in place, positioning is confirmed by radiologic scanning. Hollow cannulas, coagulating electrodes, and other instruments are used to perform specific procedures, including thalmotomy, cingulotomy, electrostimulation, radiofrequency retrograde rhizotomy, cryohypophysectomy, removal of intracranial neoplasms, interstitial radiation, and coagulation of intracranial vascular lesions.

Cerebrospinal Diversion Procedures

Cerebrospinal diversion procedures involve the shunting of cerebrospinal fluid away from the ventricles of the brain by the insertion of a valve system or catheter to another location in the body, for example, ventriculoperitoneal (abdomen), ventriculoatrial (heart), or lumbarperitoneal.

Procedure
Ventriculoperitoneal Shunt (VP shunt)

CDC Classification: I (unless a systemic infection is present).

Discussion: Shunting the ventricular fluid to a body cavity outside the cranium is usually performed to treat hydrocephalus (congenital, neoplastic, traumatic, or infectious).

The distal end of the shunt is placed in the peritoneal cavity unless contraindicated by diseases involving the peritoneal cavity. If peritoneal placement cannot be used, the shunt may be placed indirectly in the right atrium via the internal jugular vein or directly into the atrium via a thoracotomy (Fig. 14-21).

The advantages of peritoneal over atrial placement of the distal catheter are (1) avoidance of vascular and cardiopulmonary complications, (2) faster and simpler placement, (3) space to place a longer catheter (prolonging intervals between revisions in the child), and (4) easier replacement of the distal catheter, if necessary.

Positioning: Supine, right arm tucked in at the patient's side, left arm extended on an armboard. Patient's head is slightly elevated and turned to the left; a head-rest may be used (doughnut). (See Pediatric unit for additional positional precautions.)

Skin Preparation/Packs/Drapes: See Craniotomy, p. 550

Instrumentation: Craniotomy tray
   Power drill/cord
   Shunt, ventricular/peritoneal catheter
   Long passing (tunneling) instrument
   Small cardiovascular set (optional)
Supplies/Equipment:
   Basin set
   ESU/bipolar unit/suction
   Headrest (optional)
   Power source for drill
   Blades—(1) No. 10, (1) No. 15
   Needle counter
   Plastic adhesive drape sheet (optional)
   Shunt (e.g., Rickham, Holter valve, and catheter)
   Cottonoids—variety of sizes
   Medications—hemostatic agents, antibiotics
   Solutions—saline, water
   Sutures—surgeon's preference

PROCEDURAL OVERVIEW

The incision line, for a right-sided shunt, is marked above and posterior to the ear, and a transverse right upper-quadrant incision is made in the abdomen. The scalp is incised and reflected on its base. A burr hole is created and enlarged as necessary, to accommodate the reservoir of the system. A straight ventricular catheter is passed into the posterior aspect of the lateral ventricle; the stylet is removed and the opening pressure recorded. A premeasured catheter is advanced anterior to the foramen of Munro.

The transverse abdominal incision is carried down to the anterior rectus sheath. A distal catheter is passed subcutaneously from the scalp incision to the abdominal incision. The reservoir is attached to the proximal end of the valve with a connector and sutures. The valve mechanism is placed in the subgaleal space behind the ear. A longitudinal incision is made in the anterior rectus sheath; the rectus abdominis muscle is split. The peritoneum is grasped and incised. The peritoneal catheter is attached to the reservoir.

The wounds are irrigated and the abdominal incisions are closed. The valve is compressed, and the scalp incision is closed.

PERIOPERATIVE NURSING CONSIDERATIONS

- For pediatric considerations, refer to pp. 631–632.
- A reservoir may be inserted into the system between the valve and the catheter.
- Check valve patency and pressure with normal saline before use. Flush unit with saline/Ringer's solution; do not allow air into the unit.
- Handle the shunt as little as possible, avoiding contact with lint or other foreign materials. Avoid

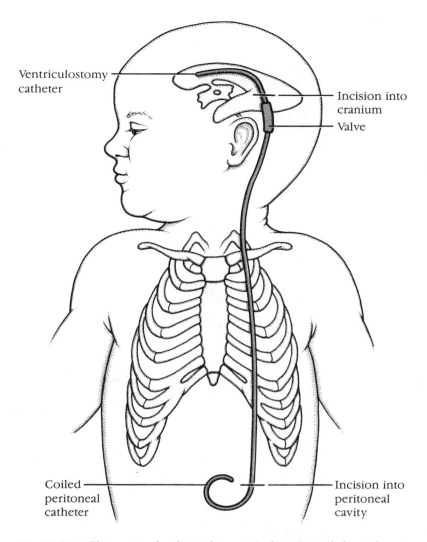

Ventriculostomy catheter

Incision into cranium

Valve

Coiled peritoneal catheter

Incision into peritoneal cavity

Fig. 14-21. Placement of catheter for ventriculoperitoneal shunt diversion

placement on gauze sponges. Unit should be placed in a clean basin.

- The valve must be properly oriented to allow only a one-way passage of fluid.
- Notify radiology department before surgery starts.

Related Procedures: Ventriculoatrial Shunt
Lumbarperitoneal Shunt

SPINAL SURGERY

Spinal surgery is performed (1) to relieve intractable pain, (2) to remove tumors and lesions from the spinal cord, and (3) to replace diseased or injured vertebral disks.

There are three approaches to surgery involving the spine:

1. *Cervical Approach*—anterior, posterior
2. *Thoracic Approach*—posterior, posterolateral, anterior
3. *Lumbar Approach*—posterior, anterior

Positioning for Spinal Surgery

Depending on the location of the injury/lesion, the basic body positioning and their modifications are used for neurosurgery. Four positions are the most commonly used:

1. *Supine*—indicated for supratentorial craniotomy, anterior cervical, and/or subtemporal decompression
2. *Prone*—indicated for lumbar, thoracic, and cervical laminectomy and/or posterior fossa craniotomy

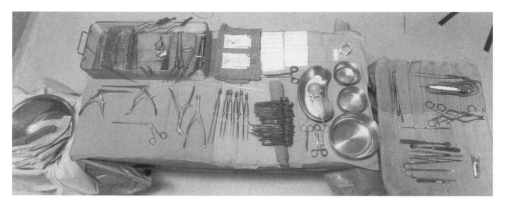

Laminectomy set-up

3. *Sitting*—indicated for cervical laminectomy, posterior fossa craniotomy, temporal craniotomy, and ventriculography
4. *Lateral*—occasionally used for thoracic and lumbar laminectomies and for lumbar sympathectomy

Procedure
Laminectomy

Definition: The creation of an opening in the lamina to expose spinal cord and/or disk.
CDC Classification: I
Discussion: Indications for a laminectomy and/or interlaminar procedures include the need for (1) removal of a herniated disk, (2) excision of a spinal cord tumor, (3) coagulation/repair of an aneurysm, or (4) repair of the spinal cord injured by trauma.
Positioning: depends on the type of laminectomy being performed
Skin Preparation: See pp. 337–338
Packs/Drapes: Laparotomy pack with fenestrated sheet
    Adherent plastic drape sheet (plain or Ioban)
    Microscope drape (optional), laser drape (optional)
Instrumentation: Laminectomy tray
    Kerrison/pituitary rongeur tray
    Microneurosurgical instruments (optional)
    Power drill/cord/drill bits (optional)
Supplies/Equipment:
    Basin set
    ESU/bipolar unit/suction
    Blades—(3 to 4) No. 10, (1) No. 15
    Needle counter
    Bone wax, cottonoids
    Asepto syringe
    Medications—hemostatic agents, antibiotics
    Fiberoptic headlight and power source (optional)
    Microscope or magnifying loops (optional)

    Positioning aids
    Special laminectomy frame, headrest (optional)
    Solutions—saline, water
    Sutures—surgeon's preference
    Cell saver (available)
    Laser (optional)

PROCEDURAL OVERVIEW—Lumbar Laminectomy for Herniated Disk

After induction of anesthesia, the patient is placed on a laminectomy frame or other positional aid in the prone position.

A midline vertical incision may be used. The wound is deepened to the level of the fascia, which is then incised. A self-retaining retractor is placed into the wound. The paraspinous muscles and periosteum are reflected on the side of the involved disk. Sponges are packed along the vertebrae with a periosteal elevator to aid in blunt dissection and to effect hemostasis.

The surgeon will use a large rongeur to bite off the protruding bony spinous process and expose the lamina. Smaller rongeurs are used close to the cord to remove the lamina and create access to the disk. Hemostasis is achieved with bone wax, and the ligamenta flava are incised, with care being taken to avoid injury to the epidural vein. Moistened cottonoids are placed to protect the dura. Nerve roots are carefully retracted, exposing the herniated disk, which is removed with a small rongeur and curettes. The wound is irrigated. The area is examined to ensure that there are no bony prominences protruding and that hemostasis is achieved. The wound is closed in layers.

PERIOPERATIVE NURSING CONSIDERATIONS

- Have previous x-ray films in the room.
- Check with the blood bank for available units if cell saver is not available.
- The patient is put to sleep in supine position, on

the stretcher/bed, then "log-rolled" over to the operating table. Have adequate help when moving/lifting the patient to the operating table following induction.

- When positioning, protect bony prominences from pressure.
- Place moistened cottonoids and bone wax within the surgeon's reach.
- For microdisectomy: a microscope is required and must be draped and positioned.

Related Procedures: Cervical/thoracic laminectomy
Laminectomy—extradural tumor
Laminectomy—meningocele

Procedure
Anterior Cervical Fusion (Cloward Technique)

Definition: Excision of one or more herniated cervical intervertebral disks, and the placement of bone graft(s) between the vertebrae to fuse them together for stabilization of the cervical spine.

CDC Classification: I

Discussion: The procedure is indicated when nerve deficit and/or pain caused by spondylosis or herniated disk persists despite conservative treatment. Fusion is usually accomplished with a bone graft from the iliac crest.

Positioning: There are two approaches to the diseased cervical vertebrae: the anterior and the posterior. The approach used depends on the location of the diseased disk. When a posterior approach is used, the patient is placed in a modified Fowler's position. For the anterior approach, the patient is placed in supine position with head turned slightly to the left; the right hip is elevated on a sandbag.

Skin Preparation: See pp. 337–338

Packs/Drapes: See Laminectomy, p. 554

Instrumentation:
Laminectomy tray
Kerrison/pituitary rongeur tray
Cervical fusion instruments (e.g., Cloward instrument tray)
Power drill/drill bits/cord
Hudson brace, mallet, depth gauge
Hemoclips/surgiclips—variety of sizes

Supplies/Equipment:
Basin set
ESU/bipolar unit/suction
Blades—(2) No. 10, (1) No. 15, (1) No. 11
Fiberoptic headlight/power source
Microscope or magnifying loops
Fiberoptic headlight and power source (optional)
Needle counter
X-ray cassette drape

Medications—hemostatic agents, antibiotics
Cottonoids
Solutions—saline, water
Sutures—surgeon's preference
Power source for drill

PROCEDURAL OVERVIEW

A transverse incision is made in the skin crease of the neck at the level of cricoid cartilage. The incision is deepened, severing the platysma muscle. A self-retaining retractor is placed in the wound and the anterior longitudinal ligament is incised, exposing the intervertebral disk. X-ray films may be taken at this time with a needle used to confirm the correct disk.

The bone graft may be taken at this time or after the surgeon has removed the diseased bone. The graft is usually taken from the iliac crest using either an osteotome or a dowel cutter. All bone chips are kept moist and saved for later packing of the fusion site. The iliac crest site is closed after hemostasis is achieved. The diseased disk is incised and removed piecemeal with rongeurs. The intervertebral space is packed with the bone graft (and chips). After hemostasis is achieved, the cervical wound is irrigated and closed in layers.

PERIOPERATIVE NURSING CONSIDERATIONS

- Have all x-rays in the room.
- Notify radiology of the need for films during the procedure. Observe all x-ray precautions.
- The donor site and incision site are prepared and draped at the same time. The bone graft site is covered with a sterile towel until the surgeon is ready to take the graft. The cervical incision site should be covered while the bone graft is being taken.
- When moving the patient after the procedure, care must be taken to keep the head in alignment with the body to prevent the graft from dislodging.
- Cervical and iliac areas may be prepped separately; two nurses may be required.

PERIPHERAL-NERVE PROCEDURES

Peripheral-nerve surgery is performed to repair injured or diseased peripheral nerves, and/or to restore near-normal function to the structure and/or involved area.

General Discussion

Descriptions of Involved Pathology

1. *Traumatic Injury*—Nerves can be severed, avulsed, contused, or rendered ischemic because of injury.

A neurorrhaphy may be needed to restore normal function.

2. *Intractable Pain*—Pain that occurs in advanced stages of some diseases (e.g., cancer, occlusive arterial disease, myelinating, or degenerative diseases) that are nonresponsive to chemotherapy without severe side effects (e.g., addiction, incapacitating sedation)
3. *Tumors*—(a) Nerve sheath—neuromas, neurofibroma, neurofibrosarcoma; (b) nerve cell—ganglioneuromas, gangliogliomas, paraganglionic tumors

Major Pathologic Locations

Diseases involving the peripheral-nerve structures are often located in the brachial plexus, involving the axillary, median, radial, and ulnar nerves; facial nerves; anterior fibial nerves; or sympathetic nerve chain.

Anesthesia Techniques

Most peripheral nerve procedures can be performed under local anesthesia with monitored anesthesia care or regional block technique (e.g., Bier block, axillary block).

Positioning

For hand, wrist, or upper-extremity surgery, the surgical team will sit at a hand table, which is extended from the side of the operating table, and the affected arm is extended out onto the table. A tourniquet is often used during this type of surgery.

Selected Peripheral Nerve Procedures

Repair Procedures

Most peripheral nerve surgery is performed to repair traumatic nerve injury of an extremity. However, dissection is also performed to remove tumors or relieve pain. The etiology will determine the location and length of the incision.

1. *Neurorrhaphy*—The anastomosis of a severed nerve, usually in the hand or forearm, providing precise approximation of the nerve ends in order to restore function.
2. *Sympathectomy*—The interruption of the sympathetic nerve fibers and ganglia of the autonomic nervous system. In particular, a lumbar sympathectomy is commonly performed to relieve arterial spasm due to vascular disease. Sympathectomies may be done in other locations along the spinal column to treat intractable pain (e.g., upper

cervical, cervicothoracic, thoracic, thoracolumbar, and lumbar).

Carpal Tunnel Syndrome

Carpal tunnel syndrome is a condition of the hand in which the median nerve is compressed by the transverse carpal ligament or by displacement of the lunate bone or volar carpal ganglion. Symptoms may include numbness and tingling of fingers and weakness of intrinsic thumb muscles. These symptoms are usually relieved with a procedure that divides the deep transverse carpal ligament.

Procedure
Carpal Tunnel Release

Definition: A decompression of the median nerve on the volar surface of the wrist.
CDC Classification: I
Positioning: Supine, affected arm extended on a hand table, unaffected arm may be placed on an armboard. A tourniquet is applied to the upper affected arm.
Skin Preparation: See pp. 337–338
Packs/Drapes: Basic pack with extremity sheet, or
  Extremity pack
  Extra drape sheets
  Impervious stockinette
  Towels
Instrumentation:
  Hand/plastic tray
  Hayers metacarpal retractors, pediatric deaver retractors (optional)
  Microneurosurgical instruments (optional)
Supplies/Equipment:
  Basin set
  Esmarch bandage
  Tourniquet and insufflator
  Needle counter
  ESU/suction (optional)
  Blades—(1) No. 10, (1) No. 15
  Solutions—saline, water
  Medications—antibiotics, local agents (optional)
  Sutures—surgeon's preference

PROCEDURAL OVERVIEW

A curved incision is made parallel to the thenar crease, angled toward the ulnar side of the wrist. Care must be taken to avoid injury to sensory branches of the median nerve. A small self-retaining retractor (e.g., Weitlander) is placed in the wound. The transverse carpal ligament is divided. The incision is irrigated and closed with fine silk/nylon, and a compression dressing or a splint is applied.

PERIOPERATIVE NURSING CONSIDERATIONS

- For tourniquet precautions, see Chapter 11, pp. 337–338.
- Circumfuncial prep of extremity is required.
- Do not allow prep solutions to "pool" under the tourniquet.

- If performed under local anesthesia, follow monitoring guidelines (Chap. 6, p. 107)
- Be prepared to assist with application of splint/cast.

Related Procedures: Reduction of carpal bone fracture
Excision of a Ganglion

Self-assessment Exercise 33

Directions: *Complete the following exercises. The answers can be found at the end of this module.*

1. An autogenous bone graft is described as one taken from the patient.

    True   False

2. A common power source for drills, saws, etc. used during orthopedic and neurosurgery would be _____.

3. Routine instrumentation for orthopedic surgery would include soft tissue instruments, and
    a.
    b.
    c.
    d.

4. An exploration of a joint is called an _____.

5. Special sponges used during neurosurgical procedures are called cottonoids.

    True   False

6. Methods for controlling bleeding during a craniotomy may include:
    a.
    b.
    c.

7. A burr hole procedure is usually performed to _____.

8. A Putti-Platt procedure is performed on the _____ to _____.

9. When preparing for a traumatic open fracture, the perioperative nurse should anticipate the need for (1) copious normal saline irrigation and (2) _____.

10. Hydrocephalus is caused by an excessive CSF absorption in the lateral ventricles. The procedure performed to reduce the fluid by diverting it to the abdominal area is called a/an _____.

THORACIC AND CARDIOVASCULAR SURGERY

Thoracic and cardiovascular procedures involve the *heart* and associated structures (*great vessels*), the peripheral vascular system, and pulmonary structures (the *lungs*).

The primary aim of thoracic surgery is to diagnose and treat diseases associated with the lungs through endoscopic procedures and resection or revision of diseased tissue. The primary aim of cardiovascular surgery is to correct congenital and/or acquired defects of the heart and vascular structures in the hopes of improving systemic circulation and tissue perfusion throughout the body.

The specific procedures, outlined in this unit, are divided into two major groups:

Thoracic Surgery
Cardiovascular Surgery
    Peripheral Vascular Procedures
    The Heart and Great Vessels

Surgical Anatomy Review

The Thoracic Cavity

The thoracic cavity consists of a right and left *pleural cavity* and a mid-portion called the *mediastinal cavity.* Fibrous tissues form a wall around the mediastinum, completely separating it from the pleural sacs, in which the right and left lungs reside.

Organs located in the mediastinal cavity include the heart, enclosed in a *pericardial sac,* a portion of the trachea, the right and left bronchi, various blood vessels, including the great vessels, lymph nodes, and nerves (Fig. 14-22).

The Heart

Cardiac Layers Considered by some to be a "living pump," the heart is a hollow, muscular organ, the walls of which are formed of three distinct layers:

1. *Epicardium:* the outermost layer of the heart wall that also serves as the lining of the pericardial sac.

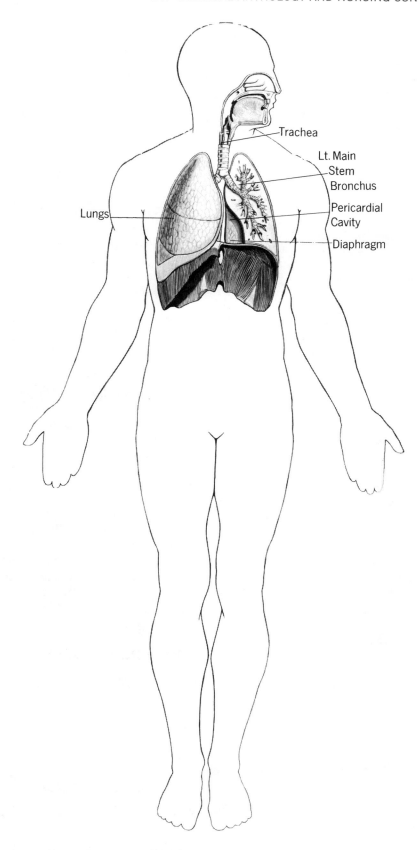

Trachea

Lt. Main
Stem
Bronchus

Lungs

Pericardial
Cavity

Diaphragm

Fig. 14-22.   Thoracic cavity structures (with heart) with pericardial cavity (pericardial sac)

2. *Myocardium:* the muscular layer of the heart; much thicker than the other layers, and responsible for the heart's pumping action.

3. *Endocardium:* a smooth layer of cells that resemble squamous epithelium. This membrane lines the interior of the heart, and is also the material of which the valves of the heart are formed.

Chambers and Valves The heart has four chambers, each divided by a *septum.* The upper chambers are called *atria* (singular, atrium), and these chambers act as the receiving chambers for blood into the heart from either the body or the lungs. The two lower chambers, called *ventricles,* function as the pumping chambers of the heart, sending the blood out of the heart to either the lungs for oxygenation (right side), or to the body for systemic circulation (left side).

There are four valves located at the entrance and exit of each chamber: *tricuspid, pulmonic, mitral,* and *aortic.* The function of the valves is to prevent backflow of blood into the chambers, thus facilitating effective cardiac circulation.

Great Vessels of the Heart The large vessels surrounding the heart have a vital role in both cardiac and systemic circulation.

The *vena cava,* considered the largest vein in the body, brings blood into the heart from the upper (*superior*) and lower (*inferior*) sections of the body. This blood is deoxygenated, since it has not passed through the cardiac cycle to the lungs.

The *pulmonary artery* serves as a conduit for blood as it leaves the right side of the heart, on its way to the lungs for oxygenation.

Oxygenated blood, returned to the left side via the *pulmonary veins,* leaves the heart through the *aorta,* the largest artery in the body. The aorta is divided into three sections, related to its anatomic location: the *aortic arch,* the *ascending aorta,* and the *descending aorta.* Three branches arise directly from the aortic arch: the *innominate artery,* the *left common carotid artery,* and the *left subclavian artery.* These branches and their tributaries carry blood to the upper portion of the body.

The descending aorta, subdivided into the *thoracic aorta* and the *abdominal aorta,* and its tributaries carry the oxygenated blood to the lower portion of the body.

Peripheral Vascular Structures

The peripheral vascular system is a complex network of vessels whose major function is to transport blood and vital substances to all parts of the body.

The major components of this system consist of *veins,* which carry blood to the heart, and *arteries,* which carry blood away from the heart.

The arterial system is a branching network whose vessels decrease in size as they traverse the body. Beginning with the largest artery, the aorta, each branches into smaller and smaller tubules until it reaches the cellular level, the smallest being the *capillary,* which is attached to a *venule,* the smallest vessel of the venous network.

The venous network carries deoxygenated blood from body tissues to the vena cava, where it enters the heart. Each vein is unidirectional, with internal valves that prevent backflow and pooling in the vessel.

Occasionally, debris is caught within a vessel, reducing its ability to transport effectively the blood to its specific location. When this occurs and causes a significant reduction in systemic perfusion, surgical intervention becomes necessary.

The Lungs and Associated Structures

In addition to the heart and great vessels, the thoracic cavity also contains the *lungs.*

The lungs are situated in the mid-thoracic cavity, and are contained within two separate *pleural cavities.* The lungs are surrounded by a membrane, the *pleura,* which further divides into the *visceral pleura* and the *parietal pleura.*

Each lung is divided into *lobes.* The left lung consists of two lobes, whereas the right lung has three.

The entire thoracic cavity is flexible, capable of expanding and contracting along with the lungs. Its interior is well sealed off from the outside by its layer of membrane, and this feature is part of the primary mechanism of breathing and the exchange of gases through inhalation and exhalation. It is imperative, therefore, that an air-tight pleural cavity be restored and negative pressure maintained for maximum pulmonary function following thoracic and/or cardiac surgery, since these procedures require entrance into this sealed cavity.

THORACIC SURGERY

Surgical intervention involving the thoracic area is centered around the lungs and associated structures, and involve procedures that can *diagnose* specific abnormalities and procedures that can *repair/revise* injured or diseased tissue.

Diagnostic Procedures

Endoscopic procedures are frequently performed in surgery prior to corrective surgery or as a separate procedure, in order to make a preliminary diagnosis. Procedures pertinent to thoracic surgery include a bronchoscopy and a mediastinoscopy.

Procedure
Flexible Bronchoscopy

Definition: This procedure involves the insertion of a *fiberoptic bronchoscope* into the respiratory tree, allowing direct visualization of respiratory structures within the lung and bronchus, and the extraction of tissue for pathologic studies. The procedure can also be used to extract foreign objects that a patient may have accidentally aspirated. Bronchoscopy can be performed using a flexible or a rigid scope, depending on the surgeon's preference.

Technique: Aseptic (masks should be worn for protection)

Position: Supine, with shoulders just above the top break in the table (to allow the head to be lowered). (If general anesthesia is used, the anesthesiologist will move to the side of the patient's head.)

Instrumentation/Supplies:
Basic pack with split sheet, gloves, gown
Flexible fiberoptic bronchoscope
Endotracheal adapter (for general anesthesia)
Fiberoptic light source/cord
Small basin with saline
Suction tubing
Leukens tube (for specimen) (opt.)
Lubricant
Telfa/Needle (for biopsy specimen)
Accessory items: Biopsy forceps, brush, slides, culture jar for slides, 10-ml syringe (2) (for saline irrigation)

PROCEDURAL OVERVIEW

1. Following intubation, a well-lubricated bronchoscope is inserted through the adapter/endotracheal tube.
2. The respiratory structures are examined.

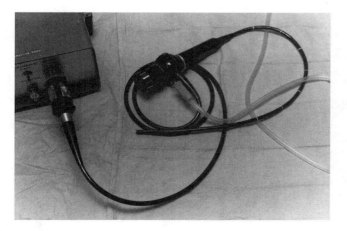

Flexible fiberoptic bronchoscope and light scope

3. A biopsy or other diagnostic procedure is performed (e.g., bronchial washings, bronchial brushings, cultures, etc.) for microscopic examination.
4. The patient is well suctioned, and the scope is slowly withdrawn.

PERIOPERATIVE NURSING CONSIDERATIONS

- Prior to the procedure, check that all equipment and supplies are available and in proper working order.
- A plastic mouthpiece may be used to protect the patient's lips and teeth, or a dampened sponge may be placed on the lips.
- Room lights may be dimmed during the procedure. Use the x-ray view box if more illumination is necessary.
- Have all chest x-rays available in the room.
- A scrub nurse may be needed to assist the surgeon during the procedure by:
  1. Managing the suction/specimen collection apparatus.
  2. Keeping syringes filled with saline.
  3. Passing and guiding biopsy forceps and other instruments into the scope as requested.
  4. Handling the specimens obtained.
- Label all specimens properly. Take care not to crush the specimen; use a needle to remove tissue from biopsy forceps, and place specimen on Telfa.
- Dispatch specimens promptly.
- Clean and disinfect the scope and accessory instruments according to manufacturer's recommendations (see pp. 193–195 for disinfection procedures).

Related Procedure: Rigid Bronchoscopy

Procedure
Mediastinoscopy

Definition: This procedure involves the endoscopic visualization and examination of the mediastinal space, including the bronchi, aortic arch, and regional lymph nodes. The procedure is usually performed when a malignancy is suspected, as a final diagnostic examination.

CDC Classification: II

Positioning: Supine, with neck extended on rolled towel under shoulders. Anesthesia personnel will be positioned at the side of the patient's head.

Skin Preparation: Begin at the suprasternal notch; include neck and shoulders; chin to nipple line

Instrumentation/Supplies:
Laparotomy pack with towels
ESU/suction

Mediastinoscopy tray
Fiberoptic light source/cords
Basin set
Blades—(1) No. 10, (1) No. 15
Telfa and needle (for specimen removal)

PROCEDURAL OVERVIEW

1. A transverse incision is made over the suprasternal notch and extended down to the pretracheal fascia.
2. The mediastinoscope is introduced into the space.
3. The anatomy is visualized and identified.
4. Any suspect lymph nodes are removed for examination.
5. The scope is removed; hemostasis is achieved; the wound is closed (and dressed if an open procedure is not scheduled to follow).

PERIOPERATIVE NURSING CONSIDERATIONS

- The approach is both endoscopic and surgical. Sterile technique must be maintained.
- Check all equipment and power sources prior to beginning procedure.
- A sponge count is required before the scope is removed and at the closing of the wound.
- Remove the specimen from biopsy forceps with a needle only; place on Telfa.
- If procedure is performed in conjunction with an open procedure, mediastinal set-up is kept separate from open case, and should be removed upon completion. The patient is reprepped and draped for the open procedure; gowns and gloves should be changed.

General Considerations—Surgical Procedures

Surgical Approach

The type of incision is determined by the operative procedure being proposed. Two basic approaches are associated with thoracic surgery procedures:

1. *Thoracotomy* (anterolateral or posterolateral)
2. *Median Sternotomy*

The most frequently used approach is the *posterolateral thoracotomy* (for surgeries not directly involving the heart), which can be adapted for a lobectomy, pneumonectomy, decortication, and drainage of empyema.

Positioning

The patient is positioned in such a manner as to provide adequate exposure of the operative site, efficient respiratory and cardiac function, and maintenance of proper alignment.

The *lateral* and *supine* positions are most frequently used, depending on the surgical approach.

The lateral position permits a full posterolateral incision, giving access to both the anterior and posterior surfaces of the lung and associated vascular structures. A *Vac-Pack* (bean bag) and/or kidney rests are used to support the torso in this position. The supine position is used for a sternotomy incision and the anterolateral thoracotomy approach. Sandbags or towels may be placed under the scapula, on the operative side, when an anterolateral incision is used.

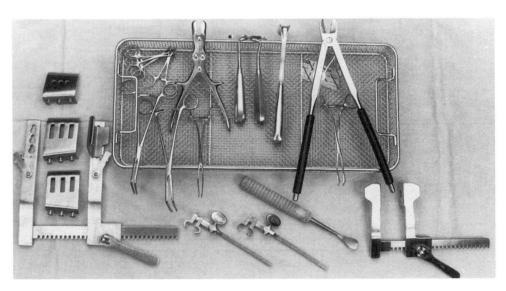

Chest instrumentation tray

Special Equipment

Chest Drainage System A sterile closed-chest drainage system is essential when the thoracic cavity has been opened by either surgery or trauma, except when a pneumonectomy is performed. Chest drainage systems provide an avenue for drainage of air, blood, and other fluids from the intrapleural or mediastinal space, in addition to reestablishing negative pressure in the thoracic cavity.

Several disposable systems are currently available, with or without an automatic transfusion system attachment. The units can be *dry* or *wet*, depending on the surgeon's preference, and can either be used as straight drainage or attached to suction.

Chest Tubes Chest tubes come in a variety of sizes, both straight and angled, and are anchored to the chest wall with suture and tape. A single tube may be used; however, two tubes are usually preferred. If two tubes are used, a Y-connector is used to connect the two chest tubes to the chest drainage system. All connections should be banded or otherwise secured to ensure an intact system.

Instrumentation The thoracic instrumentation includes a basic laparotomy instrument set and specialty instruments that can accommodate the depth of the incision and the handling of delicate structures (e.g., lung clamps, bronchus clamps, etc.). Vascular, bone, and special retractors may be added to the tray to create a chest tray that is generic to most open chest procedures.

Surgical Technique Because the *bronchus* is considered "dirty," a no-touch technique is used whenever the bronchus is encountered during a thoracic procedure. The instruments are isolated from the rest of the set-up to reduce the possibility of cross-contamination.

Additional Counts If cavity-within-a-cavity is entered, as in most thoracic procedures, an additional closing count of sponges, sharps, and instruments is required. The first count is performed prior to closure of the internal cavity, the second prior to closure of the major cavity, the third prior to closure of skin.

Chest Injuries

Trauma to the chest may result in injury to the thoracic wall and/or internal structures, such as the heart and lungs.

Chest trauma is categorized as either *blunt* or *penetrating*. Blunt trauma may not reveal any overt evidence of chest injury, even though there may be internal bleeding; therefore, a careful assessment of the patient must be made immediately upon arrival in the emergency department. Blunt trauma does not usually require surgical intervention unless sharp edges or bone fragments puncture the pleural cavity, creating a "sucking wound." If this occurs, a pneumothorax may occur, requiring immediate attention.

Penetrating trauma, on the other hand, may be caused by a high- or low-velocity-like missile, such as a bullet or a knife, in which case, an operative exploration is usually required. If an open wound is present, it must be converted to a closed chest wound before a pneumothorax occurs, which is usually followed by a mediastinal shift, producing added complications for the patient and the attending physicians.

Emergency treatment for penetrating chest wounds usually involves stabilization of the patient followed by a *thoracocentesis* (surgical puncture of the chest wall to remove fluids) and/or a *thoracotomy* for insertion of chest tubes.

The insertion of one or more chest tubes is performed following any severe chest injury to prevent cardiac tamponade. They may be inserted in the emergency department before the patient's transfer to surgery to effect the repair of the injured structure. The following outlines the procedure for chest tube insertion.

Procedural Overview: Insertion of Chest Tube(s)

1. The chest wall is incised.
2. A tube-pulling clamp (e.g., long Pean) is inserted into the intercostal space. The tapered end of the tube is placed into the jaws of the clamp, and the tube is pulled through the tissue layer.
3. The tube is positioned, x-rays are taken to confirm proper positioning, and the tube is sutured to the skin; the incision is closed.
4. The tube is connected to a sealed drainage unit.

General Nursing Considerations

- Aseptic surgical technique must be established and maintained during the insertion procedure.
- An emergency chest tray should be available to facilitate the insertion procedure.
- The sealed drainage unit should be set up according to physician's specifications (gravity or suction).
- Fluid measurement should be obtained prior to the patient's leaving the emergency department and documented for reference by the surgical team and/or nursing staff who will care for the patient after stabilization.

Selected Surgical Procedures

Procedure
Thoracotomy

Definition: A surgical approach into the thoracic cavity for exploration.
CDC Classification: II, depending on involved pathology
Discussion: This incision approach is used to provide access to the organs of the chest, particularly the lungs, heart, and aorta.
Position: Specific to incision site; lateral or supine
Skin Preparation: See pp. 337–338
Packs/Drapes: Laparotomy pack or basic pack
  Extra drape sheets
  Transverse fenestrated sheet (opt.)
  Plastic incise drape sheet (opt.)
Instrumentation:
  Chest tray
  Specialty tray (for specific procedure)
Supplies/Equipment:
  Positioning aids (e.g., Vac-Pack; sandbags)
  Basin set
  ESU suction
  Blades—(2) No. 10
  Needle counter
  Asepto syringe (2)
  Chest tubes and drainage unit (e.g., Pleurovac; Argyle chest tubes)
  Solutions—saline, water
  Sutures—surgeon's preference
  Bone wax

PROCEDURAL OVERVIEW—
Posterolateral Approach

Opening Sequence
The skin is incised and the subcutaneous tissue and muscle layers are divided. The appropriate intercostal space is identified and an incision is made and extended. If a rib is removed, the surgeon will incise the periosteum along its anterior surface. A periosteal elevator is used to free the periosteum from the bone, and the rib is severed from its attachment to the spine and sternum with rib shears. Sharp edges are trimmed to prevent possible trauma to underlying tissue. Lap sponges or towels are placed along the edges of the bone structure, and an appropriate-size self-retaining retractor is inserted between the ribs. The chest is now open for examination and specific surgical intervention.

Closing Sequence
Following the completion of the specific surgical procedure, and after chest tubes have been inserted (if required), pericostal sutures are placed around the two rib surfaces to hold them together. A rib approximator is used to bring the ribs tightly together, and the pericostal sutures are tied securely. The periosteum between the two ribs is closed and various muscle layers are approximated individually using a running suture. Hemostasis is achieved and the wound is closed according to the surgeon's preference. The chest tube(s) is connected to a sealed drainage unit.

PERIOPERATIVE NURSING CONSIDERATIONS

- The chest drainage unit is passed off the sterile field to the circulating nurse. If water is used, the water chamber is filled to the appropriate level and suction is applied to activate the unit, unless otherwise directed by the surgeon.
- All connections are secured to avoid the possibility of disconnection during transport. The chest drainage system must never be elevated higher than the chest to avoid backflow of water or blood into the pleural space.
- A portable chest x-ray should be taken postoperatively to assess correct tube placement.
- Refer to specific procedures for additional nursing considerations.

Procedure
Segmental Resection of the Lung

Definition: Excision of a section of a lobe of the lung that contains the diseased or suspected tissue.
CDC Classification: II
Special Technique: No-touch technique
Discussion: Indications for this procedure include bronchiectasis, cysts, benign or metastatic tumors, and tuberculosis.
Positioning: Lateral, with affected side up. The arm on the unaffected side is on an armboard; the arm on the affected side is placed on a padded Mayo tray or overhead arm holder attachment.
Skin Preparation: See pp. 337–338
Packs/Drapes: Laparotomy pack with transverse fenestrated sheet
  Plastic adhesive incise drape (opt.)
Instrumentation:
  Major laparotomy tray
  Chest tray
  Vascular tray (opt.)
  Internal stapling device (opt.)
  Hemoclips/surgiclips
Supplies/Equipment:
  Basin set
  ESU/suction
  Needle counter
  Blades—(3) No. 10, (1) No. 15

Dissector sponges (e.g., Kittners)
Asepto syringe
Vessel loops
Umbilical tape
Bone wax
Solutions—saline, water
Sutures—surgeon's preference
Chest tubes
Chest drainage unit

PROCEDURAL OVERVIEW

The affected lung is exposed through a posterolateral thoracotomy incision. The diseased segment is identified. The visceral pleura is dissected free from blood vessels and bronchi of the appropriate bronchopulmonic segment. Segmental branches of the pulmonary vein and artery are ligated; segmental bronchus is isolated, double clamped, and transected. The bronchial stump is stapled or sutured, and the suture/staple line is tested for air leaks. The wound is irrigated, hemostasis is verified, and chest tubes are inserted. The wound is closed, and the chest tube is connected to a sealed drainage unit.

PERIOPERATIVE NURSING CONSIDERATIONS

- Have all the patient's chest x-rays in the room.
- Set up the chest drainage system according to instructions and preference of surgeon (gravity/suction).
- Instruments contacting the bronchus are isolated and not returned to the field (no-touch technique).
- See Thoracotomy procedure (p. 564) for additional information.

Related Procedure: Wedge Resection of the Lung (excision of a small wedge-shaped section from the periphery of the lung)

Procedure
Lobectomy

Definition: Excision of one or more lobes of the lung.
CDC Classification: II
Special Technique: No-touch technique
Discussion: This procedure is usually performed when the lesion is limited to a lobe.
Positioning, Skin Preparation, Packs, Drapes, Instrumentation, Supplies, Equipment: See Segmental Resection of the Lung, p. 564

PROCEDURAL OVERVIEW

The affected lung is exposed through a posterolateral thoracotomy incision. The diseased lobe is identified,

and the visceral pleura dissected free from the hilus. The affected pulmonary artery and vein are ligated and divided. The bronchus is isolated, double-clamped, and transected; the bronchial stump is stapled/sutured closed. The suture/staple line is tested for air leaks. The pleural cavity is irrigated; hemostasis is confirmed. Chest tubes are inserted and the chest is closed in layers. The chest tubes are connected to a sealed chest drainage unit.

PERIOPERATIVE NURSING CONSIDERATIONS

- See Segmental Resection of the Lung, p. 564.

Procedure
Pneumonectomy

Definition: Removal of an entire lung.
CDC Classification: II, unless infection is present
Special Technique: No-touch technique
Discussion: The primary reason for performing a pneumonectomy is bronchogenic carcinoma. Additionally, some benign tumors, bronchiectasis, multiple lung abscess, and extensive unilateral tuberculosis may also be indications for this procedure. Since the affected pleural cavity will be empty following the procedure, special measures may need to be taken to stabilize the mediastinum and prevent central circulatory compromise resulting from a mediastinal shift.

The insertion of a chest tube is not required postoperatively as the entire lung has been removed, making the possibility of a pneumothorax nonexistent.
Positioning, Skin Preparation, Packs, Drapes, Instrumentation, Supplies, Equipment: See Segmental Resection of the Lung, p. 564.

PROCEDURAL OVERVIEW

The affected lung is exposed through a posterolateral thoracotomy incision. The chest is explored, and the feasibility of the procedure is determined, since advanced metastasis is a contraindication for the proposed procedure. If this is found, chest tubes are inserted, the wound is closed, and the chest tubes are connected to a sealed drainage unit.

If the surgeon proceeds with the procedure, the mediastinal pleura is dissected free. The bronchus, pulmonary artery, and superior and inferior pulmonary veins are isolated. The pulmonary artery and veins are ligated and the bronchial stump is double-clamped, transected and stapled/sutured closed.* Lymph node-

---

* Pleural space is flooded with normal saline to check for air leaks on inspiration.

bearing tissue is excised as necessary. Hemostasis is achieved, and the chest is closed in interrupted layers.

PERIOPERATIVE NURSING CONSIDERATIONS

- A chest tube may be inserted to assist with stabilization of the mediastinum by creating slight negative pressure in the affected pleural space.
- See Segmental Resection of the Lung (p. 564) for additional considerations.

Procedure
Decortication of the Lung

Definition: The stripping of a restrictive membrane on the visceral and parietal pleura that interferes with respirations.
CDC Classification: II, if no infection is present
Discussion: Indications for this procedure include chronic empyema, clotted hemothorax, and tuberculosis.
Positioning, Skin Preparation, Packs, Drapes, Instrumentation, Supplies, Equipment: See Segmental Resection of the Lung, p. 564.

PROCEDURAL OVERVIEW

The affected lung is exposed through a posterolateral thoracotomy incision. Rib resection may be necessary for adequate exposure. The fibrous membrane is carefully pulled away from the visceral pleura. Hemostasis is achieved and chest tubes are inserted. The wound is closed in layers and the chest tubes are connected to a sealed drainage unit.

PERIOPERATIVE NURSING CONSIDERATIONS

- See Segmental Resection of the Lung, p. 564.

PERIPHERAL VASCULAR PROCEDURES

Peripheral vascular procedures encompass procedures of the *arteries* and *veins*, excluding those in or near the heart. In many instances, the diseased vessel is completely bypassed with a synthetic or biologic vascular graft, depending on the location of the diseased vessel and the availability of an appropriate graft.

An alternative to *bypass surgery* involves the opening of a vessel and the removal of diseased tissue (*plaque*) within a vessel (*endarterectomy*).

Diagnostic Procedures

Peripheral arterial and vascular structures are assessed using two techniques: noninvasive and invasive.

Invasive Techniques

Selective *arteriography* allows the study of a specific arterial network or artery of the aorta. The use of dye injected into a vessel permits visualization of the vessel to determine the exact cause of the disease and the possible treatment that may follow. *Aortography* is a radiologic visualization of the aorta using a radiopaque substance.

A *venogram* uses the same principle as arteriography, but is used to visualize the veins and the venous network. Since these procedures are invasive, they may require special permits signed by the patient before the procedure.

In addition, selective angiography can be performed intraoperatively, to confirm the patency of a repaired vessel and/or graft.

Noninvasive Studies

A *Doppler ultrasound detection device* is applied to the skin surface to determine segmental arterial pressures and venous patency in the extremities.

It is not unusual, during either the intraoperative or postoperative phase, to test the patency of these vessels using the Doppler. A special electrode can be sterilized for use during a surgical procedure, while postoperatively, the nonsterile electrode is used to confirm peripheral pulses following reconstruction of a vessel (e.g., femoral-popliteal bypass).

General Considerations

Arterial Vascular Grafts

Prosthetic grafts are divided into two groups—synthetic and biologic—depending on their composition.

Synthetic grafts are tubular structures designed to replace or *bypass* diseased vessels. They are available in a variety of sizes (lengths and diameters) (e.g., 14–22 mm for abdominal procedures and 4–10 mm for the extremities), shapes (straight and bifurcates), and materials (knitted and woven).

Knitted polyester (Dacron) grafts are porous and softer than woven grafts, and are usually preferred for small-vessel anastomosis. Some knitted grafts require a *preclotting* process—that is, the graft is soaked in the patient's own blood before insertion, in order to make the walls of the graft impervious to blood by filling in the spaces with fibrin.

Knitted velour grafts have a uniform porosity for easy preclotting, and may be preferred by the surgeon, depending on the location requiring repair.

Woven polyester is a tight, leak-proof graft that does not require preclotting before insertion. Because such grafts are more flexible in construction, their use is limited to aortic replacement or bypass of large-caliber arteries.

Polytetrafluoroethylene (PTFE) is a microporous material that serves as an open framework (lattice) into which cells grow to become a surface for contact with blood. Like the woven graft, PTFE grafts do not require preclotting, and are usually used for small and/or medium-size vessels.

Biologic vascular grafts may be *autografts, allografts, homografts,* or *heterografts,* and can be used for both arterial and venous grafting. These grafts include saphenous vein (autograft); venous allograft (from a donor); modified human umbilical vein grafts (homograft); and bovine (carotid and aortic) arterografts (for shunts and fistulas).

Vascular Shunts/Fistulas

A prosthetic vascular shunt may be inserted to establish an external route for the diversion of blood flow through a mechanical device. An alternative to vascular shunting by a prosthetic device is the creation of an artificial *arteriovenous fistula,* between an artery and a vein for extracorporeal dialysis via the artificial kidney machine. The creation of a fistula is usually preferred over shunting because there is less chance of complications (e.g., thrombosis, infection), since the fistula is created internally.

Fogerty Catheters

Fogerty catheters are used to restore blood flow to an artery or vein by inserting the catheter into the lumen of the vessel and either (1) inflating a balloon at the tip and withdrawing the embolic material (*embolectomy catheter*), or (2) irrigating the vessel with an open-tipped catheter that has a small syringe attached to the distal opening, usually filled with heparinized saline (*irrigation catheter*).

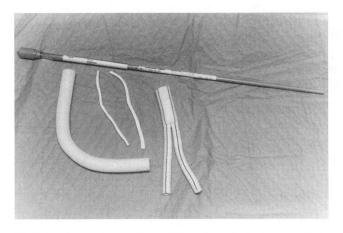

Variety of vascular grafts and Fogerty embolectomy catheter

Anticoagulant Therapy

Anticoagulant therapy has a vital role in maintaining adequate blood flow throughout the cardiovascular system. The anticoagulant used almost exclusively is sodium heparin, which prevents clot formation.

The medication may be administered systemically via the IV route, by the anesthesiologist, or it may be added to irrigation solution to be used by the surgical team during the procedure. Systemically, the dose is calculated according to the patient's *kilogram* body weight. For irrigation, the amount of heparin will be specified by the surgeon (usually 250 ml or 500 ml of IV normal saline), depending on the dilution preference.

Selected Surgical Procedures

Bypass Surgery

Bypass surgery involves the establishment of a detour around or in place of a blockage using a *bypass graft,* either synthetic or biologic, as previously discussed. The use of an *autograft,* such as the saphenous vein, is preferable, but may not be practical, depending on the anatomy involved.

Most bypass procedures closely resemble each other, except for their differences in location and choice of material. Once the basic technique, equipment, and supplies have been learned, these principles can be applied to other procedures involving the insertion and *anastomosis* of a graft.

Procedure
Femoral–Popliteal Bypass

Definition: The implantation of an artificial or autogenous graft from the common femoral artery to the popliteal artery.
CDC Classification: I
Discussion: The procedure is indicated for the treatment of occlusive atherosclerotic disease. Patency of the popliteal artery should be well established by arteriography prior to surgery.
Positioning: Supine, with the affected leg externally rotated and abducted and knee slightly bent
Skin Preparation: See pp. 337–338
Packs/Drapes: Laparotomy pack
   Extra drape sheets
   Adhesive incise drape (opt.)
   Towels (fashioned in a boot around the foot)
Instrumentation:
   Minor procedure tray
   Vascular procedure tray

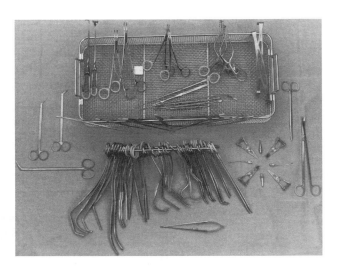

Peripheral vascular instrument

Hemoclips/surgiclips
Tunneling instruments
Supplies/Equipment:
Leg holder (for prep) (opt.)
ESU/suction (Frazier tips; extra)
Basin set
Blades—(2) No. 10, (1) No. 15, (1) No. 11
Umbilical tape
Penrose drain
Vessel loops
Medication—heparinized saline solution, antibiotics, hemostatic agents
Needle counter
Dissector sponges (e.g., Kittner)
Graft (if autograft not used)
Suture—surgeon's preference
Solution—saline, water

PROCEDURAL OVERVIEW

The groin area is incised and the incision deepened to the femoral artery. A self-retaining retractor (e.g., Weitlander; Gelpi) is placed in the wound.

The femoral artery is mobilized; a moist umbilical tape is placed around the artery (for traction). A second incision is made on the medial side of the knee. The subcutaneous, fascial, and muscle layers are dissected. A tunneling instrument is used to make a passage from the femoral triangle to the popliteal space.

The saphenous vein is harvested (unless contraindicated), dividing and ligating its multiple branches. The harvested segment is flushed with heparinized saline solution, placed in a basin, and covered with a moist sponge. If the saphenous vein cannot be used, an appropriate-size graft is chosen by the surgeon, and if the graft requires preclotting, it is performed at this time.

The Anastomosis

To perform the anastomosis, a vascular clamp is placed across the femoral artery, and a small incision (*arteriotomy*) is made (No. 11 blade or vascular scissors). The vein or graft is sutured to the common femoral artery, making certain that the distal portion of the vein is used—that is, a reversed anatomic position. An endarterectomy and patch angioplasty may be performed at the origin of the deep femoral artery. The vein/graft is passed through the tunnel and anastomosed to the popliteal artery. Before placing the final sutures, the vein/graft is flushed with blood, and an intraoperative angiogram may be performed to determine patency (Fig. 14-23A).

After the x-rays have been taken, the anastomosis is completed, and hemostasis is achieved. The wound is irrigated with plain saline, and the incisions are closed.

PERIOPERATIVE NURSING CONSIDERATIONS

- Have the patient's x-ray films, including angiographic studies, in the room.
- If a prosthetic graft is used, confirm the size, type, and preparation with the surgeon.
- If intraoperative angiography is performed, radiologic precautions must be observed (see p. 360).
- A Doppler will be needed postoperatively to confirm patency via pedal pulses.

Related Procedures:
Femoral Crossover
Axillary–Femoral/Autobifemoral Bypass

Procedure
Abdominal Aortic Aneurysmectomy

Definition: An excision and/or internal bypass of an aneurysm on the wall of the abdominal aorta that requires the insertion of a prosthetic graft to reestablish vascular continuity.
CDC Classification: I, unless traumatically induced
Discussion: An *aneurysm* is a sac-like bulging or weakening in the wall of an artery, which may be the result of arterosclerotic disease, trauma, infection, or a congenital defect in the artery. Aortic aneurysm surgery is usually performed as an elective procedure; however, should the aneurysm begin to dissect (blood flows around the vessel instead of through the lumen), or if it ruptures, a life-threatening situation occurs, which requires **immediate** surgical intervention.
Positioning: Supine, with arms extended on armboards

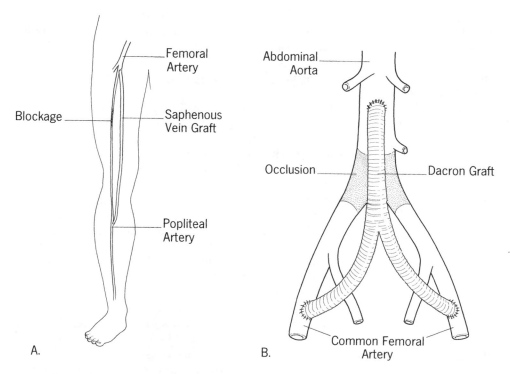

Fig. 14-23. Restorative procedures. (A) Femoral-popliteal bypass; (B) aorto bi-femoral bypass (Adapted from Linton, R. *Atlas of Vascular Surgery.* Philadelphia: WB Saunders, 1973.)

Skin Preparation: See pp. 337–338. If dissecting, the scrub sequence may be eliminated and only the antimicrobial solution applied

Packs/Drapes: Universal pack or
  CV pack/laparotomy pack
  Plastic adherent incise drape (plain/Ioban)

Instrumentation:
  Major procedure tray
  Major CV tray
  Hemoclips/surgiclips
  Harrington/Weitlander retractors

Supplies/Equipment:
  Basin set
  ESU/suction (2)
  Headlight
  Fiberoptic light source (opt.)
  Blades—(2) No. 10, (1) No. 15, (1) No. 11
  Foley catheter with urimeter
  Thermal blanket with control unit
  Needle counter
  Penrose drain
  Umbilical tape
  Vessel loops
  Dissector sponges (e.g., Kittners)
  Medications—hemostatic agents, protamine sulfate, heparinized saline solution, antibiotics
  Graft—surgeon's preference

  Solutions—saline, water
  Sutures—surgeon's preference
  Disposable syringes (3)
  Cell saver (opt.)
  Hemodynamic monitoring lines (e.g., A-line; CVP; Swan–Ganz catheters) (anesthesia preference)

PROCEDURAL OVERVIEW

The patient is placed on a thermal blanket, and the hemodynamic lines are inserted.

The abdomen is entered in a routine fashion, and the incision extended to the peritoneal cavity. The intestines are mobilized, and either pushed out of the way or placed in a special intestinal pouch (with a small amount of saline in the pouch). The posterior peritoneum over the aneurysm is incised, and the aorta is exposed, taking care to protect the inferior vena cava and uterus. Following systemic heparinization by the anesthesiologist, the surgeon is ready to incise the aneurysm.

The aorta is cross-clamped with a large atraumatic vascular clamp (e.g., Statinsky; Crafoord); the anesthesiologist is notified at the time of crossclamp. The aneurysm is opened, and the clot is evacuated. If the aneurysm sac is almost completely filled with *plaque,* it may be removed manually and passed off with the clot as specimen.

The anterior portion of the sac is removed; the back (posterior) side of the aneurysm is left intact (to prevent injury to the vena cava, which may be attached to the aorta).

The graft is prepared according to the surgeon's and/or manufacturer's instructions. The aorta is connected to the iliac or femoral vessels, chosen according to their degree of patency. Using a running suture (3-0 vascular suture), the upper end of the graft is secured to the aorta. When this anastomosis is complete, the iliac/femoral arteries are anastomosed to the bifurcated ends of the graft (Fig. 14-23B).

During the anastomoses, the wound is irrigated frequently with heparinized saline solution. To test the suture lines and evacuate clots, the vascular clamps are slowly released periodically. When bleeding is controlled, the wound is irrigated with plain saline and closed in a routine fashion.

PERIOPERATIVE NURSING CONSIDERATIONS

- Have the patient's x-rays in the room.
- Verify the type and size of the graft with the surgeon.
- Have a variety of Fogerty catheters (embolectomy and irrigation) available.
- The skin prep should be performed gently, to lessen the possibility of rupture. If emergent, speed is essential while maintaining aseptic principles.
- Verify with the blood bank the number of available units.
- Monitor urinary output.
- Maintain accurate account of irrigation solution used and blood loss.
- Be available to assist with insertion of hemodynamic monitoring lines.
- Verify possible usage of cell-saver unit.
- Moistened umbilical tape and vessel loops should be passed on a clamp (e.g., tonsil; right angle).

Embolectomy/Endarterectomy Procedures

Procedure
Arterial Embolectomy

Definition: An incision into the affected artery to facilitate removal of a plaque (debris) from the vessel wall.
CDC Classification: I
Discussion: An *embolus* may be caused by a foreign body, tumor, or traumatic injury to a vessel. The goal of this surgery is to remove the clot and restore the circulation to the limb. The most common site for an embolus is in the femoral or popliteal arteries.

Positioning, Skin Preparation, Packs, Drapes, Instrumentation, Supplies, Equipment: See Femoral–Popliteal Bypass, pp. 567–568

PROCEDURAL OVERVIEW

The appropriate incision is made and carried deeper with cautery or sharp dissection. Two self-retaining retractors (e.g., Gelpi; Weitlander) are placed in the wound. The affected artery is identified and mobilized. A moistened umbilical tape is placed around the artery for traction. A small vascular clamp is placed on the artery, and a small incision is made into the vessel.

A common method of embolectomy uses a Fogerty embolectomy catheter with a balloon at its tip. The catheter is threaded into the incision and advanced beyond the clot. The balloon is inflated with a tuberculin syringe, and the catheter is withdrawn. The balloon forces the clot from the artery, which is immediately clamped to prevent the backflow of blood. If the artery must be dilated, vascular dilators will be needed.

When the embolectomy is complete, the wound is irrigated with heparinized saline, hemostasis is achieved, and the arterial incision is closed. The wound is irrigated with plain saline, and closed in layers in a routine fashion.

PERIOPERATIVE NURSING CONSIDERATIONS

- See Femoral–Popliteal Bypass, p. 567

Procedure
Arterial Endarterectomy

Definition: Excision of an arteriosclerotic plaque from an obstructed artery.
CDC Classification: I
Discussion: The procedure is performed to restore arterial blood flow, thereby enhancing systemic circulation. There are several sites in the body where arteriosclerotic plaques commonly form. These are usually just above and below the bifurcation of a major artery.

A carotid endarterectomy will be outlined to illustrate this group of procedures.
Positioning: Supine, with head slightly extended and turned toward the opposite side. The head may be supported on a doughnut or small pillow, with a rolled towel placed between the scapula.
Skin Preparation: See pp. 337–338
Packs/Drapes: Laparotomy pack or basic pack with split sheet
  Towels
Instrumentation:
  Minor procedure tray

Small vascular instrument set or fistula/shunt tray
Hemoclips/surgiclips
Supplies/Equipment:
Basin set
ESU/suction (bipolar cautery may be used)
Blades—(2) No. 10, (1) No. 15, (1) No. 11
Umbilical tape
Vessel loops
Dissector sponges (e.g., Kittners)
Disposable syringes
Medications—hemostatic agents, antibiotics
Solutions—saline, water, heparinized saline
Sutures—surgeon's preference
Shunt (e.g., Javid) (opt.)

PROCEDURAL OVERVIEW

An incision is made along the anterior border of the sternomastoid muscle, exposing the carotid sheath, which is then incised. Small dissector sponges are used to divide the tissue so as not to damage the cranial nerve branches.

The carotid artery and both branches are mobilized with fine vascular tissue forceps and fine scissors. A moist umbilical tape is placed around the vessel; the two ends are clamped together.

If used, a prosthetic internal shunt is prepared at this time, allowing the blood to continue circulating during the procedure. Before making the arterial incisions, heparin is given intravenously to the patient by the anesthesiologist. As the team waits for the heparin to circulate, the scrub person should make sure that all instruments and equipment are properly prepared, since timing is often critical once the procedure begins.

To begin the endarterectomy, the artery is clamped above and below the bifurcation; the anesthesiologist is notified when the clamps are applied. An arteriotomy is performed (No. 11 blade; Potts scissors). A prosthetic intraluminal shunt from the common carotid artery to the internal carotid artery may be inserted and secured with sutures or shunt clamps.

The arterial plaque is identified, and grasped with a straight clamp; the plaque is dissected from the artery and passed off as a specimen.

Prior to placement of the final sutures, the shunt, if used, is removed, and the lumen is flushed with heparinized saline to remove any residual debris or air bubbles. The arterial incision is closed and the wound is irrigated with plain saline and closed.

PERIOPERATIVE NURSING CONSIDERATIONS

• See Femoral–Popliteal Bypass, p. 567.

Related Procedures: Aortoiliac
Femoral Endarterectomy

Vascular Access Procedures

Vascular access procedures are indicated when an artificial access to the circulatory system is required. This may be accomplished by the creation of a fistula or shunt or by the insertion of a multilumen catheter for the purpose of long-term nutritional support and/or the administration of medications.

Procedure
Arteriovenous Shunt/Fistula

Definition: The establishment of a communicating prosthetic loop (*shunt*) or a direct anastomosis between an artery and a vein (*fistula*).
CDC Classification: I
Discussion: Several techniques may be used to create a communication between an artery and a vein, including a buried synthetic prosthesis, a natural anastomosis, or an external prosthesis (the least frequently used). The most common site for the anastomosis is usually the *radial artery* and the *cephalic vein* of the proximal forearm; however, the lower extremity can be used if previous surgery eliminates the use of the forearm.
Positioning: Supine, with the nondominant arm extended on a hand table; the other arm may be placed on an armboard
Skin Preparation: See pp. 337–338
Packs/Drapes: Impervious stockinette
Laparotomy pack or extremity pack
Extra drape sheets
Instrumentation:
Shunt/fistula tray
Coronary artery dilators
Supplies/Equipment:
Basin set
ESU/suction
Magnifying loops (opt.)
Needle counter
Blades—(1) No. 10, (1) No. 15, (1) No. 11
Solutions—saline, water, heparinized saline
Sutures—surgeon's preference
Synthetic/biologic prosthesis (for shunt)

PROCEDURAL OVERVIEW

The appropriate incision is made over the selected arterial and venous site on the forearm. Vascular clamps or bulldog clamps are used to control the vessels. An incision is made into the lumen of the artery, which may be dilated with coronary dilators. The venous side is ligated distally.

If a shunt is used, the shunt is anastomosed to the artery and the vein. Heparinized saline is instilled into the graft. If a fistula is created, the selected artery is anastomosed to an adjacent vein. The wound is irrigated and closed and a protective dressing is applied.

PERIOPERATIVE NURSING CONSIDERATIONS

- The procedure is usually performed under local anesthesia or local with monitored anesthesia care.
- Before and during the prepping procedure, the extremity should be elevated. The full hand should be part of the prep.
- If an external shunt is used, two shunt clamps are to be attached to the gauze dressing. Should the connector become separated from the cannula, both ends must be clamped immediately.

Procedure
Insertion of Venous Access Catheter

Definition: Placement of an indwelling catheter into the superior vena cava or right atrium for longterm therapy.

CDC Classification: I

Discussion: The Broviac, Hickman, or Groshong catheter is primarily used for total parenteral nutrition, using the cephalic vein or external jugular vein. The procedure is usually done under local anesthesia and fluoroscopy. The procedure can be accomplished by a cutdown or percutaneous approach.

Positioning: Supine, with arms extended on armboards

Skin Preparation: See pp. 337–338

Packs, Drapes, Instrumentation, Supplies, Equipment: See A-V Fistula/Shunt, p. 571

PROCEDURAL OVERVIEW

1. Local anesthesia is injected into the selected area.
2. An appropriate incision is performed (cutdown), and the vein is identified and isolated.
3. A tunnel is made subcutaneously from the cutdown site to the identified exit site of the catheter (usually medial to the breast). A small incision is made over the exit site.
4. The catheter is introduced into the exit site and advanced through the tunnel to the cutdown incision. The catheter is filled with heparinized saline.
5. The vein is distally ligated and a venotomy is made; the catheter is introduced into the vein and advanced into the SVC. The catheter is aspirated, and should reveal dark blood (venous). An x-ray is taken to confirm proper placement.
6. The incisions are closed, and a dressing applied. The catheter is taped to the chest.

PERIOPERATIVE NURSING CONSIDERATIONS

- Confirm with the surgeon the type and length of the catheter to be used.
- Observe all radiologic precautions during the procedure.
- An instrument count is not required; however, sponges and sharps are to be counted according to protocol.
- Procedure can also be accomplished through percutaneous approach.

THE HEART AND GREAT VESSELS

Delicate, yet durable, this eleven ounce pump sustains the body's 60,000 mile cardiovascular system.

G.P. Davis (1967)

Cardiac surgery involves the heart and associated great vessels. Surgery performed to correct congenital malformations and acquired heart disease is discussed in this section.

Diagnostic Procedures

Cardiac surgery is preceded by an extensive cardiovascular assessment utilizing both *noninvasive* and *invasive* studies that can assist in determining the proper course of treatment.

Noninvasive Studies

Routine examinations and electrocardiography are just two of the noninvasive studies that can be used to assess the heart and its function. Other studies, including *echocardiography, pulmonary function studies, computed axial tomography,* and *radionuclide imaging (MUGA scan),* are used to determine the type and extent of the damage or deficit, in addition to measuring myocardial blood flow, which can aide in diagnosing a myocardial infarction.

Invasive Studies

Invasive studies consist of *angiography,* as previously described, and cardiac catheterization.

Cardiac Catheterization *Angiocardiography* is the most efficient diagnostic tool that can provide extensive information regarding the heart's anatomical structure and its functional capabilities.

Cardiac catheterization procedures can reveal the pressures in the heart's chambers and associated vessels, determine the oxygenation saturation and cardiac output, and calibrate the injection fraction of

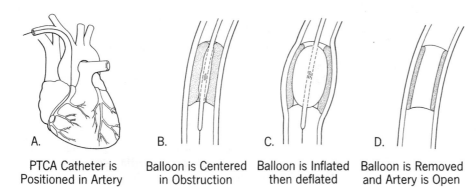

A.	B.	C.	D.
PTCA Catheter is Positioned in Artery	Balloon is Centered in Obstruction	Balloon is Inflated then deflated	Balloon is Removed and Artery is Open

Fig. 14-24. Percutaneous transluminal angioplasty

the major arteries that sustain the heart's functional capabilities.

Additionally, it can be used to visualize and diagnose coronary artery disease, valvular heart disease, or congenital anomalies, as well as determine the extent of ischemic heart disease in selective arteries by providing values related to cardiac output, cardiac index, preload and afterload, contractility, and ejection fraction.

The cardiac catheterization suite has also become the site for new, aggressive therapies, including *percutaneous transluminal coronary angioplasty* (*PTCA*).

Percutaneous Transluminal Coronary Angioplasty (PTCA) (Fig. 14-24) Depending on the extent of the severity involving a coronary artery, and the location of the obstruction, an alternative treatment that, if successful, will not require open heart surgery is a procedure referred to as PTCA (see Fig. 14-24). The procedure is performed in the cardiac catheterization laboratory, under fluoroscopy, and involves the insertion of a specially designed balloon-tipped catheter into the affected artery. The balloon is inflated, compressing the obstructing plaque against the wall of the artery and opening the vessel so that normal blood flow can be reestablished. Since the procedure is not without risk, including arterial spasms and severe arrhythmias, the patient is prepared preoperatively for possible surgical intervention should open heart surgery become necessary.

During the procedure, the cardiac surgery team remains on stand-by, to avoid losing time initiating the corrective surgical procedure if cardiac damage occurs.

General Considerations

The principles of thoracic and peripheral vascular surgery are closely associated with cardiac surgery; with additional features exclusive to this specialty.

Surgical Approach

For procedures involving the thoracic aorta or pulmonary vessels, a posterolateral thoracotomy is usually preferred (see p. 562). For procedures directly involving cardiac structures (e.g., valve replacement, coronary artery surgery), a median sternotomy incision is preferred.

Procedure
Median Sternotomy Approach

Definition: An incision of the chest, at the midline, through the sternum. This approach provides access to the organs in the mediastinal cavity, particularly the heart. It is the most common incision used for cardiac surgery procedures.

PROCEDURAL OVERVIEW

Opening Sequence
A midline incision is made from the level of the sternal notch to approximately 2 to 3 inches below the xyphoid. The subcutaneous and fascial layers are divided. The underlying tissue is separated from the sternal notch and the xyphoid using blunt dissection, and the xyphoid is divided in the center with a curved Mayo scissors. A sternal saw blade (knife) is placed in the center of the divided xyphoid (or sternal notch), and the sternum is divided in half.

The cut edges of the sternum are elevated, and hemostasis is controlled by applying bone wax to the marrow and cauterizing the periosteum and subcutaneous tissue layers.

The edges of the sternum are covered with sterile towels or laparotomy pads to protect the bone marrow, and a chest retractor (e.g., Himmelstein or Ankeney sternal retractor) is inserted and slowly opened to expose the subcutaneous tissue. The subcutaneous layer is divided with sharp dissection, elevating the tissue with a smooth tissue forceps or special clamp (e.g., Schnidt) to prevent injury to the heart. The pericardium is incised, extending the incision to expose the heart and aorta. Silk traction sutures may be placed through the edges of the pericardium and the aorta may be encircled with a moistened umbilical tape. The heart and aorta are then *cannulated*, according to the surgeon's preference, in preparation for *cardiopulmonary bypass.*

Closing Sequence
Upon completion of the specific procedure, hemostasis is achieved and chest tubes are inserted. The sternum will be closed with six to eight wire sutures (No. 5) through each sternal edge (through-and-through). As the needles are brought through, a wire cutter is used to cut the needle off, and clamps are placed on the end of each wire. Care must be taken not to allow the wire suture to kink, as this could be a cause for infection in the sternum. The sternal edges are approximated by tightening the wires, then twisting each wire together until it is snug against the sternum. The wires are further tightened with a wire twister, and the ends are bent over, to be buried in the periosteum.

The fascial and periosteal layers are approximated with interrupted suture (2-0 silk), or a running suture (0-prolene or chromic). The subcutaneous tissue and skin are closed in the surgeon's preferred manner.

Positioning
For a median sternotomy, the patient is placed in the supine position, on a thermal blanket. For coronary artery surgery, a small wedge or pillow is placed under the knees to maintain slight flexion. This will provide access to the proximal greater saphenous vein. After the hemodynamic monitoring lines (e.g., Swan, A-Line; CVP) have been inserted and secured, the arms are padded and tucked at the patient's side. A special Foley catheter (with a thermistor probe) is inserted and attached to a urimeter. The thermistor probe will be connected to the heart–lung machine for continuous monitoring of internal body temperature. The dispersive electrode is placed either on the posterior side of the thigh or on the buttocks. The positioning for a thoracotomy was discussed earlier in this unit.

PERIOPERATIVE NURSING CONSIDERATIONS
- Assemble the sealed chest drainage unit and attach to suction as directed. Two chest tubes with a Y-connector are generally used. Should a mediastinal tube be used, a sealed underwater drainage unit may not be required since the tube does not lie in the pleural cavity.
- When working with wire sutures, a clamp should be placed on the free end, and the needle holder is passed to the surgeon, while the clamped end is passed to the assistant. In this way, kinks are avoided as in accidental contamination of the wire end.
- An additional closing count is required when the pericardial cavity has been entered.

Special Equipment

In addition to the special supplies and equipment mentioned earlier in this chapter, cardiac surgery procedures require the use of hemodynamic monitoring equipment (see Chap. 7, p. 127), and the use of extracorporeal perfusion, or cardiopulmonary bypass.

Extracorporeal Perfusion

Extracorporeal perfusion via the heart–lung machine was first introduced by John Gibbons in 1953, as a means to divert the patient's blood to an artificial lung, where it could be oxygenated, and then returned to the patient, during the repair of intracardiac structures (Fig. 14-25).

Before the heart–lung machine was developed, all intracardiac procedures had to be guided by the sense of touch, unaided by direct vision, and performed under prolonged total body hypothermia. The perfusion machine made it possible to operate under direct vision, since the majority of blood within the heart had been removed and recirculated through an extracorporeal circulatory network.

Today, *cardiopulmonary bypass*, as it is frequently called, has a major role in cardiac surgery, allowing the surgeon to perform the repair without depriving the body tissues and the brain of oxygenated blood for any period of time.

Major Principles   During cardiopulmonary bypass, all venous blood ordinarily returning to the right atrium is diverted to an outside circuit. It is then passed through an artificial lung, where it takes up oxygen and gives off carbon dioxide. After passing through the artificial lung, the refreshed blood is pumped into the patient's arterial system. Thus, the heart and lungs contain no blood, except for that small quantity which enters the pulmonary vessels from the bronchial arteries. When the heart is opened, this blood is gently but continuously aspirated and returned along with venous blood to the heart–lung machine.

Cannulation Techniques   There are several anatomic sites at which cardiopulmonary bypass can be established, including the femoral vein, the inferior vena cava, and the right atrium. Blood is returned to the patient through the femoral artery, subclavian artery, or ascending aorta. The surgeon's preference, the nature of the surgery, and the condition of the vessels

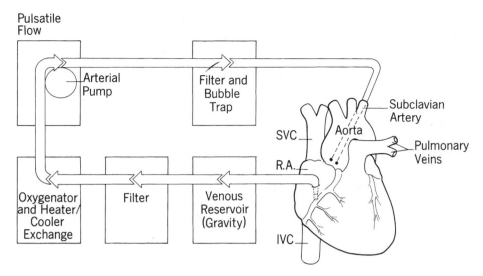

Fig. 14-25. Extracorporeal circulation principles

will determine the site chosen for each patient. For example, a common configuration is the cannulation of the right atrium by a multiholed cannula, the tip of which is inserted into the inferior vena cava. A cannula inserted into the ascending aorta returns the blood to the patient from the pump.

Prosthetic Heart Valves

The use of prosthetic heart valves to replace diseased ones has been available for nearly 40 years. Heart valves are available in two formats: *mechanical* and *bioprosthetic*

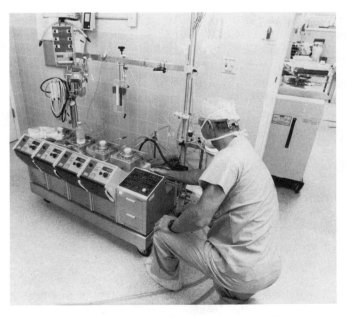

Cardiovascular perfusionist setting up heart and lung machine

(porcine). The early heart valves of the 1950s (Harkin; Starr) were made of a small metal or silicone ball that floated up and down inside a metal cage. A Teflon or Dacron skirt covered the metal ring to enable the surgeon to stitch the valve into the heart muscle. The 1960s produced other types of mechanical valves, such as the disk-and-cage valve, hinged valve, and sutureless valve, which was surrounded by tiny metal teeth that lodged directly in the heart tissue. Some mechanical valves can last for more than 20 years without needing replacement, but they can also cause blood clots, so long-term anticoagulant therapy is required. To circumvent this problem, the bioprosthetic heart valve (e.g., St. Jude; Edwards; Hancock) was designed, and for most younger patients it is the valve of choice. The most common criticism of tissue valves is their lack of long-term durability as compared with the mechanical heart valve. The choice of valves is based on the patient's physiologic condition and the surgeon's preference.

Profound Hypothermic Technique

First used for cardiac surgery in 1952, profound hypothermia reduces the patient's core temperature to as low as 27°C via the heart–lung machine, thereby reducing the metabolic needs for oxygenated blood in the tissues.

Local hypothermia is accomplished by the application of iced saline slush around the heart, and by using this solution for irrigation during the corrective phase of the procedure.

Once the repair has been completed, the patient is gradually rewarmed internally (heart–lung and irrigation) and externally by the activation of the thermal blanket under the patient.

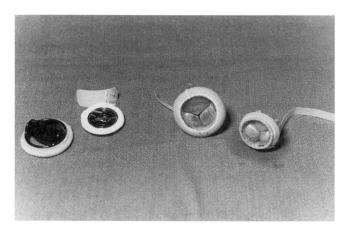

Prosthetic heart valve: mechanical and bioprosthetic models

Pharmacologic Agents

In addition to the pharmacologic agents mentioned earlier in this unit (anticoagulants, hemostatic agents, antibiotics, etc.), cardiac surgery requires the use of a specialized solution created to arrest the heart so that repairs can be performed. This solution is called *cardioplegic solution.*

Cardioplegic solution can be commercially manufactured or prepared by the hospital pharmacist, according to the surgeon's preference for specific ingredients. The solution is designed to arrest the heart during total bypass surgery. Cardioplegic solution usually contains such additives as potassium chloride, xylocaine, dextrose, insulin, albumin, tromethamine, plasmanate, or any other combinations, depending on the desired effect. The solution is administered "cold" (4°C–10°C), and can be administered either intravenously or through a special cannula via the heart–lung machine, allowing continuous infusion as needed

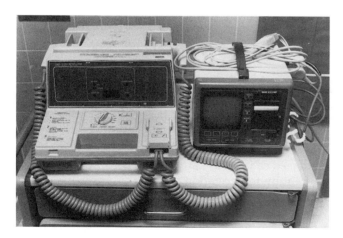

Defibrillator unit and portable monitor (internal and external defibrillator paddles)

throughout the procedure. (The latter is the preferred technique.) During this infusion period, the surgical repair is performed, and when completed, the infusion is stopped, allowing the heart to resume its normal pattern.

Emergency cardiac drugs should also be available in the procedure room, selected according to the preference of the department of anesthesia and/or the hospital pharmacy committee.

Internal Defibrillator Paddles

Defibrillator paddles must be kept readily available in the sterile field to convert the induced fibrillation to a normal sinus rhythm should the heart not convert on its own following the repair sequence. The perioperative nurse is responsible for managing this equipment, and should be thoroughly familiar with the required settings and proper operation of the unit.

Intraaortic Balloon Pump/Catheter

An increasingly performed adjunct to cardiac surgery involves the insertion of an intraaortic balloon catheter, which is generally used to increase coronary artery flow and to assist peripheral perfusion. The indication for the use of this device is usually following a myocardial infarction or cardiopulmonary bypass when left ventricular function is inadequate. After insertion of the balloon catheter, it is attached to an intraaortic balloon pump. The pumping action is coordinated with the patient's ECG so that the balloon inflates during diastole, thus improving oxygenation to the myocardium, increasing peripheral blood flow, and diminishing the workload of the heart. A critical care nurse, from the ICU/CCU area, or a cardiovascular technician from the cardiac cath laboratory is usually assigned to monitor and manage the pump during surgery; however, the perioperative nurse should be familiar with the general principles of how the equipment is used. The insertion of this specialized catheter can also be performed independent of cardiac surgery.

Selected Surgical Procedures

Procedures
Cardiac

Two representative cardiac procedures will be discussed in the section:

1. *Valvular Surgery:* The excision, replacement, and repair of the diseased mitral or aortic valve.
2. *Coronary Artery Bypass Surgery:* The grafting of either the internal mammary artery or segments

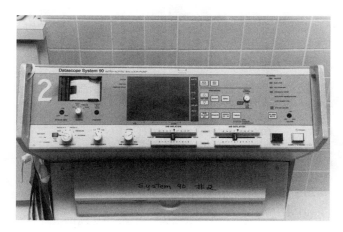

Intraaortic balloon pump (IABP) unit

of the greater saphenous vein to bypass coronary artery obstruction.

CDC Classification: I, if previous surgery has not been performed

Discussion: Intracardiac procedures will necessitate the use of cardiopulmonary bypass. To fully comprehend cardiac abnormalities and the function of extracorporeal perfusion, knowledge of the anatomy of the heart and the circulatory system is mandatory. The team concept is of utmost importance, since extra minutes are not often available, and seconds can save a life.

Incision Site/Positioning: See pp. 573–574

Skin Preparation: See pp. 337–338

Packs/Drapes:
   CV pack, universal pack, or custom CV pack
   Adhesive incise drape sheet (plain/Ioban)
   Extra drape sheets

Instrumentation:
   Cardiac procedure tray
   Sternal saw/cord
   Specialty tray (valve, coronary artery)
   Vein harvesting tray (opt.)
   Hemoclips/surgiclip applies

Supplies/Equipment:
   Thermal blanket with control unit
   Cardioverter with internal paddles
   Cell-saver unit
   Heart–lung machine
   Mayfield overhead table (opt.)
   Hemodynamic monitoring lines and transducer
   IABP machine with catheter (opt.)
   Basin set
   Large graduated pitcher (2)
   Blades—(2) No. 10, (2) No. 15, (2) No. 11
   Beaver blade
   Assorted syringes and needles

Asepto Syringes (2)
Foley catheter (thermistor probe) with urimeter
Medications—hemostatic agents, antibiotics
Solutions—saline, water, iced sterile saline slush, heparinized saline
Pacemaker wire with external pacemaker
Chest tube (2) with Y-connector
Sealed chest drainage unit with ATS attachment or capability (e.g., Pleurovac-ATS; atrium)

Note:

1. If a custom pack is used, some of the supplies may be incorporated in the pack.
2. Supplies needed for cardiopulmonary bypass will be assembled by the clinical perfusionist assigned to the case.

PROCEDURAL OVERVIEW

Aortic Valve Replacement (AVR)

The patient is properly positioned and a median sternotomy incision is performed in the routine manner. Cannulation for cardiopulmonary bypass is achieved. The aorta is occluded distal to the valve, and cardioplegia solution is infused through the aortic root into the coronary arteries. An aortotomy is performed, and the valve is excised and passed off as a specimen. The annulus is measured with valve sizers (specific to the selected prosthetic valve), and the appropriate valve is selected, inserted, and sutured into place. The aortotomy is closed. Air is vented from the left ventricle

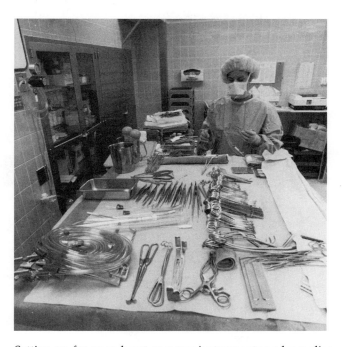

Setting up for open-heart surgery: instruments and supplies

and the aorta. The aorta is gradually unclamped and cardiopulmonary bypass is discontinued. The wound is irrigated with warm saline with or without antibiotics; temporary pacemaker electrodes are sutured to the heart. Chest tubes are inserted and the wound is closed in the routine manner. The chest tubes are connected to a sealed drainage unit and suction is applied.

Mitral Valve Replacement (MVR)

The patient is properly positioned and a median sternotomy incision is performed. Cannulation for cardiopulmonary bypass is achieved. The ascending aorta is occluded and cardioplegia solution is introduced through the aortic root to the coronary arteries. A left atriotomy is performed to expose the mitral valve. The valve is excised, and the annulus is measured with the appropriate valve sizer. The prosthesis is selected, inserted, and sutured in place. The aortic cross-clamp is gradually removed and air is aspirated from the aorta. Cardiopulmonary bypass is discontinued. The wound is irrigated; temporary pacemaker wires are sewn to the heart and chest tubes are inserted. The wound is closed in the routine manner. The chest tubes are connected to a sealed drainage unit.

Alternative Procedures

1. *Mitral Commissurotomy:* May be performed instead of valve replacement to alleviate the stenosis. The valve cups are separated by incising between them with a knife blade or breaking them apart with a mitral valve dilator (e.g., Gertode; Tubbs).
2. *Mitral Annuloplasty:* An insufficient mitral valve may require only that sutures be taken in the annulus to allow the valve leaflets to come together more efficiently.

Both alternative procedures are initially performed in a manner similar to that for mitral valve replacement.

Coronary Artery Bypass Graft (CABG)

The patient is properly positioned, and a median sternotomy incision is performed. The internal mammary artery and/or a segment of the greater saphenous vein is harvested and properly prepared for reimplantation (Fig. 14-26). Cannulation for cardiopulmonary bypass is achieved. The aorta is occluded and the cardioplegia solution is infused.

The occluded coronary artery is isolated and dilators may be inserted. The graft is anastomosed to the coronary artery and tested for leaks. Multiple grafts may be necessary, and are placed sequentially. The aortic cross-clamp is gradually released, and a portion of the aorta is then occluded. The graft(s) are measured, cut, and anastomosed to the aorta. The clamp on the aorta is removed.

Note: Some surgeons prefer to perform the aortic anastomosis prior to the coronary artery anastomoses. The sequence of anastomoses will vary, particularly if multiple grafts are required.

The grafts are again inspected for leaks. All sources of air bubble accumulation are vented. Cardiopulmonary bypass is discontinued. The wound is irrigated with warm normal saline, with or without antibiotics. Temporary pacemaker electrodes are sewn to the heart. Chest tubes are inserted and the wound is closed

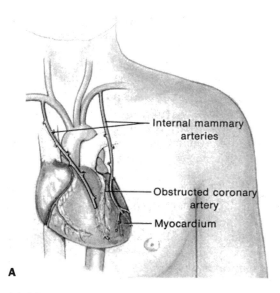

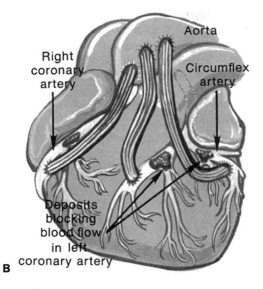

14-26. (A) CABG using mammary artery implantation; (B) triple coronary artery bypass using asephenous vein graft

in a routine manner. The chest tubes are connected to a sealed drainage unit and suction is applied.

Occasionally, coronary artery bypass may be performed in conjunction with a valve replacement procedure.

PERIOPERATIVE NURSING CONSIDERATIONS

- Circulating nurses and scrub personnel must be thoroughly familiar with the sequence of events and the routine of the surgeon since time is crucial.
- All instruments must be kept clean and free of tissue debris. An orderly arrangement is mandatory for efficient assisting during the procedure.
- Sterile iced saline slush should be available and transferred to the field in an aseptic manner before and during cardiopulmonary bypass.
- Once the patient is on the pump, urinary output is measured every 15 minutes, with amount and color noted.
- Warm saline solution is used during the closing sequence once the patient is off the pump. The thermal blanket should be turned on at this time to assist in surface warming.
- Follow specific protocol for required laboratory studies during the procedure (e.g., hemoglobin and hematocrit, potassium, arterial blood gases, etc.).
- A separate tray of instruments for the vein harvesting may be requested.
- Cardiac procedures require an additional closing count since the pericardial cavity has been entered.
- Notify the appropriate postoperative area nursing personnel (HICU/CCU) at least 30 minutes before transferring the patient in order to allow time for proper preparation of the area.
- If a bioprosthetic valve is used, follow the manufacturer's recommendations concerning the initial preparation of the valve (e.g., rinsing, etc.).
- Communication with the family and significant others should be continual throughout the procedure, since anxiety levels are extremely high owing to the nature of the procedure.
- The circulating nurse should accompany the team to the postoperative unit. Emergency equipment (e.g., ECG, transport monitor, etc.) should be sent with the patient and team in the event of any unusual occurrences.

Procedures Involving the Thoracic Aorta

Procedure
Thoracic Aortic Aneurysmectomy

Definition: Surgical removal of an aneurysmal segment of the descending thoracic aorta with insertion of a prosthetic graft.

CDC Classification: I

Discussion: Aneurysms, regardless of their location, can be categorized according to their morphology (shape).

1. *Saccular*—a sac type of formation with a narrow neck projecting from the side of the artery
2. *Fusiform*—a spindle-shaped formation with complete circumferential involvement of the artery
3. *Dissecting*—blood passes between the layers of the wall to form a false channel; usually caused by a splitting of the intima of the aorta

Surgical intervention becomes necessary when presenting symptoms indicate a compromise in circulation or there is danger of rupture. An alternative to placing the patient on the heart–lung machine is the use of a shunt (Gott) designed to divert arterial blood flow around the aneurysm. The shunt is inserted in the aorta, proximal and distal to the aneurysm. In an emergent situation, however, the use of cardiopulmonary bypass is preferred.

Surgical Approach/Positioning: Two surgical approaches may be used: median sternotomy or posterolateral thoracotomy. The positioning will depend on the surgical approach selected.

Packs, Drapes, Instrumentation, Supplies, Equipment: See Abdominal Aortic Aneurysmectomy, pp. 568–569. If cardiopulmonary bypass is used, add supplies and instrumentation for extracorporeal circulation.

PROCEDURAL OVERVIEW

A thoracotomy (median sternotomy) is performed in a standard fashion. The edges of the pleura are retracted with suture (2-0 silk) to help expose the aneurysm. The intercostal veins are clamped and ligated.

The aneurysm is dissected free from the surrounding tissue. The manner in which the dissection is continued depends upon whether an assist device (shunt) or cardiopulmonary bypass is used. The aneurysm is completely dissected and a prosthetic graft is sutured in place. The pleura is closed, and chest tubes are inserted. The chest wound is closed in a routine manner for the appropriate incision.

PERIOPERATIVE NURSING CONSIDERATIONS

- See Abdominal Aortic Aneurysmectomy, pp. 568–569.

Procedure for Permanent Pacemaker Insertion

Procedure
Insertion of a Permanent Pacemaker—Transvenous Approach

Definition: Placement of an electrode lead into the endocardium through the cephalic, subclavian, or jugular

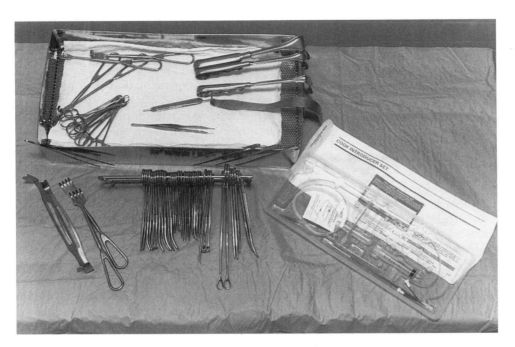

Pacemaker instrument tray with introducer set

vein, under fluoroscopy, and attaching the lead to a pulse generator.

CDC Classification: I

Discussion: Permanent pacemakers are necessary when heart block exists. A temporary pacemaker may be used until the patient can receive a permanent device. The procedure is often performed under local anesthesia, with or without the presence of anesthesia personnel.

Types of Pacemakers: A variety of pacemakers are available for the surgeon to choose from, depending on the individual needs of the patient.

1. *Asynchronous*—stimulates ventricular contraction when specified rate of pacing is required
2. *Demand*—stimulates ventricular contraction only when the heart rate falls below a preset rate
3. *Physiologic*—synchronizes atrial and ventricular activity to improve overall cardiodynamics

Positioning: Supine, with head turned slightly to the left. The left arm is usually restrained at the side; the right arm may be extended on an armboard.

Skin Preparation: See pp. 337–338

Packs/Drapes: Laparotomy drape
 Impervious stockinette (opt.)
 Image intensifier drape
 Extra drape sheets

Instrumentation:
 Pacemaker tray
 Hemoclips/surgiclip appliers

Supplies/Equipment:
 Basin set
 ESU/suction
 Image intensifier (C-arm) and monitor
 External pacemaker analyzer (usually brought by pacemaker technician/representative)
 Internal pacemaker with leads (usually brought by pacemaker technician/representative)
 Defibrillator/crash cart (available)

PROCEDURAL OVERVIEW

A cutdown is performed to expose the selected vein; the right side is usually preferred. Through a venotomy, a pacing electrode is inserted and advanced under fluoroscopy into the right ventricle. The electrode is attached to an external pacemaker for testing.

A subsequent incision is made in the chest and deepened to the fascia, creating a "pocket" for the pulse generator. A tunneling instrument is used to make a path for the electrode, which is attached to the pulse generator. The pulse generator is placed into the pocket, and the pacemaker is tested again. Once proper positioning of the lead has been reconfirmed, both incisions are closed.

PERIOPERATIVE NURSING CONSIDERATIONS

*   Special radiopaque table for fluoroscopy is necessary. Maintain radiologic safety.
*   Lead aprons must be worn throughout the procedure.

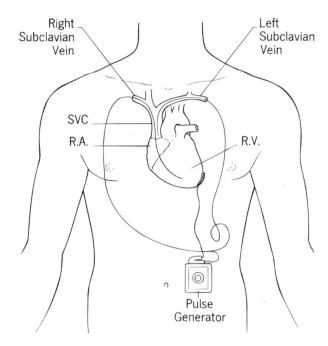

Fig. 14-27. Placement of automaticinternal cardioverter defibrillator

- Verify with the surgeon regarding the availability of generator and leads (usually brought by the pacemaker technician/representative).
- Instrument table is positioned on the patient's right side. Scrub person assists from the same side. An assistant may or may not be present.
- Have emergency defibrillator and crash cart outside the room in case of any unusual developments.
- Complete all appropriate documentation that accompanies the pacemaker. Document serial number, type, and preset rate on the intraoperative record.

Related Procedures: Insertion of AICD (Internal Defibrillator) (Fig. 14-27)
    Insertion of a Temporary Pacemaker
    Change of Generator Procedure

Self-assessment Exercise 34

Directions: Complete the following exercises. The answers are given at the end of this module.

1. The surgical intervention for a penetrating chest wound may include the _____.

2. Excessive amounts of _____ slow the heart rate, while _____ reduces the contractility.

3. A procedure performed on a newborn, which does not require the use of the heart–lung machine, is called a PDA Ligation.

                                    True   False

4. Open heart surgery requires _____ counts. List the specific intervals for each count.

5. List the types of specimens that may be obtained through a fiberoptic bronchoscope.
    a. _____
    b. _____
    c. _____

6. The procedure performed to remove an obstructive clot on the wall of an artery is called an __.
    _____

7. When collecting the supplies and equipment necessary for a segmental resection of a lung, a _____ should be added to the set-up.

8. An arteriovenous fistula is created by an anastomosis between the _____ artery and the _____ vein.

9. List the variety of grafting material commonly used for a bypass procedure (noncardiac).

10. Two pharmaceutical agents commonly used in vascular surgery are _____ (anticoagulant), which is reversed by _____.

11. An arteriogram may be performed following a femoral–popliteal bypass to _____.

Congenital Anomalies: Heart and Great Vessels

Pediatric cardiac surgery is a specialty within the field of cardiac surgery; therefore, only a brief description of specific procedures will be given. For persons who choose to work within this specialty, additional knowledge concerning specific surgical techniques is mandatory. Figure 14-28 illustrates each of the congenital anomalies. The perioperative nursing concerns associated with pediatric surgery are discussed later in this chapter.

Procedure
Closure of Patent Ductus Arteriosus (PDA Ligation)

Description: This procedure involves the closure of an unnatural communication between the pulmonary artery and the descending thoracic aorta.

The procedure may be performed in the neonatal intensive care unit (NICU) or in the OR, and does not require the use of cardiopulmonary bypass, since the heart is not directly involved (see Fig. 14-28A).

Procedure
Correction of Coarctation of the Thoracic Aorta

Description: The surgical correction of a congenital stenosis in the thoracic aorta, usually just below the origin of the left subclavian artery. The procedure does not require the use of cardiopulmonary bypass, and may be performed on an infant or an adult, since this type of anomaly is compatible with life for a considerable period of time. With an adult, however, severe hypertension is associated with this anomaly, and may necessitate surgical intervention if the condition becomes medically unmanageable (Fig. 14-28B).

Procedure
Closure of Atrial/Ventricular Septal Defect (ASD/VSD)

Description: This procedure involves the surgical correction of a congenital anomaly that involves a defective formation of either the *interatrial* or *interventricular* septum.

With an ASD, blood from the left atrium flows across the defect into the right atrium, creating a *left-*

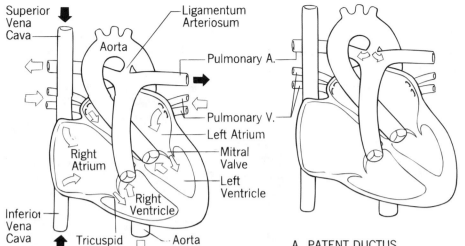

Superior Vena Cava
Aorta
Ligamentum Arteriosum
Pulmonary A.
Pulmonary V.
Left Atrium
Mitral Valve
Left Ventricle
Right Atrium
Inferior Vena Cava
Tricuspid Valve
Right Ventricle
Aorta
Normal Heart

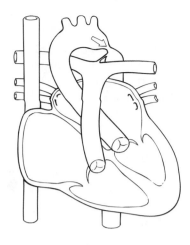

A. PATENT DUCTUS ARTERIOSUS

A vascular connection that during fetal life, provides direct access from the pulmonary artery to the aorta. Functional closure of the ductus normally occurs soon after birth. Failure to close creates a massive left to right shunt.

B. COARCTATION OF AORTA

Characterized by a narrowing of the aortic lumen, producing an obstruction to the flow of blood through the aorta, causing an increased left ventricular pressure and workload.

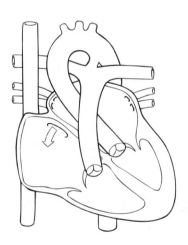

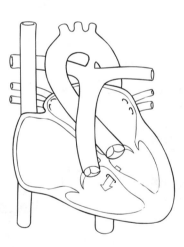

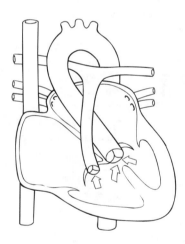

C. ATRIAL SEPTAL DEFECTS

Abnormal opening between the right and left atria, creating a left-to-right shunting of blood causing hypertrophy of both the right atrium and ventricle and enlargement of the pulmonary artery.

D. VENTRICULAR SEPTAL DEFECTS (VSD)

An abnormal opening between the right and left ventricles creating a left-to-right shunt. If pulmonary vascular resistance produces pulmonary hypertension, the shunt of blood is then reversed (right-to-left) resulting in cyanosis.

E. TETRALOGY OF FALLOT

Characterized by the combination of four defects: 1) pulmonary stenosis, 2) VSD, 3) overriding aorta, and 4) hypertrophy of right ventricle. It is the most common defect causing cyanosis and severity of symptoms is determined by the size and extent of the four defects. The surgical procedure is either palliative (for the very young) or a corrective procedure (for the older child).

Fig. 14-28. Congenital anomalies (Adapted from Ross Laboratories, Columbus OH, *Congenital Anomalies*)

to-right shunt. When a VSD is present, the high pressure in the left ventricle causes blood to flow through the defect into the right ventricle (*left-to-right shunt*).

Surgical correction usually is performed during infancy or childhood, but could be performed on an adult depending on the systemic effect of the defect. The correction is accomplished by suturing (ASD) or by the insertion of a patch graft (VSD). The use of cardiopulmonary bypass is required for both corrective procedures (see Fig. 14-28C and D).

Procedure
Correction of Tetralogy of Fallot

Description: The surgical repair of a congenital anomaly involving four separate defects: (1) pulmonary stenosis, (2) VSD, (3) overriding of the aorta, and (4) right ventricular hypertrophy.

The correction of the pulmonary stenosis alleviates the cyanotic condition, while closure of the VSD prevents heart failure. Until the correction can be accomplished, a systemic pulmonary shunt is performed to increase blood flow to the lungs. This will improve oxygenation of blood and body tissues, allowing the infant to survive and grow to a stage at which total correction is possible.

Four commonly performed systemic-pulmonary shunt procedures are the Blalock (subclavian artery to pulmonary artery), the Potts (descending thoracic aorta to pulmonary artery), the Waterson (ascending aorta to pulmonary artery), and the Glenn (vena cava to pulmonary artery).

The use of cardiopulmonary bypass is required for these corrective procedures. Should an additional defect be present (ASD), the condition is referred to as pentralogy of Fallot (*pent* meaning five) (see Fig. 14-28E).

Procedure
Correction of Transposition of the Great Vessels

Description: In this anomaly, the aorta arises from the right ventricle, and the pulmonary artery from the left ventricle. In order to sustain life, there must be communication between the left and right sides of the heart or major vessels (e.g., patent foramen ovale, PDA or ASD/VSD).

Palliative procedures performed on an infant that can improve intracardiac mixing include Blalock-Hanlon and Rashkind atrial septostomy, both of which result in an increase in the oxygen content of the systemic blood, thus sustaining life until the infant's growth is sufficient to tolerate the corrective procedure (e.g., Mustard procedure). These procedures require the use of cardiopulmonary bypass.

Procedure
Repair of Tricuspid Atresia

Description: In tricuspid atresia there is an absence of communication between the right atrium and the right ventricle, which is always accompanied by an ASD or patent foramen ovale. Other anomalies may also be present with this condition.

A palliative procedure that enlarges the ASD (Blalock-Hanlon) or the creation of a systemic-pulmonary shunt is performed to sustain life. This condition, if not immediately corrected, can cause severe rapid heart failure. This procedure requires the use of cardiopulmonary bypass.

Procedure
Repair of Truncus Arteriosus

Description: Truncus arteriosus is a retention of the embryologic bulbar trunk. It results from failure of the normal separation of this trunk into an aorta and pulmonary artery.

At birth, a single great vessel leaves the base of the heart through a single semilunar valve situated just above a VSD, and receives blood from both ventricles. The vessel gives rise to the coronary arteries, which supply the entire pulmonary and systemic circulations.

Total correction of this anomaly consists of the insertion of a small extracardiac valve–conduit that creates a pulmonary artery. Without this correction, infants show signs of severe congestive heart failure with cyanosis and failure to thrive.

The procedure requires the use of cardiopulmonary bypass.

CARDIAC TRANSPLANTATION

A unit on cardiac surgery cannot be complete without mentioning cardiac transplantation.

Although the technical aspects of cardiac transplantation have been a reality since 1967, through the work of Dr. Christian Barnard in South Africa and Drs. Shumway and Lower in the United States, its therapeutic value may be continuously evaluated over a period of time.

Cardiac transplantation techniques may vary, but the general procedure leaves part of the patient's atria intact, along with the major veins bringing blood back to the left and right sides of the heart. The donor heart is then anastomosed to the remaining section of the patient's atria, and connected to the pulmonary artery and aorta (Fig. 14-29).

Preparation for this procedure involves two operat-

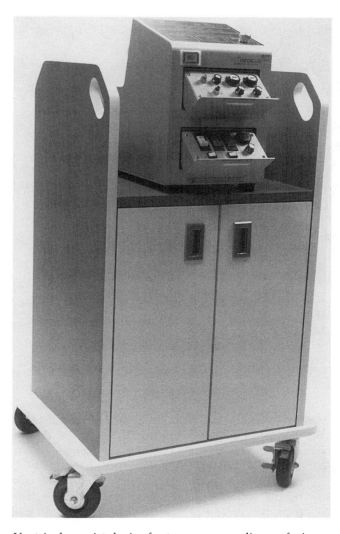

Ventricular assist device for temporary cardiac perfusion

take medication (e.g., antithymocytic globulin; Cyclosporin-E), usually for the rest of his or her life, to prevent rejection (the body's immune system attacking what it thinks is a foreign body).

Psychologically, extensive support services must be activated and available for the patient, family, and significant others during the initial adjustment phase and postoperatively. Special transplant centers, staffed with a full complement of clinical psychologists, psychiatrists, previous recipients, and medical and nursing staff, have been created around the country, to enhance awareness of transplantation surgery and to tend to the holistic needs of both the donor and recipient patient and their families.

New advances are being discovered and successfully implemented each year, including the development of a total artificial (prosthetic) heart (Jarvik-7), which could someday offer a desperately ill patient a new chance for life while awaiting a donor heart for transplantation. The creators of the artificial heart, however, readily acknowledge that their prosthetic heart is no substitute for the real thing, and in an age of biomedical miracles and technologic advances, the heart still remains one of the most durable and fascinating miracles of all.

ing rooms (for simultaneous harvesting and transplantation) fully set up for cardiopulmonary bypass surgery. The preparation of the operative site, draping, incision, and instrumentation are similar to those for procedures described in the cardiac surgery section of this chapter. Once the donor heart has been removed, it must be reimplanted within 6 hours to retain its full physiologic function. When the transplantation is performed in a hospital removed from the donor procedure, continuous communication and exact coordination of all activities are critical for a successful outcome. For severely ill patients, the use of a ventricular assist device may be needed to support heart function until the time of transplantation.

Following the transplant procedure, the real challenge begins. For a long time after the operation, the patient must undergo heart biopsies (using a small forceps through a jugular venotomy). The patient must

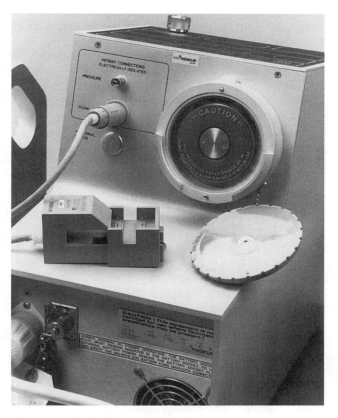

Close-up of left ventricular assist device pump-head

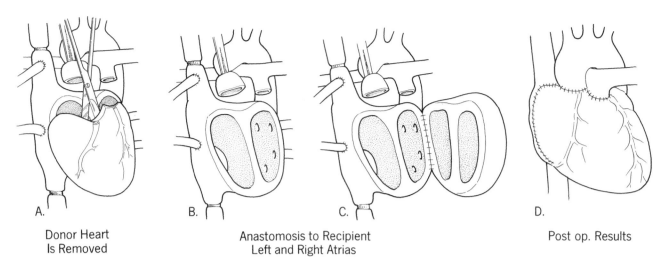

A. Donor Heart Is Removed

B. C. Anastomosis to Recipient Left and Right Atrias

D. Post op. Results

Fig. 14-29. Heart transplantation

OPHTHALMIC AND OTORHINOLARYNGOLOGIC SURGERY

Commonly referred to as *sense organs*, the eye, ear, nose, and throat make up a section of surgical services known as EENT (ophthalmic and ENT) surgery.

The body has millions of sense organs. All of its receptors—that is, the distal ends, or *dendrites*, of all its sensory neurons—are its sense organs.

The word *sense* might be defined as the ability of specialized areas of the cerebral cortex to interpret an impulse occurring in and/or around a receptor.

This unit discusses the primary sense organs, which occasionally, because of disease or traumatic injury, require surgical intervention: the *eye*, the *ear*, the *nose*, and the *throat*. The unit is divided into two sections: ophthalmic procedures and ENT procedures.

OPHTHALMIC SURGERY

The goal of ophthalmic surgery is centered around the restoration of vision lost from disease, injury, or congenital defects. Essential to this restoration is a thorough understanding of the anatomic structures and their relationship to visual capabilities.

Surgical Anatomy Review

External Structures of the Eye

In the embryo, the eye develops as an *outpocketing* of the brain. The eye, like the brain, is a very delicate organ; therefore, nature has carefully protected the eye by means of the following structures:

1. The skull bones that form the eye *orbit* (cavity) serve to protect more than one half of the eyeball (*globe*) posteriorly at its most vulnerable points: the *optic nerve* and the *retina*. There are seven bones that form the orbit: the *maxilla, palantine, frontal, sphenoidal, zygomatic, ethmoidal,* and *lacrimal* bones.
2. The *lids* and *eyelashes* aid in protecting the eye anteriorly. The lids consist of several layers, and distribute secretions, keeping the *cornea* moist. The tears, produced by the *lacrimal glands,* and secreted through a set of ducts in the *conjunctival sac,* are responsible for washing away small foreign objects that may enter the lid area.
3. A sac lined with an epithelial membrane separates the front of the eye from the globe, and aids in the destruction of some of the pathogenic bacteria that may enter from the outside.

Internal Structures of the Eye

Layers (Coating) of the Eyeball   The *globe* has three separate coats, or *tunics:*

1. *Sclera*—the outermost layer; made of firm, tough connective tissue. Commonly referred to as the "white" of the eye.
2. *Choroid*—the middle layer; heavily pigmented, preventing light rays from scattering and reflecting off the inner surface of the eye.
3. *Retina*—the innermost coating; includes 10 different layers of nerve cells, including the end organs called *rods* and *cones.* These structures act as the receptor for the sense of vision.

Additional layers of the eyeball include the *cornea*, a transparent membrane that covers the front of the globe; the *ciliary body*, an extension of the choroid layer, made of ligaments that hold the eye in place; the *iris*, or colored portion of the eye, which closes and opens to exclude or omit light; and the *pupil*, which lies in the center of the iris, and dilates and contracts according to the action of the iris.

Muscles of the Eye Eye muscles are divided into two groups: intrinsic (inside the eyeball), and extrinsic (attached to the bone and sclera).

Intrinsic muscles include the iris and ciliary bodies. The six intrinsic muscles include four rectus muscles and two oblique muscles. These muscles are responsible for moving the globe around various axes, and allow binocular focus (the ability to focus on one subject with both eyes).

Nerve Supply to the Eye The two sensory nerves associated with the eye are the *optic nerve*, which carries visual impulses received by the rods and cones in the retina to the brain (cranial nerve II), and the *ophthalmic nerve*, which carries impulses of pain, touch, and temperature from the eye and surrounding parts (a branch of the cranial nerve V).

The optic nerve is connected with the eyeball toward the medial (nasal) side of the eye, in the back. Since there are no rods or cones located in this region, the white circular area is called the "blind spot," or *optic disk*. There is a tiny depressed area in the retina called the *fovea centralis*, which is the clearest point of vision.

Three nerves carry motor fibers to the muscles of the eyeball: the *oculomotor*, which supplies voluntary and involuntary motor fibers, the *trochlear*, and the *abducens*, both of which supply one voluntary muscle each.

Lacrimal Apparatus and Conjunctiva The lacrimal gland produces tears and is located above the eye toward one side (superior and lateral) of the eyeball. Tiny tubes (ducts) carry the tears to the front surface of the eyeball; the tears serve to bathe continuously the sac that separates the front part of the eyeball from the larger posterior section. This sac is lined with mucous membrane, and is called the *conjunctiva*.

The conjunctiva is a thin membrane that lines each eyelid and is doubled back over the eyeball to protect it from dust and debris. It is kept moist by tears flowing across the front of the eye. From these openings, tears are carried by tubes that drain into the nose via the *nasolacrimal duct*, a passageway between the lacrimal sac and the inferior meatus of the nose.

The Eye's Chambers The eye contains several chambers that are filled with a nourishing fluid. The iris divides into two chambers that lie in front of the lens: the *anterior chamber*, directly in front of the iris and the *posterior chamber*, directly behind the iris. Both chambers are filled with *aqueous humor*, a substance secreted by the ciliary processes. Since the fluid is constantly being manufactured, a means of emptying has been established: the *canal of Schlemm* serves as the exit for this fluid.

The large posterior chamber, located behind the lens, is filled with a jelly-like substance, *vitreous humor*, which serves both as a means to maintain the shape of the eye and as a protective cushion.

The Lens The lens lies directly behind the iris, and is biconvex in shape. The lens is covered by a transparent capsule, which is held in place by suspensory ligaments attached to the capsule, where the ciliary bodies and choroid meet. These ligaments help to change the shape of the lens to bend the light that passes through it and to focus images projected onto the retina.

General Considerations for Ophthalmic Surgery

Patient Preparation and Education

Most patients undergoing ophthalmic surgery will enter the hospital or ambulatory surgery facility the morning of surgery, and will usually be discharged to home care following a brief postanesthesia recovery period. The patient may be a child or an adult; therefore, the perioperative nurse must be prepared to meet the individual physiologic and psychosocial needs of a highly diverse patient population.

Preparation for surgery for this patient population begins in the surgeon's office or clinic, when the decision to have surgery has been reached. Effective communication between the preadmission area and surgery concerning the planned surgical experience increases the efficiency of the process and provides continuity of patient care during the perioperative period. Arrangement for home care, if required with an outside agency, should be made as soon as possible, so that follow-up care will begin as soon as possible following surgery.

Patient education is important, since the majority of these patients will recuperate at home without the aid of direct nursing supervision. Written materials, audiovisual presentations, and formal education sessions in which questions and/or concerns can be addressed will alleviate much of the anxiety associated with the surgical event, and allow the nurse to strengthen any postoperative instructions for the patient and the family. Documentation of this teaching process should appear on all records, along with a contact person's name and phone number, should any unforeseen events occur.

Environmental Atmosphere

Ophthalmic surgery requires close attention to details; minor break of technique or a disturbance in the room could potentially lead to complete or partial loss of vision of the operated eye. It is vitally important, therefore, that the operating room remain quiet and subdued during the procedure. All extraneous noises and movement should cease once the procedure begins, with limited usage of intercoms, telephones, and pocket pagers.

Anesthesia Techniques

For the majority of ophthalmic procedures, local infiltration by the surgeon with IV sedation and monitoring by the anesthesia clinician is the technique of choice. There are occasions, however, that will require the use of general anesthesia.

The awake patient has specific needs in addition to the needs standard for all surgery, and the perioperative nurse must be aware of the patient's individuality by establishing a rapport of trust prior to the beginning of the procedure. Instructions should be precise, with questions answered promptly to manage any possible patient confusion due to sensory deprivation and/or medications.

Regional Block Anesthesia Techniques

The type of regional nerve block used will depend on the specific procedure being performed.

1. *Field Nerve Block:* Used for surgery of the eyelids. The injection begins at the outer corner of the eye, extends toward the nose; upper or lower eyelids.
2. *Retrobulbar Block:* Commonly used for achieving anesthesia and immobility of the eye. The injection is made behind the globe (eyeball) into the muscle cone to block the branches of cranial nerves III, V, and VI. Digital compression of the eyeball is then applied to aid in diffusion of the anesthetic agent.

Ophthalmic Pharmacology

Specific drugs used to diagnose and treat eye disorders are numerous and require a thorough understanding of the major classifications of the agents and their expected effects.

The patient should be well informed about the specific agents prescribed during the recovery period and when to notify the physician concerning any problems associated with the agents.

The following list provides the general categories of the agents frequently associated with ophthalmic surgery and patient care during the perioperative period (Table 14-1). The perioperative nurse should be familiar with these drugs and their preparation and dispensation method during surgery. All medications and solutions should be labeled.

Special Equipment/Supplies

Operating Microscope

The operating microscope plays a vital part in ophthalmic surgery. It is the primary tool for visualization used by the surgeon during all operative procedures involving the internal structures of the eye.

Eye Sutures

Eye sutures are available in a wide range of materials and in sizes ranging from 4-0 to 12-0. Those of small gauge must be handled gently and carefully, with the appropriate needle holder. Needle points should be protected from injury. The scrub nurse should check for *burrs* before using the suture. Eye sutures come single- and double-armed. A needle count is required during ophthalmic surgery.

Ophthalmic Sponges

Ophthalmic sponges are spear-shaped and made of a lint-free cellulose material. They are mounted on a plastic rod for easy usage. Although a sponge count is not required, the scrub person should keep track of the number used during the procedure.

Cautery Unit

Ophthalmic cautery units may be handheld, single-use items, powered by a household battery, or may be a conventional bipolar unit. The disposable unit must never be resterilized and used again, unless it is specifically designated as a multi-use item and specific instructions as to the number of uses are available in writing from the manufacturer.

Phacoemulsifier Unit

This electrical unit is used to assist in the removal of an opaque lens by means of sound waves. The unit can irrigate and aspirate the lens material following emulsification through a very small incision. More detail concerning this unit appears in the section on selected surgical procedures.

Cryoextractor and Power Source

Primarily used for intracapsular lens extraction, the cryoextractor, or miniaturized cryoprobe, freezes onto

Table 14-1   Drugs Used for Ophthalmology

Type of Agent	Comments	Examples
Miotic	Used to constrict the pupil and to reduce intraocular pressure. Used in cataract surgery to help prevent loss of vitreous humor.	Miochol, Pilocarpine HCl, Miostat 0.01%, Carbochol, DFP, Floropryl
Mydratic/Cycloplegic	Causes the pupil to dilate and facilitates examination of the retina and lens removal.	Mydriacyl, Cyclogyl, Neosynephrine (2%, 5%, or 10%)
Enzymatic	Used during cataract surgery to dissolve the zonule fibers that attach the lens of the eye.	Alpha Chymar, Zolace, Wydase
Irrigant	Used to keep eye tissue moist during surgery.	Balanced saline solution (BSS)
Topical anesthetic	Applied to reduce pain sensation in and on the eye.	Tetracaine HCl, Ophtanie, Lidocaine (1% or 2%)
Antiinflammatory	Used to reduce inflammation and help prevent edema.	Decasone, Celestan
Antibiotic	Used to help reduce infection.	Neosporin Ophthalmic
Osmotics	Used preoperatively to reduce osmolarity or to treat uncontrolled glaucoma (angle-closure glaucoma).	Glyrol, Osmologyn
Viscoelastic	Maintains a separation between tissues, thus providing support; used to protect the corneal endothelium or as a vitreous substitute during retinal or vitreous surgery.	Healon, Amisc, Viscot
Diagnostic	Used to stain the cornea to reveal under an ultraviolet light any interruptions in the normal surface of the cornea.	Fluorescein

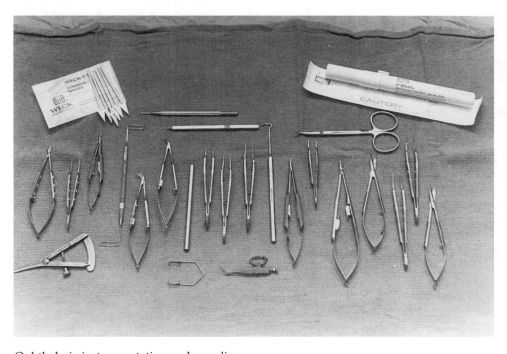

Ophthalmic instrumentation and supplies

the surface of the cataract, obtaining secure adherence, and the lens is removed en bloc. The cryoprobe is available as a disposable unit, self-contained, or as a reusable tip requiring an outside power source.

Ophthalmic Instruments

Instruments used during eye surgery are delicate and costly. Special care must be taken by all surgical personnel to ensure that the edges and tips of these instruments are examined frequently and protected from damage or careless handling. A small ultrasonic unit is frequently used to clean these instruments; if an ultrasonic unit is not available they are hand cleaned. Ideally, the instruments should be gas sterilized to preserve the life of the instrument. During surgery, the instruments can be placed on a rolled lint-free paper drape to protect the tips. Two generic trays are usually created: a cataract extraction tray and a muscle tray (Fig. 14-30).

Positioning, Skin Preparation, and Draping

The supine position, slightly elevated or flat, is used for all ophthalmic procedures. The arms are usually tucked and restrained with soft restraints. A special eye stretcher, which may also serve as the operating table, can prevent unnecessary movement of the patient during the pre- and postoperative phases, in addition to providing a headrest for the patient and arm supports for the surgeon.

A special concern for eye surgery draping is the use of lint-free materials. Towels, therefore, should be used only as part of the head drape and never placed on the Mayo or instrument table. An ophthalmic pack, complete with a special eye fenestrated sheet, may be used; however, a basic pack or head and neck pack with a small adhesive opening may be all that is required.

The drape should be kept off the patient's nose and mouth, if possible, and/or if general anesthesia is administered, since a clear path to the endotracheal tube is mandatory. Intravenous lines should be accessible at all times. If a microscope drape is used instead of sterile handgrips, the microscope should be draped before the patient.

The surgical skin prep usually includes hairline to mouth, ears, and nose:

- Use a soft cloth or cotton balls
- Start the prep from the inner aspect of the eye to the outer corner
- Eyelashes may or may not be cut (surgeon's preference). If cutting is necessary, moisten the lashes with a petroleum substance first to prevent lashes from getting into the eye, and to make cutting easier.
- Iodine and chlorhexidine gluconate are not recommended for facial preps. Check with the surgeon for solution of choice.

Selected Surgical Procedures

Surgery Involving External Structures

Procedure
Correction of Ectropin/Entropin

Definition: Correction of an eversion (*ectropin*) or inversion (*entropin*) of the lower eyelid, margins, and eyelashes.
CDC Classification: I
Discussion: The method of correction depends on the type and severity of the deformity.

Ectropin usually occurs bilaterally, and may be caused by *involution* (a relaxation of the orbicularis muscle, which may occur as a result of aging); may be *congenital* (e.g., associated with Down syndrome); or may be *paralytic* (in which the orbicularis oculi has lost its tone due to cranial nerve VII paralysis.

Entropin usually affects the lower lid. The condition may be *congenital,* owing to hypertrophy of the marginal and pretarsal orbicularis oculi muscle, causing the eyelid margin to be pushed up against the globe; *involutional* (most common), in which the canthal tendons retain their rigidity but the apposition of the lid to the globe is changed, resulting in the inversion of the eyelid; or may appear as the result of weakness of the retractor muscles of the lower lid.
Positioning, Skin Preparation, Draping: See General Considerations, p. 587
Instrumentation:
    Basic eye procedure tray or special tray (eyelid; plastic; conjunctiva)
Supplies/Equipment:
    Basin set
    Headrest (e.g., Shea; horseshoe) if not part of the stretcher/bed
    Sitting stool with back support
    Ophthalmic sponges (e.g., Weck-Cel)
    Blades—(1) No. 15 or (1) No. 11
    Cautery—ophthalmic
    Sterile saline solution (e.g., BSS; Tru-Sol)
    Topical anesthetic drops (e.g., Tetracaine) (opt.)
    Local anesthetic (e.g., Xylocaine 2% with epinepherine)
    Antibiotic ointment (opt.)

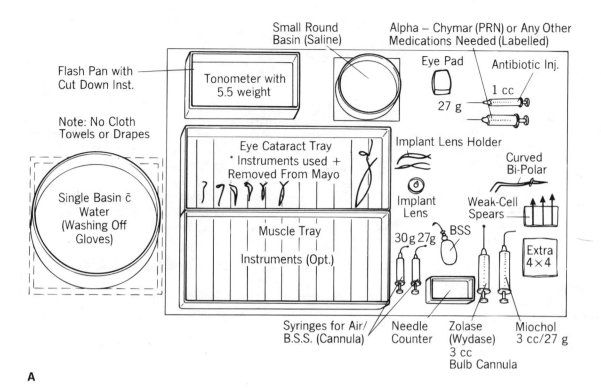

A

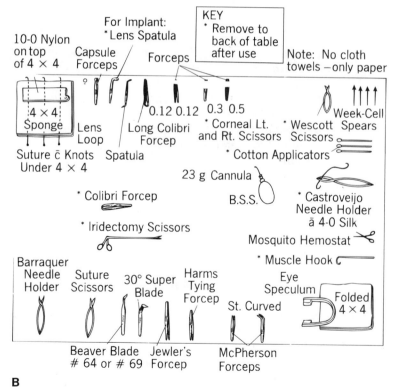

B

Fig. 14-30.   (A) Back table set-up; (B) Mayo tray set-up

Marking pen
Sutures—surgeon's preference

PROCEDURAL OVERVIEW

Ectropin

The surgeon will usually mark the area of incision in the lid with a marking pen. The skin incision is made below the lid margin, extending from the outer corner to just beyond the lateral canthus, creating a triangle-shaped wedge. Tissue may be cauterized with the ophthalmic cautery. The scrub person should continuously irrigate the eyeball to keep it moist. The wedge tissue is removed, and the closure begins. The surgeon places one or more sutures (4-0 absorbable, swedged to a spatula-type needle) through the tarsal plate and canthal ligaments. This prevents the ectropin from recurring. The deep tissue layers are closed (4-0 or 5-0 absorbable) and the skin is closed (5-0 or 6-0 silk). Antibiotic ointment may be instilled into the eye, and a patch may or may not be applied (surgeon's preference).
Note: This is only one example of a technique available to correct this condition.

Entropin

The most common technique used to treat this condition consists of an incision of a base-down tarsoconjunctival triangle. The lid is retracted downward. The incision is made and small bleeders are controlled with cautery. The eye should be irrigated to prevent the cornea from drying out. Once the triangle has been incised, three or four interrupted absorbable sutures (5-0 or 6-0 swedged to a spatula-type needle) are used, leaving the ends untied. When the last suture is placed, a tying forceps is used to tie the sutures in place. Hemostasis is achieved; antibiotic ointment is instilled into the eye, and the eye is dressed with an eye patch taped in place.

PERIOPERATIVE NURSING CONSIDERATIONS

- Eyelashes are not usually cut; if requested, it is performed prior to the skin prep.
- Eyes are always irrigated from the inner corner to the outer corner.
- Powder is meticulously removed from gloves by use of a wet towel, which is discarded after use.
- The scrub person should be ready to irrigate the eye with solution and a blunt needle.
- Precautions are taken to keep lint off the field and instruments; check instruments and needles for burrs or damage.
- Ophthalmic drops are instilled into the conjunctiva sac.
- See General Considerations (p. 587) for additional information.

Surgery Involving Internal Structures

Procedure
Cataract Extraction

Definition: The removal of an opaque ocular lens.
CDC Classification: I
Discussion: A cataract may be a congenital defect or may be caused by trauma or certain medications. At an appropriate time in the maturation of the cataract, and with sufficient loss of vision, surgical intervention becomes necessary. A cataract is one of the most common causes of gradual, painless loss of vision.
Types of Cataract Extraction Procedures:

1. *Intracapsular*—removal of the opaque lens within its capsule
2. *Extracapsular*—removal of the opaque lens by irrigation and expression, leaving the posterior capsule in situ
3. *Phacoemulsification*—a variation of the irrigation/aspiration technique. The contents of the lens capsule are fragmented with ultrasonic energy as the lens material is simultaneously irrigated and aspirated.

The procedure may be followed by the implantation of an intraocular lens (IOL). The lens prosthesis is selected by the surgeon prior to the surgery, and may either be purchased by "consignment" with a company, or kept in stock in the operating suite.
Positioning, Skin Preparation, Packs, Drapes: See General Considerations, p. 587
Instrumentation:
    Basic eye procedure tray
    Cataract extraction tray (IOL instrument) (opt.)
    Phacoemulsification tray (specific to the brand used)
    Intraocular lens implant
Supplies/Equipment:
    Basin set
    Balanced saline solution (BSS)—500 mL
    Irrigation/aspiration (I/A) pack (for phacoemulsification)
    Ophthalmic sponges (e.g., Weck-Cel)
    Ophthalmic cautery
    Microscope drape (or handgrips)
    Headrest (e.g., Shea; horseshoe) (opt.)
    Sitting stool with backrest
    Cryoextractor
    Phacoemulsifier—I/A unit (e.g., SITE)
    Honan intraocular pressure reducer cuff
    Beaver blade (No. 69)
    Super blade (30°)

Multipore filter (for Miochol)
Medications—surgeon's preference
Sutures—surgeon's preference

PROCEDURAL OVERVIEW

Intracapsular

A lid speculum is placed and traction sutures are placed in the sclera. The conjunctiva is reflected from the superior cornea. Bleeders are cauterized. The anterior chamber is entered; an iridotomy is performed as the cornea is retracted by suture traction.

An enzymatic solution (e.g., Alpha-Chymar) is instilled into the anterior chamber to dissolve the zonule fibers suspending the lens. After a short time (approximately 2–3 minutes), a cryoextractor is applied to the lens, which adheres to it, and the lens is withdrawn from the eye. The corneal incision is closed; traction sutures are removed, and the conjunctival flap is approximated.

If an intraocular lens implant (IOL) is used, it will be implanted following the extraction of the lens. The prosthesis is either sutured to the iris or simply held in place (by its shape) by the iris, depending on the type of prosthesis.

Ophthalmic ointment may be instilled, and an eye dressing and patch is applied.

Extracapsular

This procedure is similar to the intracapsular procedure, except that the lens capsule is incised, and the lens is exposed or irrigated out leaving the posterior capsule, which remains as a barrier to the vitreous humor.

When phacoemulsification is used, the anterior lens capsule is excised, the lens nucleus is prolapsed into the anterior chamber, and the ultrasonic probe is inserted into the capsule. Alternatively, the probe is set to irrigate/aspirate and then fragment the remaining lens substance. After the "phaco" procedure, the wound is closed as described in the section on intracapsular cataract extraction. An intraocular lens may be inserted in the manner previously described.

PERIOPERATIVE NURSING CONSIDERATIONS

- If a floor model microscope is used, it should be draped and brought in over the field on the opposite side of the affected eye.
- Thorough familiarity with all equipment used is mandatory for a smooth surgical procedure. Check all equipment before use.
- Follow hospital protocol for documenting the IOL, if used, and complete the lens package information.
- The circulator will usually be responsible for changing the settings on the phacoemulsifier unit. The surgeon should be advised as to each setting change.

Procedure
Iridectomy

Definition: Excision of a section of the iris.
CDC Classification: I
Discussion: This procedure is usually indicated for primary angle-closure glaucoma, secondary angle-closure glaucoma, and occluded angle glaucoma. The creation of a new communication (or channel) for aqueous chamber is the basic goal of the procedure; to relieve the pupillary block and reestablish the flow of aqueous through Schlemm's canal.
Positioning, Skin Preparation, Draping: See General Considerations, p. 591
Instrumentation:
  Basic eye procedure tray
  Glaucoma procedure tray
  Handgrips (or drape) for microscope
Supplies/Equipment:
  Headrest (opt.)
  Sitting stool with backrest
  Microscope (or loops)
  Basin set
  Ophthalmic sponges (e.g., Weck-Cel)
  Blade (Beaver No. 69 or No. 67)
  Multipore filter (for Miochol)
  Cautery
  Balanced saline solution (BSS)
  Medications—surgeon's preference
  Sutures—surgeon's preference

PROCEDURAL OVERVIEW

A small periotomy (2 mm) is made at the superior limbus. The epithelium is scraped away from the corneoscleral junction. Preplaced sutures are placed in the cornea. Prolapse of the iris is facilitated by gentle traction of the sutures. The iris is grasped, and the excision is performed. BSS is used to flush away the remaining pigmented epithelium. The preplaced sutures are tied. Additional sutures may be necessary. Topical corticosteroids and antibiotic ointment may be instilled, and an eye pad is applied.

PERIOPERATIVE NURSING CONSIDERATIONS

- See General Considerations, pp. 587–591.

Surgery Involving Repair of Congenital Defects

Procedure
Lateral/Medial Rectus Muscle Resection

Definition: Alignment of the visual axes of the eyes to correct the condition known as strabismus.

CDC Classification: I

Discussion: Muscle surgery is performed to correct the condition known as *strabismus,* in which the eye (one or both) cannot focus on an object because the muscles lack coordination. One eye (the *fixing* eye) looks directly at an object, while the other (the *deviating* eye) does not. Complete restoration to normal alignment cannot always be achieved.

1. *Lateral Rectus Resection*—the shortening of the extraocular muscle by removing a portion of the muscle and the reanastomosis of the cut ends
2. *Medial Rectus Resection*—the lengthening of the extraocular muscle by detaching it from its original insertion and reattaching it more posteriorly on the sclera

The procedure is generally performed on children to improve vision, and usually requires general anesthesia.

Positioning, Skin Preparation, Draping: See General Considerations, p. 591

Instrumentation:
Basic eye procedure tray
Basic eye muscle procedure tray

Supplies/Equipment:
Headrest
Loops (opt.)
Sitting stool with backrest
Basin set
Ophthalmic sponges (e.g., Weck-Cel)
Cautery
Balanced saline solution (BSS)
Needle counter
Medications—surgeon's preference
Sutures—surgeon's preference

PROCEDURAL OVERVIEW

Lateral Rectus Resection

The eye speculum is inserted. An incision is made in the conjunctiva at the limbus to expose the lateral rectus muscle. Two traction sutures (4-0 silk) are placed in the conjunctiva. The conjunctiva is freed from underlying tissue by blunt and sharp dissection, which is carried back well over the muscle. After locating the muscle's insertion, a muscle hook is passed under the muscle to ensure that it is free of adhesions.

A caliper is used to measure the amount of muscle to be resected. A muscle clamp is placed over the rectus muscle and the measured portion is excised with a straight tenotomy scissors, and the measured portion is passed off as a specimen. The end of the muscle is reattached to the original point of insertion. Hemostasis is achieved; the conjunctiva is closed. Antibiotic

ophthalmic ointment may be instilled and an eye pad and metal shield is applied.

Medial Rectus Resection

The procedure is identical to that for a lateral rectus resection to the point of the conjunctival incision. The surgeon uses a tenotomy scissors to expose the conjunctiva. Using a previously adjusted caliper, the distance from the original insertion point to its new one is measured.

Two absorbable sutures (5-0 or 6-0) are placed in the end of the muscle, but left untied. A straight mosquito hemostat may be placed across the muscle, between the sutures and the insertion site, to compress small blood vessels and discourage oozing. The clamp is removed after a short time and a muscle hook is passed under the muscle. The muscle is cut and cautery is applied as needed to achieve hemostasis.

The muscle is attached at the point of insertion further back on the eyeball with the previously placed sutures. The conjunctiva is closed. An antibiotic ophthalmic ointment is instilled and the eye is dressed with an eye pad and a metal shield.

PERIOPERATIVE NURSING CONSIDERATIONS

• See General Considerations, pp. 587–591.

Surgical Procedures Associated with Traumatic Conditions

Procedure
Eviscceration of the Eye

Definition: Removal of the entire contents of the eye within the scleral shell.

CDC Classification: II

Discussion: The sclera and muscles attached to the sclera remain intact to accommodate a prosthesis.

An indication for evisceration is a hopelessly traumatized eye in a young person with no history of previous eye disease. The cosmetic result is superior to the result of enucleation because the extraocular muscles remain attached to the scleral shell, resulting in a moveable implant very similar to that of natural eye movement.

Positioning, Skin Preparation, Draping: See General Considerations, p. 591

Instrumentation:
Basic eye procedure tray
Globe/orbit prosthesis tray (opt.)
Curettes

Supplies/Equipment:
Basin set
BSS irrigation solution
Cautery, disposable

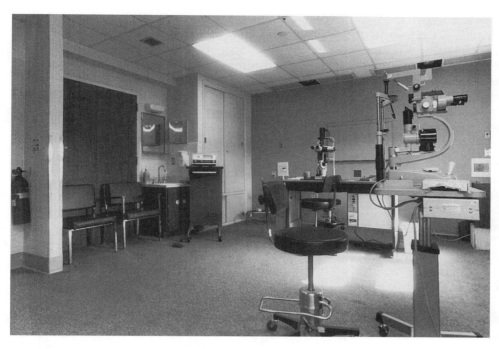

Eye laser surgical suite for outpatient surgical procedures

Ophthalmic sponges (e.g., Weck-Cel)
Suction tubing
Antibiotic ophthalmic ointment (surgeon's preference)
Blade—(1) No. 11
Sphere prosthesis and conformer

PROCEDURAL OVERVIEW

A periotomy is made superiorly from the 3 o'clock to the 9 o'clock position. An incision (same length) is made in the exposed sclera through to the uvea. The entire uvea is separated from the sclera by an evisceration spoon and is completely removed. The remaining uvea may be removed with a gauze sponge on a hemostat rotated within the scleral shell or with a special curetite (e.g., Chalazion). The wound is irrigated and hemostasis is achieved.

The scleral edges are held open by tagged sutures while the implant is inserted with a sphere introducer. The posterior surface of the cornea is removed (to reduce sensitivity), and the sclera is closed with interrupted sutures. The conjunctiva is approximated; a conformer is placed in the cul-de-sac. Antibiotic ointment is instilled and an eye pad and metal shield are applied.

PERIOPERATIVE NURSING CONSIDERATIONS

- See General Considerations, pp. 587–591.
- Have the prosthesis ready to implant.
- Follow hospital protocol regarding documentation of the prosthesis, and complete the enclosed manufacturer's form.

Use of the Optical Laser

The use of an optical laser is often a safe alternative to conventional surgery involving the eye. Clinical application for selective uses of various optical lasers will be reviewed in this section; however, the perioperative nursing implications should be reviewed for safe and effective use.

The blue-green argon laser is effective in treating retinal holes or tears. In addition, one of its major usages is the treatment of diabetic retinopathy. Other conditions include central serous retinopathy, angiomas, and hemangiomas; hemostasis (to seal vessels); aneurysms; laser trabeculoplasty (to lower intraocular pressure and facilitate aqueous drainage); laser iridotomy (make a small hole in the iris) to allow aqueous to enter the anterior chamber.

The pulsed neodymium (ND:Yag) laser can also be used for selected ophthalmic procedures, such as preoperative capsulotomy (prior to extracapsular cataract extraction); capsulotomy of the posterior capsule (post-cataract extraction); and lysis or severing of vitreous strands and/or fibrous binds that can cause macular edema. In some cases, visual problems not previously responsive to laser treatment can now be treated with the ND:Yag medium.

The Red-Yellow Krypton laser is often used for blood aberrations of choroid, which is common with senile macular disease in which normal vessels damage adjacent nerve tissues; for lesions in the premacular region, laser burn passes through cloudy vitreous hemorrhage.

Advantages of Laser Therapy

The optical laser delivery system uses the binocular microscope of the *slit lamp*, thus giving stereopsis and greater magnification in addition to allowing the procedure to be performed in an office or special eye laser suite within the hospital.

There are several advantages of laser therapy, including

1. Minimal possibility of tissue infection
2. Minimal pain (anesthesia, except topical, is eliminated)
3. Performed as an outpatient procedure, eliminating the need for hospitalization
4. Useful in poor-risk patients or for those who may have had previous unsuccessful operative procedures

Laser surgery also has its disadvantages; for example, it is not effective in correcting severe retinal damage or detachment. For these patients, surgical intervention, often a vitrectomy, is indicated.

ENT PROCEDURES

The Ear

Surgical procedures of the middle and inner ear are performed to restore the patient's hearing, which may be lost owing to disease or injury. Hearing loss can be classified into two major groups based on the physiologic cause:

1. *Conductive:* a mechanical obstruction of the external or middle ear, caused by a tumor or fixation of the ear bones.
2. *Sensorineural:* caused by a lesion in the nerve tissue or sensory pathways to the brain.

Surgical Anatomy Review

The ear is divided into three distinct parts: the external, the middle, and the internal ear.

The External Ear

The *external ear* has two divisions: (1) the flap, or modified trumpet (*auricle* or *pinna*), and (2) the tube leading from the auricle into the temporal bone (*external acoustic meatus* or *ear canal*). This canal is approximately 1.5-inches long and is positioned inward, forward, and downward, although the first portion of the tube slants upward and then curves downward. Modified sweat glands in the auditory canal secrete *cerumen,* a waxlike substance; if the secretion becomes excessive, it could produce pain and/or deafness.

The *tympanic membrane* (ear drum) stretches across the inner portion of the auditory canal, separating it from the middle ear.

The Middle Ear (Tympanic Cavity)

The *middle ear* contains three auditory *ossicles:* the *mallus,* the *incus,* and the *stapes.* There are several openings in the middle ear cavity; one from the ear canal, two into the internal ear (*oval/round windows*), and one into the *eustachian tube.*

Posteriorly, the middle ear cavity is continuous with a number of mastoid air spaces in the temporal bone. The clinical importance of these areas is related to infection, since they provide a route for bacteria to enter and travel freely in this area. Head colds in children, for example, can lead to middle ear infections (*otitis media*) or mastoid infections (*mastoiditis*).

The eustachian tube (*auditory tube*) is composed partly of bone and partly of cartilage and fibrous tissue, and is lined with mucosa. Its major function is to equalize pressure between the inner and outer surfaces of the tympanic membrane, thus preventing rupture of the membrane.

The Internal Ear (Labyrinth)

The *internal ear* consists of two main parts: a bony labyrinth and a membranous labyrinth. The bony labyrinth consists of three parts, or sections: the *vestibule,* the *cochlea,* and the *semicircular canals.* Some of the receptors for the vestibular branch of the cranial nerve VIII lie in the semicircular canal (*ampulla*). Like all receptors for both vestibular and auditory branches of the nerve, these receptors lie in contact with a supporting structure. In addition to aiding in hearing, the semicircular canals help control equilibrium and the body's ability to sense its position in relation to other objects.

General Considerations

Positioning, Skin Preparation, and Draping

For most otologic procedures, the patient is supine with the head positioned at the edge of the table; affected ear up. The other ear should be well padded to avoid nerve damage due to pressure. The surgeon is usually seated at the side of the patient's head; anesthesia is on the side, toward the foot.

Depending on the type of microscope and operating table, the patient's head may be placed at the foot of the table to allow the microscope to be properly positioned.

The skin preparation for most procedures requires the removal of hair around the site of the incision (above and behind the ear); a cap is secured with tape to create a waterproof covering, and the prep is performed over the tape. A cotton ball may be placed in the ear canal, and the face may be included in the prep on the opposite side (to the nose). Postprocedure, the face is washed clean before the application of the dressing.

The draping procedure usually consists of folded towels and adherent plastic drape sheet of special ear drape. If the microscope is used, it should be draped away from the field, then moved into position once the patient has been draped.

Power Equipment

Power drills are needed during many ear procedure to remove bony tissue. Two drills are commonly used: the Jordon-Day and the Stryker, each with special attachments, drill bits, and so on to fit a specific surgical procedure. Since most of the drill bits are not interchangeable, *careful* attention must be paid to these pieces to avoid mismatching the instruments and their parts.

Microscope

For middle and inner ear surgeries, the microscope will always be required. The lens of choice is usually a 300-mm lens, but refer to the physician's preference card before setting up the equipment.

Suction/Irrigation Equipment

A special suction/irrigation system is commonly used during ear surgery, allowing the surgeon adequate access and visualization of the operative structures simultaneously. Follow the manufacturer's recommendations for proper set-up, and test the equipment prior to use.

Instrumentation

A basic ear tray consists of instruments needed to work with bone and tissue in an extremely delicate area. Special microsurgical instruments are added to the instrumentation for selected procedure, including knives, curettes, delicate sharps, forceps, and probes (Fig. 14-31).

Medications

Three categories of medications are generally used for ear surgery: anesthetics, hemostatic agents, and irrigation fluids.

Epinepherine is usually applied to *pledgets* to control bleeding, in addition to Gelfoam. Irrigation solution is administered in a small syringe with a blunt tip or, more popular, a small bulb syringe. The solution can

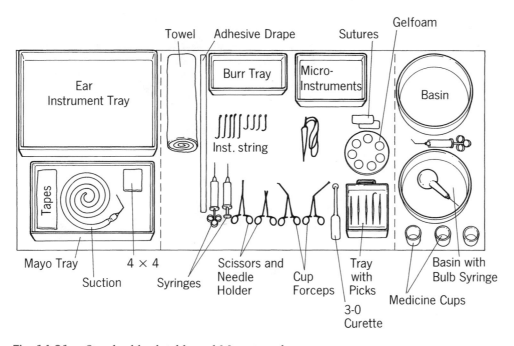

Fig. 14-31. Standard back table and Mayo tray for ear surgery

be either lactated Ringers or saline, depending on the surgeon's preference, and should be warm (not hot) to avoid trauma.

A local anesthetic agent (e.g., Xylocaine with epinepherine) is often the drug of choice, although, general anesthesia may occasionally be needed for selected procedures.

Dressings

Two types of dressings may be used:

1. Simple packing of the ear canal and antibiotic ointment.
2. Mastoid dressing (protective)—fluffed gauze, with Kerlix or Kling over the fluffs and around the head.

The choice will depend on the extent of the surgery and the amount of protection required postoperatively.

Selected Surgical Procedures

Procedure
Myringotomy

Definition: Incision into the tympanic membrane to remove fluid accumulation.
CDC Classification: II
Discussion: A myringotomy is indicated in *acute chronic otitis media.* The procedure may include the insertion of drainage tubes in the myringotomy site. In children, the procedure is performed under general anesthesia.
Positioning: Supine, with affected ear up (see General Considerations, pp. 596–598)
Skin Preparation: May or may not be required, depending on surgeon's preference
Packs/Drapes:
 Head and neck or basic pack with special ear sheet
 Towels
 Gloves (gowns may be optional)
Instrumentation:
 Basic ear tray or myringotomy tray
Supplies/Equipment:
 Small basin
 Microscope (with handgrips or drape)
 Suction/cautery (opt.)
 Myringotomy tubes (e.g., Bobbin-type)
 Culture tubes (aerobic/anaerobic)
 Sitting stool with back support

PROCEDURAL OVERVIEW

An ear speculum is inserted into the ear canal. Wax, if present, is softened and removed. The inferior poste-

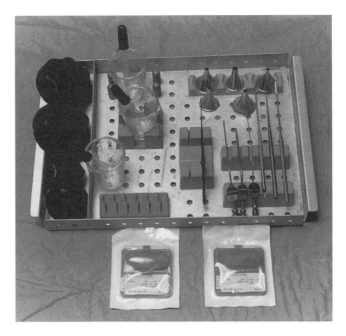

Myringotomy instruments and myringotomy drainage tubes

rior portion of the tympanic membrane is incised. A culture is taken of the fluid and then it is suctioned. The myringotomy prosthesis (drainage tube) may be inserted. A small amount of cotton may be placed in the ear canal, and a dressing may be applied (surgeon's preference).

PERIOPERATIVE NURSING CONSIDERATIONS

- Quietness and immobility of the patient are necessary for ear procedures. Careful restraint of the patient can ensure a safe procedure.
- If skin prep is required, do not allow solution to pool in the ear.
- Remove wax from curette, alligator forceps, etc., with moistened saline sponge. Guide suction tips and instruments into speculum as necessary when the microscope is used.
- Use an alligator forceps to pass the drainage tube to the surgeon.
- Follow hospital protocol for documenting an implantable device.
- The back of the surgeon's chair should be draped with a sterile drape sheet.

Procedure
Tympanoplasty

Definition: Surgical restoration of a diseased or injured tympanic membrane and/or middle ear structure.

CDC Classification: II

Discussion: Tympanoplasty restores or improves hearing in patients with a conductive-type hearing loss and may be performed in conjunction with a mastoidectomy. An autograft may be taken from the postauricular fascia.

A tympanoplasty is classified according to the extent of the disease or injury to the ossicles:

1. Malleus, incus, and stapes are intact and mobile
2. Malleus is eroded
3. Malleus and incus are absent; stapes are intact and mobile
4. All ossicles are absent, except a mobile stapes footplate
5. All ossicles are absent, except an immobile stapes footplate

Positioning: Supine, with head positioned on headrest with operative side up. Hair is secured out of the field.
Skin Preparation: See p. 596
Packs/Drapes:
  Head and neck pack
  Microscope drape (opt.)
  Plastic adhesive drape sheet (opt.)
  Towels; split sheet (for basic pack)
Instrumentation:
  Basic ear tray
  Drill (e.g., Micro-stryker), burrs, cord
  Mastoid tray (opt.)
Supplies/Equipment:
  Microscope with handgrips or drape
  Sitting stool with back support
  Power source for drills
  Basin set
  Blades—(1) No. 15, (1) No. 10
  Needle counter
  ESU/suction
  Bulb syringe (for irrigation)
  Medications—hemostatic agent, local anesthetic with epinephrine (opt.)
  Control syringe (for local) with 1½-inch, 25-gauge needle
  Solutions—saline, water
  Sutures—surgeon's preference

PROCEDURAL OVERVIEW

An endaural approach is used. The tympanic membrane (if not widely perforated) is incised and retracted. The pathology is assessed. (If a mastoidectomy is required, refer to p. 599.)

Diseased tissue and damaged ossicles are excised as needed. The ossicular chain is reconstructed using autograft or artificial materials. A myringoplasty is performed using the temporalis fascia, perichondrium, a vein, or periosteum. The edges of the perforation are separated and the graft is placed on the inner surface of the drum remnant. Small pledgets of Gelfoam or a paper patch may be used to hold the graft in place. Skin flaps, if used, are sutured; the wound is closed and a protective dressing is applied.

PERIOPERATIVE NURSING CONSIDERATIONS

- See General Considerations, pp. 596–598.
- New blades must be used on the graft.
- The graft (if not an autograft) must be used according to the manufacturer's recommendations. It should be smoothed over a flat surface (overturned basin) before implantation, and handled with smooth tissue forceps.

Procedure
Mastoidectomy

Definition: Removal of bony partitions forming the mastoid air cells.
CDC Classification: II
Discussion: This procedure eradicates infected tissue to obtain an aseptic dry ear. Until this is achieved, procedures such as tympanoplasty are not likely to be successful. There are three types of procedures involving the mastoid:

1. *Simple:* removal of the air cells only
2. *Modified Radical:* removal of air cells and posterior external auditory canal wall
3. *Radical:* removal of air cells and tympanic membrane and the malleus, incus, tensor tympanic muscle, and mucoperiosteal lining

Positioning, Skin Preparation, Draping, Instrumentation: See Tympanoplasty, p. 598
Supplies/Equipment:
  Headrest (e.g., Shea)
  Microscope with handgrips or drape
  Sitting stool with back support
  Power source for drill
  Suction—electrocoagulator/cord (opt.)
  Blades—(1) No. 15
  Needle counter
  Medications—hemostatic agent, local anesthetic, antibiotic (opt.)
  Solutions—saline, water
  Sutures—surgeon's preference
  Bulb syringe
  Eye patch (opt.)

PROCEDURAL OVERVIEW—Radical Mastoidectomy

An endaural and/or postauricular incision is performed. Hemostasis is achieved with electrocautery. The skin of the auditory canal is incised with an angled and straight canal knife. A mental flap is created and the mastoid area is then exposed with a narrow periosteal elevator and curved scissors. A self-retaining endaural retractor is placed in the wound. The malleus, incus, tympanic membrane, tensor muscle, and mucosa of the middle ear are excised. A strip of temporalis muscle may be used to fill the cavity. The cavity may be left to heal by secondary intention. The wound is packed and dressed with a protective dressing.

PERIOPERATIVE NURSING CONSIDERATIONS

- See General Considerations, pp. 596–598.
- Some surgeons use continuous irrigation. Equipment for this procedure includes irrigation solution, suction tubing, Y-connector, irrigation set, and straight tubing. Confirm with surgeon if this equipment is needed.

Procedure
Stapedectomy

Definition: The surgical removal of the stapes and the insertion of a prosthesis to reestablish the link between the incus and the oval window.
CDC Classification: I
Discussion: A stapedectomy reestablishes the chain of sound transmission in *otosclerosis*. The prosthesis used to cover the oval window may be an autologus vein graft, a perichondrium graft (from behind the ear), or an artificial prosthetic device. Part or all of the stapes footplate may be removed, and sound transmission may be reestablished using a wide variety of materials, including the crus of the stapes, Teflon, stainless steel wire, platinum prosthesis, fat, and carved autogenous bone prosthesis.
Positioning, Skin Preparation, Packs, Drapes, Instrumentation, Supplies, Equipment: See Mastoidectomy, p. 599

PROCEDURAL OVERVIEW

A tympanomeatal flap is created and the incision is completed with a Billucci scissors. The bone is excised, to visualize the oval window, using burrs or curettes. The tympanic membrane is reflected. A cotton pledget soaked in epinephrine may be used to maintain hemostasis and protect the flap. The extent of the pathologic process is assessed to determine the extent of the incision and the type and dimension of the prosthesis to be used. The crus of the stapes and the footplate are transacted and removed (completely and partially).

The stapedal tendon is cut and the remaining footplate is extracted; the oval window is sealed by connective tissue and the stapes is replaced. In a total stapedectomy, following the removal of the stapes, a wire or other prosthesis is attached to the incus and placed on the oval window graft. A dry field is established; the skin flap is replaced. Gelfoam may be placed over the flap and cotton is placed in the canal. Antibiotic irrigation and/or systemic antibiotics may be used.

PERIOPERATIVE NURSING CONSIDERATIONS

- At the end of the procedure, the surgeon may use a tuning fork to determine the patient's hearing status.
- Gelfoam may be moistened with epinephrine (e.g., 1:1000) to aid in hemostasis.
- The prosthesis package should not be opened until the surgeon determines the type and size needed.
- If a graft is needed, check with the surgeon regarding the donor site.

The Nose and Throat

Procedures of the nose and throat are generally performed by the surgeon specializing in *otorhinolaryngology*, although some general surgeons may perform a tracheostomy, radical neck procedures, or even a tonsillectomy.

Surgical Anatomy Review

The Nose

The nose consists of an internal and external portion, which lies over the roof of the mouth. The interior nose is hollow, separated by a partition—the *septum*—into the right and left cavity. The *palatine bones,* which form both the floor of the nose and the roof of the mouth, separate the nasal cavities from the oral cavity. When they fail to unite, it produces a condition known as *cleft palate.*

Each nasal cavity is divided into three passageways (superior, middle, and inferior meati) by the projection of the *turbinates* (*conchae*) from the lateral walls of the internal portion of the nose. The superior and middle turbinates are processes of the *ethmoid bone,* whereas the inferior turbinates are separate bones.

The external openings into the nasal cavities have a technical name of *anterior nares* (nostrils). They open into an area just below the inferior meatus called the *vestibule.* The posterior nares open from an area of the internal nasal cavity above the superior meatus called the *sphenoethmoidal recess* into the *nasopharynx*.

The Pharynx

The pharynx (throat) is a tubelike structure approximately 12.5 cm (5 inches) long that extends from the base of the skull to the esophagus, and lies just anterior to the cervical vertebrae. It is made of muscle, is lined with mucous membrane, and has three anatomic divisions: the *nasopharynx*, the *oropharynx*, and the *laryngopharynx*. The *adenoids*, or pharyngeal tonsils, are located in the nasopharynx on its posterior wall opposite the posterior nares.

Two pairs of organs are located in the oropharynx: the *palantine tonsils* and the *linguinal tonsils*. The palantine tonsils are the ones most commonly removed by a tonsillectomy. Rarely are the linguinal tonsils removed.

The Larynx

The larynx (voice box) lies between the root of the tongue and the upper end of the *trachea*, just below and in front of the lowest part of the pharynx. It normally extends between the fourth, fifth, and sixth cervical vertebrae, but is often somewhat higher in females and during childhood.

The larynx consists largely of cartilage and muscles lined with mucous membranes that form two pairs of folds which jut inward into its cavity. The upper pair is called the false vocal folds; the lower pair serves as true vocal cords (*glottis*) and is the narrowest part of the larynx. An edematous condition can produce an obstruction resulting in asphyxiation.

Nine cartilages form the framework of the larynx; the three largest are the *thyroid cartilage*, the *epiglottis*, and the *cricoid*. Three other pairs of smaller cartilages complete the laryngeal structure.

The Trachea

The trachea (windpipe) is a tube about 11 cm (4½ inches) long that extends from the larynx in the neck to the *bronchi* in the thoracic cavity (cervical vertebra VI to thoracic vertebra V).

The trachea is composed of three layers of tissue: (1) the mucosa (lining), (2) the submucosa (cartilaginous layer), and (3) an outside connective tissue layer (adventitia). The main structure of the tracheal wall is composed of a series of C-shaped rings. They give firmness to the wall, preventing it from collapsing and shutting off the vital airway.

At the level of the second, third, and fourth tracheal rings lies the thyroid gland. This gland is situated on the anterior side of the trachea, and is composed of

two lobes connected by a narrow bridge known as the *isthmus* (Fig. 14-32).

General Considerations

Nasal procedures, including the Caldwell-Luc or SMR (submucosal resection of the nasal septum) are performed to establish a patent airway by removing and/or reconstructing bone and cartilage in the nasal cavity and sinuses.

More extensive procedures, such as radical neck dissection, are performed following tissue biopsy through the laryngoscope or by examination of suspect tumors in the neck and mouth area, and are aimed at eradicating any cancerous tissue.

Surgical Procedures of the Nose and Sinuses

General Considerations

Nasal surgery is sometimes performed with the patient under local anesthesia with IV sedation, with or without the presence of an anesthesia clinician. Close attention should be paid to the perioperative assessment, including possible allergies, cardiac and respiratory status, and any physical limitations that may need to be addressed and planned for during the intraoperative phase.

Generalized information concerning the sequence of events should be shared with the patient to reduce anxiety that is normally present but that may be exaggerated in a patient undergoing surgery while awake.

The surgeon will often perform a topical nasal preparation before the skin preparation is performed, so a separate, nonsterile set-up is prepared according to the surgeon's preference. The preparation tray usually consists of

- Packing (e.g., ½-inch plain or cotton balls)
- Cotton-tipped applicators
- Medicine cups
- Topical anesthetic (e.g., cocaine solution)
- Local anesthetic with epinephrine
- Syringes (Leur-Lock control, 10 cc) and 25- or 27-gauge needle
- Nasal atomizer
- Scissors (e.g., straight Mayo)
- Bayonet forceps (for packing)

Positioning The patient is usually placed in the supine position, with slight reverse Trendelenberg. Arms may be tucked in at the side and secured. The patient's head may be on a headrest or a small pillow for comfort during the procedure.

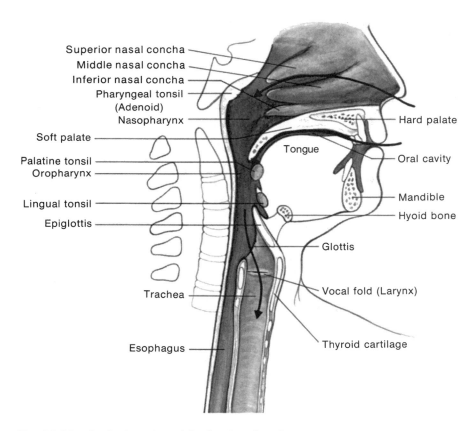

Fig. 14-32. Sagittal section of the head and neck

Instrumentation The nasal tray consists of small instruments ranging from delicate scissors and nasal rongeurs to septum cutting forceps and bone instruments. There may be two trays, one for bone and one for soft tissue, or they may be combined into one tray.

Selected Surgical Procedures

The following procedures are representative of procedures performed on the nose and/or sinuses.

Procedure
Submucosal Resection of the Nasal Septum (SMR)

Definition: Excision of a portion of the cartilaginous or osseous nasal septum beneath the flaps of mucous membrane, perichondrium, and/or periosteum.
CDC Classification: I
Definition: An SMR is performed to provide a clear airway by establishing an adequate separation between the left and right nasal cavities. The procedure may be combined with a rhinoplasty, and is often asso-

ciated with a condition referred to as a *deviated septum.* A local preparation tray should be prepared (see pp. 601–602).
Positioning: Supine, with slight reverse Trendelenberg
Skin Preparation: Check with the surgeon as to solution of choice. The face may be prepped, although the nose is considered a contaminated area

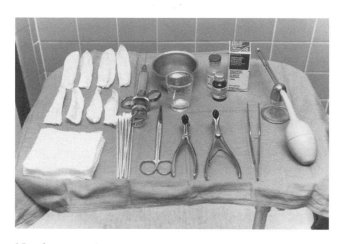

Nasal preparation tray

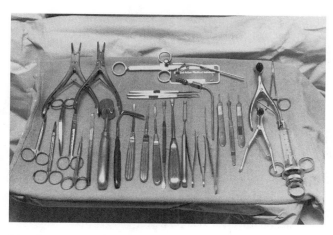

Nasal instrument tray

Packs/Drapes:
   Head and neck pack or basic pack with split sheet
   Towels
Instrumentation:
   Basic nasal tray (or rhinoplasty tray)
   Beaver knife handle
Supplies/Equipment:
   Headrest (e.g., Donought; Shea)
   Egg crate mattress
   Fiberoptic headlight and power source
   Basin set
   Blades—(4) No. 15; Beaver Blade (No. 69)
   Needle counter
   Suction/ESU (opt.)
   Syringes (2) for local nasal packing
   Solutions—saline, water
   Sutures—surgeon's preference
   Nasal splint
   Antibiotic ointment (opt.)

PROCEDURAL OVERVIEW

An incision is made anteriorly over the septum, including the mucous membrane and the perichondrium, which is reflected with elevators beyond the septal area to be resected. The septal cartilage is excised, carefully avoiding penetration of the opposite mucoperichondrium. A rongeur is used to remove any spurs from the nasal bone.

   The mucoperichondrium of the opposite side is elevated to avoid later communication that may result in a fistula. Retracting the flaps, the cartilage is excised. Excessive cartilage should not be removed, to prevent postoperative deformity. Occasionally, a cartilage graft may be placed within the flaps. A punch rongeur or cutting forceps is used to excise bony fragments of the ethmoid and deviated *vomer* (lower, posterior portion of the nasal septum).

A gouge and mallet may be used for the vomer. The intranasal incisions are sutured. A gauze packing is inserted to join the membranes in the midline and to aid in hemostasis. An external splint may be applied and a dressing is placed under the nose.

PERIOPERATIVE NURSING CONSIDERATIONS

- Do not allow the prep solution to pool in and around the eyes or ears.
- A nasal preparation tray (for topical instillation of anesthetics) should be prepared and maintained a safe distance from the sterile field.
- The operating table may be turned for easier access, and slightly flexed for patient comfort.
- A "Moustache Dressing" under the nose is commonly used for nasal procedures.

Procedure
Caldwell-Luc Antrostomy

Definition: Drainage of the antrum of the maxillary sinuses, creating a passageway between the nasal sinuses to establish drainage.
CDC Classification: II
Discussion: Chronic infection and sinusitis can cause extensive scarring within the nasal sinuses. This procedure creates a new opening into the *antrum* of the maxillary sinus, through the canine fossa, to permit evacuation of a diseased sinus and scar tissue under direct vision.
Positioning: Supine, with arm on affected side tucked; the other arm is extended on an armboard. Table is in slight Trendelenberg.
Skin Preparation: See pp. 337–338. A nasal preparation is usually performed first.
Packs/Drapes:
   Head and neck pack or basic pack with split sheet
   Towels may be wrapped around the head, over the eyelids
Instrumentation:
   Maxilla or nasal procedure tray
Supplies/Equipment:
   Fiberoptic headlight and light source (opt.)
   ESU (bipolar) and Suction (Frazier tip)
   Basin set
   Blades—(2) No. 15
   Medication—hemostatic agent (opt.)
   Needle counter
   Bulb syringe
   Solutions—saline, water
   Sutures—surgeon's preference
   Nasal packing (e.g., ½-inch plain or Iodoform)
   Preliminary nasal tray

PROCEDURAL OVERVIEW

Retracting the patient's upper lip, an incision is made just above the patient's canine tooth and premolars. Once the gum has been incised, a periosteal elevator is used to strip the periosteum from the maxilla. To gain access into the inner nasal sinuses, the bone is perforated with a chisel and mallet; the perforation is enlarged with a small rongeur (e.g., Kerrison, up and down biting), and osteotomes are used to remove dead tissue. Irrigation and suction remove debris and keep the area clean.

When adequate drainage has been established, the gingival incision is closed (plain catgut suture). The nasal sinuses may be packed with a hemostatic agent, or a standard nasal packing may be used, according to the surgeon's preference.

PERIOPERATIVE NURSING CONSIDERATIONS

- See General Considerations, pp. 601–602, for additional information.
- Check with surgeon as to preference of prep solution. Do not allow solution to pool in or around the eyes and ears.
- The table may be turned to facilitate access.

Surgical Procedures of the Throat and Neck

Procedure
Laryngoscopy

Definition: An endoscopic examination of the larynx via either flexible or rigid instrumentation.

CDC Classification: II

Discussion: Laryngoscopy is performed as a diagnostic procedure to determine the presence of disease and/or to take tissue biopsies of the suspected area. Additionally, laryngoscopy may be performed to assess laryngeal trauma, to remove foreign objects, or to aspirate thick secretions that cannot be removed by conventional suctioning methods. The use of a microscope facilitates visualization, and the procedure is then referred to as a *microlaryngoscopy.*

In a *suspension laryngoscopy,* a self-retaining laryngoscope holder gives the surgeon freedom to handle instruments while maintaining effective visual contact with the area. A carbon dioxide laser may be used in conjunction with microlaryngoscopy to remove benign lesions or early malignant tumors. However, the lesion may be vaporized, making histologic examination impossible.

Positioning: Supine; arms may be tucked in at the patient's side. The head may or may not be hyperextended.

Skin Preparation: None required

Packs/Drapes: Basic pack
  Gloves
  Drape sheet (split)
  Folded towels (to stabilize the laryngoscope holder) (for suspension laryngoscopy)

Instrumentation:
  Laryngoscope with cord (e.g., Jackson)
  Laryngoscope holder (e.g., Levy)
  Topical anesthesia preparation tray (clean set-up)
  Topical anesthetic spray (e.g., Cetacaine)
  Laryngeal spatula
  Laryngeal mirrors
  Small basin with warm water
  Gauze sponges
  Laryngeal syringe with straight and curved cannula
  Medication cup
  Cotton-tipped applicators

Supplies/Equipment:
  Bite block
  Positioning aids (sandbag; small roll)
  Fiberoptic headlight with power source
  Fiberoptic light source (for laryngoscope)
  Suction
  Microscope with 400-mm lens (for microlaryngoscopy)
  Carbon dioxide laser (opt.)
  For Microlaryngoscopy, add (if not in combined tray):
  Double-barrel scope (e.g., Jako, Dedo) and cord
  Microlaryngeal forceps (assorted)
  Scissors
  Knife
  Hook
  Aspiration tube
  Vocal cord retractor

PROCEDURAL OVERVIEW

The patient's head is tipped back and the laryngoscope is inserted. The larynx and associated structures are viewed. A self-retaining laryngoscope holder and microscope may be used. Tissue may be biopsied and secretions aspirated as needed. (It is usually more convenient for the scrub person to work directly off the instrument table rather than from a Mayo stand.)

If the carbon dioxide laser is used, a micromanipulator is used to direct the laser beam attached to the microscope. A special vocal cord retractor with suction may be used to clear the smoke from tissue evaporation. A smoke evacuator should be used when plume is evident.

PERIOPERATIVE NURSING CONSIDERATIONS

- Protective eye wear must be used.
- All laser precautions must be in force when laser is anticipated.

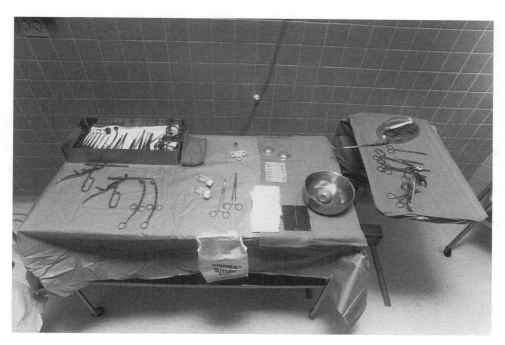

T&A instrumentation and set-up

- Following intubation, the table is turned so that the surgeon is at the patient's head; anesthesia is on the side of the patient's head.
- General anesthesia is usually preferred for a micro-laryngoscopy.
- When passing a biopsy forceps, pass with the tips closed. Guide the suction tip and forceps into the scope as required.
- The biopsy specimen should be removed with a needle and placed on a piece of Telfa.

Procedure
Tonsillectomy and Adenoidectomy (T&A)

Definition: The excision of the palantine tonsils, and if applicable, the removal of the nasopharyngeal tonsils (adenoids).

CDC Classification: II

Description: Chronic tonsillitis associated with otitis media and nasal obstruction due to enlarged (hypertrophied) adenoid glands are indications for a T&A procedure. The adenoids are usually absent in patients over 15 years of age.

In children, the procedure is relatively simple. However, the older the patient, the more fibrosis there is and the more difficult the procedure, with a greater incidence of postoperative complications (e.g., hemorrhage).

Positioning: Supine; arms may be extended on armboards or tucked at the patient's side and restrained.

The table is placed in slight Trendelenberg position. A rolled towel is placed under the shoulder to hyperextend the neck.

Skin Preparation: None required

Packs/Drapes:
    Head and neck or basic pack with split sheet

Instrumentation:
    T&A tray
    Suction/cautery with cord (opt.)
    Bayonet coagulating forceps with cord (opt.)

Supplies/Equipment:
    Basin set
    ESU/suction (bipolar or monopolar)
    Blade—(1) No. 12
    Tonsil sponges
    Medications—hemostatic agents
    Sutures—surgeon's preference
    Solutions—saline, water

PROCEDURAL OVERVIEW

The surgeon will usually sit during the procedure. The mouth is retracted open with a self-retaining mouth gag (e.g., Jennings), or a Davis model, which attaches to Mayo stand. The adenoids are removed first with an adenotome and/or a curette.

A tonsil is grasped with a small tenaculum or tonsil-grasping forceps, and the mucosa is dissected free, preserving the posterior tonsil pillar. The capsule of the tonsil is separated from its bed. Suction should be immediately available. A tonsil snare is then looped over the tonsil and snapped over the pillar, thus releasing the tonsil. The fossa may be packed with a tonsil sponge to aid in hemostasis. One or two plain catgut sutures (3-0) may be placed over the tonsillar fossa. The procedure is repeated on the opposite side. An alternative method of hemostasis may be use of a combined suction-cautery unit.

It is important to remember that the snare wire can only be used *once*, and is replaced for the removal of the other tonsil. The specimen should be separated, and one of the tonsils (usually the right tonsil) is tagged with a suture for identification.

PERIOPERATIVE NURSING CONSIDERATIONS

- The suction tip and tubing are never dismantled until the patient is completely out of the room.
- The patient is placed on his or her side before being transported to the postanesthesia care unit.
- Have ties mounted on a tonsil clamp ready in advance.
- For pediatric considerations, refer to pp. 631–632.
- Sponges and needles are counted at routine intervals.

Procedure
Tracheostomy (Tracheotomy)

Definition: The creation of a temporary or permanent opening into the trachea, with the insertion of a cannula to allow air to enter the bronchi and lungs.

CDC Classification: II

Discussion: A tracheostomy may be performed as an emergency or as an elective procedure (e.g., when an endotracheal tube is no longer tolerated by a conscious patient or when long-term respiratory support is required).

Several techniques and types of tracheostomy tubes are available. These tubes range from size five to size seven for an adult. The tube has three parts: (1) the *obturator,* (2) the *inner cannula,* and (3) the *primary tube,* with or without a cuff. The surgeon's preference card should state the preferred tube, and the circulator should verify the size and type prior to the start of the procedure. If a cuff tube is used, the scrub person must test the cuff prior to insertion.

In many instances, owing to severity of illness, the patient may require only minimum sedation during the procedure.

Positioning: Supine, with neck hyperextended with small sandbags or rolled towels under the shoulders

Skin Preparation: See pp. 337–338

Packs/Drapes: Basic pack with small fenestrated sheet
  Towels
  Extra drape sheet

Instrumentation: Tracheostomy tray

Supplies/Equipment:
  Basin set
  Suction/ESU
  Blades—(1) No. 10, (2) No. 15, (1) No. 11
  Tracheostomy tubes (assorted variety)
  Suction catheters (for trach)
  Umbilical tape
  Sutures—surgeon's preference
  Solutions—saline, water
  10-mL syringe (to inflate cuff)
  Local anesthetic with syringe; 25- or 27-gauge needle

PROCEDURAL OVERVIEW

One of two approaches may be used. The first is a transverse incision, made just above the sternal notch, and the second is a horizontal incision in the midline of the neck. The subcutaneous tissue and platysma muscle are divided and retracted using a Senn retractor. The deeper tissues and muscles are divided; the thyroid isthmus is retracted superiorly and the superior tracheal rings are exposed. An anterior disk of the third and fourth tracheal rings is excised (or incised). The end of the cannula is moistened with saline, and with the obturator in place, the surgeon inserts the tube into the opening. The obturator is removed, and the inner cannula is inserted and locked in place. Several sutures are used to approximate the skin. The tracheostomy tube is held in place with umbilical tapes (or special tracheostomy tube tape) tied in a square knot behind the patient's neck. A split gauze dressing (tracheostomy) is placed around the tube and lightly taped to the neck.

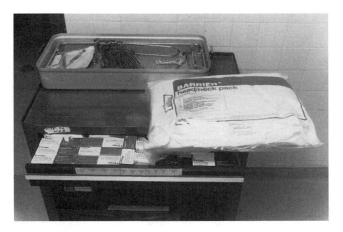

Tracheostomy instruments, head and neck linen pack, and variety of trach tubes

PERIOPERATIVE NURSING CONSIDERATIONS

- If the procedure is performed under general anesthesia an endotracheal tube is inserted. As the tracheostomy tube is being inserted, the endotracheal tube is removed. Ventilation is continued via the tracheostomy tube.
- The obturator should be cleaned and must accompany the patient out of the room. Tape the obturator to the top of the stretcher for immediate access.
- The emergency cart (crash cart) should be located outside the room.
- The tracheostomy ties should be secured after the patient's head is in normal position rather than when it is hyperextended.
- Special tracheostomy dressings may be applied.

Procedure
Radical Neck Dissection

Definition: This procedure involves the en bloc removal of lymphatic chains and all nonvital structures of the neck.

CDC Classification: I

Discussion: A radical neck dissection is indicated when the patient has had a previous tumor of the tongue, larynx, lip, or another area of the mouth removed and/or when metastasis has occurred via the lymphatic system.

It may be performed as an independent procedure, or in conjunction with a primary tumor resection of local structures whose lymph nodes drain into the cervical lymph nodes (e.g., thyroid, larynx, or jaw). When combined with more extensive resections around the pharynx and larynx, a tracheostomy is indicated.

Positioning: Supine, with affected side of the neck facing upward. The neck is slightly hyperextended with a rolled bath blanket or towel.

Skin Preparation: See pp. 337–338

Packs/Drapes: Head and neck pack
  Plastic adherent drape sheet or fenestrated sheet

Instrumentation:
  Major Lap tray
  Tracheostomy tray (opt.)
  Thyroid tray

Supplies/Equipment:
  Basin set
  ESU/suction

Foley catheter with urimeter
Thermal blanket (opt.)
Blades—(2) No. 10, (3) No. 15
Needle counter
Asepto syringe
Dissector sponges (e.g., Kittners)
Umbilical tape
Vessel loops
Suction drainage unit (e.g., Hemovac)
Solutions—saline, water
Sutures—surgeon's preference
Tracheostomy tubes (variety available)

PROCEDURAL OVERVIEW

Various incisions are used, including an H, T, Y, and double-Y. The incision site begins in the lateral neck, usually from beneath the jaw to the supraclavicular region.

The electrosurgical pencil is usually used to deepen the incision and to create skin flaps that are turned back with retractors.

The external jugular vein is severed and the deep cervical fascia is incised. Moist Laps should be available during the dissection. The dissection is continued, removing the tumor, lymph, and muscle tissue. A large rake retractor (e.g., Israel) is often used for retraction of the wound edges.

When the dissection is complete, the surgeon may elect to perform a tracheostomy. This is usually performed when extensive postoperative swelling is anticipated. At the completion of the procedure, the wound is irrigated with warm saline and hemostasis is achieved. Suction drains are placed, and the wound is closed in a routine manner. Following closure, the drainage system is activated, and a bulky dressing is applied.

PERIOPERATIVE NURSING CONSIDERATIONS

- Check with the blood bank for available units.
- Measure fluid status, intake, and output accurately.
- It a tracheostomy is required, have all necessary equipment and supplies assembled before the start of the procedure (see Tracheostomy, p. 606).

Related Procedure: Laryngectomy (removal of larynx, strap muscles, and hyoid bone)

Self-assessment Exercise 35

Directions: Complete the following exercises. The answers are given at the end of this module.

1. A cataract is described as a _____.

   Following its removal it may be replaced by an

   _____.

2. List the three basic methods used to extract a cataract lens.

3. The procedure that creates a nasoantral window for permanent drainage is called an anthrostomy (Caldwell-Luc).

   True   False

4. Which major muscle group is transected in a radical neck dissection?

5. An adenoidectomy is not usually necessary in the

   adult because _____.

6. Postoperatively, a _____ should always accompany patients who undergo a jaw wiring (arch bar) procedure for traumatic injury to the jaw.

7. A myringotomy may be performed as an aseptic rather than a sterile procedure.

   True   False

8. Describe the common usage for the following ophthalmic drugs
   a. Tetracaine HCl
   b. Alpha Chymar
   c. Miochol
   d. Mydriacyl

PLASTIC AND RECONSTRUCTIVE SURGERY

Plastic surgery deals with the *restoration of wounded, disfigured,* or *unsightly parts of the body.* Plastic surgery can be performed for cosmetic correction that may or may not be related to the physical health of the patient. Reconstructive surgery, on the other hand, is usually performed when traumatic injury causes disfigurement (e.g., burns) or when needed to correct congenital abnormalities (e.g., cleft lip repair).

Plastic surgery has been practiced for thousands of years. Artificial noses and ears have been found on Egyptian mummies, while other medical records show that the ancient Hindus reconstructed noses by using skin flaps lifted from the cheek or forehead—a technique that was often practiced, since it was a custom to mutilate the nose of a person who had broken the law.

Frequently referred to as *aesthetic* surgery, plastic surgery today is practiced by surgeons who specialize in creating something beautiful in order to improve the patient's self-image and thereby improve the quality of life.

Reconstructive surgery is largely the refinement of techniques developed during World Wars I and II to restore men disfigured by the ravages of war.

Regardless of the reasons for the surgery, however, physical appearance has always been emphasized in our society, and for this reason, aesthetic and reconstructive surgery is apt to make the patient extremely apprehensive about the outcome, as much or more than any other type of planned surgical intervention.

Categories of Plastic and Reconstructive Surgery

Four main problems are effectively treated by plastic and reconstructive surgery:

1. Correction of congenital anomalies, especially of the hands and face
2. Improvement of appearance (aesthetic surgery), especially of the face or breast
3. Resection of benign and malignant tumors that leave large soft-tissue deficits
4. Repair of traumatic injuries, especially ones involving the face, including burns, facial fractures, and so on. The goal of this type of surgery is to reconstruct and restore function as well as improve the overall image of the body.

This unit is divided into two major sections:

Aesthetic (cosmetic) surgery
Reconstructive surgery

General Considerations

Positioning, Skin Preparation, and Draping

Most plastic and reconstructive surgical procedures are performed with the patient in the supine or modified semi-Fowler's position. In some instances, the table may be turned for ease of access and slight Trendelenberg may be used.

A colorless skin preparation solution is usually preferred so that the surgeon can observe the true skin color. Careful attention must be paid to avoid pooling of solutions around or in the eyes or ears during a facial prep.

A head and neck pack, in combination with a head drape (drape sheet and two towels under the head with the uppermost towel wrapped around the head and clipped) is used for all facial surgeries. A basic pack or any other suitable pack may be used for surgeries of the breast or other areas.

Instrumentation

A variety of very fine instruments are used to perform plastic and reconstructive surgery. Delicate scissors, skin hooks, forceps, and special needle holders, designed to handle very fine suture, are part of the plastic instrumentation. It is not uncommon for the plastic surgeon to bring his or her own instruments, which will need to be processed before use.

An instrument count may not be required, depending on the procedure being performed and/or the institution's specific protocols governing counts.

Sutures

Most plastic surgery sutures are swaged to fine cutting needles. Sizes range from 4-0 to 7-0, and may be nylon, prolene, or silk, depending on the anatomic area in-

volved. For microsurgery, sizes 8-0 to 11-0 are frequently used, in both synthetic absorbable and nonabsorbable polymer materials.

A needle count is required on all procedures, regardless of the depth of the incision (superficial or deep).

Sponges

Raytec (4 × 4 gauze) is the sponge of choice since the area usually does not merit the use of laparotomy sponges. Breast surgery, however, will require both types since the area involved is deeper and wider than superficial surgeries.

Additionally, facial surgery, especially involving the eyes, may use cellulose sponges, similar to those used in ophthalmic surgery (e.g., Weck-Cel), since they can accommodate small, delicate areas.

Sponges should be counted for all procedures, according to hospital protocol.

Dressings

Dressings are often an essential element for both plastic and reconstructive procedures. A fine mesh gauze may be used for the initial dressing. The mesh may be impregnated or may be plain. Pressure dressings may be used following extensive procedures to act as a splint over soft tissue to prevent contractures. A small closed-wound drainage system (e.g., Hemovac; Jackson-Pratt) is often used in place of the pressure dressing to eliminate dead-space and prevent hematoma formation.

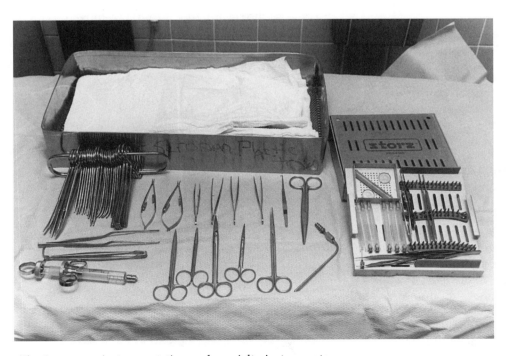

Plastic surgery instrumentation and specialty instruments

Anesthesia

Most plastic (aesthetic) surgeries can be performed under local with conscious IV sedation. An anesthesiologist or anesthesia clinician may or may not be present, depending on the type of surgery being performed. For reconstructive procedures, the choice of anesthesia will depend largely on the type of procedure and the extent of the injury.

Special Equipment/Supplies

Silastic and Teflon Materials

Many plastic and reconstructive procedures require the use of *Silastic* or *Teflon* implants. Although these materials are inert, they are foreign to the body, and special techniques must be used to prevent them from causing a foreign body reaction in the patient.

Most implantable materials come sterile. However, if they are not sterile, they should be washed first in a mild soap solution, dried carefully, and sterilized according to the manufacturer's instructions.

To avoid dust particles settling on the implant before use, cover it with a paper drape sheet, since linen towels could contain lint that may adhere to the implant, possibly causing an unfavorable reaction. Additionally, implants should be handled as little as possible and *never* with bare hands, since the oil from the handler's skin could rub off onto the material.

Silicone and Teflon materials are available in various sizes and shapes, and may be used to reconstruct soft tissue and cartilage defects. They are contraindicated for use in an infected area.

Dermatomes

A dermatome is a special cutting instrument designed to excise split-thickness skin grafts. The thickness of the graft can be calibrated by adjusting the depth gauge. The width of the graft is determined by the width of the cutting blade.

Blades may be reusable, but many are disposable; both are available in a variety of sizes. Extreme caution must be used when removing and replacing the blade to avoid injury. The length of the graft may be limited by the type of dermatome used.

The power source is either electric or air-driven, depending on the type of dermatome. If an electric dermatome is used, give the foot pedal to the surgeon, and as soon as the graft is taken, remove the foot pedal. Air-powered dermatomes cannot be immersed in water or placed in a washer-sterilizer or ultrasonic cleaner, and so must be cleaned by hand and processed according to the manufacturer's recommendation.

Additional Equipment

Depending on the procedure, selected equipment and supplies frequently associated with plastic and reconstructive surgery include:

- Bipolar coagulation unit
- Handheld (battery operated) cautery unit (e.g., Concept cautery)
- Fiberoptic headlight and power source
- Magnifying loops
- Pneumatic tourniquet with cuff
- Pneumatic power instruments (e.g., Hall drill, etc.)

Grafting Techniques

A technique frequently used in plastic and reconstructive surgery is skin grafting. Soft-tissue *autografts* are preferred by most plastic surgeons, because of compatible skin color and texture to the area of tissue being replaced.

Skin grafts are classified by the source of their vascular supply, which is essential for viability, and are categorized into three main types: (1) free graft, (2) pedicle flap, and (3) free flap (Fig. 14-33).

1. *Free Graft:* The tissue is removed from the donor site and transplanted to the recipient site. Vascular supply is from the capillary ingrowth of the recipient site. The depth of the graft is usually determined by the area to be covered and/or its purpose (see Fig. 14-34):
    a. *Split-thickness graft*—The epidermis and half of the corium (0.3–1 mm) is removed. Widely

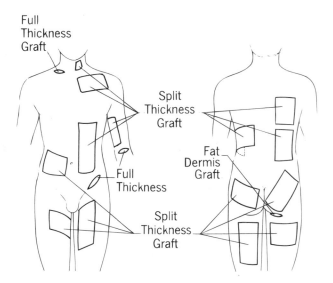

Fig. 14-33. Sites for donor autografts (Adapted from Converse, IM (ed.). *Reconstructive Plastic Surgery*, 1977.)

used to cover large denuded areas of the trunk, back, and legs. Healing is uneventful unless infection occurs.

    b. *Full-thickness graft*—The epidermis, corium, and subcutaneous fat, at a depth greater than 1 mm, is removed or elevated. Preferred for the face, neck, hands, elbows, axillae, knees, and feet.

2. *Pedicle Flap:* In this technique, the tissue remains attached at one or both ends of the donor site during transfer to the recipient site. Vascular supply is maintained from vessels preserved in the pedicle of the donor site.

    The pedicle flap technique is used most often for grafts from the palm to the finger or from the trunk or abdomen to a limb.

3. *Free Flap:* The tissue, including its vascular bundle, is detached from the donor site and transferred to the recipient site. Vascular supply is regained with microvascular anastomosis between the arteries and veins in the flap, or autograft, which establishes viability.

    This technique is frequently used with severance of digits or limbs or to cover denuded areas, restore function, or restore body contour.

    The technique used will depend largely on the area involved and the surgeon's preference related to the viability of the proposed graft.

AESTHETIC (COSMETIC) SURGERY

Selected Surgical Procedures

Procedure
Blepharoplasty

Definition: Excision of a protrusion of periorbital fat, and resection of excessive redundant skin of the eyelids.

CDC Classification: I

Discussion: The procedure may be performed on both the upper and lower lids, and may be both cosmetic and functional, since sagging skin from the upper lids may interfere with the patient's eyesight. The amount of tissue removed depends on the severity of the deformity and the age of the patient. Local anesthesia with conscious IV sedation is usually the anesthesia method of choice.

Positioning: Supine with arms tucked in at the sides. Surgeon may mark the eyelids prior to skin preparation. Table may be placed in slight Trendelenberg.

Skin Preparation: See p. 608.

Packs/Drapes: Head and neck pack or basic pack with split sheet and head drape

Instrumentation: Basic plastic tray

Supplies/Equipment:
    Small basin set
    ESU (monopolar, battery-operated handheld, or bipolar); suction
    Local anesthetic with epinephrine
    10-mL Control Leur-lock syringes (2)
    25- or 27-gauge needles (for local infiltration)
    Blades—(3 or 4) No. 15
    Needle counter
    Cotton-tipped applicators or cellulose sponges (e.g., Weck-Cel)
    Solutions—saline, water
    Sutures—surgeon's preference

PROCEDURAL OVERVIEW

An elliptical incision is made in the recess of the upper eyelid, following the premarked lines. Grasping the subcutaneous fatty tissue with a fine forceps, the tissue is gently dissected with a small scissors and removed. The upper lid incisions are covered with moist saline sponges (or eye pads) while the resection of a portion of the lower lid is performed. Small bleeders are controlled with cautery. The skin edges are approximated and closed with fine interrupted sutures. A topical antibiotic ointment or dressing (nonpressure) is applied.

PERIOPERATIVE NURSING CONSIDERATIONS

- Do not allow the prep solution to pool in or around the eyes or ears.
- A head drape should be used for all facial surgery (see General Considerations, pp. 608–612)
- The table may be flexed for added patient comfort; a foam mattress (e.g., egg crate) should be used for extra support.

Procedure
Rhytidectomy

Definition: The removal of excess skin of the face and neck area, and the tightening of underlying support structures, such as muscle and superficial fascia.

CDC Classification: I

Discussion: A rhytidectomy is often performed in combination with a blepharoplasty. As the natural aging process takes place, skin around the face and neck begins to lose its tone and will sag. This procedure, commonly called a *facelift* if performed to improve the appearance of the patient, provides both emotional and social benefits. The procedure may be performed under general or local anesthesia, depending on the preference of the patient and the surgeon.

Positioning, Skin Preparation, and Draping: See Blepharoplasty, p. 612
Instrumentation: Basic plastic tray
    Small Deaver retractors
Supplies/Equipment:
    Headrest (e.g., doughnut) (opt.)
    Restraints (padded)
    ESU/suction
    Sitting stools (2)—surgeon and scrub (opt.)
    Basin set
    Blades—(4–6) No. 15
    Needle counter
    Local anesthetic with epinephrine
    Syringes and needles (2)
    Drain (e.g., Hemovac; Jackson-Pratt) (opt.)
    Solutions—saline, water
    Sutures—surgeon's preference

PROCEDURAL OVERVIEW

The incisions are made close to the hairline or in the hair so that the resulting scars are unnoticeable. A small amount of hair may need to be shaved from the hairline; in most cases, this is performed by the surgeon. The skin and subcutaneous tissue are mobilized by *undermining* (separation of skin and subcutaneous tissue from their attachments underneath). Care is taken to avoid injury to nerves (e.g., facial nerve branches; greater auricular nerve). After hemostasis is secured, plication sutures are placed in the musculofacial tissues. Tension is placed on the flap and traction sutures are used to pull the flap superiorly and posteriorly. The excess skin is trimmed. Wound closure is completed with fine interrupted sutures. A closed-suction drainage unit (e.g., Hemovac; Jackson-Pratt) may be inserted before closure. A light pressure dressing is then applied, padding the ears.

PERIOPERATIVE NURSING CONSIDERATIONS

- See Blepharoplasty, p. 611.

Procedure
Rhinoplasty

Definition: Cosmetic reconstruction of the external nose.
CDC Classification: I
Discussion: In addition to the cosmetic effect, a rhinoplasty can be performed to alleviate nasal airway problems usually caused by a *deviated septum* or nasal trauma not corrected by the closed method. Five interrelated steps may be used: (1) tip remodeling and alar wedging (if indicated), (2) hump (bridge) removal and/or (3) narrowing, (4) septoplasty, and (5) turbinectomy.

The procedure must always be modified to meet the individual needs of the patient, and crucial to success is the maintenance of proper shape, symmetry, and proportion according to the size and shape of the face. The procedure is usually performed under local anesthesia with conscious IV sedation.
Positioning: Supine with arms tucked in at the sides. The head may be supported on a headrest. A nasal preparation is usually performed prior to beginning the prep (see pp. 601–602).
Skin Preparation: See pp. 608–609
Packs/Drapes: See Blepharoplasty, p. 611
Instrumentation: Nasal procedure tray
    Basic plastic tray
    Beaver knife handle
Supplies/Equipment:
    Headrest (e.g., doughnut; Shea) (opt.)
    Fiberoptic headlight and light source (opt.)
    ESU/suction
    Basin set
    Blades—(4) No. 15
    Beaver blades—(1) No. 64
    Needle counter
    Solutions—saline, water
    Sutures—surgeon's preference
    Nasal preparation tray (see p. 602)
    Nasal splint (opt.)
    Antibiotic ointment

PROCEDURAL OVERVIEW

The surgeon operates within the nose, making an intercartilaginous incision along the rim of the upper lateral cartilage bilaterally, freeing the skin from over the dorsal septum, and anteriorly, freeing the columella. Prominent septal lateral and alar cartilage is excised and, following reassessment, the cartilage is trimmed as needed.

The nasal bones are then *osteotomized* laterally, medially, and horizontally (if needed), and compressed to infracture the bones, creating a more normal contour. Rasping will smooth any existing irregularities, and alignment of the septum is achieved. The anterior septum and columella and the alar incisions are sutured, in addition to the marginal incisions of the rim of the lower lateral cartilage. Intranasal packing is inserted, usually consisting of a Gelfoam material or petrolatum-impregnated gauze. An external splint made from plaster or other materials may be applied and the outside of the nose is taped for additional support.

PERIOPERATIVE NURSING CONSIDERATIONS

- Do not allow prep solutions to pool in or around the eyes and ears.

- Keep tissue specimens moistened in saline solution.
- The table may be turned and flexed for ease of access and patient comfort.
- The nasal preparation tray may be set up on a clean, nonsterile Mayo tray, according to surgeon's preference.

Procedure
Otoplasty

Definition: Correction of a congenital defect that causes the ears to protrude prominently from the side of the head (*lop ears*).

CDC Classification: I

Discussion: The procedure is usually performed bilaterally, but it can involve only one ear. The procedure may also refer to the correction of *microtia* and other congenital deformities of the ear. The ideal time for the corrective procedure to be performed is usually around 4 years of age or before the child enters school, in order to prevent ridicule by the child's peers.

Positioning: Supine; arms may be tucked in at the side. If unilateral, the affected ear is up, and the other is supported on a soft headrest to avoid damage. For a bilateral otoplasty, the head is placed in an accommodating position by the surgeon.

Skin Preparation: See p. 608.

Packs/Drapes: Head drape with ears exposed
  Split sheet with basic pack

Instrumentation:
  Plastic procedure tray
  Small rasps

Supplies/Equipment:
  Headrest (e.g., doughnut, Shea) (opt.)
  Basin set
  ESU (needle tip); suction
  Blades—(2) No. 15
  Needle counter
  Local anesthetic with epinephrine (for hemostasis)
  Syringes—(2) with needles
  Solutions—saline, water
  Sutures—surgeon's preference

PROCEDURAL OVERVIEW

A variety of techniques are used to correct this defect. A common approach involves incising the skin on the posterior side of the concha. The underlying cartilage is then incised or scored. Interrupted sutures (absorbable or nonabsorbable) are placed through the cartilage to tighten it. The resulting effect "pins" the ears closer to the head. The incision is closed with fine interrupted sutures and a bulky dressing is applied.

PERIOPERATIVE NURSING CONSIDERATIONS

- For a unilateral procedure, keep the lowermost ear well padded to avoid pressure injury.
- The table may be turned for easier access.
- Do not allow prep solution to pool in or around the ear. A sterile cotton pledget may be placed in the ear to avoid solution dripping into the ear. It is usually removed at the conclusion of the prepping procedure.

Related Procedure: Microtia (using Silastic ear implant)

Breast Procedures

Procedure
Reduction Mammoplasty

Definition: Removal of excess breast and skin tissue with reconstruction of breast tissue.

CDC Classification: I

Discussion: The principal indication for this procedure is the alleviation of symptoms associated with heavy, pendulous breasts (larger than 1 lb), which can result in both physical and psychological problems. In extreme cases, the patient may suffer from backache because of the added weight that constantly pulls the body forward, in addition to possible interference with effective respiration. The condition may involve one or both breasts.

The technique used is determined by the size of the breast and the surgeon's preference. Two categories of procedures are performed: lateralizing procedures, in which no scar is left medially, and procedures that result in an inverted T scar. Proper symmetry, including nipples and areolar position, must be maintained to achieve a good cosmetic effect.

Positioning: Supine or modified Fowler's

Skin Preparation: See p. 608.

Packs/Drapes: Basic pack with transverse Lap sheet

Instrumentation: Basic plastic tray
  Freeman areolar marker
  Basic procedure tray

Supplies/Equipment:
  Basin set
  Scales (for weighing specimens)
  ESU/suction
  Blades—(4–6) No. 10
  Needle counter
  Drainage unit (e.g., Hemovac; Jackson-Pratt) (opt.)
  Solutions—saline, water
  Sutures—surgeon's preference
  Surgical support bra (opt.)

PROCEDURAL OVERVIEW

The incisions are marked, usually circumscribing the areola, which is usually left attached to underlying tissue as a pedicle graft, or removed when indicated. The nipple may be removed and transplanted. Flaps are developed that excise a wedge of excessive skin and adipose tissue inferiorly; a Freeman areolar marker may be used. The breast is reconstructed by approximating the medial and lateral breast tissue with skin flaps inferior to the nipple site, and transversely in the inframammary fold, which creates an inverted T. A bulky dressing is applied and a surgical bra may be used.

PERIOPERATIVE NURSING CONSIDERATIONS

- Keep the tissue removed from each breast separated.
- Weigh and record the amount of tissue taken from each breast.
- A closed drainage system may be inserted before wound closure.
- A surgical bra may be applied over the dressing; the nipples are usually left undressed for observation of viability.

Procedure
Augmentation Mammoplasty

Definition: The insertion of an implant behind or under the breast tissue, to increase its size.
CDC Classification: I
Discussion: This procedure may be performed (1) after a subcutaneous mastectomy, (2) on a patient whose breasts are asymmetrical, (3) for postpartum involution, or (4) for patients whose breasts are smaller than desired (aesthetic). The approach may be inframammary, periareolar, or transaxillary. The prosthesis may be gel-filled, inflatable, or filled with gel and saline.
Positioning, Skin Preparation, Draping, Instrumentation: See Reduction Mammoplasty, p. 613
Equipment/Supplies:
   Basin set
   ESU/suction
   Fiberoptic headlight with light source (opt.)
   Blades—(2) No. 10, (2) No. 15
   Needle counter
   Solutions—saline, water
   Sutures—surgeon's preference
   Breast implant (surgeon's preference)
   Surgical support bra

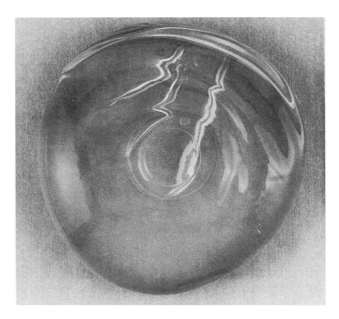

Breast implant

PROCEDURAL OVERVIEW

1. *Inframammary Approach:* The line of the incision is marked. A 3- to 4-cm incision is made just above the inframammary crease. A percutaneous flap is developed inferiorly to the pectoralis fascia. A plane is developed between the pectoralis fascia and the posterior capsule of the breast. A pocket is created by blunt dissection to accommodate the implant. Meticulous hemostasis is obtained, and the implant is inserted and adjusted as needed. The subcutaneous flap is approximated, and the skin is closed in a manner preferred by the surgeon.

2. *Periareolar Approach:* The line of the incision is marked circumferentially. The incision is made along the inferior border of the areola. The subcutaneous tissue is dissected to the inferior border of the breast. The retromammary space is enlarged by blunt dissection to accommodate the prosthesis. Hemostasis is accomplished, and the prosthesis is inserted. The inferior border of the breast is sutured to the pectoralis fascia; the incision is closed according to the surgeon's preference.

3. *Transaxillary Approach:* The incision line is marked in the axilla, and a vertical or oblique incision is carried down through the subcutaneous tissue. Using blunt dissection, a pocket over the upper poles of the sternum is created; hemostasis is achieved and the prosthesis is inserted. The wound is closed in layers according to the surgeon's preference.

PERIOPERATIVE NURSING CONSIDERATIONS

- For dressing application, see Reduction Mammoplasty, p. 613.
- For care and handling of prosthesis, see General Considerations, p. 609.

Procedure
Abdominoplasty/Abdominal Lipectomy

Definition: Removal of loose, redundant abdominal skin and underlying subcutaneous fat, and repair of the rectus muscles as necessary.

CDC Classification: I

Discussion: The procedure is performed for cosmetic purposes, to reduce a disproportionately large collection of fat in the abdomen. It should not be performed for weight reduction. A variety of techniques can be used according to the fat distribution and the surgeon's preference.

Positioning: Supine, with arms extended on armboards

Skin Preparation: See pp. 337–338

Packs/Drapes: Basic pack with transverse Lap sheet

Instrumentation:
Basic plastic tray (extra Criles/Kochers may be needed)

Supplies/Equipment:
Basin set
ESU/suction
Scales (for weighing specimens) (opt.)
Blades—(4) No. 10
Needle counter
Drainage unit (e.g., Hemovac; Jackson-Pratt) (opt.)

PROCEDURAL OVERVIEW

An incision is made just above the inguinal fold, "a W," which is extended to the umbilicus, creating a diamond shape. The umbilicus is preserved for later replacement under the flap. Dissection is usually begun at the lower portion of the W incision and progresses upward, leaving a fine layer of areolar tissue over the fascia. Each lateral branch of tissue is excised; the amount predetermined before removal so that the defect can be closed with moderate tension.

If there is a separation of the rectus muscle, it is repaired by taking "tucks" to shorten the muscle. If a large ventral hernia is present, it may be repaired with synthetic mesh. The wound is closed with heavy absorbable suture (deep fat) and a running subcutaneous suture. The vertical branches are closed first, and the umbilicus is repositioned in the vertical scar. The use of drains is according to the surgeon's preference.

PERIOPERATIVE NURSING CONSIDERATIONS

- Weigh and record the weight of the specimen.

Related Procedure: Liposuction (removal of subcutaneous fat using a high-pressure vacuum-suctioning device)

RECONSTRUCTIVE SURGERY

Correction of Congenital Defects

Procedure
Cleft Lip Repair

Definition: Correction of a congenital split (*cleft*) in the upper lip that may extend to include the palate and/or nose.

CDC Classification: I, if it does not involve the palate

Discussion: Cleft lip results from a malfusion during the embryonic process. Each lip deformity varies, but four common descriptions can best describe the condition:

1. *Unilateral incomplete cleft* with nasal deformity
2. *Unilateral incomplete cleft* with nasal deformity
3. *Bilateral incomplete cleft* with or without an adequate nasal tip or septum
4. *Bilateral complete cleft* on one side with an incomplete cleft on the other

The cleft can be closed shortly after birth, but a repair at 3 months is usually preferred. Palatal and alveolar deformities may also be present. The procedure is usually performed under general anesthesia.

Positioning: Supine, with headrest or support (see Pediatric Considerations, pp. 631–632, for additional information)

Skin Preparation: See pp. 337–338

Packs/Drapes: Basic pack with head drape and split sheet or head and neck pack

Instrumentation:
Plastic tray
Lip clamp
Beaver knife handle

Supplies/Equipment:
Headrest (e.g., doughnut) (opt.)
Thermal blanket with control unit (for pediatric patient)
Bipolar cautery, suction
Basin set
Blades—(1) No. 15, (1) No. 11
Beaver blades—(1) No. 64, (1) No. 65
Needle counter

A

CLEFT LIP

Unilateral
Incomplete

Unilateral
Complete

Bilateral
Complete

B

CLEFT PALATE

Soft Palate
Only

Unilateral
Complete

Bilateral
Complete

C

CLEFT LIP AND CLEFT PALATE

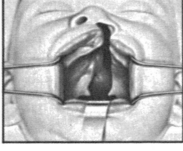

Unilateral
Complete

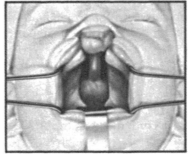

Bilateral
Complete

Fig. 14-34. Surgical repair of cleft lip and cleft palate. (A) Cleft lip repair; (B) cleft palate; (C) cleft lip and cleft palate repair (Courtesy of Ross Laboratories, Columbus, OH: Clinical Educational Aid, #11 G167, © Ross Laboratories.)

Antibiotic ointment (opt.)
Local anesthetic with epinephrine (for hemostasis)
Logan's bow
Solutions—saline, water
Sutures—surgeon's preference

PROCEDURAL OVERVIEW

A simple closure may not always be sufficient, but may permit easier restoration in subsequent stages of the reconstructive process (Fig. 14-34). To repair a simple defect, an incision is made in the upper lip and carried through the full thickness of the lip, allowing the edges to approximate in a cosmetically appealing and functional manner. The muscle, subcutaneous, and skin layers are closed separately.

Secondary repairs are performed according to individual situations a month or even a year later. Similarly, palatal and alveolar deformities are repaired in due time to ensure feeding requirements and to take advantage of tissue growth.

Postoperatively, the child's arms are restrained. The incision is protected with antibiotic ointment, and the cheeks are splinted with a Logan bow, to counter the effects of crying.

PERIOPERATIVE NURSING CONSIDERATIONS

- Refer to pp. 337–338 for special considerations for pediatric patients.
- Do not allow prep solution to pool in or around the eyes and ears.

Procedure
Cleft Palate Repair

Definition: A congenital deformity that results in a *cleft* in the hard palate, soft palate, or both.
CDC Classification: II (oral cavity)
Discussion: Like the cleft lip, a cleft palate deformity is the result of a nonunion of the palate during embryonic development. Multiple combinations of defects may exist, and in severe defects, both nursing and respiratory problems may be present.

To minimize speech pattern difficulties and provide adequate nutrition during the developmental years, repair is desirable when the patient is between one and two years of age. The repair may be done in stages, and the secondary repairs are usually performed to correct a residual fistula, to correct speech problems, and/or to facilitate dental restoration. The procedure is performed under general anesthesia.
Positioning, Draping: See Cleft Lip Repair, p. 616
Skin Preparation: None is required
Instrumentation:
Plastic procedure tray
Power drill (small), cord, drill bits (opt.)
Supplies/Equipment:
Power source for drill
Bipolar cautery unit with bayonet forceps
Suction
Thermal blanket with control unit (for pediatric patients)
Blades—(1) No. 15, (1) No. 11, (1) No. 12
Local anesthetic with epinephrine (for hemostasis)
Needle counter
Solutions—saline, water
Sutures—surgeon's preference

PROCEDURAL OVERVIEW

There are many different types of procedures for the repair of a cleft palate. All procedures use flaps raised from adjacent mucosal tissue to close the defect. If needed, bone grafts may be employed and holes may be drilled in the hard palate for suture placement.

PERIOPERATIVE NURSING CONSIDERATIONS

- For pediatric considerations, see pp. 631–632.
- Table may be turned to facilitate easier access.
- Visualization for the scrub person may be compromised owing to the anatomical area. Knowledge of sequential pattern is essential for effective assistance.
- The procedure may be performed in a semi-Fowler's position. A stool with a back support should be draped and the instrument table positioned accordingly. The Mayo stand, if used, may be positioned over the patient's chest to facilitate access to the instruments.

Maxillofacial and Oral Reconstruction

Traumatic injury to the face and mouth often requires the combined efforts of a multidisciplinary team, headed by the plastic surgeon. Injury may involve the mandible, maxilla, zygomatic bone, and soft tissue. The desired aesthetic and functional results can only be accomplished after careful dissection and reconstruction of damaged bone, and total cooperation of the entire surgical team is essential for successful results.

Procedure
Reduction of a Mandibular Fracture

Definition: The correction of a fractured lower jaw by either the closed or open method.
CDC Classification: II (oral cavity)
Discussion: Repair of a fractured mandible, like the majority of facial fractures, may require a multidisciplinary approach, including dental, nasal, and orthopedic surgery, with appropriate instrumentation.

Numerous presentations occur and all must be reduced and stabilized as soon as possible after the injury. The reduction, like any other fracture, may be corrected by either the open or the closed method. When the fracture is anterior (teeth are on either side of the fracture), intermaxillary fixation may be all that is necessary. For fractures occurring posterior to the teeth, intermaxillary fixation and open reduction is usually required.

- *Closed Method:* Application of *arch bars,* used by themselves or applied in conjunction with an open reduction procedure.
- *Open Method:* Incision into the mandible; reduction of the fracture with jaw wiring and application of arch bars.

Positioning: Supine (for both open and closed); arms may be tucked in at the sides; head positioned on a headrest

Skin Preparation:

Closed reduction—none is required

Open reduction—See p. 337

Packs/Drapes:

Closed reduction—procedure is considered "clean," not sterile; therefore, only the instrument table or Mayo tray must be draped with sterile drape sheets, and only gloves are required. A towel is used to cover the eyes and a sheet to cover the patient.

Open reduction—A sterile set-up is required; head drape with a basic pack and split sheet.

Instrumentation:

Closed Reduction and Application of Intermaxillary Wiring

Minor orthopedic tray (available)

Plastic tray

Power drill (Mini-Stryker; Hall) (opt.)

Arch bars (latex bands or other intermaxillary wiring device)

Wire cutter

Open Reduction

Minor orthopedic tray

Power drill (Mini-Stryker; Hall)

Plastic tray (opt.)

Supplies/Equipment:

Closed Reduction

Headrest

ESU/suction

Power source for drill

Open Reduction

Basin set

Power source for drill

Stainless steel wire (25-, 26-, or 27-gauge)

Blades—(2) No. 15

Needle counter

Solutions—saline, water

Sutures—surgeon's preference

Drain (e.g., ¼-inch Penrose) (opt.)

Nerve stimulator (e.g., Concept) (opt.)

PROCEDURAL OVERVIEW

Closed Reduction

An arch bar, available in precut lengths, is bent to fit the contour of the patient's maxillary and mandibular arches. The bars are attached by passing short lengths of 25- or 26-gauge stainless steel wires between the teeth and around the bar. Additional wires or small elastic bands are looped around the bars to occlude the jaw.

Open Reduction

Access is gained to the fracture site by sharp dissection through the skin and muscle layers of the lower jaw (mandible). A small rake retractor is used to retract the wound edges, and two small bone-holding clamps are used to stabilize the fracture site. Using a small drill point, mounted on a power drill, small holes are made through each of the bone fragments, and the wires are passed through the holes to maintain alignment. The wire is grasped with a blunt needle holder and twisted; the ends are cut. The periosteum and muscle layers are closed with interrupted absorbable suture (2-0 or 3-0), and the skin is closed.

A small drain may be placed in the wound, and arch bars may be applied prior to or following the open reduction.

PERIOPERATIVE NURSING CONSIDERATIONS

- It is crucial that a wire cutter be sent with the patient to the PACU in the event the jaw must be freed in an emergency.
- If arch bars or other intermaxillary wiring devices are applied first, a separate set-up is required for the open reduction (clean, sterile).
- The table may be turned to facilitate access; do not allow prep solution to pool in or around the eyes or ears.
- A method for patient communication, e.g., a wipe-off writing tablet and call bell, must be made available since verbal communication will not be possible as long as the jaw remains wired.

Related Procedures:

Reduction of Zygomatic Fracture with stainless steel wiring

Repair of Fractured Maxilla with stainless steel wiring and arch bars

Revision of Scars and Irregularities

Procedure
Dermabrasions

Definition: Dermabrasions consist of the removal of the epidermis and as much of the superficial dermal layer as necessary, with preservation of the epidermal adnexa in sufficient quantity to allow for reepithelialization with minimal or no scarring.

Surgical abrasion, as it is often referred to, is performed to smooth irregularities and discolorations on the surface of the skin (e.g., for treatment of facial cancer) or revision of scar tissue, pox marks, or pits of acne.

Healing of abraded areas is similar to that of donor

areas of a split-thickness graft, and usually by the fifth day (five to seven days), the epidermis is completely regenerated, showing signs of developing hair follicles and sebaceous glands.

CDC Classification: I
Positioning: Supine, with arms tucked in at the side
Skin Preparation: See p. 337
Instrumentation, Supplies, and Equipment:
   Dermabrader with wire brush and sanding cylinder and cord (e.g., Stryker)
   Basin set
   Local anesthetic with epinephrine
   Marking pen
   A plastic tray or selected instruments should be available. A basic pack with head drape and split sheet is usually appropriate for this procedure.

PROCEDURAL OVERVIEW

The skin is stretched by hand and the epidermis is abraded by means of a dermabrader. If the area to be treated is on or near the cheek, the surgeon may wish to pack the patient's mouth with gauze to stretch the skin taut. The area is irrigated copiously with saline during (and after) the procedure. The wound may be dressed with a nonadherent gauze dressing (e.g., Owens; Xeroform) or Telfa moistened with saline. A light compression bandage may be applied.

PERIOPERATIVE NURSING CONSIDERATIONS

- Do not allow preparation solution to pool in or around the eyes or ears.
- Table may be turned to facilitate easier access, and slightly flexed for patient comfort.
- Do not leave loose sponges near the dermabrader; they may get caught in the mechanism.
- Keep distractions in the room to a minimum.

Procedure
Chemabrasions (Chemical Peels)

Definition: Chemical peeling refers to the application of a *cauterant* to the skin for the purpose of causing a superficial destruction of the epidermis and upper layers of the dermis. After healing, the treated area has a new epithelium and a somewhat more youthful appearance.

Several agents can be used to perform the chemical peel, including phenol and trichloroacetic acid, and may be used in a combination formula (e.g., phenol, glycerin, distilled water, and croton oil), depending on the preference of the surgeon.

The cauterant acts in a way similar to surgical derm-abrasion; it destroys the entire epidermis and upper portion of the dermis by chemical coagulation (rather than by mechanical removal), with dermal regeneration occurring in two to three weeks postoperatively.

If corrective surgery on the eyelids and face is planned, the surgical procedure should be performed; at that time, only one area of the face should be treated by chemical application (e.g., forehead and perioral region), with the remainder of the face and eyelids treated after an interval of at least 8 to 12 weeks (surgeon's discretion).

Chemical peeling is not a substitute for corrective surgery, but is considered an excellent supplement for a finished look. Contraindications for this procedure generally include (1) areas devoid or deficient of epithelial elements, (2) dark-skinned individuals, (3) patients with poor nutritional status, and (4) diabetics. Since the procedure is considered *clean* and not sterile, a full sterile set-up may not be required.

CDC Classification: None (no incision is created)
Positioning, Skin Preparation, Draping: See Dermabrasion, p. 618
Supplies/Equipment:
   Chemosolution (surgeon's preference)
   Syringes (Leur-lock control)
   Impervious (waterproof) dressing tape (opt.)

PROCEDURAL OVERVIEW

The face (or selected area) is painted with the chemosolution, which burns and erodes the area to which it is applied. Small strips of impervious (water-proof) tape are precut and applied to the area, and allowed to dry. A light dressing may be applied.

PERIOPERATIVE NURSING CONSIDERATIONS

- Heavy conscious IV sedation is usually used for the procedure; therefore, constant physiologic monitoring is required.
- A PCA pump may be used for postoperative pain management.
- The surgeon will usually formulate the solution. A table containing the solutions and syringes should be created according to preference.
- The procedure may or may not require a sterile set-up depending on the surgeon's preference.
- The skin preparation solution is only used to degrease the skin.
- The circulator will cut the tape as directed by the surgeon; the tape usually stays on approximately 48 hours. The patient should be cautioned to avoid any excessive talking, which could adversely affect the aesthetic results of the procedure.

Surgical Treatment of Burns

It is not unusual for a plastic surgeon to become involved with the surgical treatment of burn patients, since a great majority of the reconstructive treatment involves skin grafting. Depending upon the extent of injury, the area in need of grafting may be limited to the skin or it may involve other superficial tissue.

Classification of Burns

One way of classifying burns is by the depth at which tissue destruction has occurred:

1. *First-degree Burns*—involves only the outside layer of the epidermis, and usually heals spontaneously after a few days (e.g., sunburn).
2. *Second-degree Burns*—resulting in injury to the entire epidermis and a portion of the dermis. The area of destruction forms a brown crust, which separates from the underlying tissue within a few weeks as new epithelium begins to develop.
3. *Third-degree Burns*—results in destruction of the entire skin thickness. Within a few days, the burn area develops a thick, black, leathery crust called *eschar*. In this type of burn, there is no possibility of spontaneous regeneration of the epithelium.

First- and second-degree burns are called *partial-thickness* burns, while third- and fourth-degree burns are called *full-thickness* burns.

Methods of Surgical Treatment

Patients with third- and fourth-degree burns may be brought to the operating room for *debridement* of the area and for dressing changes under anesthesia.

An *escharectomy*—the excision of a full-thickness eschar down to the fascia—allows more viable tissue, which is not visible, to heal. The procedure is usually not performed on the hands, face, or neck. All denuded (stripped) areas created by the procedure are usually covered with a biologic dressing for three to five days. They are frequently grafted with a full-thickness *autograft*. If sufficient skin is not available for autografting, a homeograft or heterograft may be used as a biologic dressing for a short time, and changed every three to five days.

Other operative procedures involving the burn patient include escharotomy and fasciotomy. Of primary concern is the prevention of infection and the promotion of healing. The probability of infection increases in greater proportion to the percentage of the body surface burned; therefore, strict adherence to aseptic technique is mandatory during any treatment involving a burn patient.

Hypothermia must be prevented; therefore, the operating room temperature must be adjusted to between 80°F and 90°F with low relative humidity (30 percent). A thermal blanket should be used, and all solutions warmed prior to irrigation or infusion.

If special beds are used to transport the patient to the operating room, the patient is put to sleep on the bed, then moved very carefully to the operating table.

The psychological support provided to the patient during this time is essential for the healing process to be effectual. Although it may be difficult to hide, facial expressions and body language can become a sign of rejection, so special attention must be made toward preserving a therapeutic environment by all persons involved with the patient.

Because of the nature of the burn, reconstructive surgery may be performed in stages to avoid any traumatic shock to the already compromised system.

THE PEDIATRIC PATIENT IN SURGERY

Children are not little adults, nor should they be viewed in that light . . . —E. Erickson

It is important for the surgical team members to realize that children respond very differently to their fears and anxieties than adults. In most cases, children cannot understand the surgical environment or the reason for the planned surgical intervention, and the perioperative nurse and surgical team members must approach children with an awareness of these fears, to protect the child from an experience that may be emotionally damaging.

Anxiety related to separation from the family is the child's most overwhelming feeling. They can feel abandoned, alone, and afraid while awaiting surgery, or worse, they can feel that the separation is a form of punishment for something he or she has done that was "bad." To help overcome these fears, the perioperative nurse who cares for the child during the surgical experience needs to be near the child and provide reassurance that he or she will be reunited with the family after surgery, and that the family is waiting for the child in the child's room or outpatient surgery area.

Classification of Pediatric Patients

Pediatric patients are generally grouped according to the following age groups (biologic grouping):

1. Neonate	Birth to 1 month
2. Infant	Up to 1 year
3. Toddler	1 to 3 years
4. Preschooler	3 to 6 years
5. School age	6 to 11 years
6. Adolescent	11 to 18 years

Pediatric Surgical Procedures

Pediatric surgery involves all specialty areas and is usually classified into three major divisions:

1. *Surgery Involving Congenital Anomalies:* A congenital anomaly involves any deviation from normal anatomy and/or location of an organ or any part of the body.

Mortality rates in the neonate are influenced by three uncontrollable factors usually associated with congenital anomalies: (1) multiplicity of anomalies, (2) premature birth, and (3) low birth weight (failure to thrive).

2. *Surgery Associated with an Acquired Disease Process:* Systemic and/or specific organ infections or disease, malignant tumors, or benign lesions can occur in children as they do in the adult, and like the adult, the condition may be treated surgically, usually without further difficulty to the child, depending on the pathophysiologic cause and location.

3. *Surgery Performed for Repair of Traumatic Injuries:* Accidental injury is the leading cause of death or disfigurement in children. Injury can occur during the birth process or any time thereafter, to any part of the body. It is imperative that diagnosis be made quickly to minimize long-term effects of the injury, since the margin for error in diagnosis and treatment of a child is less than that in an adult with a similar injury.

Technical advancements and a greater understanding of the special needs of the child in surgery have advanced pediatric surgery so that the anomalies and injuries that may not have been treated in previous years can now be treated with a successful outcome for the patient.

Pediatric surgery is a specialty within the field of surgery, and the surgeons who perform pediatric procedures have an expanded understanding of not only the technical aspects of the procedures, but also the unique psychological and pathophysiologic problems involving the child from birth through adolescence.

General Nursing Considerations

Because of the uniqueness of the child, the perioperative nurse should be aware of several crucial factors affecting the outcome of the surgical event. These include, but are not limited to, metabolism, fluid and electrolyte balance, temperature regulation, cardiovascular and pulmonary responses, infection, safety, and pain management during the preoperative and postoperative phases.

Perioperative nursing considerations for pediatric surgical care should include the following areas as part of a standard care plan (Table 14-2).

Maintenance of Body Temperature and/or Prevention of Heat Loss Considerations

- Transport neonates and infants in a heated isolette.
- Adjust operating room temperature at least 10 minutes before the start of the procedure.
- Use thermal blankets (e.g., K-Pad), head covering, radiant heat lamps, or a combination of these for all pediatric procedures.
- Use a soft roll or other means to cover the extremities to assist in preserving body heat.
- Warm all IV, irrigation, and skin prep solutions prior to administration and/or use.
- Continuously monitor external and/or internal body temperature throughout the procedure.

Monitoring of Fluid and Electrolyte Status

- Accurately measure all irrigation solutions used.
- Weigh sponges if significant blood loss is anticipated. Immediate weighing of sponges reduces the evaporation factor.
- Report all fluid and blood loss to anesthesiologist for prompt intervention.

Proper Use of Restraints to Aid in Position and Provide Immobility

- Use a mummy-like wrap for newborns and small infants.
- Use soft, well-padded, nonconstricting extremity restraints.
- Prevent cardiovascular compromise or respiratory embarrassment while restrained.

Adherence to Skin Care Precautions to Avoid Chemical Burns or Skin Breakdown

- Avoid pooling of solutions in or under the patient.
- Avoid the use of direct application of adhesive tape whenever possible. Use hypoallergenic tape (e.g., Durapore; Micropore), or create a double-sided tape
- Pad pressure points (e.g., sacrum, elbows, heels, and knees) to avoid skin breakdown and nerve injuries.

Avoidance of Injury Related to Positioning and Safety

- For small infants and neonates, drop the foot and/or head of the operating table to facilitate easier access to the patient.
- Avoid hyperextension and/or hyperflexion of jointed areas.

Table 14-2   Operative Standard Care Plan for Pediatric Surgery—Generic

INITIATED   DISCONTINUED
DATE: _____   DATE: _____
TIME: _____   TIME: _____
RN: _____   RN: _____

Nursing Diagnosis Patient Care Problem	Expected Patient Outcome	Nursing Interventions	Evaluating RN's Initials
Knowledge deficit related to: a. Hospitalization b. Unfamiliar environment c. Sequence of events	The patient, family, and/or significant others will verbalize and/or demonstrate their understanding of the environment, routing admission orders, and particulars relating to the surgical event.	1. Determine how much teaching will be required. 2. Conduct preoperative teaching program with patient, parents, siblings, and significant others present. 3. Relate sequence of events during all three phases of surgical intervention. 4. Conduct tour of OR and associated areas whenever possible. 5. Discuss discharge planning and home care activities specific to the planned surgical procedure.	
Anxiety/fear related to: a. Separation from family b. Fear of the unknown c. Pain	The patient will verbalize/communicate specific fears related to the hospitalization and/or planned surgery.	1. Explain to the child, in the child's language, what he or she will feel, smell, touch, taste, see, etc. 2. Encourage the child to bring a familiar object to the OR (e.g., toy, blanket, etc.). 3. Explain to the child that he or she will leave the parent(s) during the surgery, but that they will be waiting for him or her when surgery is finished. Be specific as to where the family will be waiting. 4. Allow the child to express feelings (e.g., crying, anger, etc.). 5. Communicate anxiety levels to appropriate personnel (e.g., holding area nurse, PACU nurse, etc.).	
Potential for injury related to: a. Positioning b. Chemical, electrical, or physical hazards c. Retained foreign object d. Transportation	The patient will remain free from injury.	1. Provide and monitor all safety factors related to patient care. 2. Select supplies consistent with the size of the child. 3. Apply soft, nonconstrictive restraints after child has been anesthetized to reduce anxiety level related to immobility.	

Table 14-2 *(continued)*

Nursing Diagnosis Patient Care Problem	Expected Patient Outcome	Nursing Interventions	Evaluating RN's Initials
		4. Carry the child to the OR and transport in a wagon, if appropriate age, to holding area.	
		5. Encourage parent(s) to accompany the child to the holding area.	
		6. If a crib is used, maintain siderails in the up position.	
		7. Use dispersive (ground pad) electrodes appropriate for the size of the child.	
		8. Perform sponge, sharp, and instrument counts as required.	
		9. Avoid pooling of prep solutions under the child.	
		10. Never leave the child unattended, even if restrained.	
		11. Avoid hyperextension or hyperflexion of joint areas.	
		12. Pad all pressure points (e.g., elbows, heel, sacrum, etc.).	
Potential for alteration in body temperature.	The patient will remain normothermic for age and size.	1. Adjust room temperature 70°F at least 10 minutes before the arrival of the patient.	
		2. Place a thermal blanket on the table and set control so as not to exceed 100°F, to prevent surface burns.	
		3. Utilize warm blankets, head coverings (infants), thermal sheets, etc. to preserve body temperature.	
		4. Expose only those areas directly related to preparation of the incision site. Wrap all extremities with a soft roll if not covered by drapes, blankets, etc.	
		5. Warm all IV, irrigation, and prep solutions before administration or use.	
		6. Continuously monitor external and/or internal temperature throughout the procedure.	
		7. Be aware of protocol for malignant hyperthermia crisis.	

(continued)

Table 14-2   *(continued)*

Nursing Diagnosis Patient Care Problem	Expected Patient Outcome	Nursing Interventions	Evaluating RN's Initials
Potential imbalance of fluid and electrolytes related to: a. NPO status b. Fluid/blood loss	The patient will exhibit an adequate hydration status for age and size.	1. Accurately measure intake and output throughout the procedure. 2. Weigh sponges if excess blood loss is anticipated. 3. Weigh sponges immediately to reduce evaporation factor for a more accurate reading. 4. Use pediatric urimeters when indicated. 5. Record and communicate fluid and blood loss to appropriate personnel.	
Anxiety of parent(s)/significant others related to: a. Separation from the child b. Unknown diagnosis c. Surgical treatment	The parent(s) and/or significant others will be able to verbalize feelings of anxiety or fears and apply effective coping mechanisms.	1. Encourage parents/ significant others to verbalize concerns and ask questions. 2. Maintain frequent communication during the procedure and following transfer of the child to the PACU. 3. Communicate to surgeon and/or appropriate persons concerns or questions that may arise.	

- **Never leave a child unattended on the operating table,** even if he or she is restrained.
- Restrain the child with your body, covering the patient during induction of anesthesia if necessary.
- Remain with the anesthesiologist until the child is stable and all monitoring and IV lines are secure.
- For small children and infants, carry the child to the operating room instead of transporting him or her in a crib.
- When transporting a child in a crib, keep the side-rails up at all times.

Preoperative Preparation

Preoperative teaching is most important for pediatric patients and their families. A formal program should be designed to meet the unique needs of the patient through "Show and Tell" with objects from surgery (e.g., masks for the child to play with and/or a tour of the holding area). If possible, a tour or view of an operating room accompanied by the parent and the perioperative nurse, in addition to seeing and talking with the team members in OR attire, can reduce the anxiety of seeing strange people in strange clothing.

The child should be allowed to bring his or her favorite toy or stuffed animal with them to surgery, and whenever possible let the parents remain with the child in the holding area prior to surgery.

The shave prep should not be needed except for cranial surgery or surgery in the adolescent, and because of skin sensitivity, a depilatory is not recommended.

Special Equipment/Supplies

Instrumentation

Specific instruments, designed to accommodate the size of a child, include those normally found on an adult tray. Size and weight are more critical factors; very small and delicate instruments must be used to protect and preserve anatomic structures. For example, hemostats with fine points, noncrushing vascular clamps that permit occlusion of major vessels, and lightweight instruments that will not inhibit respirations should be part of a basic pediatric tray. In addition, instruments should never be laid on top of the

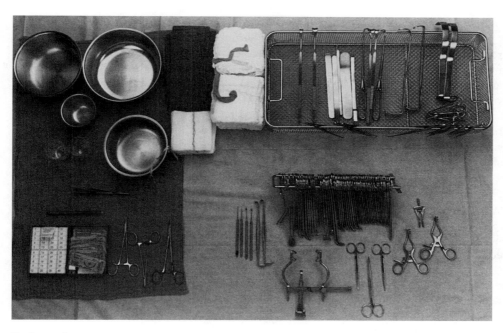

Pediatric laparotomy set-up

patient when they are not in use (which is often done with adults), since it could restrict circulation to that area or cause a bruise.

Surgery performed on adolescents usually requires the use of an adult instrument tray. However, discussion by surgical team members to determine the appropriate tray for the age and weight of the patient will provide an effective surgical outcome.

Supplies/Equipment

Disposable drape sheets without a fenestration are often advantageous, since the surgeon can create the opening to fit the proposed surgical approach, especially for neonates and small infants. Towels with small towel clips and a pediatric drape sheet may be used for most surgical procedures involving children, while adult drape sheets are usually preferred for adolescents.

Raytec (4 × 4) sponges are frequently used with small Laps or "tapes" (4 × 18) in place of the large laparotomy sponges. Dissector sponges (e.g., Kittners) are frequently used for blunt dissection, preserving surrounding structures.

The *ESU* may be replaced by a handheld battery-operated cautery unit for neonatal and infant surgery, or a fine-tipped bipolar cautery forceps may be used.

Should the ESU be preferred, a pediatric ground pad (dispersive electrode) is chosen based on the size of the patient. An adult ground pad should never be used unless the size of the patient is comparable to the size of the dispersive electrode surface area.

Sutures, ranging from size 0-0-0 to 5-0, are most common for delicate, fragile tissue. The material can be either absorbable or nonabsorbable depending on the wound need, swedged to a ½-inch or ⅜-inch circle needle. A subcuticular closure is usually performed with small Steri Strips used to help approximate the skin edges, while small skin staples may be preferred for the adolescent patient.

Catheters as small as size eight French are available if needed for neonates and infants. For urinary retention, a Foley catheter with a 3-mL balloon is preferred, and a pediatric urimeter will provide a more accurate measurement of urinary output. If a stomach tube is needed, a plain or whistle-tipped catheter may be used, depending on the surgeon's preference.

Since adhesive tape is often abrasive to young, tender skin, an adhesive spray, or *collodion,* is frequently used with Steri Strips over a small incision (especially when a subcuticular closure has been used). A stockinette, placed over the dressing of an extremity, can protect it from soil and help keep the dressing in place, yet facilitate an easy dressing change when needed.

Ambulatory Surgery and the Pediatric Patient

Since separation can produce the greatest anxiety for the child, many pediatric patients are now being safely managed as either ambulatory (same-day) or short stay (23-hour) surgery patients, depending on the type of surgery, the individual need of the patient, and the set-up of the institution.

Procedures such as hernia repair, circumcision, cystoscopy, and corrective eye muscle surgery are just a few of the procedures that can be accommodated by ambulatory surgery, while tonsillectomies or open/closed reduction of fractures may require additional monitoring and therefore a short-stay procedure may be the safest method. Either way, the child is less traumatized since separation is shortened, eliminating a traumatic hospitalization.

During the preoperative period, the child should undergo the routine preoperative laboratory studies, a medical history, and a physical examination either as an outpatient or in the physician's office, and receive an explanation of the proposed surgical procedure by the surgeon. The nursing assessment and preoperative teaching program should include home care instructions, with specific emphasis related to diet, activity restrictions, and adverse signs and symptoms related to the procedure to be alert for during the recovery phase.

Postoperatively, the child should be taken to the PACU for close monitoring until physiologic signs and symptoms are stable. The child can then be transported to the respective second-stage recovery area for observation, and any additional teaching or discharge instructions for the parent(s) can be discussed during this time. The child is usually ready for discharge one to two hours postoperatively. For infants and younger children, the criteria for discharge should usually include the ability to drink fluids and/or to urinate, assuring the full recovery of the swallowing reflex and adequate kidney function. If short-stay is recommended, a rooming-in arrangement may be available for the parent to avoid any trauma or fear during the postoperative period.

Selected Surgical Procedures

The following is a representation of a variety of surgical procedures in all services, commonly associated with the pediatric surgical patient.

Procedure
Inguinal Hernia Repair

Definition: Ligation of the patent processus vaginalis, through which intraabdominal viscera have passed into the inguinal canal.
CDC Classification: I
Discussion: Most pediatric inguinal hernias are indirect, therefore correction is accomplished by a high li-

gation of the *patent processus vaginalis* (sac) without repair of the inguinal floor. In the male patient, care must be taken to avoid injury to the *spermatic cord* structures. A *hydrocele* (undescended testicle) may be associated with the hernia, and is usually corrected at the same time.

In the female patient, the ovary and fallopian tubes may be encountered within the hernial sac. Routinely, both groin areas will be explored, since it is not unusual for small children to have bilateral hernias owing to the close proximity of the involved anatomic structures.
Positioning: Supine, with arms restrained at the side
Skin Preparation: See pp. 337–338
Packs/Drapes: Pediatric transverse Lap sheet or basic pack and sheet with small fenestration
Instrumentation:
 Pediatric laparotomy tray
Supplies/Equipment:
 Thermal blanket and/or heating lamp
 Head covering
 Extremity wrap or thermal sheet
 ESU; handheld cautery or bipolar cautery
 Suction (Frazier tip)
 Basin set
 Blades—(2) No. 15
 Needle counter
 Dissector sponges (e.g., Kittners)
 Solutions—saline, water
 Sutures—surgeon's preference

PROCEDURAL OVERVIEW

A transverse incision is made over the inguinal area in the direction of the skin crease, exposing the external oblique *aponeurosis* (a fibrous sheet of connective tissue), which is then incised. The contents of the inguinal canal are explored, and the sac is identified.

If a hydrocele is present, the sac is ligated and the excess sac is removed. The external oblique aponeurosis is closed; the skin is closed using a subcuticular technique.

If a sliding hernia (in females) is present (e.g., part of the sac wall is the broad ligament or mesentery), the sac is transected and ligated as close as possible to the sliding portion, including the round ligament. The transversalis fascia is closed over the defect prior to closure of the external oblique aponeurosis. A subcutaneous closure with Steri Strips or collodion dressing is performed.

PERIOPERATIVE NURSING CONSIDERATIONS

- To avoid hypothermia, do not start the skin prep until the surgeon is in the room and ready to begin.
- Use warm preparation solutions, exposing only the immediate area involved with the incision site.

- For further information, see General Considerations, pp. 620–626.

Related Procedure: Repair of Umbilical Hernia—Pediatric

Procedure
Repair of Congenital Diaphragmatic Hernia

Definition: Repair of an opening in the diaphragm through which the abdominal contents protrude into the thoracic cavity.

CDC Classification: II

Discussion: As in the adult, a hernia is caused by a weakening in the wall of a cavity or organ, creating a bulge or pouch. Several types of diaphragmatic hernias are seen in the newborn and usually require prompt repair to prevent life-threatening cardiorespiratory and obstructive phenomena. The most common type involves a hernia through the pleuroperitoneal canal. The goal of the surgical repair is to reduce the hernia, thereby repairing the defect. This type of hernia can be approached by either an abdominal approach, or a transthoracic approach for an esophageal hiatal hernia.

Positioning, Skin Preparation, Draping: See Inguinal Hernia Repair, p. 626

Instrumentation:
Pediatric laparotomy tray
Hemoclips/surgiclips (short, medium)

Supplies/Equipment:
See Inguinal Hernia Repair, p. 626
Add:
Vessel loops or umbilical tape
Infant chest drainage unit
Small chest tube (e.g., 10 Fr.) (opt.)
Hemoclips (small, medium)
Gastrostomy tube (opt.)
Silastic sheeting (for defect repair) (opt.)

PROCEDURAL OVERVIEW

To avoid confusion, the procedure will be described from the abdominal approach.

A paramedian or subcostal incision is made on the side of the hernia. The abdomen is explored for disease or conditions other than the hernia (e.g., malrotation, adhesive banding, intestinal atresia). In some instances, air is introduced intrapleurally to assist in delivering the abdominal contents out of the pleural space. The hernia is then repaired (a sac is not usually present) with interrupted sutures. Before tying the final suture, the air is removed from the pleural space as the compressed lung is inflated. If, however, the lung is *hypoplastic* (incomplete development of organ or tissue) because of prolonged compression by displaced abdominal viscera, a chest tube is left in place. The flap of the diaphragmatic edge is tacked down over the initial line of sutures with a second row of fine sutures. The chest tube is brought out through the abdominal wall, and the incision is closed.

PERIOPERATIVE NURSING CONSIDERATIONS

- See General Considerations, p. 627.

Procedure
Repair of Omphalocele

Definition: Correction of a defect of the umbilicus occurring during fetal development, resulting in the protrusion of the abdominal viscera outside the abdominal cavity.

CDC Classification: II

Discussion: The size and extent of the omphalocele can vary from one containing the greater portion of the abdominal viscera, including the spleen and liver, to one containing only a small loop of bowel or intestines. The condition results from a herniation through a midline defect in the abdominal wall around the area of the umbilicus.

Usually there is no skin covering the defect, which greatly increases the incidence of a life-threatening infection for the already compromised infant. In most cases, additional congenital anomalies are usually present in these patients, and, depending on the capability of the abdominal cavity to contain the contents of the omphalocele, a one- or two-stage procedure may be performed.

Positioning/Draping: See Repair of Inguinal Hernia, p. 626.

Skin Preparation: The surgeon may prefer to perform the skin preparation (see p. 337 for appropriate prep area)

Instrumentation:
Pediatric laparotomy tray
Hemoclips/surgiclip (short, medium)

Supplies/Equipment:
See Repair of Inguinal Hernia, p. 626
Add:
Silastic/silicone mesh (for defect repair) (opt.)
Gastrostomy tube or catheter (opt.)

PROCEDURAL OVERVIEW

Single-Stage Repair
The omphalocele is covered with a warm saline laparotomy sponge. An incision is made separating the skin from the peripheral borders of the sac. The umbilical vessels are ligated and the sac and rim of the defect are excised.

A gastrostomy may be performed, creating an artificial opening into the stomach with insertion of a gastrostomy tube or catheter, permitting the drainage of stomach contents during the healing process. The abdominal contents are reduced within the abdomen, and the abdomen is closed in a routine manner.

Double (Two-Stage) Procedure

When the defect cannot be closed and/or the abdominal cavity cannot safely accommodate the contents of the omphalocele, an attempt is made to mobilize the surrounding skin to cover the protruding viscera. If this is impossible, a synthetic material (e.g., Silastic or silicon mesh) is used to cover the defect by suturing it around and over the viscera. As growth permits (6–24 months), a complete repair procedure may be achieved, requiring one or two additional procedures.

PERIOPERATIVE NURSING CONSIDERATIONS

- Do not begin skin preparation without specific instructions from the surgeon.
- See General Considerations, pp. 620–626, for more information.

Procedure
Pyloromyotomy for Pyloric Stenosis

Definition: The incision and suturing of the muscles of the pylorus to treat congenital hypertrophy of the pyloric sphincter (pyloric stenosis) that can cause pyloric and/or gastric obstruction.

CDC Classification: I

Discussion: The *Ramsted-Fredet pyloromyotomy* is the procedure of choice to correct this defect surgically.

Signs and symptoms of high gastrointestinal obstruction usually appear at around 2 to 6 weeks of age, with the first symptom being projectile vomiting that is free of bile. As a precautionary measure, the stomach is emptied via a nasogastric tube prior to induction of anesthesia, and the nasogastric tube is then removed to prevent gastric contents from accumulating around the tube during the procedure.

Positioning, Skin Preparation, Drapes: See General Considerations, pp. 620–626

Instrumentation:
　Pediatric laparotomy tray
　Pyloric spreaders

Supplies/Equipment:
　Thermal blanket with control unit
　Thermal sheets, head covering, etc.
　Basin set
　Handheld cautery, suction
　Blades—(2) No. 15
　Needle counter

Dissector sponges (e.g., Kittners)
Solutions—saline, water
Sutures—surgeon's preference

PROCEDURAL OVERVIEW

The abdomen is opened through a right subcostal transverse incision, splitting the rectus muscle vertically and excising the peritoneum. The pylorus is delivered into the wound and rotated to expose the anterior superior border of the mass. Using a pyloric spreader, all remaining circular muscle fibers are separated to the level of the submucosa. Any lacerations of the gastric or duodenal mucosa are immediately repaired. After hemostasis is achieved, the peritoneum and posterior rectus sheath are closed with a continuous absorbable suture. The anterior rectus sheath is closed with absorbable suture and the skin is closed using a subcuticular technique. Steri Strips are applied with an abdominal dressing.

PERIOPERATIVE NURSING CONSIDERATIONS

- See General Considerations, pp. 620–626.

Procedure
Repair of Tracheoesophageal Fistula

Definition: The restoration of esophageal continuity (esophageal atresia) and the repair of an abnormal connection between the trachea and the esophagus (tracheoesophageal fistula).

CDC Classification: I

Discussion: Esophageal atresia, which may or may not be associated with a fistula, may develop during the first three to six weeks of life. The most common fistula occurs at the upper segment of the esophagus, ending in a blind pouch with the lower segment of the esophagus connected by a fistula to the trachea. Prompt surgical intervention may prevent respiratory and eating difficulties. It may be necessary to perform a gastrostomy first, to decompress the air-distended stomach.

Positioning: Lateral; right side up; a small pillow placed between the legs, left leg is straight, right is flexed.

Skin Preparation: See p. 337

Packs/Drapes: Pediatric laparotomy sheet
　Plastic adherent sheet (opt.)

Instrumentation:
　Pediatric laparotomy tray
　Pediatric thoracotomy (or chest) tray
　Hemoclip/surgiclip (short, medium)
　Small bone cutter

Supplies/Equipment:
　Thermal blanket with control unit
　Positioning aids

Basin set
ESU/suction
Scale (to weigh sponges) (opt.)
Blades—(2) No. 15
Needle counter
Vessel loops or umbilical tape
Infant chest drainage unit (opt.)
Chest tube (No. 10 Fr.) (opt.)
Hemoclips/surgiclips (small, medium)
Bone wax
Solutions—saline, water
Sutures—surgeon's preference

PROCEDURAL OVERVIEW

If a transpleural approach is used, a right posterolateral incision is made over the fifth rib and the pleura is entered via the fourth intercostal space. The mediastinal pleura is incised and the lower esophagus is exposed and mobilized. The tracheoesophageal fistula is transected, closed, and tested for air leaks (by filling the chest with a small amount of saline). Depending on the diameter and thickness of the upper and lower muscular wall segments, esophageal continuity is established by one of several one- or two-layer techniques.

A small gastrostomy feeding tube may be passed transnasally into the esophagus, across the anastomotic site, into the stomach for postoperative feeding. A chest tube is positioned, and the incision is closed.

If the chest is entered retropleurally, a chest tube is not required, but a small Penrose drain may be inserted close to the anastomosis and brought out through the lateral corner of the wound.

PERIOPERATIVE NURSING CONSIDERATIONS

- When transferring a patient with a chest tube, keep the closed drainage system below body level.
- Refer to General Considerations, pp. 620–626, for additional information.

Procedure
Repair of Intestinal Obstruction

Definition: Reestablishment of intestinal patency in any number of conditions that create a blockage of the intestinal tract.
CDC Classification: II
Special Technique: Bowel technique
Discussion: Intestinal obstruction is the most frequent gastrointestinal emergency requiring immediate surgical intervention in the newborn. Symptoms may include emesis, abdominal distention, and failure to pass flatus and meconium.

The repair of an intestinal obstruction may include

(1) untwisting of a volvulus, (2) division of an intestinal band, (3) release of an internal hernia, (4) resection of bowel with anastomosis, or (5) creation of an intestinal stoma. Surgical intervention should be performed within the first few hours of life, since delay may severely increase the risk of major complications.
Positioning, Skin Preparation, Draping, Supplies, Equipment: See Pyloromyotomy for Pyloric Stenosis, p. 628
Instrumentation:
Pediatric laparotomy tray
Hemoclip/surgiclip appliers (short, medium)

PROCEDURAL OVERVIEW

The abdomen is opened through an appropriate incision related to the anatomic area that is obstructed. With atresia or stenosis, the entire bowel is examined to rule out multiple areas of involvement.

For duodenal atresia, a paramedian or transverse incision is made in the upper abdomen. Bypass of the obstructed duodenal segment is usually preferred over resection. An *antecolic duodenojejunostomy* is usually the procedure of choice, in which a loop of the proximal jejunum is brought anterior to the transverse colon and to the side of the distended proximal duodenum. A side-to-side anastomosis is fashioned in one or two layers according to the surgeon's preference and size of the small jejunal lumen. The abdomen is closed in a routine fashion.

PERIOPERATIVE NURSING CONSIDERATIONS

- Separate all instruments associated with the anastomosis and follow bowel technique protocol.
- See General Considerations, pp. 620–626, for additional information.

Procedure
Repair of Intussusception

Definition: A telescopic *invagination* of a portion of the intestine into an adjacent part, producing mechanical and vascular impairment.
CDC Classification: II
Special Technique: Bowel technique (if bowel resection is performed)
Discussion: Invagination is the insertion of one part of a structure within another part of the same structure, which is what happens with intussusception. This defect can be relieved by either reduction via hydrostatic pressure (usually barium enema) or by a laparotomy with manual manipulation of the defected segment.

The most common site for intussusception is around the ileocecal valve, in which the terminal ileum becomes invaginated into the cecum. If not reduced, either spontaneously or by hydrostatic pressure, gangrene will ultimately ensue unless surgical intervention is prompt.

Positioning: Supine, with arms restrained at the sides
Skin Preparation: See p. 337
Packs/Drapes: Pediatric laparotomy drape with basic pack
Instrumentation:
    Pediatric laparotomy tray
    Internal stapling devices (opt.)
Supplies/Equipment:
    Thermal blanket with control unit
    ESU/suction
    Blades—(3) No. 15
    Needle counter
    Vessel loops or umbilical tape
    Internal staples (opt.)
    Solutions—saline, water
    Sutures—surgeon's preference

PROCEDURAL OVERVIEW

A transverse or low right paramedian incision is made and the peritoneum is entered. Manual manipulation is attempted to reduce the intussusception. Should the viability of the bowel be in question, however, a resection is performed in a fashion similar to that of an adult bowel resection, with a primary anastomosis or the ends of the bowel brought out as a stoma through separate incisions. With the latter, the anastomosis is performed as a secondary procedure. The abdomen is closed in a routine manner.

PERIOPERATIVE NURSING CONSIDERATIONS

* If the bowel resection is performed, isolate all instruments, following bowel technique.
* See General Considerations, pp. 620–626, for additional information.

Procedure
Resection and Pull-Through for Hirschsprung's Disease (*Aganglionic Megacolon*)

Definition: The removal of a portion of the colon and rectum, and the anastomosis of the proximal normal colon to the distal rectum or anus.
CDC Classification: II
Special Technique: Bowel technique
Discussion: In Hirschsprung's disease a segment of the colon or rectum lacks the necessary ganglion cells, resulting in decreased tone and reduced or absent peristalsis proximally. Because the colon contents cannot pass normally through the involved segment, the colon becomes distended, causing increased abdominal distention. Although the distal colon is more frequently

involved, the disease may encompass the entire colon. The problem may be recognized soon after birth or in later infancy, and may develop into *necrotizing enterocolitis*, which is often fatal in the neonate if not treated promptly. Before definitive surgery is performed, a colostomy may be created to relieve the obstruction and allow for normal bowel function.

The *Swenson Pull-Through* procedure is most often performed, but several other procedures can be used to relieve this condition, usually determined by the extent of the disease and the surgeon's preference. The procedure may use the perineal approach, the abdominal approach, or a combination similar to an abdominal-perineal resection in the adult may be employed.
Positioning: Modified lithotomy or supine with legs in a "frog-leg"–like position
Skin Preparation: See p. 337
Packs/Drapes: (will depend on the approach)
* Pediatric Lap sheet with extra fenestration created for combined approach
* Pediatric Lap sheet with abdominal opening covered and hole created for a perineal approach
Instrumentation:
    Pediatric laparotomy tray
    Small malleable retractors
    Internal stapling devices (opt.)
Supplies/Equipment:
    Additional Mayo stand and/or back table for perineal approach
    Thermal blanket with control unit
    ESU (handheld cautery)/suction
    Scale (to weigh sponges) (opt.)
    Basin set
    Hemoclips/surgiclips
    Plastic adhesive drape sheet (e.g., Vi-Drape) (opt.)
    Needle counter
    Blades—(1) No. 10, (4) No. 15
    Foley catheter with pediatric urimeter
    Dissector sponges (e.g., Kittners)
    Solutions—saline, water
    Sutures—surgeon's preference

PROCEDURAL OVERVIEW

The procedure will be described as a combined procedure. A left paramedian incision is made, and if a colostomy is present, it is excised. The sigmoid colon is mobilized, and the superior hemorrhoidal vessels are divided. Frozen section specimens may be taken to determine the presence of ganglia.

The pelvis is entered, the lateral rectal ligaments are cut, and the rectum is further mobilized, staying close to the bowel. A long clamp (Babcock or ring forcep) is inserted transanally, and a segment of the dissected colon is seized from within. Using counter pressure from the pelvis, the colon is everted and "pulled-through" the anus. Should the portion be too large, it may need to be excised abdominally before pulling the proximal portion of the intestine through the anus. The layers of the everted bowel are circumferentially incised, and absorbable suture is used to anchor the rim of the retained portion of the colon to the anal canal in either a single or double layer. The specimen is amputated and the anastomosis is performed using absorbable suture or internal staples. At the completion of this segment, gowns, gloves, and set-up should be changed, in preparation for the abdominal segment of the procedure.

The proximal edge of the muscular cuff is approximated to the seromuscular layer of the colon, completing the abdominal anastomosis. The abdomen is irrigated and closed in a routine manner, usually without the insertion of drains.

PERIOPERATIVE NURSING CONSIDERATIONS

- Check with Blood Bank for available units.
- Maintain aseptic technique during the Perineal portion of the procedure; follow Bowel Technique protocol.
- If tape is used during positioning, do not allow tape to directly contact the skin.
- Obtain and segregate specimens for multiple biopsies in separate containers as needed.
- For additional information, see General Considerations, pp. 620–626.

Procedure
Repair of Imperforate Anus

Definition: The establishment of colorectal continuity when there is absence of an anal orifice, and/or closure of a fistula, if present.
CDC Classification: II
Special Technique: Bowel Technique
Discussion: There are four classes or descriptions of imperforate anus:
  I. Stenosis at the anus or distal rectum—treated by dilation and/or incision
  II. Membranous barrier at the anal opening—treated with incision and dilation
  III. Rectum ends in a blind pouch above the perineum, usually associated with various fistulas. Correction will depend on the pathology present.
  IV. Anal canal and distal rectum end in a blind pouch proximally. The more proximal rectum ends in a blind pouch above the distal segment.

Type IV is rare and usually treated by a preliminary colostomy, with a second-stage repair several months later. Type III may also be initially treated with a colostomy, with definitive repair occurring around three months of age depending on the child's general health status.

Positioning: Modified Lithotomy or Supine with frog-leg–like position. A folded towel under the buttocks (to elevate anal area).
Skin Preparation: See p. 337
Packs/Drapes: See p. 630
Instrumentation:
  Pediatric Laparotomy Tray
  Hegar Dilators; Probes (opt.)
Supplies/Equipment:
  Thermal blanket with control unit
  ESU (handheld cautery)/suction
  Scale (to weigh sponges) (opt.)
  Basin set
  Blades—(2) No. 15
  Needle counter
  Nerve stimulator (for location)
  For extensive surgery, see Pull-Through Procedure, p. 630

PROCEDURAL OVERVIEW—*Imperforate Anus Class III*

Identification of the tract is accomplished using a small clamp inserted into the fistula. A perineal incision is then made in the midline of the tract. Dissection is carried through the skin and subcutaneous tissue. The fistula is identified and divided; the exterior end is not closed, to allow postoperative drainage.

The rectum is freed on all sides and the rectoanal repair is started using absorbable sutures. The rectum is opened and the bowel wall is trimmed back. Traction sutures are placed through the skin and the full thickness of bowel. Repeated dilation may be necessary as the opening may shrink in the next few months. For extensive procedures, see Resection and Pull-Through, p. 630.

PERIOPERATIVE NURSING CONSIDERATIONS

- See Resection and Pull-Through procedure, p. 630

Additional Pediatric Problems Requiring Surgery

Resection of Tumors

Tumors occur in children as well as in adults. As with the adult, the therapy considered is based on the type and location of the tumor. *Chemotherapy* and *radiation therapy* may be additional adjuncts to the planned surgical intervention.

Tumors commonly occurring in children are:

1. *Wilm's Tumor*—neoplasm of the kidney
2. *Neuroblastoma*—large retroperitoneal tumors associated with early childhood
3. *Sacrococcygeal Tumors (Teratoma)*—resectable in the neonate, but may undergo changes if not removed early. Found in the area of the sacrum and coccyx, but may extend into the pelvis or abdomen.

Pediatric Gastrostomy

A gastrostomy is most frequently performed to permit liquid feedings, allow for gastric drainage, or provide retrograde dilation of an esophageal stricture. A gastrostomy can be performed in conjunction with other abdominal surgeries, or as a single procedure. A gastrostomy catheter (e.g., Pezzer, Malecot, or Foley) is inserted into a purse-string opening created at the greater curvature of the stomach, and then brought out through a stab wound lateral to the incision.

Pediatric Colostomy

A colostomy is usually performed as an emergency procedure to bypass an obstructed colonic segment distally or for diversion of fecal material to minimize infection due to perforation. Most pediatric colostomies are temporary, but may be permanent when the rectum is congenitally absent or unable to be reconstructed, or in the case of neurologic and neoplastic processes.

Pediatric Orthopedic Surgery

Primarily elective and reconstructive, pediatric orthopedic surgery is performed to correct deformities of the musculoskeletal system. Fractures are treated similarly to adults. However, children do not tolerate external fixation devices as do adult patients, and closed reduction of long bone fractures is preferable to the open method. Tendon repairs, repair of congenital dislocated hip, repair of spinal deformities (e.g., scoliosis), and talipes deformity are some examples of surgery involving the pediatric patient.

Pediatric Neurosurgery

Neurosurgical procedures involving the pediatric patient are usually associated with injury or congenital malformation of neurologic structures. Examples include

1. *Encephalocele*—associated with a posttraumatic defect in the orbital roof or a congenital defect, resulting in the protrusion of brain substances through a herniation in the skull. A transcranial approach and repair of the dura with orbital roof reconstruction is the method used to repair this defect.
2. *Spina Bifida Occulta*—a defect in the bony canal that does not usually involve neural elements. It may be associated with a dermal sinus continuous with a subarachnoid space. Bony defects are usually not an operative condition.
3. *Meningocele*—a bony defect with an external sac producing herniation of the meninges through the defect. The dermal sac usually contains cerebrospinal fluid; however, the spinal cord remains intact with no neurologic deficits in most cases. Surgery involves exposure down to the spinous processes, above and below the lesion; opening the sac; exploration of the contents (to assure no nerve roots are incorporated); and amputation of the sac, with closure of the dural defect and skin. A skin graft may be required.
4. *Myelomeningocele*—a spina bifida with herniation of the meninges and cord into the dermal sac. The surgical approach is usually through an equatorial skin incision around the dermal sac, to preserve ample skin for closure. If possible, the meningeal sac is not perforated but stripped free of adjacent tissue down to the opening in the spinal canal to determine the size of the defect. The sac can then be safely opened and explored; the spinal cord is detached and replaced in the canal. The dura is closed at the level of the defect, then fascia, subcutaneous tissue, and skin are closed. Prognosis is usually rather poor.

Pediatric Urologic Surgery

Pediatric urology concerns the diagnosis and treatment of infections and correction of congenital anomalies.

Some form of an anomaly in the genitourinary tract can be found in 10 to 15 percent of newborns. Secondary infections are frequently associated with congenital anomalies and chronic diseases.

The most common procedures associated with pediatric urology are cystoscopic examinations, kidney surgery, orchiopexy, and circumcision.

Surgical problems particular to children are not limited to any one area of the body, nor to any one surgical specialty, but because the child is a special kind of patient, with needs that vary depending on his or her developmental and gestational age, each must be treated as an individual; with love, support, and caring by all members of the surgical team.

Self-assessment Exercise 36

Directions: Complete the following exercises. The answers are given at the end of this module.

1. Skin grafts are classified into three types. Name them.

    a. _____

    b. _____

    c. _____

2. A Browne dermatome is used for skin grafting procedures.

    True   False

3. Reconstructive surgery is also referred to as *aesthetic surgery.*

    True   False

4. An augmentation mammoplasty is described as an _____.

5. Define the following procedures:
    a. Blepharoplasty
    b. Rhytidectomy
    c. Dermabrasion

6. List the primary methods used to preserve an infant's body temperature.

7. The surgical technique used to correct an aganglionic megacolon consists of a(n) _____ procedure.

8. Briefly describe the five major concerns and considerations related to the pediatric patient in surgery.

Topics and Issues Affecting Practice

The key to safe practice lies in the acquisition of knowledge

INTRODUCTION

The pace and complexity of today's health-care setting demands that the professional nurse practicing in the perioperative nurse's role be aware of the current trends and issues facing today's practitioner. This chapter discusses topics and issues that directly and/ or indirectly relate to perioperative nursing practice and caring for the patient during the surgical experience. These topics include:

- Ambulatory Surgery Concepts
- QA: Monitoring the Effectiveness of Care
- Perioperative Nursing Education Process
- Perioperative Nursing Research

AMBULATORY SURGERY CONCEPTS

Introduction

During the 1980s, ambulatory health care and surgical procedures have undergone a veritable explosion in popularity and the range of services provided. In fact,

patient visits have increased in such numbers that both free-standing *same-day SurgiCenters* have been opening all across the country, and many hospitals/agencies offer ambulatory surgery (outpatient surgery) for an increased number of procedures that once required in-patient hospitalization.

The original concepts of ambulatory surgery are as old as history itself. Recorded ancient history of medicine, surgery, and nursing describes a process by which the sick visited special houses and temples to seek a cure, either medically or surgically, then returned home to recover.

In the early 1900s, one of the earliest reports of ambulatory surgery patients came from Scotland, where hemorrhoidectomies and other procedures were performed on both adults and children.

In 1986, an important milestone was reached regarding the ambulatory surgery units/facilities. *Standards of care* were developed and monitored by accreditation agencies in order to evaluate and improve the quality of health care provided in this area, and, to this end, a separate chapter, now a separate Manual, was written by the Joint Commission Organization (JCAHO). It outlines the specific aspects of care to be provided, staffing, physical plant, and the types of patients recommended for this service.[1]

In the 1995 *Ambulatory Health Care Standards Manual*, the table of contents[2] consists of 14 separate chapters, including QA; Medical Records; Surgical and Anesthesia Services; Teaching, Education, Research; and ancillary services associated with this unique service. As with any health-care service, evaluation, education, and consultation are vital elements for improving the quality of care. These elements, coupled with the commitment of dedicated professionals, provide the foundation for a successful ambulatory care program for those seeking this mode of treatment and nursing care.

Settings for Ambulatory Surgery

There are four kinds of ambulatory surgery settings: (1) the integrated or hospital affiliated model, (2) the separated facility, (3) the satellite facility, and (4) the free-standing facility.

In the *integrated model*, a hospital develops a formal ambulatory surgery program that is incorporated into an existing inpatient surgery program. Approximately 80 percent of outpatient surgery is performed in this setting.

The second, the *separated model*, can either be within the hospital itself, or on the grounds of the hospital, with dedicated ORs specifically for ambulatory surgery procedures, rather than a dual purpose as in the integrated model.

The *satellite model* is a facility separated from the hospital, yet linked in name and/or organizational structure. It may be close to the main facility, or in an area that requires medical/surgical services, yet is too small to merit a full hospital service.

The fourth kind is the *independent* or *free-standing* model. This facility is not affiliated with any hospital or health-care agency. It may have been started by a group of surgeons who deal in one specialty, for example, plastic surgery, ophthalmology, etc. This concept was brought to the attention of the public in the 1970s when Wallace Reed and John Ford, both anesthesiologists, opened their *SurgiCenter* in Phoenix, Arizona. It is this model that has been used to design and facilitate ambulatory surgery across the country.

Advantages of Ambulatory Surgery

There are several advantages of ambulatory surgery that have impact on current health care and the patient population seeking the service. These advantages include, but are not limited to, (1) decreased cost to the patient and institution, (2) increased bed availability for seriously ill patients, (3) decreased risk of acquiring a nosocomial infection during the perioperative period, and (4) less disruption to the patient's personal life, resulting in decreased psychological stress associated with the hospital experience.

Patient Selection Recommendations

It has been suggested by many members of the medical and surgical community that the requirements and patient selection for ambulatory surgery procedures should include:[3]

1. an operation of 60–90 minutes or less with minimal bleeding; procedures that have minor physiologic and psychological derangements;
2. procedures for patients who are expected to have minimal postoperative complications;
3. patients who are in good health (*ASA Classification I or II*);
4. reliable patients and support systems, for example, family and significant others (SO), willing to follow pre- and postoperative instructions;
5. patients who psychologically accept the ambulatory surgery concept;
6. cooperative surgeons, anesthesiologists, and nursing personnel.

Recommended Surgical Procedures

What kinds of procedures can be performed safely and efficiently on an ambulatory basis? In a survey conducted in 1989, of the 10 most frequently performed procedures in the United States, 7 of these would be appropriate for ambulatory surgery implementation:[4] biopsies, dilation and curettage, excision of skin lesions, tubal ligations, cataract extraction, inguinal herniorrhaphy, and diagnostic urologic procedures (e.g., cystourethroscopy). Additionally, miscellaneous orthopedic, ENT, and plastic surgeries are frequently performed on an outpatient basis. (See Table 15-1.) Today, that list has increased considerably, to include most general, gynecologic, and urologic procedures in addition to those already listed.

PERIOPERATIVE NURSING CONSIDERATIONS

The perioperative nurse's role, that of caring for the patient during the preoperative, intraoperative, and postoperative phases of surgical intervention, can be optimally practiced in the ambulatory surgery setting. The *Standards and Recommended Practices*, established

Table 15-1 Commonly Performed Outpatient Procedures

Gynecology	Thoracic surgery	General surgery
Conization of cervix	Esophageal dilatation	Breast biopsy
Dilation and curettage	Pacemaker battery replacement	Laryngoscopy
Salpingectomy	Neurosurgery	Esophagoscopy
Hymenal ring lesion excision	Carpal tunnel release	Gastroscopy
Salpingogram	Median nerve decompression	Endoscopy
Therapeutic abortion	Ulnar nerve transfer	Node biopsies
Tubal ligation	Dental/oral surgery	Herniorrhaphy
Hymenotomy	Dental extraction	Lipoma removal
Exam under anesthesia	Curettage of maxilla	Nevus removal
Culdoscopy	Intraoral biopsy	Lesion excision
Vaginoplasty	Closed reduction jaw fracture	Polyp excision
Minilaparotomy	Otolaryngology	Bronchoscopy
Bartholin cyst excision	Nasopharyngoscopy	Brachial arteriogram
Orthopedic surgery	Nasal septum repair	Pilonidal cyst excision
Arthroscopy	Otoplasty	Debridement
Nail removal	Tonsillectomy and adenoidectomy	Hemorrhoidectomy
Cast change	Adenoidectomy	Abscess incise and drain
Ligament repair	Bronchoscopy, laryngoscopy	Sigmoidoscopy
Metacarpal wire removal	Nasal fracture reduction	Urology
Plate (bone) removal	Foreign body removed from ear	Cystogram and pyelogram
Ganglion excision	Plastic surgery	Biopsy bladder tumor
Ulnar nerve transplant	Augmental mammoplasty	Transurethral resection
Median nerve decompression	Nose reduction	Circumcision
Release Dequervains hand	Blepheroplasty	Vasectomy
Release Dupuytren contracture	Skin grafts	Cystoscopy
Release trigger thumb	Redundant tissue removal	Orchiectomy
Fracture reduction	Basal cell carcinoma excision	Prostate biopsy
Bunionectomy	Contracture release	Testicular biopsy
Excision exostosis	Ganglionectomy	
Bursa removal	Otoplasty	
Tendon repair	Scar revision	
Ophthalmology	Tendon repair	
Eye cyst excision		
Exam under anesthesia		
Cataract procedures		
Ptosis		
Tear duct probe		
Enucleation		
Eyelid surgery		
Eye muscle surgery		
Chalazion		
Iridectomy		

Adapted from Katz, R. Issues in outpatient surgery, *Sem Anesth* v:258, 1987.

by AORN, are the same, except that the entire process takes place over a shorter period of time. In any event, the nursing practice requires the same commitment to quality patient care as that required in a traditional hospital setting.

Perioperative nursing practice, involving the ambulatory patient in what ever type of model or setting, is just as intense varied, and specialized as in the hospital, and includes all services and phases of surgical intervention. The nurse working in this setting must be flex-ible, capable of working in any setting, able to perform as a team member, and qualified to perform nursing activities with minimal direct supervision. All nurses working in this setting should be cross-trained for all areas, and continuing education and staff development programs should be ongoing, since the quality of patient care is of primary importance, and changes in technology, methods, and techniques present a constant challenge.

Ambulatory surgery is a safe and effective alternative for the patient requiring surgery if performed properly and patient selection is carefully observed. As innovative ways to provide low-cost, high-quality health care are explored, ambulatory surgery will increase in popularity and gain importance as one of the most valuable resources to both the patient and the health-care system.

QUALITY IMPROVEMENT: MONITORING THE EFFECTIVENESS OF CARE

What Is Quality Improvement?

Let's define the words *quality* and *improvement* in order to gain a better understanding of the merit of a *quality improvement program.*

- *Quality* a characteristic or attribute that states excellence or superior degree; related to a grade of excellence
- *Improvement* an act or process that enhances the value or excellence of actions taken

Quality improvement, therefore, could be described as a process intended to ensure a level of excellence by comparing current practices to established standards to promote and maintain quality of care.

Historical Overview

Florence Nightingale first expressed concern for quality patient care in 1858 when she wrote about her findings of living conditions of the British soldier during the Crimea War, and subsequently compared the mortality rate of the armed forces with the mortality rate of the civilian population. As part of her report, she concluded that a major problem, directly related to deplorable living conditions of the army, contributed to the high mortality rate, and suggested that immediate action be taken to correct the situation by instituting stricter housekeeping codes and sanitation practices. Through planned interventions (action), a change began to emerge within the health-care environment, including basic reforms, attitudes, and practices designed to improve the quality of patient care.

In 1863, after her major reform programs had been in practice for some time, Ms. Nightingale turned her attention to the surgical "theater," and proposed the keeping of a *log of circumstances* surrounding surgical procedures and the related patient outcomes. The purpose of this log was to monitor the quality of patient care and find new ways for improving the quality of care, thus decreasing the mortality and morbidity rate

associated with surgery. And so, the first quality assurance (QA) program for surgery was created. Since that time, QA programs have become the "watch-dog" of the medical and nursing professions, ensuring the public trust by monitoring and evaluating the *major aspects of care* within the health-care environment, including the performance of those persons and services directly or indirectly involved with the patient/client.

Continuous Quality Improvement: Concepts to Practice

In 1965, the federal government created the Professional Standards Review Organization (PSRO). This body consisted of physicians, and was charged by the government to monitor the quality of care, services, and costs provided by institutions serving the public. In 1957, the Joint Commission on Accreditation of Hospitals (JCAH) was established by the government to take over the monitoring activities through a process known as "accreditation." All hospitals and institutions wishing to receive or currently receiving federal subsidy had to be accredited by JCAH in order to continue to receive their allotted funding.

By 1979, QA standards were incorporated into the accreditation process as a means to protect the public from unsafe practices. Thus began the process of creating QA plans for all areas and all settings of health care.

Medical and nursing QA programs were also established to conduct QA audits on major aspects of care, and these audits became the major component of the evaluation (accreditation) process, as stated in the Accreditation Manual:

> There shall be evidence of a well defined, organized program, designed to enhance patient care through ongoing assessment of the important aspects of care, and the correction of identified problems.
> *(JCAHO Manual, 1990)*

In 1986, the JCAHO, as it was now called, began to look at quality assurance programs in a different light—not what was bad and how to fix it, but rather what was good and how to improve it. This new approach became known in health care as *continuous quality improvement,* or CQI.

The purpose or goal of this program is to examine the health care provided, identify problems or opportunities to improve the quality and appropriateness of care, and ultimately improve the overall quality of care. Patient outcomes became, and are, the buzz word since they directly reflect how the patient responded to the interventions provided by the health-care team and/or the institution.

Quality Improvement Standards: Perioperative Nursing

I. Assign responsibility for maintaining and evaluating activities

II. Delineate the scope of patient-care activities or services

III. Identify important aspects impacting the quality of patient care

IV. Identify quality indicators for each important aspect of care

V. Establish thresholds for evaluation of indicators

VI. Collect and organize data for evaluation

VII. Evaluate care based on cumulative data

VIII. Take actions to improve care and services

IX. Assess the effectiveness of action(s) and document outcomes

X. Communicate relevant information to organization-wide quality improvement program

Source: AORN, Standards and recommended practices, Denver, CO: The Association, 1995, Pp. 116–121.

In accordance with the new "agenda for change" initiated by JCAHO, AORN, in 1990, developed the Quality Improvement Standards for Perioperative Nursing to be used as a guide to promote continuous quality improvement throughout the perioperative period. These standards are based on the 10-point plan suggested by JCAHO.

JCAHO Monitoring Characteristics

Seven characteristics, established by the Joint Commission, formulated the initial investigation program, and are still applicable today when reviewing the QA program and activities. The QA activities:

1. are planned, systematic, and ongoing.
2. are comprehensive in scope.
3. are based on *indicators* and *criteria* that the department, service, or staff agree on, and that are acceptable to the organization/institution.

Indicator: signs, symptoms, events, or occurrences that may signal potential problems (red flag)
Criteria: key elements of care that, if met, reflect compliance to a pre-established standard

4. are accomplished by routine collection and periodic evaluation of the collected data.

5. result in appropriate actions to solve identified problems, or take other identified opportunities to improve patient care.
6. are continual and concurrent in an effort to ensure that improvements in care and performance are maintained.
7. result in information delivered from the monitors, and evaluation data, which are within the institution on a routine basis.

Four Essential Components for QA Programs

In order for a QA program to be effective, the design of the program should contain four essential elements or components.

Setting/Stating Program Objectives

QA begins with the establishment of goals and objectives. These goals and objectives will form the foundation of the QA program at all levels. The goals are usually derived from standards.

Goal: is written in futuristic terms; it is broad in definition, and gives direction for the program
Standard: defines how the attainment of the goal will occur and is stated in present tense

EXAMPLES: Management Goals for the Department of Surgery Performance Standards: Circulating Nurse

Promoting Quality: Quality Investment (QI)

The quality of a person's performance is related to his or her own standards of performance, skills in attaining them, and the support systems that reward acceptable performance.

EXAMPLES: Staff Development/Skills Training Programs
Continuing Education—Products, Technology, Personnel
Employee Performance Appraisals
Preventative Maintenance Programs
Product Evaluation Task Force
Development of positions/programs that may lead to recruitment/retention, for example, Perioperative Nursing Internship Program

Activity Monitoring

Performances should be monitored by *quality control* and *quality supervision.*

Quality Control: concurrent systems of performance monitoring and remediation when needed.

EXAMPLE: Occurrence Screening

Consists of a concurrent review of the intraoperative record or chart to identify deviations from the required procedure of documentation

Nursing Audits

Usually focuses on current clinical practice. Identifies potential or actual problems. The audits should include solutions for correction and be concurrent, requiring a follow-up for comparison.

Quality Supervision: Supervisory rounds and *incident tracking* are two formats of current monitoring, conducted and reviewed by the supervisor (nurse manager). Supervisory rounds (inspection) can encourage and maintain a high standard of performance through visibility. Incident tracking can determine if there are any trends or recurrent problems and devise the necessary action(s) or recommendations to correct the identified problems. Follow-up audits maintain the concurrent format.

Performance Assessment

Performances should undergo periodic assessment and evaluation, using the pre-established standards and corrective counseling as needed. Three aspects should be considered: (1) quality review, (2) quality evaluation, and (3) quality approval.

1. *Quality Review:* analysis of performance of employee and system, and retrospective audits that indicate the quality of care; review of previous performances; trending of actions (if any)
2. *Quality Evaluation:* audits conducted on a regular basis with follow-up as needed. Audits are criteria-based measurements of performance based on objective data; can be based on outcome standards and/or include medical audits (e.g., Physicians' Survey)
3. *Quality Approval:* retrospective survey as to performance of personnel and system from others, for example, patients, hospital personnel, or outside agencies

Implementing QA Programs in Surgery

Selecting a Sample Size

The number of audits conducted must be representative of the care provided by the department and the individual practitioners. This requires an adequate sample size, requiring reasonable homogeneous patient population in order to provide reliable and accurate results.

One of the best sampling techniques, applicable to most studies, is that of *random selection.* This method ensures that all patients in the target population have an equal chance to be included in the study. Random selection can be accomplished by either (1) drawing a patient's number or name from the proposed surgical schedule until the predetermined number has been attained, or (2) selecting one specific day to include all patients within that day.

Another method is called *systematic sampling,* which is accomplished by the selection of a predetermined number (nth patient). For example, if you want to audit 10% of the population, every 10th patient would be audited. To adequately evaluate patients from all services, systematic sampling may be required. Additionally, the person coordinating the QA program and those collecting the data should discuss the feasibility of conducting the audits on the other shifts, weekends, and so forth.

Establishment of Thresholds (Compliance Factor)

Thresholds are pre-established levels of performance related to each indicator created. Thresholds are used to initiate the evaluation of *important aspects of care.* They can be applied to a series of cases, events, or items, and fall into four categories of activities:

1. **High Risk**—exposure to chance of injury to patient and/or staff.

Established Threshold—100% or 0%
Examples include, but are not limited to:
Counts; Electrosurgical Safety; Laser Management Usage of Tourniquets; Positioning, etc.

2. **High Volume**—routine tasks which are performed on a daily basis. Usually coordinated with standards of performance.

Established Threshold—85%–95%
Examples include, but are not limited to:
Performing Surgical Skin Prep; Documentation; Creation, Maintaining, and Termination of Sterile Field; Use of Special Equipment, etc.

3. **Low Volume**—those instances or practices which rarely occur or never occur. Related to pre-established protocols/procedures

Criteria Development Sheet (Structure/Process Review)

PURPOSE: To develop review criteria from existing nursing standards for use in performing a structure/process audit or concurrent monitor. The results will be used to improve nursing performance, systems function, and patient care.

USE: Complete prior to beginning any Structure or Process review. May be completed by group process or an individual and then posted for approval by all area staff. The form should accompany each review completed.

TOPIC: ELECTROSURGICAL SAFETY MANAGEMENT

CRITERIA SOURCE: Protocol—Electrosurgical Safety Management

CRITERIA TYPE: Structure   Process

DATA RETRIEVAL METHOD: Chart Review   Observation (Staff/Patient)   Interview (Staff/Patient)
Other:

Elements	Compliance Goal (%)	Exceptions	Constitutes Compliance
1. Performance of preprocedural inspection of unit/accessory items	98	None	1. Prior to each use of the ESU, the unit is inspected and tested according to protocol.
2. Management of dispersive electrode (ground pad)	100	None	2. Selection of proper ground pad and site meets acceptable criteria: a. size appropriate to patient size b. site clean and dry c. site over large muscle mass d. maintains uniform body contact e. site rechecked if patient is repositioned f. site recorded on intraoperative record g. postoperative inspection and documentation of site appearance
3. Management of active electrode (hand piece)	100	None	3. Active electrode is properly used during procedure. a. cord length is adequate and flexible to reach operative site and generator without undue stress b. tip is kept clean and free of crusting blood/tissue c. tip is securely mounted in insertion site and checked before use d. active electrode is stored properly between usages e. if electrode not functioning properly, corrective action is taken
4. Termination of use	98	None	4. At conclusion of case, ESU is cleaned and stored according to protocol.

Source: Broward General Medical Center, Ft. Lauderdale Department of Surgical Services, Ft. Lauderdale, FL, 1991.

Established Thresholds—100%–0%
Examples include, but are not limited to:
 Death in the OR; Management of Malignant
 Hyperthermia Crisis; Cardiac Arrest, etc.

4. **General**—these activities are constant and never change. They usually coincide with standards of practice.

Established Thresholds—85%–95%
Examples include, but are not limited to:
 Aseptic Technique; OR Attire; Traffic Control;
 Employee Guidelines (Behavior)

The following pages provide an example of a *criteria development sheet* outlining one example of a QA study specifically designed for surgery.

Nursing Management and QA Programs

A successful QA program needs the cooperation and promotion of all members of the surgical staff, including management. By participating in the selection of the person(s) who will aide in the program design and selection of topics, the nurse manager can demonstrate a commitment to quality assurance while establishing an environment conducive to quality patient care.

During the planning stage, certain tasks should be performed by all members selected (volunteered) to be part of the *QA Committee for Surgery.*

1. Review the existing program
   - Determine the strengths and weaknesses of the current activities and develop a plan that can
   - Correct the weaknesses while retaining the existing strengths.
2. Designate the time for development and implementation of program activities.
   - Review the goals and objectives of the program and
   - Determine how the components fit into the three categories of nursing standards.
   STRUCTURE STANDARDS
   - People; Equipment; Environment
   PROCESS STANDARDS
   - Protocols; Procedures; Standards of Care
   OUTCOME STANDARDS
   - Quality of Results; Productivity; Patient/ Client Satisfaction
3. Selection and/or appointment of responsible person(s) for QA activities and unit-based QA committee
   - Members should include Management Staff (AHN; Team Leaders); Staff Nurses; Clinical Nurse Specialist/Educator

4. Assess changes that need to be made in order to reflect actual or current activities
   - As policies/protocols change, so too should the QA monitors, criteria, evaluation tools
5. Plan activities to create acceptance and recognize achievement of QA program
   - Staff input is vital for a dynamic program. Report studies and findings at staff meetings; ask for ways of improving findings if needed. Meetings should involve all staff members, not just nurses.

Credentialing and QA Programs

As a profession matures, it recognizes the need to be accountable for its actions by assuring the competence of the practitioner. Credentialing through licensing, as mandated by the state board of nursing, is one way of assuring the quality of nursing practice within the institution and the profession.

Certification in nursing has developed as a mechanism to provide formal recognition for excellence in the practice of nursing. ANA and AORN recognize the validity of certification, and are conducting programs to raise the level of nursing practice to one of excellence. Voluntary certification in one's speciality field, such as CNOR, is one example of this process.

Accountability is no longer a luxury, but a demand by consumers of all health-care services. It is required by federal legislation (e.g., HRS, JCAHO), and is mandated by the profession. Self-regulation and accountability are the hallmarks of a mature profession. QA programs can assist in this assurance of quality as the nursing profession expands its potential.

PERIOPERATIVE NURSING EDUCATIONAL PROCESS

GIVE a man a fish, and you feed him for a day; TEACH a man to fish and you feed him for a lifetime
—author unknown

The perioperative nursing educational process spans a vast area of educational programs and learning needs. These educational needs can be as simple as providing continuing education of new products and techniques for existing staff to a more in-depth educational offering such as an internship program for entry-level practitioners.

According to the AORN Standards for Administrative Practice (1995), "Staff development programs shall be provided for operating room personnel."[4] These programs include orientation for new employees, scientific and technical product updates, professional development programs, or programs designed to enhance the practice of perioperative nursing. Regardless of the type, one aim is always constant—to expand existing knowledge and skill thereby providing comprehensive patient care, in a safe, therapeutic environment, for both patient and staff.

The Educational Process: A Continuum

Nurses and students alike come into the perioperative nursing environment with diverse backgrounds of skill and knowledge. According to Benner (1984) in her book *Novice to Expert,* learners pass through five stages during a life-long learning process. Each person achieves these levels at a different pace, progressing from "novice to expert." Using this model, nurses enter into perioperative nursing at the same beginning level depending on their expertise and competency to practice. As they gain the necessary knowledge and skills, required to practice this specialized area of nursing, they progress on a continuum to the level of expert (mastery).[5]

Stage I: Novice

Novices are beginners who have no experience in the situations they are expected to perform. This could apply to either the new employee, unfamiliar with their new work environment, or the new graduate eager to work in the perioperative arena.

Stage II: Advanced Beginner

Advanced beginners are those who can demonstrate marginally acceptable performance. This could be applied to the nurse undergoing an orientation program, or the new graduate enrolled in a perioperative internship program. Both are learning new knowledge and skills. Both can practice nursing safely, but still require supervision or guidance from experienced nurses in the perioperative setting.

Stage III: Competent

Competent nurses are those who have been on the same or similar job 6 months to 1 year. Practice is based on considerable conscious, abstract, and analytic assessment of a problem or situation related to the environment, and/or the patient, and/or the community.

Stage IV: Proficient

A proficient nurse is one who has been in practice in the same setting or role for 1 to 2 years. This individual perceives situations as a whole rather than in terms of individual aspects. This perception is based largely on experience.

Stage V: Expert

This individual no longer relies on an analytical approach to connect an understanding of the situation to an appropriate action. Expertise is based on vast experience (beyond 3 years) along with the development of an intuitive grasp of each situation, and is able to create alternative solutions to situations or problems. Performance, therefore, becomes fluid, flexible, and highly proficient.

By using these stages as a guideline for the educational process, perioperative nurses develop on a similar continuum. This developmental process can help to form the basis for competency-based educational programs for perioperative nursing practice when applying specialized knowledge and skill to everyday situations (Fig. 15-1).

Perioperative Nursing Education Model

In addition to the developmental process, the concept of novice to expert can also be applied to the educational programs designed for perioperative nursing. There are three phases of program development, which include the *entry-level phase,* the *mastery-level (Expanded Practice) phase,* and the *advanced-practice phase.* These programs address both clinical and academic preparation, and can form the basis for a clinical ladder progression in perioperative nursing (Fig. 15-2).

Phase I: Entry-Level Phase

The Perioperative Nursing Internship Program (PNIP) is designed to provide the participant with the foundation of knowledge and technical skills required to perform in an entry-level role of the perioperative nurse during the three phases of surgical intervention: Preoperative, Intraoperative, and Postoperative. Courses include

1. Introduction to perioperative nursing concepts
2. Fundamentals of perioperative nursing practice
3. Perioperative patient care management

Additionally, courses provide a clinical component that allows the participant to apply the knowledge and skills gained to the role of the scrub and circulating nurse during the perioperative period.

Course Length and Format   May vary, but usually consists of 4 to 6 months. Can be offered as either continuing education and/or for credit depending on the affiliation.

KNOWLEDGE	SKILL
EXPERT	
↔	
Uses judgment in determining appropriate nursing actions that are in the best interest of the patient	Applies principles of physiological and psychosocial concepts to daily tasks and patient-centered activities
PROFICIENT	
↔	
Makes decisions based on scientific knowledge, nursing experience, and patient information	Knows principles and can adapt to varying situations
COMPETENT	
↔	
Makes decisions based on scientific knowledge and nursing experience	Knows principles and can apply them only in usual or routine situations
ADVANCED BEGINNER	
↔	
Makes decisions based on nursing experience	Knows principles but needs assistance in applying them appropriately
NOVICE	
↔	
Makes decisions based on assumptions about types of patients	Does not know principles but can follow directions and assist in patient care activities

Fig. 15-1. Concept to practice (Adapted from AORN. *Blueprint for Orientation: A Manual for Perioperative Educators.* Denver, CO: The Association, 1988.)

Instructional Methods The structure is both directed learning and independent study utilizing the principles of adult education. The clinical component utilizes preceptors in the surgical suite (scrub and circulators) to provide guidance and resources for the participant throughout the program. Clinical sites are arranged by the student, with approval by the faculty.

Target Audience

1. Registered Nurse (RN) licensed in the state of the program offering with minimal or no previous ex-

perience in the OR or those who have an interest or are currently working in the OR
2. RN-BSN transition students (could be used as an elective)
3. Senior nursing students (theory only)

The PNIP may also be used for perioperative nurses seeking to update their current practice or who wish to review theory and concepts as preparation for certification examination in perioperative nursing (theory only).

Phase II: Mastery-Level Phase

Two certification programs in perioperative nursing are directed toward enhancing the practice of nursing during the three phases of surgical intervention. The first is the certification in perioperative nursing practice (CNOR).

CNOR: Certification Perioperative Nursing Practice
Definition: CNOR certification is defined as the documented validation of the professional achievement of identified standards of practice by an individual RN providing care for patients before, during, and after surgery.[6]
Purpose of Certification

- To demonstrate concern for accountability to the general public for nursing practice
- To enhance quality patient care
- To identify professional nurses who have demonstrated professional achievement in providing patient care during the perioperative period
- To provide personal satisfaction for professional nurses performing in the perioperative role

Certification Process Certification depends on the successful completion of a written examination. On passing the exam, perioperative nurse may include CNOR in title.
Certification Eligibility

- Licensed as an RN in the country where they currently practice
- Minimum of 2 years in perioperative nursing practice as an RN and 2400 hours during a 2-year period before application date
- Currently employed or employed within the last 2 years in an OR setting. This practice can include administration, education, research, or general staff nurse.
- As of the year 2000 a BSN will be required to be eligible to sit for exam

The second is the expanded role of a perioperative nurse as a Registered Nurse first assistant, or RNFA.

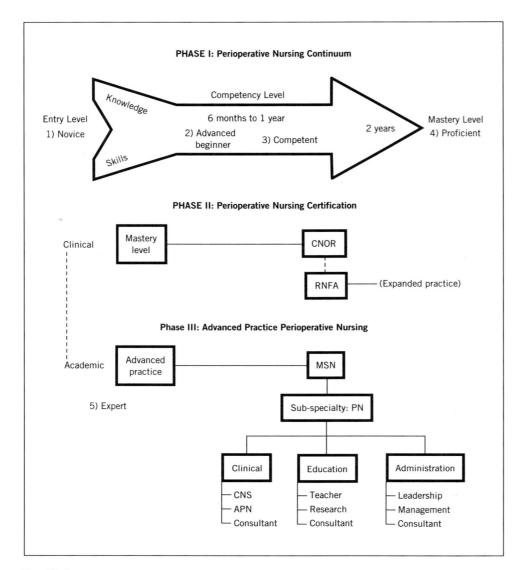

Fig. 15-2. Perioperative nursing education—a continuum model

The scope of practice of the nurse performing as first assistant is part of perioperative nursing in an expanded role.

The observable nursing behaviors within this expanded role during the intraoperative phase are:

- handling tissue
- providing exposure
- utilization of instrumentation
- suturing
- providing hemostasis

These behaviors are practiced separate and apart from the scrub role performed by perioperative nurses and/or paraprofessionals (surgical technicians).

These behaviors may vary depending on patient population, practice environments, services provided, ac-

cessibility of human and fiscal resources, institutional policy, and state nurse practice acts.

RNFA Requirements

1. Current certification as CNOR (documentation required)
2. Documentation of 2000 clinical hours are verified through a log maintained by the participant and must accompany the application. Five-hundred hours must be earned within the past 2 years.

- Classroom—4 months (45 hours) in theory, simulated lab practice, written assignments
- Clinical—4 months (120 hours) supervised internship utilizing surgeons and RNFAs as preceptors.

Clinical hours are verified through a log maintained by the participant.

Certification—CRNFA

To be certified, one must successfully complete the written examination for RNFA. As of the year 1998, a BSN will be required for eligibility to sit for the certification exam for RNFA.

State Nurse Practice Act—Florida

Acceptance of this statement, first submitted to the Board of Nursing in 1993, was approved by the board, and is recognized by the board as practice within the scope of professional nursing practice.

Phase III: Advanced-Practice Phase

Statement

The perioperative Advanced Practice Nurse (APN) is a registered professional nurse who uses specialized knowledge and skills in the care of clients and families undergoing operative and other invasive procedures. The APN possesses a graduate degree in nursing (MSN) that forms the foundation for an advanced practice role.

The perioperative APN conducts comprehensive health assessments and demonstrates autonomy and skill in diagnosing and treating complex responses of clients (i.e., patient, family, community) to actual and potential health problems that are related to the prospect or performance of operative or other invasive procedures. The perioperative APN formulates clinical decisions to manage acute and chronic illness by assessing, diagnosing, and prescribing treatment modalities, including pharmacologic agents.

The perioperative APN promotes wellness. The perioperative APN integrates clinical practice, education, research, management, leadership, and consultation into a single, comprehensive role. The perioperative APN functions in a collegial relationship with nurses, physicians, and others who influence the health-care environment.

Statement approved by: BOD-AORN 1994
House of Delegates—AORN
3/95

AORN. Standards and recommended practices. Denver, CO: The Association, 1995.

Additionally, the AORN Nursing Practice Committee has established Nursing Competency Statements for the perioperative APN.[7]

1. The perioperative APN is competent to manage client health/illness status.

2. The perioperative APN is competent in the helping/healing role.
3. The perioperative APN is competent to teach and/or coach disease prevention and health promotion.
4. The perioperative APN is competent in the organizational and work role.
5. The perioperative APN is competent to monitor and promote the quality of perioperative practice.

Perioperative Nursing Internship Program (PNIP)

As mentioned in Chapter 1 of this book, the OR experience for student nurses at one time was an important part of the generic nursing education program. But as program needs changed and the ideologies in nursing education underwent modification, the OR rotation, as a clinical learning experience, was eventually eliminated from the basic curriculum, leaving a deficit in entry-level practitioners for this specialty area.

In an effort to ensure that qualified OR nurses are providing this specialized nursing practice, several steps have been taken, including (1) the establishment, through AORN, of *Project Alpha*, created for the purpose of reinstituting a perioperative nursing component into curricula in nursing education at a variety of levels,[8] both nationally and through local AORN chapters, and (2) the creation of postgraduate courses in perioperative nursing, conducted in a variety of settings across the country. A PNIP, conducted outside the hospital environment, has recently become more cost effective than the previous one-on-one courses that were conducted in the hospital as staffing needs demanded. Through these collaborative programs, perioperative nursing, as a specialty, has again become part of the nursing education process.

Since its inception, AORN has been directly involved with promoting perioperative nursing education. Teaching has always been an intricate part of the professional nurse's role, so perioperative nurses naturally became involved with perpetuating this specialty by introducing methods to incorporate perioperative nursing practice for both entry-level students and those wishing to expand their current knowledge through formal education. The PNIP, regardless of its setting, has become one of those methods.

Characteristics of Participants

There are several reasons why a nurse and/or student would want to participate in a PNIP.

1. To work in an area they have always wanted to, but could not, due to lack of knowledge or experience.

2. To explore the role of the perioperative nurse in order to decide if this is the area they wish to practice (entry level)
3. To update skills and knowledge in order to re-enter the work force of OR nursing
4. To provide a means for nurses to change their current areas of practice
5. To provide existing practitioners a means to expand their knowledge and skills and/or review for the CNOR examination

For whatever reason, the PNIP provides both a recruitment and retention tool for hospitals, and a means to further one's formal education (e.g., RN-BSN Transitional Program) when affiliated with a university/college as an elective, or as postgraduate continuing education offering.

Curriculum Design and Development

The components for curriculum design and development of a PNIP must evolve in an organized, step-by-step manner, and must be dynamic; it must continually undergo reevaluation and change as the technology and student needs change.

The program can be designed around a limited student experience, such as a 1- or 2-day rotation in the OR, to observe the role of the perioperative nurse (perioperative experience), or a full semester program designed to teach the basic concepts of perioperative nursing practice (theory and clinical) during all three phases of surgical intervention.

A *curriculum* is described as the totality of learning activities that are designed to achieve specific educational goals. By applying the principles and practices of adult education during the planning and implementation stages, a dynamic PNIP can emerge, capable of answering to the needs of the varied student population.

The program (*course*) content should be consistent with the goals and objectives of the school and institution(s) it affiliates with including a predetermined length (hours) of clinical experience. Teaching methodologies should be selected according to the specific content to be learned, such as lecture, discussion, role-play, demonstrations, etc., and may involve individual learning modules and/or directed learning experiences, depending on the school's philosophy, the curriculum design framework, and the learning needs of the students.

Utilization of Preceptors

Clinical preceptorships have long been accepted as the most effective means of orienting new staff to an institution or new work group. Clinical preceptors can assist with bridging the gap between theory and practice. A preceptor format is a successful teaching/learning method for students and new employees. Nurses who volunteer for the preceptor role can have a positive influence on student nurses who are given the opportunity to practice techniques and to apply the concepts, theories, and knowledge of perioperative nursing learned in the classroom. A majority of PNIPs utilize the preceptor format during the clinical experience.

Definition, Characteristics, Role   A *preceptor* is an experienced RN specially selected by a direct supervisor and/or nursing educator according to established criteria of the clinical facility and/or the nursing education program. A preceptor has a specific responsibility to provide and direct the learning experience for the learner.

A perioperative nursing preceptor may be selected based on some or all of the following criteria:

1. technical knowledge and skill expertise in perioperative nursing practice
2. educational preparation (BSN or postgraduate degrees)
3. knowledge of and ability to apply principles of adult teaching and learning
4. willingness to serve in a preceptor role
5. responsibility, professionalism, organization, self-confidence, and respect for and by peers.[9]

Clinical preceptors fulfill three primary roles:

1. staff nurse role model
2. teacher/educator
3. resource person

As a role model, the preceptor provides an example of the role and responsibilities of a perioperative nurse. As a teacher/educator, the preceptor applies the principles of adult education in order to accomplish the goals and objectives of the clinical experience. This teaching/learning process includes the assessment, planning, implementation, and evaluation of the students' needs and progress throughout the clinical practicum. As a resource person, the preceptor supplies the necessary knowledge related to the policies, procedures, and expectations of the perioperative nurse within a specific environment/setting.

A perioperative nursing preceptor may be an individual assigned to direct the learner on a one-on-one basis, or may be a variety of competent persons selected for their clinical expertise in specialty areas/roles (i.e., scrub, circulating, general, gynecology, GU, orthopedics, etc.). When a perioperative nursing educator/CNS is available, this individual assumes the role of the coordinator for the clinical experience by assigning the learner to specific personnel who can best emulate the role of a scrub nurse or circulating nurse, and is aware of the needed learning experiences required to accomplish the objectives of the overall practicum for the learner.

Program Evaluation

Evaluation is an essential component for the success of any program. Specific tools, designed with input from all involved, should be established for (1) selection of surgical experiences, (2) program content and design, and (3) the program faculty, preceptors, and students.

Evaluation provides feedback necessary to both the learner and the preceptor so that the process or cycle of assessing learning needs, planning instruction to meet those needs, and implementing an educational program can continue effectively.

The evaluation should reflect the competency of the learner. Measurable criteria are the expected behaviors or outcomes that have been learned by the student. Competency is the same as a behavioral objective. Competencies are useful in the perioperative setting because of the skills necessary to perform the required tasks. The Competency Statements for Perioperative Nursing (AORN) therefore serve as the basis for the evaluation of the learner's performance. These measurable criteria, used to evaluate the learner, reflect the competency statements developed within the framework of the nursing process, and Standards of Practice for Perioperative Nursing.

Several times throughout the clinical practicum, the preceptor, student, and faculty member will meet to discuss the progress of the learner in the clinical area.

Mid-point and *final* evaluation forms will be provided to assist in evaluating the learner's progress. At the conclusion of the clinical practicum, the student will also evaluate the preceptor and the clinical experience in order to improve the teaching/learning experience.

A CLINICAL LADDER PROGRAM FOR PERIOPERATIVE NURSING

Perioperative nursing is a specialty within the discipline of nursing, but how does one recognize and promote this clinical specialty within the existing structure of the nursing profession and/or the institution? One answer is the establishment of a *clinical ladder* program specifically designed to recognize and reward clinical competence in perioperative nursing practice.

Traditionally, nursing rewards clinical competency by providing a means to move upward on the continuum to management positions, but with this move, nursing care is directed away from patient-care activities into the administrative circle, which emphasizes the managerial role of the nurse, not clinical practice. Since this role requires more time away from the bedside, the clinical performance competency level would

fall, and some nurses, who were unprepared for their new position, became frustrated as they tried to "practice" effective bedside nursing. A newer, more palatable solution to this problem would be the establishment of a clinical ladder program, designed to promote clinical competence rather than removing those nurses from bedside nursing practice.

A clinical ladder program is described as a hierarchy of criteria, intended to provide a means of evaluation and/or development of nurses providing direct patient care. The objectives of such a program should:

1. provide recognition and placement of the highly skilled nurse practitioners performing direct patient-care activities
2. identify levels of nursing competence within the institution/area
3. acknowledge the nurses' educational preparation and/or certification in a specialty area
4. provide realistic and measurable expectations for practice that can serve as a guide toward advancement within the program and/or nursing area
5. allow the practitioner to set his or her goals related to nursing practice
6. assist in recruitment and retention programs within the institution, thus promoting highly qualified practitioners within the institution.

The implementation of a clinical ladder program may be lengthy and involved, or it may be simple and self-explanatory. Whatever the format, it should provide the depth of knowledge that forms the basis for clinical decisions and the scope of practice and degree of responsibility and accountability for patient care for each level created. By utilizing the Basic Competency Statements for Perioperative Nursing Practice (Module I), a framework for the position descriptions for each level can be created, implemented, and evaluated realistically using established criteria.

The following pages outline one example of a clinical ladder series of levels designed for the perioperative nurse practitioner. By incorporating this nontraditional approach to recognizing the competent clinical practitioner, nurses striving for excellence in clinical practice can see the progress of their career and find the challenge of reaching the next level rewarding, not only for themselves, but for the patient, the institution, and their specialized nursing profession (Table 15-2).

Certification—First Step on the Ladder

Certification is described as a process by which a nongovernmental agency or association grants recognition to an individual who has met certain predetermined

Program Syllabus

COURSE: Perioperative Nursing Internship Program
COURSE HOURS: Theory: 40 hours
                       Clinical: 186 hours

CONTACT HOURS: 40

COURSE FORMAT: 14 weeks
  Theory: 3 hours/week (Wed., 5–8 PM)
  Clinical: 18 hours/week (3 days/week: 6 hours/day)*
                       (Monday, Tuesday, and Thursday)
  Clinical sites to be agreed on by faculty and student.

OFFERING: Summer term
PRE/CO-REQUISITE:
  1. Registered Nurse (RN) licensed in the state of Florida with minimal or no previous experience in the OR, or who has an interest in or is currently working in the OR.
  2. RN-BSN transition students
  3. Senior semester nursing students (theory only).

CATALOG DESCRIPTION: Introduction and exploration of perioperative nursing practice during the three phases of surgical intervention: Preoperative, Intraoperative, and Postoperative.

COURSE DESCRIPTION: This course provides the participant with foundation of concepts, theories, and technical skills required to perform in an entry-level role of the perioperative nurse during the three phases of the perioperative period. The course progresses through three sections:
  1. Introduction to perioperative nursing concepts
  2. Fundamentals of perioperative nursing practice
  3. Perioperative patient-care management
Additionally, the course provides a clinical component that allows the participant to apply the knowledge gained to the roles of scrub and circulating nurse for a variety of surgical procedures.

CONCEPTUAL FRAMEWORK
  The conceptual framework of this course is built on the definition of professional nursing as stated by the American Nurses Association (ANA) and perioperative nursing practice as defined by the Association of Operating Room Nurses (AORN). Additionally, the utilization of a nursing systems theory provides a practice model for the perioperative nurse during the perioperative period. The framework is concurrently intersected with five processes necessary for effective professional nursing practice: research, communication, change, teaching/learning, professionalism, and management. The emphasis of the course provides for the correlation of theories and concepts with the varied roles of the professional perioperative nurse.

COURSE OBJECTIVES:
  With assistance from the faculty, the student will:

  1. Compare and contrast the components of the nursing process, nursing theories, and concepts while caring for a client undergoing surgical intervention.
  2. Analyze the five roles of the professional nurse: caregiver, client advocate, leader/role model, research consumer, and teacher/educator, as they apply to perioperative nursing practice.
  3. Examine and utilize an awareness of the biophysical and psychosocial sciences associated with providing nursing care during the perioperative period.
  4. Recognize and demonstrate the principles of surgical asepsis when caring for a client during the intraoperative period.

Program Syllabus (continued)

5. Correlate the knowledge and skills acquired with the implementation of the perioperative nurses' role for a variety of surgical procedures.
6. Examine the ethical and legal boundaries of perioperative nursing practice during the three phases of surgical intervention.
7. Identify and explore research priorities associated with the practice of perioperative nursing in today's health-care setting.

TOPICAL OUTLINE:

Part I (weeks 1–4) Introduction to Perioperative Nursing Concepts

Classroom lectures with clinical skills introduced in a simulated lab setting. Emphasis is placed on concepts of perioperative nursing practice; OR Theories and Techniques, and a review of the biophysical and psychosocial sciences interrelated with those concepts, theories, and techniques.

Module I. Perioperative Nursing Concepts
A. Introduction and Orientation
B. Environmental Orientation
C. Standards of Perioperative Nursing Practice

Module II. Biophysical Science Review
A. Microbiology and Surgical Wound Healing
B. Surgical Pharmacology
C. Anesthesia and Nursing Implications
D. Intravascular Homeostasis and Hemodynamics

Module III. Asepsis and the Surgical Environment
A. OR Theory and Techniques

Part II (weeks 5–8) Fundamentals of Perioperative Nursing Practice

Clinical exposure in the OR and adjacent areas with classroom lecture interspersed at specific intervals. Emphasis is on the circulating and scrub roles and the application of acquired knowledge while performing as a member of the surgical team.

Module III. Asepsis and the Surgical Environment
B. Foundations of Surgery

Module IV. Perioperative Nursing Practice
A. The Nursing Process: A Theoretical Approach
B. Legal Aspects of Perioperative Nursing Practice

Part III (weeks 9–14) Perioperative Patient-Care Management

Selected classroom lectures and student performance in the surgical setting that includes the preoperative assessment and teaching; intraoperative nursing management (circulating and scrub roles); and postoperative follow-up, evaluation, and discharge planning for a variety of procedures and/or settings.

Emphasis is on the total care management of a client undergoing a surgical experience, and the development of independent nursing actions within a controlled, supervised environment for a variety of surgical procedures.

Module V. Implementation of Perioperative Nursing Practice
A. Selected Nursing Activities
1. Preoperative Phase
2. Intraoperative Phase
3. Postoperative Phase
B. Topics for Further Discussion

Table 15-2 Perioperative Nursing: Clinical Ladder Concepts

Position	Education	Experience	Management Responsibilities
Specialty Coordinator (original title: AHN/team leaders)	1. Currently licensed in appropriate state 2. BSN-prepared or enrolled in BSN program 3. Maintains or is eligible for AORN certification (CNOR) 4. Enrolled or completed leadership-development program 5. Active participation in AORN and/or specialty organization	1. Three to five yr clinical OR experience, including one yr as OR clinician II in a specialty area or recommendation from management group* 2. Demonstrates advanced clinical expertise in specialty area	1. Assists in the development of educational programs related to specialist service 2. Participates in the evaluation process of team members 3. Revises and updates specialty service patient-billable supplies 4. Manages inventory and budgetary activities specific to surgeon/staff needs 5. Generates ideas for research and QA studies
OR Nurse Clinician II	1. Currently licensed in appropriate state 2. Eligible for AORN certification in 2 yr 3. Eligible for management workshop with recommendation from management group* 4. Member of AORN	1. Two years clinical OR experience, including 1 yr as OR Clinician I in specialty service 2. Demonstrates current knowledge of procedures and equipment for area of specialty service 3. Eligible to serve as preceptor for new employees/students 4. Performs scrub/circulator duties with proficiency	1. Can assume relief specialty coordinator I role as needed 2. May serve as coordinator of QA studies 3. Assumes management assignments as directed
OR Nurse Clinician I	1. Currently licensed in appropriate state 2. Maintains professional competence through continuing education 3. Member of AORN	1. One yr clinical OR experience including 6 mo to 1 yr as staff nurse 2. Ability to scrub/circulate with competence for a variety of surgical procedures	
Staff Nurse	1. Currently licensed in appropriate state 2. Successful completion of recognized perioperative internship program 3. Member of AORN	1. Previous OR experience (new employee) 2. Graduate-perioperative nursing internship program	

* The following people comprise the *management group*: Director—Surgical Services Ad Hoc; OR Supervisor (Nurse Manager)—Surgery; Clinical Nurse Specialist/Educator Surgical Service; and specialty coordinators.

qualifications that have been specified by that agency or association.

In 1950, the ANA proposed a means of formal recognition of superior performance in nursing through a voluntary certification program. In response to this program, in 1977, AORN's House of Delegates voted to develop a voluntary certification program that would recognize clinical competence in perioperative nursing practice, and in 1979 the first National Certification Examination for Perioperative Nursing Practice was administered. In that year, 688 nurses became certified in perioperative nursing practice and were entitled to add the initials CNOR to their credentials. By January of 1990, 13 years later, 13,317 perioperative nurses had become certified,[10] which helped to establish the first level of advanced clinical practice for a clinical ladder program.

Through the national certification program, perioperative nurse practitioners have been able to enhance the quality of patient care, identify those nurses who have demonstrated professional achievement in perioperative nursing, and provide a means for self-evaluation and self-satisfaction. Certification has also created a sense of awareness, both within and outside the nursing profession, demonstrating professional achievement of identified standards of practice during the perioperative period.

Advanced Practice Role: Clinical Nurse Specialist (CNS)

The Perioperative CNS is the last step on the clinical ladder series, since the role not only signifies advanced clinical competence, but the candidate has, in addition to certification, attained an advanced degree in nursing as defined by the ANA.[11] The CNS is a nurse prepared at the graduate level, with focus in a specific clinical area. The CNS role incorporates clinical, administrative, and educational aspects of professional nursing practice, with a goal of coordinating and managing the specific needs of the patient and/or family.

The interest and need for the perioperative CNS has been explored and requested by many across the country, but since this is a comparatively new role, in relation to other clinical nurse specialties, support from not only other clinical nurse specialists but universities offering a master's program with emphasis in perioperative nursing practice can assist in fostering this goal: to advance clinical nursing through higher education within their chosen field. For the perioperative CNS, certification in perioperative nursing practice (CNOR) would become a requirement, since it signifies a mastery level in perioperative nursing practice as specified for the CNS role.

The next logical step in the development of a perioperative CNS role is to create a realistic position description that can evolve and develop as the specialty progresses, and in this way, the perioperative CNS role will become an innovative and vital component of the health-care system and the professional practice of nursing during the perioperative period.

Could this eventually lead toward the establishment of an ARNP specializing in perioperative nursing practice? Only time, interest, and commitment to this specialized profession will provide the answer.

PERIOPERATIVE NURSING RESEARCH

Since its earliest beginnings, nursing, and perioperative nursing specifically, has been based on practice handed down from one generation to another using formal and informal education. Nursing is a learned, service-oriented profession, and must therefore constantly seek scientific data to assist in not only expanding existing knowledge, but in creating safer, more efficient methods for delivery of this service. Perioperative nursing research has become the tool to find these answers, and to help guide current practices.

Research . . . The Heart of Knowledge Acquisition

Research is "a studious inquiry, examination, investigation or experimentation . . . aimed at revising accepted theory or laws in the light of new facts, or a practical application of revised theories and laws."[12]

Research is the heart of knowledge acquisition. Without on-going research, concepts, theories, and laws cannot evolve beyond their present interpretations. Nursing research has experienced remarkable growth in the past two decades. During this time, the focus of nursing research has been directed toward problems relating to the practice of professional nursing. Today, that focus is slowly shifting to the desired patient outcomes as a direct result of nursing intervention.

Professional accountability demands that nurses utilize the findings of research to perform their roles, in addition to evaluating methods used to carry out research projects currently being conducted. Perioperative nurses may not conduct formal research studies, but they must become involved in the research process by identifying clinical problems, participating in data collection and research projects, and reading research studies to determine how they might apply these findings to daily practice.

Importance of Perioperative Nursing Research

The ultimate goal of any profession is "to improve the practice of its members . . . to provide the best benefit to its recipients."[13] As a specialty within the profession of nursing, perioperative nursing must continue to enhance its professional image and expand its body of knowledge through scientific inquiry to foster the commitment and accountability to health-care consumers. Research has an important role to play in helping perioperative nurses establish a scientific base for its practice. By establishing a scientific base, perioperative nurses will be able to make more informed decisions in their practice by using the information gained from research to initiate changes in the practice setting resulting in improvement of the quality of patient care and the practice of professional nursing.

Methodology for Perioperative Nursing Research

A distinction is usually made between two broad types of research methods associated with nursing research. These are quantitative and qualitative research methods. *Quantitative research* involves the "systematic collection of numerical information . . . under conditions of considerable control . . . with the analysis of the data using statistical procedures."[14] *Qualitative research* involves the collection and analysis of subjective narrative material using procedures that require minimal control. Most of the perioperative nursing research studies are quantitative in nature, although the qualitative method is being used more frequently today than in the past. The choice of research method will depend largely on the nature of the research question being asked, and the personal preference of the nursing researcher.

Scientific research can also be categorized in terms of its function or its objective: (1) description, (2) exploration, (3) explanation, and (4) prediction and control. Additionally, research studies can be either *experimental* or *nonexperimental*, depending on the nature of the research problem. Experimental studies command more powerful results, however, when experimentation is not feasible or when the research problem does not lend itself to an experimental (or quasi-experimental) design, the nonexperimental design is an appropriate method for investigative purposes.

Impact of Research to Practice

Regardless of the design used to conduct scientific research, for perioperative nursing to mature as a profession and be recognized as a profession, perioperative nurses must continue to be active in the research process related to clinical issues and patient problems. Over the past several years, research related to perioperative nursing practice has increased in amount as well as depth of subject matter. Today, all of the revised recommended practices for perioperative nursing are based on strong scientific research, conducted by perioperative nurses around the country, eliminating a practice based on hunches, hearsay, and tradition.

Nurses in all specialties of nursing and all levels of nursing education have a responsibility to develop an awareness of the research process, but more importantly, to transfer this knowledge to the daily practice of nursing. To achieve its rightful place in the arena of professions, perioperative nursing practice must be supported by scientific research to meet the criteria of a "true" profession.

Today, more than ever before, nurses are required to be accountable for the quality of care they give in a variety of settings. This accountability includes the documentation of the effectiveness of the services they are providing to the health-care consumer. Perioperative nursing, as a specialty within the nursing profession, has an obligation to the patients, the profession, and the community they serve to improve and *validate* the quality of practice through ongoing clinical research.

Perioperative nurses need to educate not only their peers, but agency administrators and surgeons, as to the professional benefits derived from clinical research, including cost-effectiveness, employee satisfaction, and efficiency, and the continuation of quality patient care during the perioperative period.

THE END IS THE BEGINNING

> I like the dreams of the future better than the history of the past.
>
> *Thomas Jefferson*

Perioperative nursing has come full circle. From its beginnings as a task-oriented practice with very little nursing to care delivered to a variety of patients in a variety of settings by a nursing specialist—a perioperative nurse.

Through research, education, and commitment to quality patient care, this specialist delivers the most comprehensive nursing care through the most difficult times for both the patient and family. This nurse is part psychologist, part surrogate mother, part friend, part caregiver, part teacher, part researcher, all rolled into one extraordinary person.

Perioperative nurses are indeed *specialists in caring*—for patients, family, colleagues, and associates they work with on a daily basis. In order to maintain this quality practice, perioperative nurses, both expert and novice, must work together to find a better way to improve and update the standards of care. By doing so, we ensure continuous quality improvement of patient care while simultaneously improving the professional practice of perioperative nursing. We owe it to ourselves, our profession, and to the patient entrusted to our care.

But by far, the most important benefit is the feeling of self-satisfaction of the practitioners as they realize the accomplishment of their ultimate goal: *to render to all quality patient care*, and through a desire to improve that quality, perioperative nurses will continue to be *Specialists in Caring*.

References

1. Joint Commission. Accreditation manual for ambulatory health-care standards. Chicago: JCAHO, 1990. P. vii.
2. Ibid., p. v.
3. Katz Ronald. Issues in outpatient surgery. *Sem Anesth* V: 258, 1987.
4. Ibid., p. 260.
5. National Certification Board: Perioperative Nursing, Inc. CNOR and CRNFA certification and recertification policy manual. Denver, CO: NCB: PNI, 1996.
6. Ibid.
7. AORN Standards and recommended practices. Denver, CO: The Association, 1993. P. 102.
8. AORN Standards and recommended practices. Denver, CO: The Association, 1995. P. 17.
9. Ibid., pp. 87–92.
10. AORN. Project alpha handbook (rev. ed.). Denver, CO: The Association, 1990. P. 1.
11. ANA. Advanced practice nursing: a new age in health care. Nursing facts. Washington, D.C.: ANA, 1993.
12. Merrian-Webster collegiate dictionary. 10th ed., 1993. P. 995.
13. Polit D and Hungler B. Nursing research: principles and methods (14th ed.). Philadelphia: Lippincott, 1991. P. 4.
14. Ibid., p. 24.

Questions for Review for Module V

Provide the correct answers to the following questions. The answers are given at the end of this module.

1. Selected procedure(s) that require(s) isolation of instruments from the rest of the operative field include
   1. transverse colectomy
   2. common duct exploration
   3. esophagogastrostomy
   4. gastrojejunostomy
   5. appendectomy
   a. 1, 3, 5
   b. 2, 5
   c. 1, 2, 3
   d. 3, 4, 5

2. The surgical procedure for Carcinoma of the Head of the Pancreas is a _____ procedure.
   a. Heller
   b. Roux-en-Y
   c. Hofmeister
   d. Whipple

3. An anastomosis between the small intestine and the colon is called a(n)
   a. gastroenterostomy
   b. ileocolostomy
   c. ileojunostomy
   d. ileocecostomy

4. The placement of a purse-string suture in the submucosal layer of the cervical os to prevent spontaneous abortion during the second trimester of pregnancy is known as a
   a. colporophy
   b. Manchester procedure
   c. Shirodkar procedure
   d. colpotomy

5. The needle holder used by a surgeon to close the vaginal cuff following an abdominal hysterectomy must be
   a. a Heaney needleholder
   b. on a vaginal set-up instead of an abdominal tray
   c. considered contaminated and separated from other instruments
   d. standard length

6. Besides the routine two closing counts that occur in a laparotomy, when is an additional count performed during a cesarean section?
   a. immediately after the baby and placenta have been delivered
   b. before closure of the uterus
   c. at the time of peritonealization
   d. as fascia is being closed

7. Following a TUR-P, the surgeon may leave a three-way Foley catheter inserted for the purpose of
   a. drainage
   b. continuous irrigation of the bladder to assist in blood clot removal
   c. injection of dye
   d. injection of a hemostatic agent

8. Saline and sterile water are *not* the irrigation solution of choice for a TUR-P operation because they are
   a. nonelectrolytic and nonhemolytic
   b. hypertonic and hypotonic
   c. electrolytic and hemolytic
   d. isotonic and autogenous

9. Intramedullary rods are used to correct which type of fracture?
   a. intertrochanteric
   b. shaft fractures of long bones
   c. greenstick
   d. comminuted fracture of long bones

10. For which of the following complications following a fracture must a patient be closely observed?
    a. shock
    b. fat embolism
    c. thromboembolism
    d. all of the above

11. A special *fracture table* may be requested when performing a _____ procedure.

12. Compression of the median nerve or its blood supply in a canal at the wrist is known as
    a. a ganglion
    b. De Quervain's tenosynovitis
    c. carpal tunnel syndrome
    d. Dupuytren's contracture

13. Mr. A.'s preoperative diagnosis is *torn semilunar cartilage*. He is scheduled for a
    a. Putti-Platt procedure
    b. arthrotomy of the ankle
    c. arthroscopy; possible menisectomy
    d. Keller procedure

14. In corrective surgery for coronary artery disease, a *saphenous vein* or *mammary artery* graft is inserted as a bypass between the coronary artery and the _____ and attached to the _____.
    a. aorta; left ventricular myocardium
    b. pulmonary artery; right ventricular myocardium
    c. left ventricle; aorta
    d. aorta; right ventricle

15. A lobectomy of the lung is described as a _____ and will require a _____ postoperatively.

16. Specimens can be obtained through a fiberoptic bronchoscope by means of
    a. washings
    b. brushings
    c. biopsy
    d. all of the above

17. The *intraaortic balloon pump* is used to treat _____ ventricular failure. It is inserted in the _____ aorta and increases coronary perfusion by inflating during _____.
    a. left; descending; diastole
    b. right; ascending; systole
    c. left; ascending; systole
    d. right; descending; diastole

18. For a CABG procedure, an additional count is required
    a. after completing the graft anastomosis
    b. prior to closing the pericardial cavity
    c. before closing the thoracic cavity
    d. before closing the fascia

19. The patient with which of the following diagnoses would require priority emergency surgery?
    a. epidural hematoma
    b. subdural hematoma
    c. intracerebral hemorrhage
    d. cerebral thrombosis

20. The procedure of choice for *otosclerosis* is:
    a. stapedectomy
    b. tympanoplasty
    c. myringotomy
    d. anthrostomy

21. The removal of an opaque ocular lens and the insertion of an implant describes a procedure referred to as a(n) _____.

22. The body temperature of infants may be preserved during surgery by
    a. wrapping extremities with soft cotton wadding
    b. using a thermal blanket under the child
    c. using warmed irrigation and intravenous solutions
    d. all of the above

23. The most common congenital anomaly of the neonate incompatible with life and requiring immediate surgical intervention is
    a. imperforate anus
    b. club foot
    c. hydrocephalus
    d. ventricular septal defect

24. Anxiety in toddlers is stimulated by
    a. separation from family
    b. fear of death
    c. previous experience
    d. fear of pain

25. The primary goal of the perioperative nurse's preoperative visit to a pediatric patient is to _____.

Bibliography for Module V

Chapter 13

Anderson, PD. *Human Anatomy and Physiology Coloring Workbook and Study Guide.* Boston: Jones and Bartlett, 1990.

Grey, H. *Anatomy of the Human Body,* 37th ed. Philadelphia: Lea and Febiger, 1989.

Thibodeau, GA. *Anthony's Textbook of Anatomy and Physiology,* 13th ed. St. Louis: Mosby, 1990.

Thomas, CL, ed. *Tabor's Cyclopedic Medical Dictionary,* 14th ed. Philadelphia: Davis, 1981.

Stanfield, PS and Hui, YH. *Medical Terminology: Principles and Practices.* Boston: Jones and Bartlett, 1989.

Snell, R. *Clinical Anatomy for Medical Students,* 5th ed. Boston: Little, Brown and Co., 1995.

Chapter 14

Arciniegas, E. *Pediatric Cardiac Surgery*. Chicago: Year Book Medical Publishers, 1985.

Atkinson, LJ and Kohn, ML. *Berry and Kohn's Introduction to Operating Room Technique,* 7th ed. New York: McGraw-Hill, 1992.

Chapman, MW. *Operative Orthopedics*. Philadelphia: Lippincott, 1988.

Cooley, DA. *Techniques in Cardiac Surgery,* 2nd ed. Philadelphia: Saunders, 1984.

Converse, JM, ed. *Reconstructive Plastic Surgery: Principles and Procedures,* 4th ed. Philadelphia: Saunders, 1983.

Conway-Rutowski, BL. *Carini and Owens' Neurological and Neurosurgical Nursing,* 8th ed. St. Louis: Mosby, .

Crenshaw, AH, ed. *Campbell's Operative Orthopedics—Volumes I and II,* 7th ed. St. Louis: Mosby, 1987.

Davis, JH, et al. *Clinical Surgery—Volume 2.* St. Louis: Mosby, 1987.

Dillard, DH and Hillet, DW. *Atlas of Cardiac Surgery.* New York: MacMillan, 1983.

Fairchild, S. Perioperative nursing. In B. Kozier, G. Erb, K. Blais, and J. Wilkinson (eds.), *Fundamentals of Nursing,* 5th ed. Menlo Park, CA: Addison-Wesley, 1995: Pp. 1398–1424.

Froom, D. *Gastrointestinal Surgery.* New York: Churchill-Livingstone, 1985.

Gregory, B. *Orthopedic Surgery* (Perioperative Nursing Series). St. Louis: Mosby, 1994.

Graff, WK and Smith, JW. *Plastic Surgery: A Concise Guide to Clinical Practice,* 3rd ed. Boston: Little, Brown and Co., 1980.

Gruendemann, B, et al. *Alexander's Care of the Patient in Surgery,* 8th ed. St. Louis: Mosby, 1987.

Hallmark, G and Findlay, M. Cesarean birth in the operating room, *AORN J* 36:978, 1982.

Hilt, N, ed. *Arthroscopy of the Knee* (special ed.). National Association of Orthopedic Nurses, 1983.

Hoerenz, P. The operating microscope III: Accessories. *J Microsurgery* 2:22, 1980.

Lewis, SM and Collier, IC. *Medical-Surgical Nursing: Assessment and Management of Clinical Problems,* 3rd ed. New York: McGraw-Hill, 1994.

Liechty, RD and Soper, RT. *Synopsis of Surgery,* 5th ed. St. Louis: Mosby, 1985.

Lyons, RD and Coren, DA. The head and neck patient: a team approach to rehabilitation, *AORN J* 40:751, 1984.

May, DR and Adams, MA. Ventricular assist devices: a bridge to cardiac transplantation, *AORN J* 46:633, 1987.

Meeker, R and Rothrock, J. *Alexander's Care of the Patient in Surgery,* 10th ed. St. Louis: Mosby, 1995.

Moncada, G. Special nursing considerations for the craniofacial patient, *Plas Surg Nurs* 5:14, 1985.

Potter, P and Perry, AG. *Fundamentals of Nursing,* 3rd ed. St. Louis: Mosby, 1993.

Proximate ILS Disposable Stapler System: Reference Manual. Sommerville, NJ: Ethicon, Inc., 1990.

Ricci, M. *Core Curriculum for Neuroscience Nursing, Volumes I and II.* Park Ridge, IL: American Association of Neurosurgical Nurses, 1984.

Sabiston, Jr., DC, ed. *Davis-Christophers Textbook of Surgery: The Biological Basis of Modern Surgical Practices,* 3rd ed. Philadelphia: Saunders, 1986.

Saunders, WH, et al. *Nursing Care in Eye, Ear, Nose, and Throat Disorders.* St. Louis: Mosby, 1986.

Schwartz, SI, et al. *Principles of Surgery,* 4th ed. New York: McGraw-Hill, 1983.

Seifert, P. *Cardiac Surgery* (Perioperative Nursing Series). St. Louis: Mosby, 1994.

Thibodeau, GA. *Anthony's Textbook of Anatomy and Physiology,* 13th ed. St. Louis: Mosby, 1990.

U.S. Surgical Corporation. *Stapling Techniques in General Surgery Using Autosuture,* 3rd ed. Norwalk, CT: U.S. Surgical Corporation, 1988.

Walsh, PC, et al. *Campbell's Urology—Volume 3,* 5th ed. Philadelphia: Saunders, 1986.

Welsh, KJ, et al. *Pediatric Surgery,* 4th ed. Chicago: Year Book Medical Publishers, 1986.

Wells, MP and Villano, K. Total abdominal hysterectomy: perioperative patient care, *AORN J* 42:368, 1985.

Whaley, LF and Wong, DL. *Essentials of Pediatric Nursing,* 2nd ed. St. Louis: Mosby, 1985.

Zollinger, RM and Zollinger, Jr., RM. *Atlas of Surgical Operations,* 5th ed. New York: MacMillan, 1983.

Chapter 15

AORN. *Standards and Recommended Practices.* Denver, CO: The Association, 1995.

———. *Project Alpha Handbook,* rev. ed. Denver, CO: The Association, 1990.

———. *Quality Improvement in Perioperative Nursing.* Denver, CO: The Association, 1992.

———. *Practice Resources: Ambulatory Surgery.* Denver, CO: The Association, 1994.

———. *Practice Resources: Orientation, Education, and Preceptors in Perioperative Nursing.* Denver, CO: The Association, 1994.

———. *Practice Resources: RN First Assistant.* Denver, CO: The Association, 1994.

———. *Core Curriculum for the RN First Assistant.* Denver, CO: The Association, 1994.

American Hospital Association. *AHA/90—Accreditation Manual for Hospitals.* Chicago: Joint Commission on Accreditation of Healthcare Organizations, 1990.

———. *Ambulatory Health Care Standards Manual.* Chicago: JCAHO, 1990.

American Nurses Association. *Advanced Practice Nursing.* Washington, DC: The Association, 1993.

Bevis, EO. *Curriculum Building in Nursing: A Process,* 3rd ed. New York: National League for Nurses, 1989.

deTournay, R and Thompson, M. *Strategies for Teaching Nursing,* 3rd ed. New York: John Wiley and Sons, 1987.

Groah, LK. *Operating Room Nursing: The Perioperative Role.* Reston, VA: Reston Publishing Co., 1983.

Gruendemann, BJ. Ambulatory surgery: impact on nursing. In *Ambulatory Surgery Anthology.* Denver, CO: AORN, 1987.

Gruendemann, B. Dare to excel in ambulatory surgery, *AORN J* 41:330, 1985.

Joint Commission on Accreditation of Health Care Organizations. *Transitional Strategies for Quality Improvement in Nursing.* Chicago: JCAHO, 1991. Chs. 2 and 3.

Larkin, MA. Quality assurance: a system for surgical services, *AORN J* 51:456, 1990.

Kelly, LY and Joel, LA. *Dimensions of Professional Nursing,* 7th ed. New York: McGraw-Hill, 1995.

Mackie, RJ, Peddie, R and Pendelton, R. Quality assurance: a design for perioperative nurses, *AORN J* 42:55, 1985.

Marker, CGS. The Marker model for nursing standards: implications for nursing administration, *Nurs Admin Q* 12:2, 1987.

Mauldin, BC, ed. *Ambulatory Surgery: A Guide to Perioperative Nursing Care.* New York: Grune and Stratton, 1983.

Pendarvis, JH. The value of the OR experience in nursing education, *Surg Rounds* (November 1990): 84.

Polit, D and Hungler, B. *Nursing Research,* 4th ed. Philadelphia: Lippincott, 1991.

Rothrock, J. *The RN First Assistant: An Expanded Perioperative Nursing Role.* Philadelphia: Lippincott, 1987.

Roth, R, ed. *Perioperative Nursing Core Curriculum.* Denver, CO: AORN, 1995.

Wilson, C. *Hospital-wide Quality Assurance Models for Implementation and Development.* Philadelphia: Saunders, 1987.

Additional Resources

For technical support and a current resource list of products and equipments mentioned in this text, consult the *Operating Room Product Directory Guide* published by AORN, Inc. at: AORN, Inc., Customer Service, 2170 So. Parker Road, Suite 300, Denver, CO 80231-4511.

Answers for Module V

Chapter 13

Self-assessment Exercise 1, Anatomic Directions/Planes

A. Cranial (superior)
B. Caudal (inferior)
C. Anterior (ventral)
D. Posterior (dorsal)
E. Lateral
F. Medial

1. Transverse
2. Median
3. Coronal (frontal)
4. Proximal
5. Distal
6. Sagittal

Self-assessment Exercise 2, Body Cavities

1. Cranial
2. Spinal
3. Thoracic
4. Abdominal
5. Pelvic
6. Pleural
7. Mediastinal
8. Abdominopelvic

Self-assessment Exercise 3, Areas and Regions of the Body

1. Right upper quadrant (RUQ)
2. Left upper quadrant (LUQ)
3. Right lower quadrant (RLQ)
4. Left lower quadrant (LLQ)
A. Right hypochondric
B. Epigastric
C. Left hypochondric
D. Right lumbar
E. Umbilical
F. Left lumbar
G. Right iliac
H. Suprapubic (hypogastric)
I. Left iliac

Self-assessment Exercise 4, The Cell

1. Endoplasmic reticulum
2. Mitochondria
3. Cell membrane
4. Golgi complexes
5. Nucleolus
6. Nucleus

Self-assessment Exercise 5, Tissues and Muscles

A. Connective tissue
B. Cuboidal
C. Cardiac/striated
D. Visceral/smooth
E. Skeletal/striated

Self-assessment Exercise 6, The Integumentary System

1. Epidermis
2. Papilla
3. Sweat gland
4. Hair follicle
5. Sebaceous gland
6. Pilometer muscle
7. Subcutaneous muscle
8. Dermis

Self-assessment Exercise 7, The Skeleton (AX = axial skeleton)

A. Cranium (AX)
B. Facial bones (AX)
C. Mandible (AX)
D. Clavicle
E. Scapula
F. Sternum (AX)
G. Humerus
H. Costal cartilage (AX)
I. Vertebral column (AX)
J. Ilium
K. Pelvis
L. Radius
M. Ulna
N. Carpals
O. Metacarpals
P. Phalanges
Q. Sacrum (AX)
R. Knee joint
S. Femur
T. Patella
U. Tibia
V. Fibula
W. Ankle
X. Calcaneus/Tarsals
Y. Metatarsals
Z. Phalanges

LONG BONES
1. Epiphyseal line
2. Medullary cavity
3. Diaphysis
4. Periosteum
5. Epiphysis

Self-assessment Exercise 8, The Skull

1. Occipital bone
2. Parietal bone
3. Frontal
4. Temporal bone
5. Zygomatic bone
6. Maxilla
7. Mandible
8. Nasal bone
9. Lacrimal bone
10. Sphenoid bone

Self-assessment Exercise 9, The Muscles

Anterior View
A. Frontalis
B. Orbicularis oculi
C. Zigomaticus
D. Orbicularis oris
E. Trapezius
F. Sternocleidomastoid
G. Deltoid
H. Pectoralis major
I. Biceps brachii
J. Serratus anterior
K. Rectus abdominis sheath
L. Brachioradialis
M. External oblique
N. Extensor digitor
O. Flexor carpi radialis
P. Satorius
Q. Adductor longus
R. Gracillis
S. Rectus femoris
T. Vastus medialis
U. Vastus lateralis
V. Tibialis anterior
W. Gastrocnemius

Posterior View
1. Epicranial aponeurosis
2. Occipitalis
3. Trapezius
4. Triceps brachii
5. Teres major
6. Latissimus dorsi
7. Gluteus maximus
8. Biceps femoris
9. Gastrocnemius
10. Achilles tendon

Self-assessment Exercise 10, The Heart

1. Right atrium
2. Right ventricle
3. Left atrium
4. Left ventricle
5. Vena cava (superior/inferior)
6. Aorta
7. Pulmonary artery
8. Pulmonary veins
9. Aortic valve
10. Pulmonic valve
11. Tricuspid valve
12. Mitral valve

Self-assessment Exercise 11, The Systemic Circulation

Venous System
A. External jugular
B. Internal jugular
C. Rt. subclavian
D. Lt. innominate
E. Superior vena cava
F. Axillary
G. Basilic
H. Hepatic
I. Inferior vena cava
J. Renal
K. Common iliac
L. External iliac
M. Femoral
N. Popliteal
O. Anterior
P. Ulnar
Q. Internal iliac
R. Great saphenous
S. Posterior tibial

Arterial System
1. Common carotid
2. Left subclavian
3. Aortic arch
4. Axillary
5. Brachial
6. Sup. mesenteric
7. Inf. mesenteric
8. Abd. aorta
9. Radial
10. Ulnar
11. Common iliac
12. External iliac
13. Femoral
14. Popliteal
15. Ant. tibial
16. Dorsalis pedis
17. Peroneal
18. Post. tibial

Self-assessment Exercise 12, The Respiratory System

1. Glottis
2. Trachea
3. Bronchus—lt. main stem
4. Bronchioles
5. Visceral pleura
6. Pleural cavity
7. Respiratory bronchioles
8. Alveolar sacs
9. Pulmonary capillary
10. Rt. upper lobe
11. Rt. middle lobe
12. Rt. lower lobe

Self-assessment Exercise 13, The Brain

A. Cerebrum
B. Frontal lobe
C. Parietal lobe
D. Occipital lobe
E. Cerebellum
F. Temporal lobe
1. Central sulcus (Rolando)
2. Lateral sulcus (Sylvius)
3. Pons
4. Medulla
5. Spinal cord

Self-assessment Exercise 14, The 12 Cranial Nerves (S = sensory, M = motor)

I. Olfactory (S)
II. Optic (S)
III. Oculomotor (M)
IV. Trochlear (M)
V. Trigeminal (S)
VI. Abducens (S)
VII. Facial (M, S)
VIII. Acoustic (S)
IX. Glossopharyngeal (M, S)
X. Vagus (M, S)
XI. Accessory (M)
XII. Hypoglossal (M)

Self-assessment Exercise 15, The Eye

1. Sclera
2. Pupil
3. Lens
4. Posterior body (vitreous chamber)
5. Anterior chamber
6. Cornea
A. Fovea centralis
B. Optic disk
C. Retinal arteries and veins
D. Retina
E. Choroid
F_1. Superior rectus muscle
F_2. Inferior rectus muscle
G. Conjunctiva
H. Ciliary muscles
I. Iris

Self-assessment Exercise 16, The Ear

1. Pinna
2. External auditory canal
3. Tympanic membrane (ear drum)
A. Auditory meatus
B. Internal auditory canal
C. Middle ear
D. Inner ear

4. Malleus (hammer)
5. Incus (anvil)
6. Stapes (stirrups)
7. Oval window
8. Internal jugular vein
9. Tympanic cavity
10. Semicircular canal
11. Vestibular nerve
12. Auditory nerve
13. Cochlear nerve
14. Cochlea

E. Temporal bone
F. Eustachian tube
G. Organ of Corti

Self-assessment Exercise 17, The Alimentary Tract

1. Oral cavity
2. Pharynx
3. Parotid gland
4. Esophagus
5. Diaphragm
6. Cardiac stomach
7. Liver
8. Spleen
9. Pyloric sphincter
10. Pyloric stomach
11. Gallbladder
12. Duodenum
13. Transverse colon
14. Jejunum
15. Ascending colon
16. Descending colon
17. Sigmoid colon
18. Ileum
19. Cecum
20. Ileocecal valve
21. Rectum
22. Appendix
23. Anal sphincter

Self-assessment Exercise 18, The Biliary Circuit

1. Liver
2. Gallbladder
3. Duodenum
4. Stomach
5. Jejunum
6. Pancreas
7. Lt. hepatic duct
8. Rt. hepatic duct

Self-assessment Exercise 19, The Liver and Surrounding Organs

1. Common hepatic duct
2. Cystic duct
3. Common bile ducts
4. Pancreas
5. Pancreatic duct
6. Duodenum
7. Gallbladder
8. Liver
9. Left/right hepatic ducts
10. Ampulla of Vater

Self-assessment Exercise 20, The Endocrine Glands

1. Hypophysis (pituitary)
2. Thyroid
3. Parathyroid
4. Thymus (in a child)
5. Pancreas
6. Adrenal glands
7. Gonads: testes (male)
8. Gonads: ovaries (female)

Self-assessment Exercise 21, The Urinary System

A. Lt. kidney
B. Rt. kidney
C. Ureters
D. Bladder
1. Inferior vena cava
2. Adrenal gland
3. Abdominal aorta
4. Renal artery
5. Renal vein
6. Common iliac vein
7. Common iliac artery
8. External iliac artery
9. External iliac vein

E. Prostate gland
F. Urethra (penile)
G. Bladder trigone

Self-assessment Exercise 22, The Kidney

1. Fibrous capsule
2. Cortex
3. Medulla
4. Hilus
5. Major calyx
6. Opening of calyx
7. Renal pelvis
8. Minor calyx
9. Ureter
10. Pyramids

Self-assessment Exercise 23, The Male Reproductive Organs

1. Urinary bladder
2. Vas deferens
3. Ureter
4. Seminal vesicle
5. Corpus cavernosum
6. Penis
7. Urethra
8. Sigmoid colon
9. Prostate gland
10. Rectum
11. Bulbourethral gland
12. Anus
13. Prepuce
14. Glans penis
15. Urethral meatus
16. Epididymis
17. Testis
18. Scrotum

Self-assessment Exercise 24, The Female Reproductive Organs

1. Body of uterus
2. Ovarian ligament
3. Fallopian tube
4. Ovary
5. Myometrium
6. Broad ligament
7. Endometrium
8. Cervix
9. Vagina
10. Hymen
A. Mons pubis
B. Labia majora
C. Glans clitoris
D. Labia minora
E. Opening—urethra
F. Opening—vagina
G. Perineum
H. Anus

Self-assessment Exercise 25, The Breast and Mammary Glands

1. Clavicle
2. Ribs
3. Areola
4. Nipple
5. Intercostal muscles
6. Fat
7. Alveolus
8. Lactiferous duct
9. Ampulla
10. Lobe

Self-assessment Exercise 26, Prefixes and Suffixes

A. Suffix
1. -rrhaphy
2. -algia
3. -ic; -al
4. -otomy
5. -ectomy
6. -oscopy
7. -oscope
8. -plasty
9. -tripsy
10. -ostomy

B. Prefix
1. endo-; intra-
2. dys-
3. sub-; infra-
4. a-; an-
5. inter-
6. supra-

C. Medical Terms
1. Colitis
2. Rhinoplasty
3. Bronchoscopy
4. Hysterectomy
5. Cholelithiasis
6. Herniorrhaphy
7. Cystoscopy
8. Salpingectomy
9. Thoracotomy
10. Colostomy

Self-assessment Exercise 27, Working with Terminology

A. Directions of the Body
1. L
2. G
3. D
4. K
5. A
6. I
7. C
8. F
9. J
10. H
11. B
12. E

B. Body Relationships
1. F
2. D
3. E
4. B
5. A
6. C

C. Body Movements
1. C
2. B
3. A
4. I
5. F
6. D
7. E
8. G
9. J
10. H

D. Terms and Meanings
1. B
2. F
3. E
4. H
5. A
6. D
7. C
8. G

Self-assessment Exercise 28, Applying Medical Terminology

A. Common Terms
1. Abdomen
2. Umbilicus
3. Axillary
4. Clavicle
5. Scapula
6. Digits; phalanges
7. Sublinguinal

Parts of the Spine
8. Cervical
9. Thoracic
10. Lumbar
11. Sacrum
12. Coccyx

Anatomic Parts
13. Subcostal
14. Retropubic
18. Arthro-
19. Cranium

15. Tympanic membrane
16. Trachea
17. Osteo-
20. Gastrointestinal
21. Otorhinoesophago-
22. Larynx

B.
1. Adhesions
2. Hemisphere
3. Meninges
4. Cystocele ·
5. Ligament
6. Meniscus
7. Colostomy
8. Peritoneum
9. Anastomosis
10. Parietal pleura
11. Hypophysectomy
12. Myringoplasty

Self-assessment Exercise 29, Working with Vocabulary

1. TUMORS
   *Lypo*sarcoma
   *Adeno*sarcoma
   *Osteo*sarcoma
   *Lympho*sarcoma
   *Fibro*sarcoma

2. INSTRUMENTS
   *Opthalmo*scope
   *Oto*scope
   *Broncho*scope
   *Cysto*scope
   *Esophago*scope
   *Gastro*scope
   *Laryngo*scope
   *Procto*scope
   *Colono*scope
   *Laparo*scope
   *Mediastino*scope
   *Arthro*scope
   *Choledocho*scope
   *Nephro*scope

3. CORRECT SPELLING
   1. (A) Ovary
   2. (B) Nose
   3. (B) Fallopian tubes
   4. (B) Throat (pharynx)
   5. (C) Ureter
   6. (C) Cold
   7. (C) Skull
   8. (A) Paralysis
   9. (C) To suture
   10. (C) Sacrum

4. DEFINE THE FOLLOWING TERMS
   1. Removal of the gallbladder through a laparoscopic approach
   2. Excision of tissue surrounding a draining sinus tract in the area of the anus
   3. Surgical incision and removal of a kidney stone
   4. Formation of an opening into the membranous covering of the heart for the purpose of drainage
   5. Removal of an obstructive clot in a blood vessel
   6. Surgical removal of old scars or age wrinkles by sanding the skin
   7. Radiographic examination of the blood vessels and lymphatics using radiopaque substances
   8. Excision of a bone(s) in a posterior arch of the vertebra (spinal column)
   9. Surgical formation or reformation of a joint
   10. Visual examination of the esophagus and the stomach via a flexible (or rigid) fiberoptic endoscope
   11. Removal of the meniscus cartilage of the knee

12. Incision into the thoracic (chest) cavity
13. Plastic revision of the nose
14. Removal of an entire mass or part of the eyeball without rupture
15. Removal of a segment of the large intestine with restoration of bowel continuity through anastomosis
16. Cutting through (into) a fibrous valve
17. Radiographic procedure to examine the common duct during gallbladder surgery
18. A diversion of portal venous blood to the systemic venous system
19. Visual examination of the urinary bladder and adjacent structures via the urethra using a telescopic instrument
20. An opening made into the maxillary sinus for the purpose of drainage

Self-assessment Exercise 30, Common Abbreviations

1. Dilation and curettage
2. Term used to designate fluoroscopic x-ray unit or image intensifier (related to its shape)
3. Tonsillectomy and adenoidectomy
4. Abdominal aortic aneurysm
5. Cataract extraction with intraocular lens implant
6. Termination of pregnancy
7. Therapeutic vacuum curettage
8. Cholecystectomy with common duct exploration
9. Anterior and posterior repair
10. Transurethral resection of the prostate
11. Percutaneous transluminal coronary angioplasty
12. Percutaneous nephrolithopaxy (nephrolithotomy)
13. Exploratory laparotomy
14. To follow
15. Diagnosis
16. Open reduction, internal fixation
17. Frozen section with biopsy
18. Fracture
19. Foley catheter to continuous bladder irrigation
20. Above-knee/below-knee amputation
21. Closed reduction right wrist
22. Coronary artery bypass graft
23. Mitral valve/aortic valve replacement
24. Atrial septal defect/ventricular septal defect
25. Total abdominal hysterectomy with bilateral salpingo-oophorectomy
26. Within normal limits
27. Normal sinus rhythm
28. Computerized axial tomography
29. Intravenous cholangiogram; inferior vena cava
30. Culture and sensitivity

Self-assessment Exercise 31, Putting It All Together

1. a. Examination of the kidney (noninvasive), which demonstrates the organ at a specific depth
   b. Multilevel radiographic visual presentation using computerized imaging

   c. Injection of radiopaque dye intravenously to assist in visualization of the kidney pelvis
   d. A tissue sample removed for pathologic examination
   e. Removal of a kidney
2. a. Complete blood count
   b. Blood urea nitrogen
   c. Within normal limits
   d. Hematocrit
   e. Hemoglobin
   f. Diagnosis
   g. Normal sinus rhythm
3. a.   6. b
4. b   7. c
5. a   8. Bronchoscope
                                      Colonoscope
                                      Cystoscope

Chapter 14

Self-assessment Exercise 32

1. C
2. True
3. Gastrojejunostomy
4. Foley, regular; Foley 3-way; ureteral (for retrograde studies)
5. True
6. McBurney
7. Percutaneous nephrolithopaxy
8. Cystic duct and artery
9. Ascending
10. C
11. Transurethral; suprapubic; retropubic; perineal
12. Bakelite obturator and sheath
    Foroblique telescope
    Resectoscope and cutting loops
13. 4: Preincisional
    Before closure of uterus
    Before closure of peritoneal cavity
    Before closure of skin
14. C
15. Tubal Pregnancy; Salpingectomy

Self-assessment Exercise 33

1. True
2. Nitrogen
3. Curettes and osteotomes
    Drills and drill bits; blades; saws
    Periosteal elevators
    Lowmen bone-holding clamp
4. Arthroscopy
5. True
6. Bone wax; hemostatic agents; cautery
7. Relieve pressure on brain tissue (trauma); to begin a craniotomy procedure
8. Shoulder; prevent recurrent anterior dislocation of the shoulder
9. X-ray equipment and lead aprons
10. Ventriculoperitoneal (VP) shunt

Self-assessment Exercise 34

1. Insertion of chest tubes
2. Potassium; sodium
3. True
4. 4: Preincisional
   Before closure of the pericardial cavity
   Before closure of the thoracic cavity
   Before closure of skin
5. Washings; brushings; biopsy
6. Embolectomy
7. Chest tubes and closed drainage system
8. Radial; cephalic
9. Knitted Dacron; knitted velour; woven polyester PTFE; biologic (autogenous)
10. Heparin, protamine
11. To confirm patency of vessel anastomosis

Self-assessment Exercise 35

1. Opaque lens; intraocular lens implant
2. Extracapsular; intracapsular; phacoemulsification
3. True
4. Sternocleidomastoid
5. Adenoids usually atrophy after puberty
6. Wire cutters; emergency tracheostomy tray
7. True
8. a. Topical anesthetic
   b. Enzymes to dissolve fibers holding lens in place
   c. To *constrict* pupil and reduce intraocular pressure
   d. To *dilate* pupil to facilitate examination of the retina and lens removal

Self-assessment Exercise 36

1. Full thickness; split thickness; pedicle
2. True
3. False: *aesthetic* refers to cosmetic surgery
4. Reconstruction (enlargement) of breast with insertion of an implant
5. a. Removal of excessive periorbital fat around the eye
   b. "Face-lift": tightening of facial tissue
   c. Revision of scars and/or age lines through chemoabrasion or sanding of skin

6. Wrapping extremities in soft cotton roll
   Use of thermal blanket; artificial heat lamp
   Use of warmed IV and irrigation solutions
   Warming the operating room prior to the patient's arrival
7. "Pull-through" procedure (colorectal resection)
8. 1. Maintenance of body temperature and/or prevention of heat loss
   2. Monitoring of fluids and electrolytes with careful replacement therapy
   3. Use of immobility restraints
   4. Maintenance of skin integrity and avoidance of chemical burns
   5. Avoidance of injury and maintaining safety factors during transport, moving, and lifting

Questions for Review

1. B
2. D
3. B
4. C
5. C
6. B
7. B
8. C
9. B
10. D
11. Fractured femur or femoral head
12. C
13. C
14. A
15. Removal of a lobe of the lung; closed-chest drainage system
16. D
17. A
18. B
19. A
20. A
21. Cataract extraction with intraocular lens implant
22. D
23. A
24. A
25. Establish rapport with patient and family

Index

Index